Professional Issues in Nursing

CHALLENGES & OPPORTUNITIES

Carol J. Huston, RN, MSN, MPA, DPA, FAAN

Professor, School of Nursing
California State University, Chico
Chico, California

2007–2009 President
Sigma Theta Tau International
Honor Society of Nursing

 Wolters Kluwer | Lippincott Williams & Wilkins
Health
Philadelphia · Baltimore · New York · London
Buenos Aires · Hong Kong · Sydney · Tokyo

Acquisitions Editor: Hilarie Surrena
Project Manager: Michelle L. Clarke
Director of Nursing Production: Helen Ewan
Art Director, Design: Joan Wendt
Art Director, Illustration: Brett MacNaughton
Manufacturing Coordinator: Karin Duffield
Production Services: Aptara, Inc.

2nd Edition

9 8 7 6 5 4 3 2 1

Printed in China

Library of Congress Cataloging-in-Publication Data

Huston, Carol Jorgensen.
   Professional issues in nursing : challenges & opportunities / Carol J. Huston. — 2nd ed.
      p. ; cm.
   Includes bibliographical references and index.
   ISBN 978-1-60547-395-6 (alk. paper)
   1. Nursing—United States. I. Title.
   [DNLM: 1. Nursing—trends. 2. Ethics, Nursing. 3. Nurse's Role. 4. Nursing—manpower.
5. Professional Competence. WY 16 H972p 2009]
RT82.H87 2009
610.73—dc22   2009008823

To purchase additional copies of this book, call our customer service department at **(800) 638-3030** or fax orders to **(301) 223-2320**. International customers should call **(301) 223-2300**.

Visit Lippincott Williams & Wilkins on the Internet: at **LWW.com.** Lippincott Williams & Wilkins customer service representatives are available from 8:30 am to 6 pm, EST.

LWW.COM

CCS0409

I dedicate this book to all those volunteer nurse leaders who have inspired and supported me during my leadership tenure in Sigma Theta Tau International, Honor Society of Nursing. In particular, I owe a tremendous debt of gratitude to Dr. Patricia Thompson for her unwavering support and for being such an important part of one of the most amazing experiences in my life.

I also dedicate this book to my wonderful husband Tom, who is always by my side and who has supported me in so many ways, for so many years. How did I get so lucky?

CONTRIBUTORS

Marjorie Beyers, RN, PhD, FAAN
Consultant, Patient Care Services
Barrington, Illinois
(*Chapter 23*)

Damazo Rebekah, MSN, PNP
Rural Northern California Clinical Simulation
    Center Project Coordinator
Certified Pediatric Nurse Practitioner
Professor, School of Nursing
California State University, Chico
Chico, CA
(*Chapter 4*)

Catherine Dodd, RN, PhD, FAAN
Deputy Chief of Staff at Mayor's Office
Former District Director House Speaker Nancy
    Pelosi at U.S. House of Representatives
San Francisco, California
(*Chapter 22*)

Sherry D. Fox, RN, PhD
Director, School of Nursing
California State University
Chico, California
(*Chapter 4*)

Clarilee Hauser, PhD, RN
Assistant Professor, School of Nursing
Adelphi University
Garden City, New York
(*Chapter 22*)

Charmaine Hockley, PhD; RN; FRCNA; JP
Director, Charmaine Hockley & Associates
Workplace Relationships—International
    Consultant
Strathalbyn, South Australia
(*Chapter 12*)

Jennifer Lillibridge, PhD, RN
Professor
California State University, Chico
School of Nursing
Chico, California
(*Chapter 16*)

Jeanne Madison, PhD, RN
Associate Professor, School of Health
University of New England
Armidale, Australia
(*Chapter 8*)

Catherine Wilde McPhee, MSN, RN, FNP-C
Associate Chair of the Undergraduate School
    of Nursing
Azusa Pacific University
Azusa, California
(*Chapter 3*)

Suzanne S. Prevost, PhD, RN
Associate Dean
Practice and Community Engagement
College of Nursing
University of Kentucky
(*Chapter 2*)

Margaret J. Rowberg, DNP, APN
Certified Adult Nurse Practitioner
Associate Professor, School of Nursing
California State University, Chico
Chico, CA
(*Chapter 21*)

Sheron Salyer, RNC, DNSc
Associate Professor
Middle Tennessee State University School of
    Nursing
Murfreesboro, TN
(*Chapter 2*)

REVIEWERS

Mary Cole Campbell
Nursing Instructor
Sharon Regional Health System School of
   Nursing
Sharon, PA

Barbara A. Gilbert, RN, MSN, FN
Nursing Faculty
Excelsior College and University of Phoenix
Canton, NY

Patricia K. Lafferty, MSN, RN, Doctoral
Student
Instructor/Advisor
University of Central Florida College of Nursing
Orlando, FL

Carolyn J. Nickerson, EdD, MSN, MA, RN
Associate Professor
Duquesne University School of Nursing
Pittsburgh, PA

Susan L. Piva, MS, RN
Associate Professor/Coordinator for Sophomore
   Level Students
Brevard Community College
Cocoa, FL

Dianna Lipp Rivers, RN, DrPH, MPH(N),
BSN, CNAA, BC
Associate Professor of Nursing
Lamar University
Beaumont, TX

Donna M. Romyn, PhD, MN, RN, BScN
Director Centre for Nursing and Health Studies
Athabasca University
Athabasca, Alberta

Tricia Ryan, RN, BSN, MSN Student
Nursing Instructor/Per-diem Staff Nurse
Sharon Regional Health Systems School of
   Nursing
Sharon, PA

Sharon K. Tighe, EdD, MN, RN-BC, ARNP
Professor
Daytona Beach Community College
Daytona Beach, FL

PREFACE

As a nursing educator for more than 28 years, I have taught many courses dealing with the significant issues impacting the nursing profession. I often felt frustrated that textbooks that were supposed to be devoted to professional issues in the field instead deviated into nursing research, theory, and leadership concepts. In addition, while many of the existing professional issues books dealt with the enduring issues of the profession, it was difficult to find a book for my students that incorporated those with the "hot topics" of the time.

The first edition of *Professional Issues in Nursing: Challenges & Opportunities* was an effort to address both of these needs. The second edition maintains this precedent with content updates as well as the addition of a chapter on using simulation to teach nurses and the deletion of the chapter on differentiated practice. This edition continues, however, to be first and foremost a professional issues book. While an effort has been made to integrate research, theory, and leadership into chapters where it seemed appropriate, these topics in and of themselves are too broad to be fully addressed in a professional issues book. This book also is directed at what I and my expert nursing colleagues have identified as both enduring professional issues as well as the most pressing contemporary issues facing the profession. It is my hope, then, that this book fills an unmet need in the current professional issues text market. It has an undiluted focus on professional issues in nursing and includes many timely issues not addressed in other professional issues texts.

This book has been designed for use at both the baccalaureate and graduate level. It is envisioned that this book will be used as a primary textbook or as a supplement for a typical two- to three-unit professional issues course. It would also be appropriate for most RN–BSN bridge courses and may be considered by some faculty as a supplemental reader to a Leadership/Management course that includes professional issues. The book can be used in both the traditional classroom and in online courses because the discussion question format works well for both small and large groups onsite as well as in bulletin board and chat room venues.

The book is edited with the primary author contributing 14 chapters and guest contributors with expertise in the specific subject material, contributing the remaining nine chapters. The book is divided into five units, representing contemporary and enduring issues in professional nursing. The five sections include: *Furthering the Profession, Workforce Issues, Workplace Issues, Legal and Ethical Issues,* and *Professional Power.* Each unit has four to five chapters.

Each chapter begins with an overview of the professional issue being discussed. Multiple perspectives on each issue are then identified in an effort to reflect the diversity of thought found in the literature as well as espoused by experts in the field and varied professional nursing and health care organizations. "Discussion Points" encourage readers to pause and reflect on specific questions (individually or in groups), and "Consider" features encourage active learning, critical thinking, and values clarification by the users. In addition, at least one research study is profiled in every chapter in an effort to promote evidence-based analysis of the issue. Each chapter concludes with questions for additional discussion, a comprehensive and current reference list, and an expansive bibliography of resources for further exploration (electronic links, news media, and print resources). Each chapter also includes multiple displays, boxes, figures, and tables to help the user visualize important concepts.

This book comes with a set of instructor resources that can be accessed on thePoint, LWW's very popular web-based course and content management system. With the materials you'll find on thePoint, you'll be able to construct exams from a collection of NCLEX-style test questions, enhance your lecture with PowerPoint slides, foster in-class discussions, test your students' reading comprehension, and get them started on applied practice of their knowledge. Answers are provided for all of the tests and learning activities, all designed to make your job as instructor as easy as possible.

New to This Edition

■ A chapter on using simulation to teach nurses has been added, while a chapter on differentiated practice was deleted.

■ New or updated content has been added throughout the book to reflect cutting-edge trends in healthcare. Specifically, this edition has expanded or added the following content:

  ■ A broader discussion of the *Clinical Nurse Leader* (CNL) role.

  ■ New content on the *Doctor of Nursing Practice* (DNP) debate as entry for advanced practice nurses.

  ■ Integration of the 2008 AACN *Essentials of Baccalaureate Nursing Education* document in assessing distance education program outcomes.

  ■ Strategies for supporting evidence-based practice in the work environment.

  ■ The impact of generational diversity on the current nursing shortage and workforce issues.

■ Innovative staffing models which have been developed as an alternative to mandatory overtime.

■ Cutting edge workplace technologies including robotics, electronic health records, biometrics, smart cards, intranets, and wireless local area networking.

■ New VISA requirements, regulatory requirements, international NCLEX for migratory nurses.

■ Recent workforce projections related to the current international nursing shortage and a burgeoning shortage of qualified nursing faculty.

■ An examination of California's compliance as well as resultant patient outcomes, five years after implementation of mandatory minimum staffing ratio legislation.

■ New case studies of whistleblowers seeking financial compensation through the False Claims Act

Carol J. Huston, RN, MSN, MPA, DPA, FAAN

CONTENTS

CHAPTER 1

Entry into Practice: The Debate Rages On

• CAROL J. HUSTON •

Learning Objectives

The learner will be able to:

1. Differentiate between technical and professional nurses as outlined in Esther Lucille Brown's classic *Nursing for the Future.*
2. Identify what if any progress has been made on increasing the educational entry level for professional registered nursing since the publication of the 1965 position paper of the American Nurses Association on entry into practice.
3. Identify similarities and differences between contemporary associate and baccalaureate degree nursing programs.
4. Describe basic components of associate degree educational programs as outlined by Mildred Montag and compare those with typical associate degree programs in the 21st century.
5. Analyze how having one National Council Licensure Examination (NCLEX) for entry into practice, regardless of educational entry level, affects the entry-into-practice dilemma.
6. Identify key driving and restraining forces for increasing the educational entry level for professional nursing.
7. Analyze the potential effects of raising the educational entry level on the current nursing shortage, workforce diversity, and intraprofession conflict.
8. Examine current evidence-based research that explores the effect of registered nurse educational level on patient outcomes.
9. Explore how shifting health care delivery sites and increasing registered nursing competency requirements are affecting employer preferences for hiring a more educated nursing workforce.
10. Compare the nursing profession's educational entry standards with those of the other health care professions.
11. Identify positions taken by specific professional organizations, certifying bodies, and employers regarding the appropriate educational level for entry into practice for professional nursing.
12. Explore personal values, beliefs, and feelings regarding whether the educational entry level in nursing should be increased to a baccalaureate or higher degree.

Few issues have been as long-standing or as contentious in nursing as the entry-into-practice debate. Taylor (2008, p. 611) agreed, suggesting that "the issues surrounding entry into practice have been a rock in the shoe of nursing for many years." Although the entry-into-practice debate goes back to the 1940s with the publication of Esther Lucille Brown's classic *Nursing for the Future*, the debate came to the forefront with a 1965 position paper by the American Nurses Association (ANA) (1965a, 1965b). This position paper suggested an orderly transition from hospital-based diploma nursing preparation to nursing education in colleges or universities based on the following premises:

■ The education of all those who are licensed to practice nursing should take place in institutions of higher education.

■ The minimum preparation for beginning professional nursing practice should be a baccalaureate education in nursing.

■ The minimum preparation for beginning technical practice should be an associate education in nursing.

■ The education for assistants in the health care occupations should be short, intensive, pre-service programs in vocational education institutions rather than on-the-job training programs.

In essence, two levels of preparation were suggested for registered nurses: *technical* and *professional*. Persons interested in technical practice would enroll in junior or community colleges and earn associate degrees in 2-year programs. Those interested in professional nursing would enroll in 4-year programs in colleges or universities. Hospital-based diploma programs were to be phased out.

The curriculums for the two programs were to be very different, as were each program's focus. The 2-year technical degree was to result in an associate degree in nursing (ADN). This degree, as proposed by Mildred Montag (Fig. 1.1) in her dissertation in 1952, with direction and support from R. Louise McManus, would prepare a beginning, technical practitioner who would provide care in acute care settings under the supervision of a professional nurse.

In a typical associate degree program, approximately half of the credits would be fulfilled by general education courses such as English, anatomy, physiology, speech, psychology, and sociology and the other half would be fulfilled by nursing courses (Ellis & Hartley, 2008). The 4-year degree would result in a bachelor of science in nursing (BSN) and would encompass coursework taught in ADN programs, as well as more in-depth treatment of the physical and social sciences, nursing research, public and community health, nursing management, and the humanities. The additional course work in the BSN was intended to enhance the students' professional development, prepare them for a broader scope of practice, and provide a better understanding of the cultural, political, economic, and social issues affecting patients and health care delivery.

The ANA 1965 position statement was reaffirmed by a resolution of the ANA House of Delegates in 1978, which set forth the requirement that the baccalaureate degree would be the entry level into professional nursing practice by 1985. Institutions that administered associate degree and diploma programs responded strongly to what they viewed as inflammatory terminology and clearly stated that not being considered "professional" was unacceptable. The end result was that both ADN and diploma programs refused to compromise title or licensure. Dissension ensued both within and among nursing groups, and little movement occurred to make the position statement a reality.

CONSIDER

Titling (professional vs. technical) was and will be an important consideration before consensus can be reached on the entry into practice.

Almost 45 years later, entry into practice at the baccalaureate level has not been accomplished. Even the strongest supporters of the BSN for entry into practice cannot deny that despite efforts spanning more than 50 years, registered nurse (RN) entry at the baccalaureate level continues to be an elusive goal.

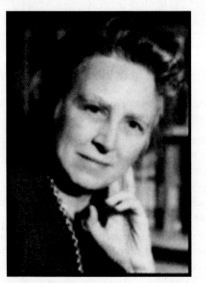

Figure 1.1. Mildred Montag.

PROLIFERATION OF ADN EDUCATION

It is doubtful that Mildred Montag had any idea in 1952 that ADN programs would some day become the predominant entry level for nursing practice or that this education model would proliferate as it did in the 1960s—just one decade after she completed her doctoral work. Although the overwhelming majority of nurses in the early 1960s were educated in diploma schools of nursing, enrollment in baccalaureate programs was increasing, and associate degree programs were just beginning. By the year 2000, diploma education had virtually disappeared, and although BSN education had increased significantly, it was ADN education that represented nearly two thirds of all nursing school graduates.

Indeed, ADN education continues to be the primary model for nursing education. As of 2007, ADN programs comprised 59% of all basic RN programs and produced 63% of RN graduates (NLN Data Reveal Dramatic Drop, 2006/2007, para 3). Currently, 42.2% of RNs enter the workforce with an associate degree, although only 33.7% of the current workforce lists the associate degree as their highest educational preparation (National Organization for Associate Degree Nursing ([NOADN], 2008). This may reflect the number of ADN nurses who have degrees in other fields or who return to school at some point to earn a BSN degree.

Yet, enrollment in baccalaureate nursing programs is also on the rise (up from 16% in the early 1960s). The American Association of Colleges of Nursing (AACN) (2007a) stated that as of 2004, 47.2% of the RN workforce held a baccalaureate or graduate degree in some field (including nursing) and that from 2000 to 2004, the number of nurses pursuing baccalaureate degrees increased by 12.9%, whereas those pursuing graduate degrees increased by 37.0%.

LICENSURE AND ENTRY INTO PRACTICE

Critics of BSN as a requirement for entry into practice argue there is no need to raise entry levels because passing rates for the National Council Licensure Examination (NCLEX) show no significant differences among ADN, diploma, and BSN graduates (Table 1.1). Although some might argue that this suggests similar competencies across the educational spectrum, the more common precept is that the NCLEX is a test that measures minimum technical competencies for safe entry into basic nursing practice and, as such, may not measure performance over time or test for all of the knowledge and skills developed through a BSN program. One must also ask why the nursing profession has not differentiated RN licensure testing based on educational preparation for RNs, just as has been done for practical nurses, registered nurses, and advanced practice nurses.

> **DISCUSSION POINT**
> Should separate licensing examinations be developed for ADN-, diploma-, and BSN-educated nurses?

Complicating the picture is that both ADN and BSN schools preparing graduates for RN licensure meet similar criteria for state board approval and have roughly the same number of nursing coursework units. All of these factors contribute to confusion about differentiations between ADN- and BSN-prepared nurses and result in an inability to move forward on implementing the BSN as the entry level for professional nursing.

> **CONSIDER**
> Critics of BSN entry into practice argue that ADN-, diploma-, and BSN-educated nurses all take the same licensing examination and therefore have earned the title of Registered Nurse. In addition, nurses prepared at all three levels have successfully worked side by side, under the same scope of practice, for more than 50 years.

Research also suggests that there are differences in the demographics of BSN and ADN graduates. A study by the Michigan Center for Nursing (2006) suggested that ADN program students tend to be older than students in BSN programs, following the trend that older graduates are more likely to seek associate degrees than bachelor's degrees. Sexton, Hunt, Cox, et al.'s (2008) study of more than 5,000 nurses also found that the BSN nurses in their convenience sampling were younger than the ADN-educated nurses, with 28% of the baccalaureate-educated nurses being born in or after 1980, as compared to 13% of the associate degree nurses.

TABLE 1.1	National Council Licensure Examination for Registered Nurses (NCLEX-RN) Passage Rate per Educational Program Type, January–March 2008	
Program Type	**Number of Graduates**	**NCLEX-RN Passage Rate (%)**
Diploma	1,056	86.6
Associate degree	17,438	86.6
Baccalaureate degree	10,937	87.9

Source: National Council of State Boards of Nursing (NCSBN) (2008). *Number of candidates taking NCLEX examination and percent passing, by type of candidate.* Retrieved May 23, 2008, from Table_Of_Pass_Rates_2008.pdf

It is also generally believed that ADN graduates represent greater diversity in race, gender, age, and educational experiences than BSN-prepared nurses. Indeed, the *2005-2006 Annual School Report* of the California Board of Registered Nursing (2007) suggested that ADN programs have the highest percentage of ethnic minorities among students enrolling in prelicensure programs for the first time. In addition, the report suggested that ADN programs had the greatest percentage of ethnic minority students who completed a nursing program.

Critics of the BSN requirement for entry into professional nursing suggest that greater diversity is needed in nursing, and this may be lost if entry levels are raised. However, a study by the Michigan Center for Nursing (2006) found only small differences in race/ethnicity between the two groups (86% of the BSN students were white, non-Hispanic, as compared to 81% of the ADN students), and there were no differences in gender representation (both groups were overwhelmingly female). In addition, the AACN (2007c) in their *Annual State of the Schools* report suggested that 24.8 percent of students enrolled in entry-level baccalaureate programs in fall 2006 represented racial/ethnic minority groups.

In addition, many employers state they are unable to differentiate roles for nurses based on education because both ADN- and BSN-prepared nurses hold the same license. Ironically, state boards of nursing have asserted their inability to develop a different licensure system, given the fact that employers have not developed different roles.

Furthermore, many employers provide no incentives for BSN education in terms of pay, recognition, or career mobility and are afraid to do so, fearing that they may be unable to fill vacant nursing positions. The starting rate of pay for ADN- and BSN-prepared nurses historically has not been significantly different, although this appears to be changing. The AACN (2007b) reported that recent surveys suggest that BSN nurses earn salaries more than 10% higher than ADN nurses. Similarly, in 2006, the state of California conducted a survey of registered nurses that showed a mean income of $75,017 for BSN-educated nurses and a mean income of $70,804 for ADN-educated nurses (Nursing Link, 2008). In addition, because many advanced positions often require a BSN, the BSN-prepared nurse often has the potential to earn more money (Nursing Link, 2008).

Graf's (2006) research also found an earnings benefit for ADN nurses who earned a BSN, but this wage increase was offset by the educational investment expenses incurred. Indeed, Graf found that, on average, the costs of the BSN degree were greater than the cumulative increased earnings over the nurse's subsequent work life. For some respondents, however, the return on investment ranged from break-even to as much as an 11% increase, and when returns on investment were higher, ADN-educated nurses were much more likely to pursue higher degrees than when returns were negative. Graf concluded that wage incentives are essential to improving overall return-to-school rates, particularly at the baccalaureate level, and that health care organizations must consistently provide a substantial wage differential for advanced preparation before ADN nurses will seek educational advancement.

EDUCATIONAL LEVELS AND PATIENT OUTCOMES

Perhaps the most common argument against raising the entry level in nursing is an emotional one, with ADN-prepared nurses arguing that "caring does not require a baccalaureate degree." Many ADN-educated nurses argue passionately that patients do not know or care what educational degree their nurse holds as long as they receive high-quality care by the nurse at their bedside. ADN nurses also frequently claim that BSN-prepared nurses are too theoretically oriented and thus are not in touch with real practice. In addition, many ADN nurses suggest that baccalaureate-prepared nurses are deficient in basic skills mastery and conclude that care provided by ADN nurses is at least as good as, if not better than, that provided by their BSN counterparts.

CONSIDER

Most ADN-prepared nurses argue that significant differences exist between their practice and that of a licensed vocational/practical nurse (LVN/LPN), despite there often being only 12 months difference in length of educational preparation. Yet, many ADN-educated nurses argue that the additional education that BSN-educated nurses have makes little difference in their practice over that of their ADN counterparts. How can this argument be justified?

Research Study Fuels the Controversy: Differences between BSN and ADN Education

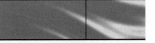

The purpose of this phenomenological study was to explore and describe the experience that associate-degree and diploma nursing graduates have when transitioning from ADN educational preparation to BSN. Twelve nurses with a variety of clinical backgrounds and completion of different RN-to-BSN programs were interviewed to elicit the lived experience of transitioning from RN to BSN.

STUDY FINDINGS

The ability to see the bigger picture was the most powerful common experience identified by the ADN-educated nurses. They suggested that BSN education allowed them to move beyond old patterns of thinking and behavior to envision the whole person, critically analyzing the complexity of the human experience. They reported that the biggest change occurred in their thought processes, although skills level also advanced for many. By the end of the program, the nurses saw their work in a different light and began recreating their everyday practice. The nurses felt that they had successfully transitioned from ADN nurses to BSNs and emerged with a renewed commitment to their profession, forever changed by the experience.

Delaney, C. & Piscopo, B. (2007). There really is a difference. Nurses' experiences with transitioning from RNs to BSNs. *Journal of Professional Nursing, 23*(3), 167–173.

An increasing number of studies, however, report differences between the performance levels of ADN- and BSN-prepared nurses. Delaney and Piscopo (2007) found that ADN nurses who returned to school for a baccalaureate degree reported improved critical thinking skills and enhanced professionalism. In addition, these students saw a direct relationship between their education and their approach to patient care (see Research Study Fuels the Controversy).

Research also overwhelmingly supports better outcomes for patients cared for by BSN-prepared nurses than for those cared for by nurses with associate degrees. In a landmark 2003 study Dr. Linda Aiken and her colleagues at the University of Pennsylvania identified a clear link between higher levels of nursing education and better patient outcomes (AACN, 2007b). This study found that "surgical patients have a 'substantial survival advantage' if treated in hospitals with higher proportions of nurses educated at the baccalaureate or higher degree level and that a 10% increase in the proportion of nurses holding BSN degrees decreased the risk of patient death and failure to rescue by 5%" (AACN, 2007b, para 8).

Research by Dr. Aiken and colleagues also showed that hospitals with better care environments, the best nurse staffing levels, and the most highly educated nurses had the lowest surgical mortality rates. In fact, the researchers found that every 10% increase in the proportion of BSN nurses on the hospital staff was associated with a 4% decrease in the risk of death (Aiken, Clarke, Sloane, et al., 2008) (see Research Study Fuels the Controversy).

Research Study Fuels the Controversy: Effect of Education on Patient Outcomes

Data from 10,184 nurses and 232,342 surgical patients in 168 Pennsylvania hospitals provided striking evidence that educational entry level makes a difference in patient outcomes.

STUDY FINDINGS

This study found that patients experienced significantly lower mortality and failure-to-rescue rates in hospitals in which more highly educated nurses were providing direct patient care. Nurses reported more positive job experiences and fewer concerns with care quality, and patients had significantly lower risks of death and failure to rescue in hospitals with better care environments.

Aiken, L., Clarke, S. P., Sloane, D. M., Lake, E. T., & Cheney, T. (2008). Effects of hospital care environment on patient mortality and nurse outcomes. *Journal of Nursing Administration, 38*(5), 223–229.

These findings are similar to those of another recent study, led by Dr. Ann E. Tourangeau, of 46,993 patients at the University of Toronto, which found that hospitals with higher proportions of baccalaureate-prepared nurses tended to have lower 30-day mortality rates. The study suggested that a 10% increase in the proportion of baccalaureate-prepared nurses was associated with 9 fewer deaths for every 1,000 discharged patients (Hospital Death Rate Study, 2007).

Finally, a meta-analysis by the Agency for Healthcare Research and Quality in 2006 found evidence from several observational studies that hospitals with higher proportions of nurses with BSN degrees (36% vs.11%) had lower mortality rates and that states with larger proportions of BSN degrees reported lower rates of fatal injuries (Kane, Shamliyan, Mueller, Duval, & Wilt, 2007).

As more outcomes research is becoming available suggesting an empirical link between the educational entry level of nurses and patient outcomes, nursing leaders, professional associations, and employers are increasingly speaking out on the need to raise the profession's entry level as a means of improving quality patient care and patient safety.

EMPLOYERS' VIEWS AND PREFERENCES

Nursing employers are divided on the issue of entry into practice. The academic requirements of associate degree, diploma, and baccalaureate programs vary widely, yet health care settings that employ nursing graduates often make no distinction in the scope of practice among nurses who have different levels of preparation.

Employers, however, appear to be increasingly aware of purported differences between BSN and ADN graduates, and this may be reflected in their hiring preferences. Many more position descriptions for nursing managers and administrators now require or at least prefer a BSN degree. Indeed, Susan Odegaard Turner, an experienced nurse and health care consultant, suggested that the BSN has become the degree employers prefer, and pointed out that it often takes about the same amount of time to complete the science prerequisites and get an ADN as it does to earn a BSN. So, in the end, the BSN gives a person "more cluck for your buck" (Vogt, 2007, para 2).

> **DISCUSSION POINT**
> If indeed employers prefer hiring BSN-prepared registered nurses, why don't more employers offer pay differentials for nurses with BSN degrees?

Indeed, the Veterans Administration (VA), with its 35,000 nurses on staff, is leading the nation in raising the bar for a higher educational entry hire level in nursing. The VA established the BSN as the minimum education level for new hires and required that all non–entry-level nurses have at least a BSN by 2005. A 2007 VA description of hiring programs and incentives suggested that VA nurses who want to advance beyond Nurse Level 1 must earn a BSN degree (U.S. Department of Veterans Affairs, 2007). As the nation's largest employer of registered nurses, the VA has committed $50 million over a 5-year period to help VA nurses obtain baccalaureate or higher nursing degrees (AACN, 2007b).

SHIFTING HEALTH CARE DELIVERY SITES AND REQUIRED COMPETENCIES

Data from the 2004 National Sample Survey of Registered Nurses show that approximately 56% of U.S. registered nurses work in hospitals (NOADN, 2008). Although hospitals continue to be the main site of employment for nurses, there is an ongoing shift in health care from acute care settings to the community and integrated health care settings. This shift will clearly require more highly educated nurses who can function autonomously. In addition, 21st-century nurses must "assume leadership roles within integrated systems, act as co-coordinators of care services, and serve as supervisors for other care providers. Their focus will be on preventative care within a financially constrained system in which cost-effective strategies will have to be identified and implemented" (Way & MacNeil, 2007, p. 164). These are all skills that are emphasized in a baccalaureate nursing curriculum.

> CONSIDER
> Baccalaureate and graduate-level skills in research, leadership, management, and community health are increasingly needed in nursing as health care extends beyond the acute care hospital.

Way and MacNeil (2007) stated that these contemporary changes in health care require nurses who have well-developed research-based clinical skills, critical thinking and decision-making abilities, interpersonal skills, and leadership abilities. They argued that rapid advances in technology, increased complexity of health care systems, and the exponential growth in nursing knowledge require nurses to have broad skill sets and that these skills are learned at the baccalaureate level.

Similarly, the National Advisory Council on Nurse Education and Practice (NACNEP) suggests that nursing's role for the future calls for RNs to manage care along a continuum, to work as peers in interdisciplinary teams, and to integrate clinical expertise with knowledge of community resources. This increased complexity of scope of practice will require the capacity to adapt to change; exhibit critical thinking and problem-solving skills; have a solid foundation in a broad range of basic sciences; have a knowledge of behavioral, social, and management sciences; and be able to analyze and communicate data (AACN, 2007b). All are integral components of BSN education. As a result, NACNEP has recommended to the U.S. Congress that at least two thirds of the nursing workforce hold baccalaureate or higher degrees in nursing by 2010 (AACN, 2007a).

The Council on Physician and Nurse Supply also released a statement in 2007 calling for a national effort to substantially expand baccalaureate nursing programs, citing the growing body of evidence that nursing education affects both the quality and safety of patient care. Consequently, the group called on policymakers to shift federal funding priorities in favor of supporting more baccalaureate-level nursing programs (AACN, 2007b). Some nurse leaders have even suggested that a BSN degree may not be adequate preparation for these expanded roles and that instead master's or doctoral degrees should be required for entry into practice for registered nursing.

DISCUSSION POINT

Would raising the entry level to the master's or doctoral degree eliminate the tension between supporters of ADN and BSN as entry levels into nursing, given that both educational preparations would be considered inadequate? Is a graduate degree currently feasible as the entry level for professional nursing? If not, what would it take to make it happen?

ENTRY LEVEL AND PROFESSIONAL STATUS

Nurses, consumers, and allied health care professionals are currently questioning why the entry level into professional nursing is so much lower than that in other health care professions. Does nursing require less skill? Is the knowledge base needed to provide nursing care skill based instead of knowledge based? Should nursing be reclassified as a vocational trade and not a profession? The answer to these questions, of course, is no. Yet, clearly, nurses have resisted the normal course of occupational development that other health care professions have pursued. As a result, nurses are now the least educated of the health care professionals, with most health care professions now requiring graduate degrees for entry. Indeed, one must question whether nursing is at risk of losing its designation as a profession because of its failure to maintain educational equity.

The primary identity of any professional group is based on the established education entry level. Attorneys, physicians, social workers, engineers, clergy, and physical therapists, to list a few examples, have in common an essential education at the bachelor's level. Advanced degrees are required in many professions for entry positions at the professional level. Only nursing continues the hypocrisy of pretending that education is unimportant and does not make a difference. Only nursing allows individuals with no college course work, or with limited college study that lacks a well-rounded global college education, to lay claim to the same licensure and identity as that held by nurses having a baccalaureate education.

Indeed, the educational gap between nursing and other health professions continues to grow (Table 1.2). Disciplines such as occupational therapy, physical therapy, speech therapy, and social work all require master's or doctoral degrees. Pharmacy has also raised its educational standards to that of a doctoral degree.

CONSIDER

"Nursing's lack of progress in advancing its educational requirements stands in contrast to other health professions, including pharmacy and physical therapy, which have moved to require doctoral-level education for the new practitioners" (Keepnews, 2006, p. 4).

TABLE 1.2	Entry-Level Degrees for the Health Professions

Health Profession	Entry Level Degree
Medicine	Doctorate
Pharmacy	Doctorate
Social work	Master's
Speech pathology	Master's
Physical therapy	Master's transitioning to doctorate
Occupational therapy	Master's
Nursing	Associate

> **DISCUSSION POINT**
> Is nursing in danger of losing its designation as a "profession" if it fails to maintain educational entry levels comparable to those of the other health professions?

Still, there are those individuals who suggest that the BSN requirement for entry to practice is elitist. Kidder and Cornelius (2006) disagreed, and suggested that although most professional disciplines are defined by the educational degree required to practice, nursing is not. Instead, they suggested that nursing's multilevel entry into practice has a negative effect on the profession's appeal to an emerging workforce and creates the misconception that licensure equates with professional status.

Failure to maintain educational parity with other health care professions also contributes to nursing being viewed as a second-class citizen in the health care arena. It is difficult to justify the profession's argument that nursing should be an equal partner in health care decision making when other professions are so much better educated, suggesting that nurses are either undereducated for the roles they assume or that the nursing role lacks complexity.

> **CONSIDER**
> Nursing is the only health care "profession" that does not require at least a bachelor's or higher degree for entry into practice.

THE TWO-YEAR ADN PROGRAM?

Many ADN-prepared nurses also express frustration when discussing the need to raise the entry level in professional nursing because they feel the ADN degree does not appropriately represent the scope of their education or the time they had to put in to earn what is typically considered to be a 2-year degree. ADN nurses argue that the "2-year" ADN program is a myth. Many ADN students follow nontraditional education paths, and almost all ADN programs now require 3 or more years of education, not 2 years, with a minimum of 12 to 24 months of prerequisites and a full 2 years of nursing education. Most associate degrees require approximately 60 semester units or 90 quarter units of coursework, although there is a great deal of variance, with some programs now requiring more than 70 semester units and more than 100 quarter units.

> **CONSIDER**
> The "2-year" ADN program is a myth.

Indeed, it is almost impossible to graduate from an ADN program in less than 3 years, and often 4 or more years are required. Given that most BSN programs require approximately 120 semester units for graduation, the question must be asked whether requiring so many units at the associate degree level, without granting the upper division credit that could lead to a BSN degree, is an injustice to ADN graduates.

This extension of educational time in ADN programs has generally been attributed to the need to respond to a changing job market, that is, the need to prepare ADNs to work in more diverse environments (nonhospital) and to increasingly assume positions requiring management skills. Although Montag clearly intended a differentiation between level of education and level of practice between ADN- and BSN-prepared nurses, many ADN programs have added leadership, management, research, and home health and community health courses to their curricula in the last 2 decades.

One must ask then what part of the associate degree curriculum should be cut to add these new experiences. What should the balance be between community and acute care experiences in ADN programs? How much management content do ADN nurses need, and what roles will they be expected to assume? If no content is deleted from the ADN programs to accommodate the new content, how can ADN education reasonably be completed within a 2-year framework?

Montag expressed concern that when ADN programs add content inappropriate for technical practice, appropriate content may have to be deleted to maintain the estimated time for completion. The question that follows then is: If ADN education now incorporates much of what was meant to be BSN content, and if the time needed to complete this education is near that of a bachelor's degree, why are ADN graduates being given associate's degrees, which reflect expertise in technical practice, rather than BSN degrees, which reflect achievement of these higher-level competencies?

SHORTAGES AND ENTRY-LEVEL REQUIREMENTS

According to Donley and Flaherty (2008, p. 2), "In times of shortage, there is usually a call to reduce educational requirements and to change licensing and accreditation standards." Indeed, Montag's original project to create ADN education was directed at reducing the workforce shortage of nurses that existed at that time by reducing the length of the education process to 2 years.

Clearly, the immediate short-term threat of raising the entry level to the bachelor's degree might be to exacerbate the existing shortage. In the long run, however, raising the entry level might elevate the public image of nursing and increase recruitment to the field because the best and the brightest might seek professions with greater academic prestige.

In addition, raising the entry level may affect retention rates in nursing. Research conducted by Sexton et al. (2008) suggested that BSN-prepared nurses generally have more positive perceptions of the work environment than colleagues educated in ADN programs. Having more BSN nurses may actually then stabilize the nursing workforce as a result of their higher levels of job satisfaction, which is a key to nurse retention.

CONSIDER
The effect of raising the entry level in nursing to the baccalaureate level on the current profound nursing shortage is not known.

The other reality is that a chronic shortage of nursing personnel has persisted despite the proliferation of ADN programs. This negates the argument that the current nursing shortage should be used as an excuse for postponing action to raise educational standards. A nursing shortage existed at the time of the 1965 ANA proposal and has occurred intermittently since that time. Clearly, nursing has been swept along by a host of social, economic, and educational circumstances that have little to do with nursing or the clients that it serves. Perhaps, then, the decision to raise the entry-to-practice level in nursing should be made because it is the right and necessary thing to do and not as a result of the influence of external communities of interest.

Taylor (2008, p. 4) agreed, going so far as to suggest that as a result of research that clearly shows a link between nurses' educational entry level and patient outcomes, "employers who hire nurses with less than a bachelor's degree are doing their patients a disservice." He went on to say that "the nursing shortage should not be an excuse to push for the continuance of associate degree programs only to graduate more nurses to fill the ever-increasing number of positions nationwide."

CONSIDER
Nurses, professional health care and nursing organizations, credentialing programs, and employers are divided on the entry-into-practice issue.

Debate over entry into practice is as varied among professional health care and nursing organizations, credentialing programs, and employers as it is among individual nurses. Getting support for the BSN as the entry-level requirement for nursing will be difficult because the overwhelming majority of nurses are currently ADN prepared, and there are inadequate workplace incentives to increase entry requirements to the BSN degree.

PROFESSIONAL ORGANIZATIONS, UNIONS, AND ADVISORY BODIES SPEAK OUT

Not surprisingly, the position statement issued by the NOADN (2006) on entry into practice reaffirms the role and value of associate-degree nursing education and practice. The position statement suggests that graduates of ADN programs are professional nurses who are essential members of the interdisciplinary health care team, that they are prepared to function in diverse health care settings, and that associate-degree education provides a dynamic pathway for entry into professional registered nurse practice.

Similarly, the position of the National League for Nursing (NLN)—the national voice for nurse educators in all types of nursing education programs—has historically been that the nursing profession should have multiple entry points (NLN, 2007). As such, the NLN suggests that instead of investing energy debating entry into the profession, the focus should turn toward opportunities for lifelong learning and progression for those who enter the nursing profession through diploma and associate-degree programs.

In addition, the Nurse Alliance of the Service Employees International Union (SEIU) Healthcare, an organization of 85,000 registered nurses, has firmly rejected any bill that would limit entry into or maintenance of practice to the BSN, arguing this would only exacerbate the current nursing shortage (SEIU, 2008). Instead, they argue that more resources must be made available to support nursing education at all levels, to give academic credit for work experience, to provide workplace support for nurses who wish to return to school, and to develop more online and hybrid programs for nurses who cannot attend traditional on-site classes to advance their education.

An increasing number of professional nursing organizations, however, are now supporting the BSN requirement for entry into professional nursing. The ANA, however, is no longer the standard bearer in this effort. Instead, organizations such as the AACN, the American Nephrology Nurses' Association (ANNA), the Association of Operating Room Nurses (AORN), and the American Organization of Nurse Executives (AONE) have published position statements supporting BSN entry.

For example, the AACN now suggests that

the primary pathway for entry into professional-level nursing, as compared to technical-level practice, is a four-year Bachelor of Science (BSN) degree in nursing and that the professional nurse with a baccalaureate degree is the only basic nursing graduate prepared to practice in all health care settings—critical care, public health, primary care, and mental health (AACN, 2008, para 5).

Similarly, the ANNA reaffirmed in 2005 its position that the minimum preparation for beginning professional nursing practice should be the baccalaureate degree in nursing, and minimum preparation for beginning technical nursing practice should be the associate degree in nursing (Minimum Preparation for Entry, 2006).

The AORN has also supported the baccalaureate degree for entry into nursing since 1979 (Taylor, 2008). AORN's current position statement on entry into practice reaffirms its belief that there should be one level for entry into nursing practice and that the minimal preparation for future entry into the practice of nursing should be the baccalaureate degree (Taylor, 2008). One participant at the 2005 AORN conference noted that the issue of the level of entry into practice demands resolution by the nursing profession, arguing that "multiple entry levels have caused confusion" and that the establishment of one entry level would reduce ambiguity and "demonstrate our responsibility to be self-regulating in establishing education requirements" (Kuehl, 2005, para 5).

In 2004, the AONE also published guiding principles suggesting that "the educational preparation of the nurse of the future should be at the baccalaureate level. This educational preparation will prepare the nurse of the future to function as an equal partner, collaborator and manager of the complex patient care journey that is envisioned by AONE" (AONE, 2005, para 3).

The National Advisory Council on Nurse Education and Practice, which advises the Secretary of the U.S. Department of Health and Human Services and the U.S. Congress on policy issues related to nurse workforce supply, education, and practice improvement, also urged that a minimum of two thirds of working nurses hold baccalaureate or higher degrees in nursing by 2010 (AACN, 2007b). Yet, federal and state regulation of entry into practice has, for the most part, not occurred.

Just one state changed its nurse practice legislation so that baccalaureate education was necessary for registered nurse licensure. That state, North Dakota, however, repealed this act in 2003, bowing to pressure from nurses and some health care organizations to once again allow non-baccalaureate entry into practice. California, however, does require a BSN for certification as a public health nurse in that state, and multiple states require a BSN to be a school nurse because that is considered to be a part of public health nursing.

In addition, state nursing associations in California, New York, and New Jersey have over the last decade called for initiatives to establish the BSN as the entry level for nursing in their state. Typically these initiatives suggested a target date for implementation (commonly 2010) and the promise of grandfathering for current registered nurses, yet for the most part these initiatives have either stalled or met such resistance that they have been discarded (Aughenbaugh, 2006).

COLLABORATION AND CONSENSUS BUILDING: IS IT POSSIBLE?

Silva and Ludwick (2002, para 7) suggested that dissension among nurses, professional organizations, and employers poses several ethical issues: "Respect for persons is violated when nurses and student nurses denigrate each other over credentials and over who are the competent nurses. Nurse educators and administrators violate respect for persons when they bicker and dispute each other over educational preparation and hiring practices."

In both cases, the principle of respect for persons, as identified in the ANA *Code of Ethics for Nurses with Interpretive Statements* (ANA, 2001), is violated. Silva and Ludwick suggested that the ethical solution is not to participate in verbal sparring, but to speak against it when it is heard and to engage in conversation about entry into practice based on mutual respect and concern for what is best for the profession.

Similarly, Silva and Ludwick (2002, para 8) argued that collaboration—another goal identified in the ANA code—has failed regarding entry into practice: "Each entry level has its proponents, and each group of proponents has tended to put forth an agenda without consideration of other groups. Each entry-level group seems to lack the trust, recognition and respect that are vital to collaboration." Silva and Ludwick suggested that ethical solutions at the individual level require becoming involved and/or staying involved with professional associations and pushing for collaboration on ending the stalemate on entry into practice.

GRANDFATHERING ENTRY LEVELS

Traditionally, when a state licensure law is enacted or when an existing law is repealed and a new law enacted, a process called "grandfathering" occurs. Grandfathering allows an individual to continue to practice his or her profession or occupation after new qualifications have been enacted into law (Ellis & Hartley, 2008). Should the entry-level requirement for nursing be raised to a bachelor's or higher degree, debate will un-

doubtedly occur as to how and when grandfathering should be applied.

> ### CONSIDER
> "Grandfathering" current ADN nurses as professional nurses would smooth political tensions between current educational entry levels but would threaten the essence of the goal.

Several professional organizations have actively advocated that all RNs should be grandfathered if the entry level is raised. Other professional organizations have argued that it should not occur at all. Still others believe that grandfathering should be conditional. For example, all RNs licensed at the time of the law would be allowed to retain their current title for a certain time but would be required to return to school to increase their educational preparation if it did not meet the new entry level.

LINKING ADN AND BSN PROGRAMS

Unfortunately, returning to school is not part of the career path for most nurses, which makes the entry level even more important. In a study of 2,418 nurses who graduated in 1983/1984, only 26% had returned to school by 20 years later (Beville, Cleary, Lacey, & Nooney, 2007). Similarly, only 17% of those who graduated in 1993/1994 had returned at the 10-year mark. Of those who had attained a master's degree in nursing or a doctorate in any field, more than 80% had begun their nursing career with a bachelor's degree. In addition, younger age at entry into nursing, male sex, and belonging to a racial or ethnic minority were associated with being more likely to pursue higher academic degrees (Beville et al., 2007).

McGrath (2008) suggested that many nonbaccalaureate RNs do not even consider returning to school. They question why anyone would want to do that, what it would get them, what effect it would have on their family, and what resources would be needed to do so. In addition, she noted that whereas employers prefer baccalaureate-educated nurses, they may overtly or covertly discourage the RN from returning to school for fear they might "lose their best staff nurses" to other institutions or other areas of nursing (p. 88).

McGrath (2008) went on to say that cost is frequently perceived as the chief obstacle to obtaining advanced education. Given that many practicing nurses are in their 40s, there are appropriate concerns regarding the cost benefit of returning to school. In addition, younger nurses considering a return to school are often advised to get more clinical experience in a specialty area first. This kind of thinking is unique to nursing, in that most professions encourage more education as soon as possible for their best and brightest.

These same concerns were cited by Megginson (2008), who asserted that approximately 70% of practicing RNs in the United States are educated at the associate-degree or diploma level, and only 15% ever move on to achieve a higher degree. Using phenomenological inquiry via focus group interviews, Megginson found that barriers for return to school included (1) time constraints, (2) fear, (3) lack of recognition for past educational and life accomplishments, (4) equal treatment of BSN, ASN, and diploma RNs, and (5) negative ASN or diploma school experience. Incentives to return to school for RNs included (1) being at the right time in life, (2) working with options, (3) achieving a personal goal, (4) believing that the BSN provides a credible professional identity, (5) receiving encouragement from contemporaries, and (6) finding user-friendly RN-to-BSN programs.

More than 620 RN-to-BSN programs nationally build on the education provided in diploma and ADN programs, including more than 340 programs that are offered at least partially online (AACN, 2007a). In addition, 149 RN-to-master's degree programs are available, which cover the baccalaureate content missing in the other entry-level programs, as well as graduate-level course work.

In addition, statewide articulation agreements exist in many states, including Florida, Connecticut, Arkansas, Texas, Iowa, Maryland, South Carolina, Idaho, Alabama, and Nevada, to facilitate credit transfer from community colleges to universities with BSN programs. According to Leighty (2007, para 3), "Generally, the pacts allow for the transfer of 60 semester credits, which is consistent with agreements between two- and four-year institutions for other academic disciplines."

CONSIDER

A broad new system, composed of direct transfer, linkage, and partnership programs, is needed between community college and baccalaureate institutions to ensure a smooth transition from ADN to BSN as the entry-level requirement for professional nursing practice. This transition will be costly.

Unfortunately, however, sometimes there is little integration, standardization, or cooperation between public systems of education. Such integration, standardization, and cooperation will be essential for transition to BSN entry levels. Transition programs or services for non–baccalaureate-prepared nurses must be designed to facilitate entry into baccalaureate and advanced education and practice programs. In addition, funding must continue to be increased for colleges and universities sponsoring baccalaureate and advanced practice nursing education programs.

Clearly, barriers for educational re-entry must be removed if the educational entry level in nursing is to be raised to a bachelor's or higher degree. Alternative pathways for RN education must be developed to create opportunities for learners who might not otherwise be able to pursue additional nursing education. For example, there is

> a trend in some states to let nursing students obtain BSN degrees at some community colleges, often in partnership with four-year institutions. In most states, however, students enter upper level programs through broad articulation agreements that insure the seamless transfer of their community college credits to the school offering the BSN (Leighty, 2007, para 2).

Finally, raising the entry level in professional nursing practice will be costly. University education simply costs more than education at community colleges, and significant increases in federal and state funding for baccalaureate and graduate nursing education will be needed. Given the significant budget deficits currently faced by almost all states, the likelihood of funding increases for nursing education is directly related to the public and legislative understanding of the complexity of roles that nurses assume every day and the educational level that they perceive is needed to accomplish these tasks.

AN INTERNATIONAL ISSUE

The entry-into-practice debate in nursing is not limited to the United States, although several countries have already established the baccalaureate degree as the minimum entry level and grandfathered all of those with a license before that date. For example, since 1982, all provincial and territorial nurses associations in Canada have advocated the baccalaureate degree as the education entry-to-practice standard, and most provincial and territorial regulatory bodies have achieved this goal. The Canadian Nurses Association (CNA) and the Canadian Association of Schools of Nursing (CASN) reaffirmed this goal in a joint statement released in 2004.

Similarly, Australia moved toward the adoption of a BSN for entry into nursing at the same time the United States began to rely heavily on 2-year associate's degree programs (Wawrzynski & Davidhizar, 2006). In South Africa, nurses who complete a 2-year course of study are called Enrolled Nurses or Staff Nurses, whereas those who complete 4 years of study attain Professional Nurse or Sister status. Enrolled Nurses can later complete a 2-year bridging program and become Registered General Nurses (The High Tech End of Training, 2007/2008).

Wales, Scotland, and Northern Ireland also only offer one entry point for nursing entry, and that is a 3-year university degree (Points of Entry and Specialization, 2007). Other one-entry-point countries include Italy, Norway, and Spain (3-year university degree), Ireland (4-year university degree), and Denmark (3.5-year degree at nursing school in the university college sector (Points of Entry and Specialization, 2007).

CONSIDER

"Outside the United States, a growing list of countries, states, and provinces (including the Philippines, Australia, Ontario, and other Canadian provinces, among others), now require baccalaureate education in nursing" (Keepnews, 2006, p. 4).

Yet, conflict continues even in countries that have adopted or are moving toward the BSN entry level. A 2006 discussion paper by the Royal College of Nursing (RCN) Australia suggested the RCN continue to recognize both registered (BSN) and enrolled (ADN) nurses as qualified and appropriately educated to provide nursing services to the community (Royal College of Nursing, 2006). Similarly, Rheaume, Dykeman, Davidson, and Ericson (2007) contended that the adoption of the baccalaureate degree in New Brunswick, Canada, in 1993 as basic preparation for entry into nursing has further complicated the lives of nurses because baccalaureate-educated nurses provide less direct care to patients and instead take on more administrative roles. As a

result, strain has developed between older and younger nurses, accentuating differences in working knowledge and work ethic. In addition, many of these nurses felt inadequately prepared to handle the increased emphasis on coordination activities as part of their BSN leader role.

CONCLUSIONS

The entry-into-practice debate in the United States continues to be one of the oldest and hottest professional issues nurses face entering the second decade of the 21st century. Graf (2006, p. 135) suggested that "nursing is a dynamic and complex discipline, one that requires skilled, knowledgeable, and autonomous practitioners." This suggests a need for more nurses prepared at the baccalaureate and advanced degree levels, yet the reality is that the majority of nursing graduates continue to be prepared at the associate level.

It appears then that little progress has been made since 1965 in creating a consensus to raise the entry level into professional nursing practice, although experts do not agree even on that issue. Donley and Flaherty (2008, p. 22) suggested that if the 1965 ANA statement is viewed as "a call to close hospital schools of nursing and move nursing education inside the walls of universities or colleges," then it was successful. If, however, the position is viewed as "a mandate for a more educated nurse force to provide better patient care, the goal has not been achieved" (p. 22).

Achieving the BSN as the entry degree for professional nursing practice will take the best thinking of nursing leaders. It will also require courage, as well as a respect for persons not seen in the entry debate, and collaboration of the highest order. It will also require nurses to depersonalize the issue and look at what is best for both the clients they serve and the profession, rather than for them individually.

Even the most patient planned-change advocate would agree that 45 years is a long time for implementation of a position. Clearly, the driving forces for such a change have not yet overcome the restraining forces, although movement is apparent. The question seems to come down to whether the nursing profession wants to spend another 45 years debating the issue or whether it wants to proactively take the steps necessary to make the goal a reality.

FOR ADDITIONAL DISCUSSION

1. What are the greatest driving and restraining forces for increasing entry into practice in nursing to a bachelor's degree or higher level?

2. Are the terms "professional" and "technical" unnecessarily inflammatory in the entry-into-practice debate? Why do these terms elicit such a "personal" response?

3. Is calling the associate degree in nursing a 2-year vocational degree an injustice to its graduates?

4. What is the legitimacy of requiring so many units at the community college level for an ADN degree? Why can't community colleges award bachelor's degrees?

5. How does the complexity of nursing roles and responsibilities compare to that of other health professions with higher entry levels?

6. What is the likelihood that nurses and the organizations that represent them will be able to achieve consensus on the entry-into-practice issue?

7. If the entry level is raised, should grandfathering be used? If so, should this grandfathering be conditional?

8. Is the goal of BSN entry a realistic goal by 2015? If not, when?

REFERENCES

Aiken, L., Clarke, S. P., Sloane, D. M., Lake, ET, & Cheney, T. (2008). Effects of hospital care environment on patient mortality and nurse outcomes. *Journal of Nursing Administration, 38*(5), 223–229.

American Association of Colleges of Nursing (AACN) (2007a). *Fact sheet. Creating a more highly qualified nursing workforce.* Retrieved May 22, 2008, from http://www.aacn.nche.edu/Media/FactSheets/NursingWrkf.htm

American Association of Colleges of Nursing (AACN). (2007b). *Fact sheet. The impact of education on nursing practice.* Retrieved May 22, 2008, from http://www.aacn.nche.edu/Media/pdf/3-07EdImpact.pdf

American Association of Colleges of Nursing (AACN). (2007c). *2007 annual state of the schools.* Retrieved May 23, 2008, from http://www.aacn.nche.edu/media/pdf/AnnualReport07.pdf

American Association of Colleges of Nursing (AACN). (2008). *Fact sheet.* Retrieved May 22, 2008, from http://www.aacn.nche.edu/Media/FactSheets/aacnfact.htm

American Nurses Association (ANA). (1965a). *A position paper.* New York: Author.

American Nurses Association (ANA). (1965b). *Educational Preparation for Nurse Practitioners and Assistants to Nurses: A Position Paper.* New York: Author.

American Nurses Association (ANA). (2001). *Code of ethics for nurses with interpretive statements.* Washington, DC: American Nurses Publishing. Retrieved May 16, 2008, from http://www.nursingworld.org/ethics/ecode.htm

American Organization of Nurse Executives. (2005). *BSN-level nursing education resources.* Retrieved May 22, 2008, from http://www.aone.org/aone/resource/practiceandeducation.html

Aughenbaugh, A. W. (2006). *Resolution seeking legislation to require a 10-year BSN passes at 2006 annual meeting preserving entry.* New Jersey Nurse. Retrieved May 22, 2008, from http://findarticles.com/p/articles/mi_qa4080/is_200605/ai_n16537323

Beville, J. W., Cleary, B. L., Lacey, L. M., & Nooney, J. G. (2007). Educational mobility of RNs in North Carolina: Who will teach tomorrow's nurses? *American Journal of Nursing, 107*(5), 60–70.

California Board of Registered Nursing. (2007). *2005–2006 annual school report.* Retrieved May 23, 2008, from http://www.rn.ca.gov/pdfs/schools/prelicensure.pdf

Canadian Association of Schools of Nursing and Canadian Nurses Association (2004). *Joint position statement. Educational preparation for entry into practice.* Retrieved May 21, 2008, from http://www.cna-aiic.ca/CNA/documents/pdf/publications/PS76_educational_prep_e.pdf

Delaney, C., & Piscopo, B. (2007). There really is a difference: Nurses' experiences with transitioning from RNs to BSNs. *Journal of Professional Nursing, 23*(3), 167–173.

Donley, S. R., & Flaherty, M. J. (2008). *Entry into practice: Revisiting the American Nurses Association's first position on education for nurses. A comparative analysis of the first and second position statements on the education of nurses.* Retrieved May 20, 2008, from http://www.nursingworld.org/mods/mod524/entry2.pdf

Ellis, J. R., & Hartley, C. L. (2008). *Nursing in today's world* (9th ed.). Philadelphia: Lippincott Williams & Wilkins.

Graf, C. M. (2006). ADN to BSN: Lessons from human capital theory. *Nursing Economics, 24*(3), 135–142.

Hospital death rate study reveals wide variations and stresses importance of Registered Nurses (2007). Press Releases. *Journal of Advanced Nursing.* Retrieved May 23, 2008, from http://www.journalofadvancednursing.com/default.asp?File=pressdetail&id=195

Kane, R. L., Shamliyan, T., Mueller, C., Duval, S., & Wilt, T. J. (2007). *Nurse staffing and quality of patient care.* Agency for Healthcare Research and Quality, U.S. Department of Health and Human Services. Retrieved June 30, 2008, from http://www.ahrq.gov/downloads/pub/evidence/pdf/nursestaff/nursestaff.pdf

Keepnews, D. M. (2006). A fresh approach to an old issue. *Policy, Politics, & Nursing Practice, 7*(1), 4–6.

Kidder, M. M., & Cornelius, P. B. (2006). Licensure is not synonymous with professionalism: It's time to stop the hypocrisy. *Nurse Educator, 31*(1),15–19.

Kuehl, N. K. (2005). Delegates define membership status, hear task force reports, and debate merits of proposed position statements at business sessions: Monday, April 4, to Thursday, April 7, 2005. *AORN Journal* (online). Retrieved June 29, 2008, from http://findarticles.com/p/articles/mi_m0FSL/is_6_81/ai_n14919322

Leighty, J. (2007). *Nursing by degrees—From ADN to BSN.* Nurse.com/Nursing Spectrum/NurseWeek. Retrieved May 23, 2008, from http://include.nurse.com/apps/pbcs.dll/article?AID=/20070930/ALL/71002002/

McGrath, J. (2008). Why would I want to do that? Motivating staff nurses to consider BSN education. *Journal of Perinatal and Neonatal Nursing, 22*(2), 880–890.

Megginson, L. (2008). RN-BSN education: 21st century barriers and incentives. *Journal of Nursing Management, 16*(1), 47–55.

Michigan Center for Nursing. (2006). *Survey of nursing education programs: 2005–2006 school year.* Retrieved May 23, 2008, from http://www.mhc.org/mhc_images/edprogramsurvey06.pdf

Minimum preparation for entry into professional nursing practice. (2006). *Nephrology Nursing Journal.* Retrieved May 20, 2008, from http:// findarticles.com/p/articles/mi_m0ICF/is_3_33/ai_n17213805

NLN data reveal dramatic drop in nursing school admissions perhaps signaling end of growth trend: Minority enrollment declines—Hispanics still underrepresented, ADN and BSN programs increase—ADN programs contribute outsize share of students (2006/2007). *Georgia Nursing, 66* (4), 26.

National Council of State Boards of Nursing (NCSBN). (2008). *Number of candidates taking NCLEX examination and percent passing, by type of candidate.* Retrieved December 22, 2008, from https://www.ncsbn.org/Table_of_Pass_Rates_2008.pdf

National League for Nursing (NLN). (2007). *Reflection and dialogue. Academic/professional progression in nursing.* Retrieved May 22, 2008, from http://www.nln.org/aboutnln/reflection_dialogue/refl_dial_2.htm

National Organization for Associate Degree Nursing. (2006). Position statement of associate degree nursing. Retrieved May 20, 2008, from https://www.noadn.org/component/option,com_docman/Itemid,250/task,cat_view/gid,87/

National Organization for Associate Degree Nursing (NOADN). (2008). *Nursing facts.* Retrieved May 22, 2008, from https://www.noadn.org/resources/nursing-facts.html

Nursing Link. (2008). *ADN vs. BSN: Which should you choose?* Retrieved May 23, 2008, from http://www.nursinglink.com/education/534-adn-vs-bsn-which-should-you-choose

Points of entry and specialization in nurse education: International perspectives (2007). Policy plus evidence, issues and options in health care. Issue 5. Retrieved

December 21, 2008, from http://www.kcl.ac.uk/content/1/c6/02/56/58/PolicyIssue5.pdf

Rheaume, A., Dykeman, M., Davidson, P., & Ericson, P. (2007). The impact of health care restructuring and baccalaureate entry to practice on nurses in New Brunswick. *Policy, Politics, & Nursing Practice, 8*(2), 130–139.

Royal College of Nursing. (2006). *Comment on discussion paper: "On a Roll—a review of the enrolled nurse scope of practice in South Australia."* Retrieved June 29, 2008, from http://www.rcna.org.au/UserFiles/nurses_board_of_south_australia_review_of_the_enrolled_nurse_scope_of_practice_in_south_australia_(june_2006)_.pdf

Service Employees International Union (SEIU). (2008). *Position statement on BSN requirement for RN practice.* Retrieved June 29, 2008, from http://www.seiu.org/health/nurses/bsn_requirement.cfm

Sexton, K. A., Hunt, C. E., Cox, K. S., Teasley, S. L., & Carroll, C. A. (2008). Differentiating the workplace needs of nurses by academic preparation and years in nursing. *Journal of Professional Nursing, 24*(2), 105–108.

Silva, M., & Ludwick, R. (2002). Ethics column: Ethical grounding for entry into practice: Respect, collaboration, and accountability. *Online Journal of Issues in Nursing.* Retrieved May 16, 2008, from http://www.nursingworld.org/ojin/ethicol/ethics_9.htm

Taylor, D. L. (2008). Should the entry into nursing practice be the baccalaureate degree? *AORN Journal, 87*(3), 611–614, 616, 619–620.

The high-tech end of training. (2007/2008). *Nursing Update, 31*(11), 42–43.

U.S. Department of Veterans Affairs. (2007). *Hiring programs and incentives.* Retrieved May 23, 2008, from http://www.va.gov/jobs/hiring_programs.asp#3

Vogt, P. (2007). *Career changes can take varied educational paths into nursing.* Monster Career Advice. Retrieved May 23, 2008, from http://career-advice.monster.com/career-change/healthcare/nursing/career-changers/Career-Changers-Can-Take-Varied-Edu/home.aspx

Wawrzynski, M. S., & Davidhizar, R. (2006). The Bachelor of Science in Nursing degree as entry level for practice: Recapturing the vision in the United States. *Health Care Manager, 25*(3), 263–266.

Way, M., & MacNeil, M. (2007). Baccalaureate entry to practice: A systems view. *Journal of Continuing Education in Nursing, 38*(4), 164–169.

BIBLIOGRAPHY

Brown, B. J. (2007). The perfect storm: Ratios, retirement, and entry into practice. *Nursing Administration Quarterly, 31*(2), 95–96.

"BSN in 10" frequently asked questions. (2008). *New Jersey Nurse, 38*(1), 7.

Corlett, S. A. (2007). I am a professional. *American Nurse Today, 2*(9), 9.

Dreher, H. M. (2008). Innovation in nursing education: Preparing for the future of nursing practice. *Holistic Nursing Practice, 22*(2), 77–80.

Entry-level education. (2007). *Nursing BC, 39*(5), 15–16.

Fealy, G., & McNamara, M. (2007). A discourse analysis of debates surrounding the entry of nursing into higher education in Ireland. *International Journal of Nursing Studies, 44*(7), 1187–1195.

Increasing RN-BSN enrollments: Facilitating articulation through curriculum reform. (2008). *Journal of Continuing Education in Nursing, 39*(7), 307–313.

Letters to the Editor. The "degree" debate continues. *American Nurse Today, 2*(10), 9–10.

Lin, L., & Liang, G. (2007). Addressing the nursing work environment to promote patient safety. *Nursing Forum, 42*(1), 20–30.

Lorentz, L. (2007). Are BSN nurses overrated? *American Nurse Today, 2*(8), 8.

McGrath, J. M. (2008). Why would I want to do that? Motivating staff nurses to consider BSN education. *Journal of Perinatal & Neonatal Nursing, 22*(2), 88–90.

Mu, K., & Coppard, B. M. (2007). The development of an entry level occupational therapy doctorate in the USA: A case illustration. *WFOT Bulletin, 56*, 45–53.

News from AACN. Moving nurses along the education continuum. (2007). *Journal of Professional Nursing, 23*(4), 187–188.

Porter-Wenzlaff, L. J., & Froman, R. D. (2008). Responding to increasing RN demand: Diversity and retention trends through an accelerated LVN-to-BSN curriculum. *Journal of Nursing Education, 47*(5), 231–235.

Raso, R. (2007). The wrong idea about BSN in ten... "10 years and counting" [May 21, 2007]. *Nursing Spectrum (New York, New Jersey Metro Edition), 19A*(13), 4.

Reams, S., & Stricklin, S. M. (2006). Bachelor of Science in Nursing completion: A matter of patient safety. *Journal of Nursing Administration, 36*(7–8), 354–356.

Rogers, L. (2007). Baccalaureate requirement would boost nursing's image [Letter]. *American Nurse Today, 2*(6), 8–9.

Rosenberg, L. (2007). Nursing academics endorse master's entry programs: Students prepare to be point-of-care nurses with leadership skills. *Nursing Spectrum (New York, New Jersey Metro Edition), 19A*(22), 8–9.

Sarachman, L. (2006). Proud diploma RN..."ADN RNs: what's in a name?" [September 11, 2006]. *Nursing Spectrum (DC, Maryland & Virginia Edition), 16*(23), 4.

Sizemore, M. H., Robbins, L. K, Hoke, M. M., & Billings, D. M. (2007). Outcomes of ADN-BSN partnerships to increase baccalaureate prepared nurses. *International Journal of Nursing Education Scholarship, 4*(1), 1–18.

Spencer, J. (2008). Increasing RN-BSN enrollments: Facilitating articulation through curriculum reform. *Journal of Continuing Education in Nursing, 39*(7), 307–313.

Staines, R. (2008). College chief criticizes training variation. *Nursing Times, 104*(4), 8.

Wendt, A., & Kenny, L. (2007). Monitoring entry-level practice: Keeping the National Council Licensure Examination for Registered Nurses current. *Nurse Educator, 32*(2), 78–80.

WEB RESOURCES

American Association of Colleges of Nursing	http://www.aacn.nche.edu/
American Association of Community Colleges	http://www.aacc.nche.edu/
American College of Nurse Practitioners	http://www.acnpweb.org/i4a/pages/index.cfm?pageid=1
American Nephrology Nurses Association	http://anna.inurse.com/
American Nurses Association	http://www.ana.org/
American Nurses Foundation	http://nursingworld.org/anf/
American Organization of Nurse Executives	http://www.aone.org/
Association of California Nurse Leaders	http://www.acnl.org/
Emergency Nurses Association	http://www.ena.org/
National Black Nurses Association	http://www.nbna.org/
National Council of State Boards of Nursing	http://www.ncsbn.org/
National League for Nursing	http://www.nln.org/
National Organization of Nurse Practitioner Faculties	http://www.nonpf.com/
National Organization for Associate Degree Nursing	http://www.noadn.org/

CHAPTER 2

Evidence-Based Practice

• SUZANNE S. PREVOST AND SHERON SALYER •

Learning Objectives

The learner will be able to:

1. Differentiate between evidence-based practice and best practices.
2. Explain why the identification and implementation of evidence-based practice is important both for assuring quality of care and in advancing the development of nursing science.
3. Identify personal, professional, and administrative strategies, as well as support systems, that promote the identification and implementation of evidence-based practice.
4. Describe the types of knowledge and education that nurses need to prepare them for conducting research and leading best practice initiatives.
5. Recognize the need to ask critical questions in the spirit of looking for opportunities to improve nursing practice and patient outcomes.
6. Delineate research and nonresearch sources of evidence for answering clinical questions.

7. Describe and compare practices that have evolved in the workplace as a result of tradition-based and research-based inquiry.
8. Compare the efficacy of the randomized, controlled trial, integrative review or meta-analysis, with practice-based evidence for continuous process improvement (PBE-CPI) to answer clinical research questions.
9. Specify institutions, units, teams, or individuals in the community that could be considered regional or national benchmark leaders in the provision of a specialized type of medical or nursing care.
10. Explore reasons for the disconnect that often exists between nurse researchers/academics studying evidence-based practice and nurses who seek to implement research into their practice.

Nurses and other health care providers constantly strive to provide the best care for their patients. As new medications and health care innovations emerge, determining the best options can be challenging. This process has become more difficult in recent years as health care administrators, insurance companies and other payers, accrediting agencies, and consumers demand the latest and greatest health care interventions. Nurses and physicians are expected to select health care interventions that are supported by research and other credible forms of evidence. They may also be expected to provide evidence to demonstrate that the care they deliver is not only clinically effective but also cost-effective, and satisfying, to patients. In light of these challenges, the term *evidence-based practice* has emerged as a descriptor of the preferred approach to health care delivery.

This chapter begins by defining the concept of evidence-based practice. Examples of when and where nurses are using evidence-based practice are provided, as are strategies for determining and applying these practices. In addition, the *who* of evidence-based practice is addressed regarding how nurses in various roles can support this approach to care. Finally, future implications are discussed.

WHAT IS EVIDENCE-BASED PRACTICE?

The term evidence-based practice is being used with increasing frequency among health care providers. Evidence-based practice has a variety of definitions and interpretations. The term evidence-based practice evolved when discussions of evidence-based medicine were expanded to apply to an interdisciplinary audience, which included nurses. David Eddy, one of the leaders of the movement, defined evidence-based medicine as "the conscientious, explicit, and judicious use of current best evidence in making decisions about the care of individual patients" (Eddy, 2005, p. 9). Sigma Theta Tau International (2008, p. 57), the honor society for nurses, expanded this definition to address a broad nursing context with the following definition of evidence-based nursing practice:

the process of shared decision-making between practitioner, patient, and others significant to them based on research evidence, the patient's experiences and preferences, clinical expertise or know-how, and other available robust sources of information.

Historically, various industries, in health care and beyond, have used the term *best practice* to describe the strategies or methods that work most efficiently or achieve the best results. This concept is often associated with the process of *benchmarking*, which involves identifying the most successful companies or institutions in a particular sector of an industry, examining their methods of doing business, using their approach as the goal or gold standard, and then replicating and refining their methods. Today, benchmarking data is one of the less scientific forms of evidence that is used, along with the results of formal research studies, to identify evidence-based nursing practices.

CONSIDER

Today, most nurse experts agree that the best practices in nursing care are also evidence-based practices.

Although this process of identifying the best evidence-based practices has become more scientific, the ultimate goal remains: to provide optimal patient care, with the goal of enhancing nursing practice and, in turn, improving patient or system outcomes.

DISCUSSION POINT

Are there any situations in which an evidence-based practice might not be considered a best practice? If yes, give an example and explain why.

WHY, WHEN, AND WHERE IS EVIDENCE-BASED PRACTICE USED?

Each week, new developments and innovations occur and are reported in health care—not only in research findings, but also in the public media. Contemporary health care consumers are knowledgeable and demanding. They expect the most current, effective, and efficient interventions.

Why Is Evidence-Based Practice Important?

In their quest to provide the highest-quality care for their patients, nurses are challenged to stay abreast of new developments in health care, even within the limits of their areas of specialization. Simultaneous with the growth of health care knowledge, health care costs have increased and patient satisfaction has taken on greater importance. Administrators expect health care providers to satisfy their customers and to do it in the most clinically effective and cost-effective manner.

Control of health care costs was one of the early drivers of the evidence-based practice movement. As discounted and prospective reimbursement systems decreased revenue to hospitals and providers, it became increasingly apparent that some providers were capable of providing high-quality care in a more efficient and cost-effective manner than their peers. The practices of these industry leaders were quickly identified and emulated. Within the current litigious and cost-conscious health care environment, there remains a sense of urgency to select and implement the most effective and efficient interventions as quickly as possible.

Nurses are increasingly accepted as essential members, and often as leaders, of the interdisciplinary health care teams. To effectively participate and lead a health care team, nurses must have knowledge of the most effective and reliable evidence-based approaches to care, and as nurses increase their expertise in critiquing research, they are expected to apply the evidence of their findings to select optimal interventions for their patients.

The processes and tools of evidence-based practice can help nurses respond to these challenges. This approach to care is based on the latest research and other forms of evidence, as well as clinical expertise and patient preferences. All of these factors contribute to providing quality care that is clinically effective, cost-effective, and satisfying to health care consumers.

DISCUSSION POINT
What type of knowledge and education do nurses
need to prepare them for leading evidence-based
practice initiatives as described?

When and Where Is Evidence-Based Practice Used?

In recent years, the implementation of evidence-based practice has been identified as a priority across nearly every nursing specialty. During the late 1990s, Sigma Theta Tau International conducted a strategic planning process to establish future directions for the organiza-

tion. In a poll of the organization's members, Sigma Theta Tau International learned that the most frequently cited request and recommendation from practicing nurses was a desire for support systems and resources to help them implement evidence-based practice. This feedback was consistent across nursing specialties and across nursing roles and positions. Initiatives to help nurses to understand and implement evidence-based practice have become a priority since that time. A review of recent literature yields case studies and recommendations for evidence-based practice implementation across several nursing specialties. These are shown in Table 2.1.

TABLE 2.1 **Evidence-Based Practice across Nursing Specialties**

Area of Specialization	Author and Year	Title or Theme	Type of Report
Administration	Shirey (2006)	Promoting evidence-based practice	Strategies for nurse managers and administrators
Critical care	Kuriakose (2008)	Endotracheal tube suctioning	Synthesizes related research and nursing recommendations
Emergency	Funderburke (2008)	Best practices for triage	Describes four strategies for an evidence-based approach to triage
Gerontology	Booth, Tolson, Hotchkiss, & Schofield (2007)	Using action research to develop evidence-based guidelines	Describes a process for gaining nursing consensus on practice guidelines
Medical-surgical	Keast, Parslow, Houghton, Norton, & Fraser (2007)	Prevention and treatment of pressure ulcers	Evidence-based guideline with literature synthesis for each intervention
Mental health	Curran et al. (2005)	Implementing research findings using opinion leaders	Report of a research study
Oncology	DiSalvo, Joyce, Tyson, Culkin, & McKay (2008)	Cancer-related dyspnea	Examines the evidence, provides recommendations, and identifies gaps in the literature
Pediatrics	Zolotor et al. (2007)	Practice-based intervention for gastroenteritis	Describes a quality improvement process for implementing evidence-based practice
Primary care	Thompson, McCaughan, Cullum, Sheldon, & Raynor (2005)	Barriers to evidence-based practice in primary care nursing	Survey of 82 primary care nurses from three institutions
Women's health	Bogdan-Lovis & Sousa (2006)`	Midwives' knowledge of evidence-based practice	Report of a research study

In addition to the universal application across nursing specialties, the concept of evidence-based practice is also valued across nursing roles and responsibilities. Nicklin and Stipich (2005) discussed the importance of preparing nurse leaders and administrators to promote evidence-based practice. Clinical nurse specialists are frequently called on to serve as leaders of evidence-based practice initiatives (Profetto-McGrath, Smith, Hugo, Taylor, & El-Haij, 2007). Melnyk, Fineout-Overholt, Feinstein, Sadler, and Green-Hernandez (2008) described the strategies of nurse educators who are incorporating evidence-based practice into nursing curricula. Last, but not least, staff nurses are frequently being expected to participate in, or lead, evidence-based practice initiatives (Phillips et al., 2006).

Evidence-Based Practice Around the World

A commitment to evidence-based practice is not limited to the United States. A few countries—in particular, Australia, Canada, and the United Kingdom—adopted this approach to care several years before it became popular in the United States. The Joanna Briggs Institute, which started at the University of Adelaide, Australia, in 1996, now has 54 centers providing evidence-based resources to health care providers in 90 countries. The Registered Nurses Association of Ontario has been developing and distributing evidence-based nursing practice guidelines for more than a decade. Lee and Huang (2006) described some of these concurrent development trends across the international nursing community. Nursing Knowledge International (NKI), a subsidiary of Sigma Theta Tau International, also serves as an international clearinghouse and facilitator to promote international nursing communication, collaboration, and sharing of resources in support of evidence-based practice.

> CONSIDER
>
> In recent years, the concept of evidence-based practice has evolved and been embraced by nurses in nearly every clinical specialty, across a variety of roles and positions, and in locations around the globe.

How Do Nurses Determine Evidence-Based Practices?

Evidence-based practice begins with questions that arise in practice settings. Nurses must be empowered to ask critical questions in the spirit of looking for opportunities to improve nursing practice and patient outcomes. In any specialty or role, nurses can regard their work as a continuous series of questions and decisions.

In a given day, a staff nurse may be called to ask and answer questions, such as "Should I give the analgesic only when the patient requests it, or should I encourage him to take it every 4 hours? Will aggressive ambulation expedite this patient's recovery, or will it consume too much energy? Will open family visitation help the patient feel supported, or will it interrupt her rest?"

A nurse manager or administrator might ask, "Who is the most qualified care provider for our sickest patient today? What is the optimal nurse-to-patient ratio for a specific unit? Do complication rates and sentinel events increase with less-educated staff? Do longer shifts result in greater staff fatigue and medication errors? Will higher-quality and more expensive mattresses decrease the incidence of pressure ulcers? What benefits promote nurse retention? How does the use of supplemental (or agency) staffing affect the morale of existing staff? Can this population be treated on an outpatient, rather than an inpatient, basis? What is the optimal length of time for a comprehensive home care assessment? How many patients can a nurse practitioner see in 8 hours?"

Likewise, a nurse educator may ask, "Is it more effective to teach a procedure in the laboratory or on an actual patient? What are the most efficient methods of documenting continued competency? Do Web-based students perform as well on standardized tests as students in traditional classrooms?"

Each type of question can lead to important decisions that affect outcomes, such as patient recovery, organizational effectiveness, and nursing competency. The best answers and consequently the best decisions come from informed, evidence-based analysis of each situation. See Box 2.1 for a list of questions to assist the nurse in the process of evidence-based decision making for various nursing scenarios.

> DISCUSSION POINT
>
> In your preferred area of nursing specialization, what are some key questions and decisions that nurses address on a daily basis?

BOX 2.1   **KEY QUESTIONS TO ASK WHEN CONSIDERING EVIDENCE-BASED PRACTICES**

- Why have we always done "it" this way?
- Do we have evidence-based rationale? Or is this practice merely based on tradition?
- Is there a better (more effective, faster, safer, less expensive, more comfortable) method?
- What approach does the patient (or the target group) prefer?
- What do experts in this specialty recommend?
- What methods are used by leading, or benchmark, organizations?
- Do the findings of recent research suggest an alternative method?
- Is there a review of the research on this topic?
- Are there nationally recognized standards of care, practice guidelines, or protocols that apply?
- Are organizational barriers inhibiting the application of evidence-based practice in this situation?

FINDING EVIDENCE TO ANSWER NURSING QUESTIONS

Nurses rely on various sources to answer clinical questions such as those cited previously. A practicing staff nurse might consult a nurse with more experience, more education, or a higher level of authority to get help in answering such questions. Institutional standards or policy and procedure manuals are also a common reference source for nurses in practice. Nursing coworkers or other health care providers, such as physicians, pharmacists, or therapists, might also be consulted. Although all of these approaches are extremely common, they are more likely to yield clinical answers that are *tradition based* rather than *evidence based*.

If evidence-based practice is truly based on "research evidence, patient's experiences and preferences, clinical expertise . . . and other available robust sources of information" (Sigma Theta Tau, 2008), then local expertise and tradition is not sufficient. However, the optimal source of best evidence is often a matter of controversy.

DISCUSSION POINT

What are the best sources of evidence for answering clinical questions?

Research is generally considered a more reliable source of evidence than traditions or the clinical expertise of individuals. However, many experts argue that some types of research are better, or stronger, forms of evidence than others. In medicine and pharmacology, the *randomized, controlled trial* (RCT) has been

considered the gold standard of clinical evidence. RCTs yield the strongest statistical evidence regarding the effectiveness of an intervention in comparison to another intervention or placebo. For many clinical questions in medicine and pharmacy, there may be multiple RCTs in the literature addressing a single question, such as the effectiveness of a particular drug. In such situations, an even stronger form of evidence is an *integrative review or meta-analysis* wherein the results of several similar research studies are combined or synthesized to provide the most comprehensive answer to the question.

In nursing literature, RCTs, meta-analyses, and integrative reviews are significantly less common than in medical or pharmaceutical literature. For many clinical questions in nursing, RCTs may not exist, or they may not even be appropriate. For example, if a nurse is considering how best to prepare a patient for endotracheal suctioning, it would be helpful to inform the patient what suctioning feels like. This type of question does not lend itself to a RCT, but rather to descriptive or qualitative research. In general, qualitative, descriptive, or quasi-experimental studies are much more common methods of inquiry in nursing research than RCTs or meta-analyses. Furthermore, the body of nursing research overall is newer and less developed than that of some other health disciplines, so for many clinical nursing questions, research studies may not exist.

Recently, a new research method has evolved that provides excellent support for evidence-based practice. Fittingly, this research method is referred to as *practice-based evidence for continuous process improvement (PBE-CPI)*. PBE-CPI incorporates the variation from routine clinical practice to determine what works best, for which patients, under what circumstances, and at what cost. It uses the knowledge of front-line caregivers, who help to develop the research questions and define variables (Horn & Gassaway, 2007). This method can provide a more comprehensive picture than a randomized, controlled study that only examines one intervention with a very limited population under strictly controlled, laboratory-like circumstances. Although research results are usually considered the optimal form of evidence, many other data sources have been used to support the identification of optimal interventions for nursing and other health care disciplines. Some of the additional sources are as follows:

■ Benchmarking data
■ Clinical expertise
■ Cost-effectiveness analyses
■ Infection control data
■ Medical record review data
■ National standards of care
■ Pathophysiologic data
■ Quality improvement data
■ Patient and family preferences

Another dilemma for the practicing nurse is the time, access, and expertise needed to search and analyze the research literature to answer clinical questions. In the midst of the current nursing shortage, few practicing nurses have the luxury of leaving their patients to conduct a literature search. Many staff nurses practicing in clinical settings have less than a baccalaureate degree; therefore, they likely have not been exposed to a formal research course. Findings from research studies are typically very technical, difficult to understand, and even more difficult to translate into applications. Searching, finding, critiquing, and summarizing research findings for applications in practice are high-level skills that require substantial education and practice.

DISCUSSION POINT

If a practicing nurse has no formal education or experience related to research, what strategies should she or he use to find evidence that answers clinical questions and supports evidence-based practice?

BOX 2.2

SUPPORT MECHANISMS TO PROMOTE EVIDENCE-BASED PRACTICE

■ Garner administrative support.
■ Collaborate with a research mentor.
■ Seek assistance from professional librarians.
■ Search for sources that have already reviewed or summarized the research.
■ Access resources from professional organizations.
■ Benchmark with high-performing teams, units, or institutions.

SUPPORTING EVIDENCE-BASED PRACTICE

In light of the challenges of providing or implementing evidence-based practice, nurses must consider some alternative support mechanisms when searching for the best evidence to support their practice. Recommended mechanisms of support are summarized in Box 2.2.

Garner Administrative Support

The first strategy is to garner administrative support. The implementation of evidence-based practice should not be an individual, staff nurse–level pursuit. Administrative support is needed to access the resources, provide the support personnel, and sanction the necessary changes in policies, procedures, and practices. Recently, nursing administrators have had increased incentives to support evidence-based practice because this approach to care is being recognized as a standard expectation of accrediting bodies, such as the Joint Commission on Accreditation of Healthcare Organizations (JCAHO). Evidence-based practice is also one of the expectations associated with the highly regarded Magnet Hospital Recognition program. Most nursing administrators who want their institutions to be recognized for providing high-quality care will recognize the value of evidence-based practice and therefore should be willing to provide resources to support it.

Collaborate With a Research Mentor

One way nurse administrators can support the use of evidence-based practice is through the provision of nurse experts who can function as research mentors. Advanced practice nurses, nurse researchers, and nursing faculty are

| **BOX 2.3** | STRATEGIES FOR THE NEW NURSE TO PROMOTE EVIDENCE-BASED PRACTICE |

- Keep abreast of the evidence—subscribe to professional journals and read widely.
- Use and encourage use of multiple sources of evidence.
- Find established sources of evidence in your specialty; don't reinvent the wheel.
- Implement and evaluate nationally sanctioned clinical practice guidelines.
- Question and challenge nursing traditions, and promote a spirit of risk taking.
- Dispel myths and traditions not supported by evidence.
- Collaborate with other nurses locally and globally.
- Interact with other disciplines to bring nursing evidence to the table.

examples of nurses who may provide consultation and collaboration to support the process of searching, reviewing, and critiquing research literature and databases to answer clinical questions and identify best practices. Most staff nurses do not have the educational background, research expertise, or time to effectively review and critique extensive research literature in search of the evidence to support evidence-based practice. Research mentors can assist with these processes, whereas staff nurses can often provide the best insight on clinical needs and patient preferences.

Laura Cullen and Marita Titler, international experts on evidence-based practice, described some of their strategies for promoting evidence-based practice, including an internship program that pairs staff nurses with advanced practice nurse mentors (Cullen & Titler, 2004). They recommended the review and adaptation of national practice guidelines for use in local agencies. They used algorithms, charts, and documentation scales as prompts to remind clinicians of the new practices. They also strongly recommended identifying opinion leaders and "change champions"—experienced and trusted clinicians in the setting—who are willing to lead by example in using the new practices. However, the adoption of evidence-based practice is not limited to expert clinicians. Box 2.3 includes a list of strategies for the new graduate nurse to promote evidence-based practice.

Seek Assistance From Professional Librarians

Another valuable type of support that is available in academic medical centers, and in some smaller institutions, is a medical librarian. A skilled librarian can save nurses a tremendous amount of time by providing guidance in the most comprehensive and efficient ap-

proaches to search the health care literature to find research studies and other resources to support the implementation of evidence-based practice.

Search Already Reviewed or Summarized Research

Another strategy nurses can use to expedite the search for evidence-based practice is to specifically seek sources that have already reviewed or summarized the research literature. For example, some journals, such as *Evidence-Based Nursing* and *WorldViews on Evidence-Based Nursing*, specifically focus on providing summaries, critiques, and practice implications of existing nursing research studies. For example, some of the topics covered in the July 2007 issue of *Evidence-Based Nursing* included the following:

- Reducing ventilator-associated pneumonia
- Delaying type 2 diabetes in people with impaired glucose tolerance
- Identifying the best research design to fit the question

The worldwide epidemic of child and adolescent obesity and the latest evidence on telehealth interventions are two of the topics that were reviewed and summarized in the 2008 issues of the journal *WorldViews on Evidence-Based Nursing*. When conducting a literature search, use of keywords, such as "research review" or "meta-analysis," can assist the nurse in identifying research review articles that have been published on the topic of interest.

The *Cochrane Collaboration* is a large international organization comprised of several interdisciplinary teams of research scholars that are continuously conducting reviews of research on a wide variety of clinical topics. The Cochrane Collaboration promotes the use of evidence-based practice around the world. The Cochrane reviews tend to focus heavily on evaluating the effectiveness of medical interventions, for example, comparing the effects of different medications for specific conditions. Therefore, many of the Cochrane review summaries are more useful for primary care providers, such as physicians and nurse practitioners, than for staff nurse clinicians. Some of the Cochrane projects of interest to nurses in direct care positions include their reviews of products designed to prevent pressure ulcers, nursing interventions for smoking cessation, interventions to help patients follow their medication regimens, and interventions to promote collaboration between nurses and physicians.

The Agency for Healthcare Research and Quality (AHRQ) is also a good resource for identifying research reviews and summaries that have been compiled by national panels of experts. One particularly helpful AHRQ resource is the *National Guideline Clearinghouse* (NGC) available at http://www.guideline.gov/. The mission of the NGC is to "provide physicians and other healthcare providers . . . an accessible mechanism for obtaining objective, detailed information on clinical practice guidelines and to further their dissemination, implementation and use" (National Guideline Clearinghouse, 2008, para 2).

All of the practice guidelines available through this site are developed through systematic searches and reviews of research literature and scientific evidence by a professional organization, health care specialty association, or government agency. Nursing organizations that have contributed guidelines to the NGC include the Association of Women's Health, Obstetric, and Neonatal Nurses, the Oncology Nursing Society, and the Registered Nurses Association of Ontario. Each guideline includes an abstract summary and a list of recommended practices, strategies, or interventions for a specific clinical condition. The NGC contains more than 2,200 unique practice guidelines. See Research Study Fuels the Controversy on page 27 for a synopsis of a study promoting practice guideline adherence.

Access Resources From Professional Organizations

Professional nursing organizations can also provide a wealth of resources to support evidence-based practice.

| BOX 2.4 | AMERICAN ASSOCIATION OF CRITICAL CARE NURSES PROTOCOLS FOR PRACTICE (2006) |

- Care of the mechanically ventilated patient.
- Creating healing environments.
- Noninvasive monitoring.
- Palliative care and end-of-life issues.

For example, the American Association of Critical Care Nurses has published several *Protocols for Practice* that are relevant to nursing care in critical care units. These protocols are based on extensive literature reviews conducted by national panels of nurse researchers and advanced practice nurses. A sampling of the topics covered in these protocols is listed in Box 2.4.

The AACN also publishes another type of resource known as *Practice Alerts*. Although the development process is similar to that of the protocols, the product is shorter and more specifically focused on areas where current common practices should change based on the latest research. Some of the topics covered in the Practice Alerts include prevention of ventilator-associated pneumonia, pulmonary artery pressure monitoring, and family presence during resuscitation.

The Association of Women's Health, Obstetric, and Neonatal Nursing (AWHONN) also provides several resources to support evidence-based practice. The AWHONN *Research-Based Practice Program* was designed to "translate research into nursing practice, ultimately advancing evidence-based clinical practice" (AWHONN, 2008, para 1). Through this program, several nationwide, multiyear projects have been completed. Topics addressed through this mechanism have included management of women in second-stage labor, urinary continence for women, neonatal skin care, and cyclic pelvic pain and discomfort management.

AWHONN also sponsored an *Evidence-based Clinical Practice Guideline Program*. Each of their guidelines includes clinical practice recommendations, referenced rationale statements, quality of evidence ratings for each statement, background information describing the scope of the clinical issue, and a quick care reference guide for clinicians. Cardiovascular health for women and perimenstrual pain and discomfort are two of the

Research Study Fuels the Controversy: Clinical Practice Guideline Adherence

The HEART Failure Effectiveness & Leadership Team (HEARTFELT) is an intervention designed to improve adherence with national practice guidelines. This quasi-experimental study compared clinician adherence with practice guidelines before and after implementation of HEARTFELT, which included an automated electronic pathway, access to evidence for clinicians and patients, self-management education tools, and ongoing feedback to providers regarding their adherence.

STUDY FINDINGS
After the intervention, clinician adherence with addressing self-management issues and patient discharge education improved. However, there were no significant differences in the provision of recommended medical interventions. Interventions such as this, which was an automated component of the electronic medical record, make good use of new developments in research and technology to facilitate evidence-based practice.

Dykes, P. C., Acevedo, K., Boldrighini, J., Boucher, C., Frumento, K., Gray, P., et al. (2005). Clinical practice guideline adherence before and after implementation of the HEARTFELT (HEART Failure Effectiveness & Leadership Team) intervention. *Journal of Cardiovascular Nursing*, 20(5), 306–314.

guideline topics produced through this program (AWHONN, 2008).

The American Association of Operating Room Nurses (AORN), the Oncology Nursing Society (ONS), and Sigma Theta Tau International also provide Web-based resources to facilitate implementation of evidence-based practice. AORN has published *Evidence-Based Guidelines for Safe Operating Room Practices*, the ONS provides an *Evidence-Based Practice Resource Center*, and Sigma Theta Tau International publishes Web-based continuing education programs and several supportive publications, including *Worldviews on Evidence-Based Nursing*. Web addresses for each of these professional organizations are included in the Web Resources at the end of this chapter, along with other Web sites that provide helpful resources.

> ### DISCUSSION POINT
> What institutions, units, teams or individuals in your community can you identify that would be considered regional or national benchmark leaders in the provision of a specialized type of medical or nursing care?

Benchmark With High-Performing Teams, Units, or Institutions

Finally, nurses can use benchmarking strategies to poll nurse experts from high-performing teams, units, or institutions to learn more about their practices for specific clinical problems or patient populations. Leaders of professional nursing organizations, such as Sigma Theta Tau International or the National Association of Clinical Nurse Specialists, can help nurses to locate and contact established nurse experts in various areas of specialization. Accrediting organizations, such as the JCAHO, can assist in identifying institutions that are known as national leaders in providing specific types of care. The University of Iowa, Arizona State University, and McMaster University of Ontario are three North American institutions that have established reputations as leaders in evidence-based nursing practice.

> ### DISCUSSION POINT
> When the investigation reveals a need for an evidence-based change in practice, what strategies are useful for implementing change?

CHALLENGES AND OPPORTUNITIES: STRATEGIES FOR CHANGING PRACTICE

Nurses use several mechanisms for incorporating new research into current practice in the pursuit of promoting evidence-based practice. Perhaps the most common mechanism is through the development and refinement of research-based policies and procedures. Fortunately, the JCAHO has mandated that health care institutions must implement formal processes for reviewing the latest research and assuring that institutional policies and procedures are consistently revised in keeping with current research findings.

Protocols, algorithms, decision trees, standards of care, critical pathways, care maps, and institutional clinical practice guidelines are additional mechanisms used to incorporate new evidence into clinical practice. Each of these formats is used by health care teams to guide clinical decision making and clinical interventions. Although nurses often take the lead in developing or revising these devices, participation and buy-in from the interdisciplinary health care team are essential to achieve successful implementation and consistent changes in practice.

In addition to consensus from the interdisciplinary team, support from patients and their families is important. This element of the process is frequently overlooked or not thoroughly considered. As previously mentioned, evidence-based nursing practice involves "the process of shared decision-making between practitioner, patient, and others significant to them based on research evidence, the patient's experiences and preferences, clinical expertise or know-how, and other available robust sources of information" (Sigma Theta Tau, 2008, p. 57).

If the review of evidence leads the health care team to recommend an intervention that is inconsistent with the patient or family's values and preferences (such as a specific dietary modification or transfusion of blood products), the recommendation may lead to poor adherence or total disregard by the patient, not to mention a loss of the patient's trust and confidence in the health care team.

> **DISCUSSION POINT**
> Can you think of situations in which the latest research may be inconsistent with the values of an individual or group of patients?

Challenges to Implementing Evidence-Based Practice

Although evidence-based practice is being discussed and pursued by nurses around the world, several obstacles continue to inhibit the movement. Funk, Champagne, Weiss, and Tornquist (1991) originally studied this problem, and Retsas (2000) used a modification of their survey to poll 400 Australian nurses. He identified several barriers that he grouped into four main factors: accessibility of research findings, anticipated outcomes of using research, support from others, and lack of organizational support, which was perceived to be the most significant limitation. In recent years, other researchers have investigated the same questions with similar results. In a 2006 study by Karkos and Peters, 275 nurses identified the setting to be the greatest perceived barrier to research use, even though these nurses were practicing in a hospital that had received Magnet Hospital designation (See Research Study Fuels the Controversy).

> **DISCUSSION POINT**
> What obstacles would limit your involvement in the process of pursuing evidence-based practice?

Research Study Fuels the Controversy: Reading to Facilitate Evidence-Based Practice

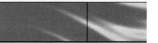

Access and familiarity with professional literature are important prerequisites for the implementation of evidence-based nursing practice. Therefore, this research team investigated reading patterns of staff nurses in relation to research and other professional journals.

STUDY FINDINGS

In this descriptive study, 20% of the nurses surveyed did not read any professional journals on a regular basis, 53% reported reading at least one general nursing journal, and 64% of the nurses reported reading seven or more journals in their area of clinical specialty. None of the nurses in the survey read a research journal on a regular basis. Nearly half of the nurses indicated that the hospital library was the most convenient place for them to conduct literature searches, but one third of the sample had limited knowledge of literature-searching procedures. Regular reading of journals can facilitate evidence-based practice. Advanced practice nurses and medical librarians can help staff nurses to gain an understanding of available literature resources and the procedures for efficiently searching the literature.

Leasure, A. R., Stirlen, J., & Thompson, C. (2008). Barriers and facilitators to the use of evidence-based best practices. *Dimensions of Critical Care Nursing, 27*(2), 74–82.

CONCLUSIONS

Many nurses are experiencing success in promoting evidence-based practice. Organizations such as the AHRQ and the Cochrane Collaboration provide support to help clinicians overcome some of the barriers, such as the difficulties in obtaining and understanding research reports, and the isolation from colleagues and consultants. The many agencies that support teams of research experts to collect, critique, and summarize the research and other forms of evidence pave the way for front-line clinicians to find and adopt evidence-based practices.

Yet challenges continue. Too few nurses understand what evidence-based practice is all about. Organizational cultures may not support the nurse who seeks out and uses research to change long-standing practices rooted in tradition rather than science. In addition, a stronger connection needs to be established between researchers and academicians who study evidence-based nursing practice and staff nurses who must translate those findings into the art of nursing practice. Nursing cannot afford to value the art of nursing over the science. Both are critical to making sure that patients receive the highest quality of care possible.

FOR ADDITIONAL DISCUSSION

1. Can decision support tools such as algorithms, decision trees, clinical pathways, and standardized clinical guidelines ever replace clinical judgment?

2. Why does at least some level of disconnect exist between nurse researchers/academics studying evidence-based practice and nurses who seek to implement such research into their practice? Is the problem a lack of communication? Do most nurses have access to evidence-based nursing research findings?

3. How static are evidence-based practice findings? Can you identify an evidence-based practice that was later found to be ineffective or inappropriate?

4. Should evidence-based practices be institution specific, or should they always be more generalizable?

5. Is evidence-based nursing research grounded more in quantitative or qualitative research? Are both needed?

6. What can be done to increase the research knowledge base of most practicing registered nurses (RNs), given that almost two thirds of the nursing workforce has been educated at the associate-degree level?

REFERENCES

American Association of Critical Care Nurses (2006). *Protocols for practice*. Aliso Viejo, CA: Author. Retrieved September 18, 2008 from http://www.aacn.org/DM/MainPages/PracticeHome.aspx#evidence

Association of Women's Health, Obstetric and Neonatal Nurses (AWHONN). (2008). *Research-based practice programs*. Retrieved September 18, 2008 from http://www.awhonn.org/awhonn/content.do?name=03_JournalsPubsResearch/3G_ResearchBasedPractice Projects.htm

Bogdan-Lovis, E. A., & Sousa, A. (2006). The contextual influence of professional culture: Certified nurse-midwives' knowledge of and reliance on evidence-based practice. *Social Science & Medicine, 62*(11), 2681–2693.

Booth, J., Tolson, D., Hotchkiss, R., & Schofield, I. (2007). Using action research to construct national evidence-based nursing care guidance for gerontological nursing. *Journal of Clinical Nursing, 16*(5), 945–953.

Cullen, L., & Titler, M. G. (2004). Promoting evidence-based practice: An internship for staff nurses. *Worldviews on Evidence-Based Nursing, 1*(4), 215–223.

Curran, G. M., Thrush, C. R., Smith, J. L., Owen, R. R., Ritchie, M., & Chadwick, D. (2005). Evidence-based medicine: Implementing research findings into practice using clinical opinion leaders: Barriers and lessons learned. *Joint Commission Journal on Quality and Patient Safety, 31*(12), 700–707.

DiSalvo, W. M., Joyce, M. M., Tyson, L. B., Culkin, A. E., & Mackay, K. (2008). Putting evidence into practice: Evidence-based interventions for cancer-related dyspnea. *Clinical Journal of Oncology Nursing, 12*(2), 341–352.

Dykes, P. C., Acevedo, K., Boldrighini, J., Boucher, C., Frumento, K., Gray, P., et al. (2005). Clinical practice guideline adherence before and after implementation of the HEARTFELT (HEART Failure Effectiveness & Leadership Team) intervention. *Journal of Cardiovascular Nursing, 20*(5), 306–314.

Eddy, D. M. (2005). Evidence-based medicine: A unified approach. *Health Affairs (Millwood), 24*(1), 9–17.

Funderburke, P. (2008). Exploring best practice for triage. *Journal of Emergency Nursing, 34*(2), 180–182.

Funk, S. G., Champagne, M. T., Weiss, R. A., & Tornquist, E. M. (1991). Barriers to using research findings in practice: The clinician's perspective. *Applied Nursing Research, 4*, 90–95.

Horn, S. D., & Gassaway, J. (2007). Practice-based evidence study design for comparative effectiveness research. *Medical Care, 45*(10 Suppl 2), S50–S57.

Karkos, B., & Peters, K. (2006). A magnet community hospital: Fewer barriers to nursing research utilization. *Journal of Nursing Administration, 36*(7/8), 377–382.

Keast, D. H., Parslow, N., Houghton, P. E., Norton, L., & Fraser, C. (2007). Best practice recommendations for the prevention and treatment of pressure ulcers: Update 2006. *Advances in Skin & Wound Care, 20*(8), 447–462.

Kuriakose, A. (2008). Using the Synergy Model as best practice in endotracheal tube suctioning of critically ill patients. *Dimensions of Critical Care Nursing, 27*(1), 10–15.

Leasure, A. R., Stirlen, J., & Thompson, C. (2008). Barriers and facilitators to the use of evidence-based best practices. *Dimensions of Critical Care Nursing, 27*(2), 74–82; quiz, 83–84.

Lee, S., & Huang, C. (2006). Concurrent development trends in the international nursing profession. *Journal of Nursing (China), 53*(3), 21–26.

Melnyk, B. M., Fineout-Overholt, E., Feinstein, N. F., Sadler, L. S., & Green-Hernandez, C. (2008). Nurse practitioner educators' perceived knowledge, beliefs, and teaching strategies regarding evidence-based practice: Implications for accelerating the integration of evidence-based practice into graduate programs. *Journal of Professional Nursing, 24*(1), 7–13.

National Guideline Clearinghouse (2008). *Mission statement.* Retrieved September 19, 2008 from http://www.guideline.gov/about/mission.aspx.

Nicklin, W., & Stipich, N. (2005). Enhancing skills for evidence-based healthcare leadership: The Executive Training for Research Application (EXTRA) program. *Nursing Leadership, 18*(3), 35–44.

Phillips, J. M., Heitschmidt, M., Joyce, M. B., et al. (2006). Where's the evidence? An innovative approach to teaching staff about evidence-based practice. *Journal for Nurses in Staff Development, 22*(6), 296–301.

Profetto-McGrath, J., Smith, K. B., Hugo, K., et al. (2007). Clinical nurse specialists' use of evidence in practice: A pilot study. *Worldviews on Evidence-Based Nursing, 4*(2), 86–96.

Retsas, A. (2000). Barriers to using research evidence in nursing practice. *Journal of Advanced Nursing, 31*(3), 599–606.

Shirey, M. R. (2006). Evidence-based practice: How nurse leaders can facilitate innovation. *Nursing Administration Quarterly, 30*(3), 252–265.

Sigma Theta Tau International position statement on evidence-based practice: February 2007. (2008). *Worldviews on Evidence-Based Nursing, 5*(2), 57–59.

Thompson, C., McCaughan, D., Cullum, N., Sheldon, T., & Raynor, P. (2005). Barriers to evidence-based practice in primary care nursing—Viewing decision-making as context is helpful. *Journal of Advanced Nursing, 52*(4), 432–444.

Zolotor, A. J., Randolph, G. D., Johnson, J. K., Wegner, S., Edwards, L., Powell, C., et al. (2007). Effectiveness of a practice-based, multimodal quality improvement intervention for gastroenteritis within a Medicaid managed care network. *Pediatrics, 120*(3), e644–e650.

BIBLIOGRAPHY

Anderson, J. A., & Willson, P., (2008). Clinical decision support systems in nursing: Synthesis of the science for evidence-based practice. *CIN: Computers, Informatics, Nursing, 26*(3), 151–158.

Carroll, D. L., Rankin, S. H., & Cooper, B. A. (2007). The effects of a collaborative peer advisor/advanced practice nurse intervention: Cardiac rehabilitation participation and rehospitalization in older adults after a cardiac event. *Journal of Cardiovascular Nursing, 22*(4), 313–319.

Cocoman, A., & Murray, J. (2008). Intramuscular injections: A review of best practice for mental health nurses. *Journal of Psychiatric & Mental Health Nursing, 15*(5), 424–434.

Estabrooks, C. A., Kenny, D. J., Adewale, A. J., Cummings, G. G., & Mallidou, A. A. (2007). A comparison of research utilization among nurses working in Canadian civilian and United States Army healthcare settings. *Research in Nursing & Health, 30*(3), 282–296.

Emerson, R. J., & Records, K. (2008). Today's challenge, tomorrow's excellence: The practice of evidence-based education. *Journal of Nursing Education, 47*(8), 359–370.

Franzini, L., Boom, J., & Nelson, C. (2007). Cost-effectiveness analysis of a practice-based immunization education intervention. *Ambulatory Pediatrics, 7*(2), 167–175.

Gawlinski, A., & Rutledge, D. (2008). Selecting a model for evidence-based practice changes: A practical approach. *AACN Advances in Critical Care Nursing, 19*(3), 291–300.

Girard, N. J. (2008). Practice-based evidence. *AORN Journal, 87*(1), 15–16.

Halcomb, E., Moujalli, S., Griffiths, R., & Davidson, P. (2007). Effectiveness of general practice nurse interventions in cardiac risk factor reduction among adults. *International Journal of Evidence-Based Healthcare, 5*(3), 269–295.

Hudson, K., Duke, G., Haas, B., & Varnell, G. (2008). Navigating the evidence-based practice maze. *Journal of Nursing Management, 16*(4), 409–416.

Jutel, A. (2008). Beyond evidence-based nursing: Tools for practice. *Journal of Nursing Management, 16*(4), 417–421.

Kline, N. E., & Thom, B. (2008). On 'evidence-based practice': Don't forget human experiences and clinical judgment. *Nursing Science Quarterly, 21*(1), 92.

Krugman, M. (2008). Is it research, evidence-based practice, or a quality improvement project? *Journal for Nurses in Staff Development, 24*(3), 137–139.

Leonard, E. E., & Wynd, C. A. (2008). Meta-analysis as a tool for evidence-based practice: An example using the Rice meta-analysis of smoking cessation interventions. *Applied Nursing Research, 21*(1), 40–44.

Malloch, K., & Porter-O'Grady, T. (2006). *Introduction to evidence-based practice in nursing and health care.* Sudbury, MA: Jones and Bartlett.

McConnell, E. S., Lekan, D., Hebert, C., et al. (2007). Academic-practice partnerships to promote evidence-based practice in long-term care: Oral hygiene care practices as an exemplar. *Nursing Outlook, 55*(2), 95–105.

Munroe, D., Duffy, P., & Fisher, C. (2008). Nurse knowledge, skills, and attitudes related to evidence-based practice: Before and after organizational supports. *MedSurg Nursing, 17*(1), 55–60.

Newhouse, R., Dearholt, S., Poe, S., Pugh, L., & White, K. (2007). Organizational change strategies for evidence-based practice. *Journal of Nursing Administration, 37*(12), 552–557.

Polit, D., & Beck, C. (2008). *Nursing research: generating and assessing evidence for nursing practice.* Philadelphia: Wolters Kluwer Health/Lippincott Williams & Wilkins.

Rauen, C. A., Chulay, M., Bridges, E., Vollman, K. M., & Arbour, R. (2008). Seven evidence-based practice habits: Putting some sacred cows out to pasture. *Critical Care Nurse, 28*(2), 98–124.

Reigle, B. S., Stevens, K. R., Belcher, J. V., Huth, M. M., McGuire, E., Mals, D., et al. (2008). Evidence-based practice and the road to Magnet status. *Journal of Nursing Administration, 38*(2), 97–102.

Schoenfelder, D. P. (2007). Innovations in community-based and long-term care. Simply the best: Teaching gerontological nursing students to teach evidence-based practice. *Journal of Gerontological Nursing, 33*(8), 6–11.

Springhouse (2007). *Best practices: Evidence-based nursing procedures.* Philadelphia: Lippincott Williams & Wilkins.

Talsma, A., Grady, P. A., Feetham, S., et al. (2008). The perfect storm: Patient safety and nursing shortages within the context of health policy and evidence-based practice. *Nursing Research, 57*(1 Suppl), S15–S21.

Thompson, D. N., & Burns, H. K. (2008). Reflection: An essential element of evidence-based practice. *Journal of Emergency Nursing, 34*(3), 246–248.

Wallace, C. J., Bigelow, S., Xu, X., & Elstein, L. (2007). Collaborative practice: Usability of text-based, electronic patient care guidelines. *CIN: Computers, Informatics, Nursing, 25*(1), 39–44.

Wood, M. J. (2008). The state of evidence-based practice. *Clinical Nursing Research, 17*(2), 71–73.

WEB RESOURCES

Agency for Healthcare Research and Quality: Evidence-Based Practice	http://www.ahrq.gov/clinic/epcix.htm
American Association of Critical-Care Nurses	http://www.aacn.org
Association of Peri Operative Registered Nurses	http://www.aorn.org
Association of Women's Health, Obstetric, and Neonatal Nurses	http://www.awhonn.org
The Cochrane Collaboration	http://www.cochrane.org/
The Joanna Briggs Institute for Promoting and Supporting Best Practice	http://www.joannabriggs.edu.au/about/home.php#
National Guideline Clearinghouse	http://www.guideline.gov/
Nursing Knowledge International	http://www.nursingknowledge.org/Portal/Main.aspx?PageID5700
Oncology Nursing Society	http://www.ons.org
Sigma Theta Tau International—Honor Society of Nursing	http://www.nursingsociety.org

CHAPTER 3

Blending the New Essentials of Baccalaureate Education and Distance Learning Education Models

• CATHERINE WILDE McPHEE •

Learning Objectives

The learner will be able to:

1. Identify the nine essentials of professional nursing education as outlined in the 2008 American Association of Colleges of Nursing (AACN) *Essentials of Baccalaureate Education* document.
2. Outline historical milestones in the development of distance education.
3. Explore advantages and disadvantages of distance education in nursing.
4. Analyze how technology-mediated teaching strategies change the way teaching and learning occurs.
5. Describe needs unique to distance learners that are not typically experienced by students in traditional classroom settings.
6. Identify skills needed by distance faculty that may not be needed or used as heavily by faculty in traditional classroom settings.
7. Identify personality characteristics and external factors that increase the likelihood of success for a distance learner.
8. Compare evidence-based learner outcomes in distance education programs with those of traditional on-site campus programs.
9. Identify sources of best practices for planning, implementing, and evaluating distance education programs.
10. Compare regulatory mechanisms for assessing the quality of nursing education programs in distance education and traditional on-campus programs.
11. Consider how distance educational programs and traditional on-campus programs may differ in providing specific content and experiences for student learners to meet the recommendations outlined in the 2008 AACN *Essentials of Baccalaureate Education for Professional Nursing Practice* document.
12. Reflect on the personal likelihood of achieving desired learner outcomes as a distance student.
13. Explore personal values, beliefs, and feelings regarding whether professional socialization needs can be met in distance learning programs.

There is little doubt that current health care trends have increased the complexity of health care delivery by nurses. Increased acuity of patient care, a rapidly enlarging geriatric population, increasing psychosocial and cultural diversity among patients, and an international nursing shortage are just a few of the factors challenging the efforts of nurses in the 21st century to deliver safe and competent care. In addition, public awareness of quality issues in health care and the risks associated with unsafe health care are increasing while spiraling health care and insurance costs result in ever-increasing num-

bers of uninsured and underinsured individuals. In fact, there are so many challenges to the health care system and to providing quality health care as we enter the second decade of the 21st century that many experts consider the health care system to be in crisis.

AACN'S *ESSENTIALS OF BACCALAUREATE EDUCATION FOR PROFESSIONAL NURSES*

In response to these dramatic changes and the increasing recognition that 21st-century health care providers

---

BOX 3.1 | **AACN'S (2008) NINE ESSENTIALS OF BACCALAUREATE EDUCATION**

---

1. Liberal Education for Baccalaureate Generalist Nursing Practice.
2. Basic Organizational and Systems Leadership for Quality Care.
3. Scholarship for Evidence-Based Practice.
4. Information/Patient Care Technology.
5. Healthcare Policy, Finance, & Regulatory Environments.
6. Communication and Collaboration.
7. Clinical Prevention and Population Health.
8. Professionalism and Professional Values.
9. Baccalaureate Generalist Nursing Practice.

Source: American Association of Colleges of Nursing (AACN) (2008). *The essentials of baccalaureate education for professional nursing practice.* Available at:
http://www.aacn.nche.edu/Education/bacessn.htm. Accessed September 21, 2008.

---

require new skill sets to face these challenges, the AACN revised their benchmark document *Essentials of Baccalaureate Education for Professional Nurses* in 2008 (AACN, 2008). Originally created in 1998, the new document is the result of a decade-long consensus-building process by nurse educators, clinicians, administrators, and researchers representing a wide range of nursing programs, specialties, and organizations. The document provides direction for the preparation of the professional nurse for practice and describes what can be expected of new nurses at the time of their graduation from a baccalaureate nursing program.

The newly prepared *Essentials* document, which was due for final AACN approval in October 2008, identifies five required components of professional nursing education: liberal education, professional values, core competencies, core knowledge, and role development. In addition, the document describes nine essentials of baccalaureate nursing education (Box 3.1), as well as the roles of the professional nurse in the 21st century, and suggests teaching methodologies and strategies. In response to this document, all schools of nursing education—traditional and distance (online)—must evaluate their programs for compliance and adjust them to achieve these expected outcomes (AACN, 2008).

DISTANCE EDUCATION PROGRAMS

Distance education, also known as *distributed learning*, uses a wide range of computing and communications

technologies to provide learning opportunities beyond the time and place constraints of the traditional classroom setting. In addition, distance education draws in students who might not otherwise be able to pursue coursework because of lack of access to a campus or because work, family, or economic considerations preclude full-time, on-site education. Indeed, many students who take online courses do so to balance work, school, and family commitments. Online distance education also meets the needs of students who prefer more independence in their learning.

Like most major changes in approaches to education, distance education has encountered responses ranging from eager anticipation to absolute refusal to consider accepting anything to be an educational modality that does not include a traditional classroom, students, and faculty. In addition, technology-mediated teaching strategies change the way in which teaching and learning occur, and thus distance education challenges the traditional relationships between students and faculty and between students and academic institutions. These changes require new ways of assessing the quality of education and new strategies regarding how to best support student learning.

To better understand the complexities of distance learning in nursing education, this chapter begins by taking a brief look at the history of distance education and then explores the use of distance education for educating the nursing professional. Next, the chapter compares distance learner outcomes with learner outcomes in traditional delivery systems and also examines the need for integration of the *Essentials of Baccalaureate Nursing Education* to produce quality program outcomes. The chapter concludes by examining what distance education offers the nursing profession, both in terms of reducing the current shortage and in terms of advancing the educational preparation of professional nurses in the 21st century.

DISTANCE LEARNING: HISTORICAL PERSPECTIVES

Although not new, distance education is certainly a change in the approach to education delivery. Distance learning is no longer just education being offered at a geographic location other than the campus where one is enrolled. It is now provided in multiple formats and is distributed in multiple ways (Table 3.1).

Distance education began with print medium and correspondence studies in the 1870s as the postal service began distributing correspondence studies to students across the United States. Radio programs of the 1920s were the first "distance education technology," followed by telephone and audio conferencing in the 1950s and television and video-

based systems that were able to provide a more classroom-like setting.

Although moving slowly for about 30 years, distance education has changed significantly in recent years due to the increased use of computer-mediated learning, the Internet, and related technologies. In response to these advances in technology, distance education now refers to any course being offered at any time and any place other than in a classroom on the campus where one is enrolled. It is not bound by time or place and typically involves teaching and learning strategies that differ from the traditional classroom setting and the traditional role of faculty (National Council for State Boards of Nursing [NCSBN], 2008).

Distance education has experienced many changes in recent years and will continue to evolve with the phenomenal growth of telecommunications technologies. The growth rate of online education in 2003/2004 (18%) was a factor of 10 greater than that projected by the National Center for Educational Statistics (NCES) for the U.S. postsecondary student population on the whole for the same time period (NCES, 2005). This growth is projected to continue at a rate similar to that demonstrated in the fall of 2005, when 3.2 million postsecondary students in the United States studied online. This represents 17% of the postsecondary population and a growth rate of 35% from the year before (Sloan Consortium, 2006).

TABLE 3.1	Historical Milestones in Distance Education
1873	Print medium and correspondence studies
1920s	Radio: the first "distance education technology"
1950s	Telephone; audio conferencing; first nursing audio conference; psychiatric course offered by the University of Nebraska
1960s–1980s	Television; video-based systems, including cable, microwave, and satellite, provide more of a "classroom feeling"
1966	First successful group of computer-assisted instruction (CAI) for continuing nursing education: Programmed Logic for Automatic Teaching Operations (PLATO)
1972	The Ohio State University initiates first CAI course
1980s	CAI expands with the availability of asynchronous and synchronous technology
1990s	Internet access proliferates

Source: Armstrong, M., Gessner, B., & Cooper, S. (2000). POTS, PANS, and PEARLS: The nursing profession's rich history with distance education for a new century of nursing. *The Journal of Continuing Education in Nursing, 31*(2), 63–70.

ACCESS TO CONTEMPORARY FORMS OF DISTANCE LEARNING

A variety of methods are used for distance learning. Courses are *Internet enabled, Web based, computer mediated, online, synchronous,* and/or *asynchronous.* The differences among these terms have to do with the extent to which the computer is required to complete course requirements, whether students are required to use the Internet to access the course or course materials, and how much flexibility students have in completing course requirements according to their personal schedules.

For example, online programs can be entirely Web based or have some required on-campus requirements or clinical experiences. Students may also be allowed to complete 100% of their course requirements at a time of their choosing (*asynchronous*) or may be required to meet at predetermined times in person or in virtual environments (*synchronous*) to speak in chat rooms, to create presentations, or to engage in video-streamed lecture interaction.

When distance learning is described as "more accessible" or "more available," it may mean that courses are available in geographic areas where institutions of higher learning do not exist and/or that course requirements are amenable to the schedule of the learner rather than that of the individual teacher or institution. It may also simply mean that more courses can be offered because the availability of educators is increased as a result of faculty members being given the flexibility to teach according to their schedules.

However, a classic document by the Institute for Higher Education [IHE] (1999) challenged the public to carefully scrutinize the notion of "easy access" and encouraged assessment of the special skills and technical support required if students are to interact fully.

The IHE also advocated that more research be done to determine whether the advantage of easier access is overshadowed by difficulties not normally encountered by students in on-campus programs. Much research has been done in this area, yet many studies have not answered this question empirically. Research must continue at a pace consistent with advances in technology.

WHY DISTANCE EDUCATION IN NURSING?

Nurses have many different motivations for attaining or furthering their education using distance education modalities. Nurses identified traveling long distances to a campus-based course as a major barrier to further education (White, Roberts, & Brannan, 2003). Precious time spent enroute to campus, coupled with high fuel and automotive costs, could also easily be perceived as a deterrent. In addition, geographic barriers to nursing education continue to exist. Many rural areas continue to be underserved by institutions of higher learning. Even now, many students and nurses drive, and even fly, hours to a university to meet their educational needs. In addition, work and family obligations, including child care, necessitate a more flexible learning environment. In fact, the University of Florida (2008) suggested that more than half of distance students are married with dependents and half are 35 years old or older. These factors clearly make distance education an excellent solution for students who want to begin or advance their educational preparation in nursing as adult learners.

Today's nurses need increased education and training to deliver complex patient care. Distance technology makes it cost-effective to run smaller, more specialized classes, which enhance the quality of learning. Specialty courses can be tailored to address geographic shortages in nursing specialties and meet specific community health needs. It is not just the inadequate number of nurses, but also the distribution and lack of preparation that are contributing to the current nursing shortage.

Fortunately, the advent of technology has expanded the capacity of educational institutions to reach far beyond their geographic areas. Educators point out that distance education courses may fight the "brain drain" from rural communities because adult students who learn within their communities can work while they go to school and may be more likely to remain in their communities once they complete their educational experiences.

The financial burden of an education in nursing is also prohibitive to many students, particularly those in minority groups. Although distance education is likely no cheaper in terms of tuition than on-campus courses, it allows learners greater flexibility in terms of maintaining jobs (income) while they go to school, reduces travel time, and may reduce costs that would have to be spent on childcare.

Compensation by employers and increased funding by private and governmental agencies for all education, including distance education, encourages people to enter nursing and to continue their nursing education. The increased use of technology in education may increase access to and ultimately lower the cost of education.

CONSIDER
Distance education may cost a student less as a result of decreased travel costs, child care cost and time, and less time missed from work.

FINANCIAL AID FOR DISTANCE EDUCATION

The Nurse Reinvestment Act, signed by President George W. Bush in 2002, directed that grants be awarded to schools of nursing and health care providers to develop programs aimed at recruiting students to enter nursing, promoting re-entry into the profession, and providing specialty training. Previously, a 1992 statute, known as the "50% rule," prevented students at colleges providing more than 50% of their courses online from obtaining certain kinds of federal loans, specifically the financial assistance authorized through of Title IV of the Health Education Act, as amended (HEA). On February 8, 2006, the Higher Education Reconciliation Act

(HERA) eliminated this rule. In recognition of the status of online education, Congress removed distance learning from the "correspondence school" category and, in doing so, equated online education more with traditional forms of education.

SCOPE OF DISTANCE EDUCATION IN NURSING

Online degree programs in nursing have multiplied rapidly in recent years, and the new reality is that distance education for nursing now exists for associate-through doctorate-level degrees. The choice of which educational program is pursued frequently depends on school preferences, cost, length of program, and access to the technologies used.

A survey conducted by the Instructional Technology Council of community colleges in 2007 reported a 15% increase from 2004/2005 for distance education enrollments, substantially ahead of overall campus enrollments, which averaged 2% nationally (Instructional Technology Council, 2008). The increase surged to 18% from 2005 to 2006, reflecting a continuing robust pace for enrollment growth.

In addition, programs for registered nurse (RN) to Bachelor of Science in Nursing (BSN), RN to Master of Science in Nursing (MSN), and MSN in many advanced practice majors are available online (Stokowski, 2004). Numerous online doctoral programs also exist, including complete or partial online Doctor of Philosophy (PhD) programs at respected universities such as Duquesne University, the University of Arizona, and the University of Colorado.

In a distance learning survey conducted by the National Council of State Boards of Nursing (NCSBN, 2004), a large majority of state boards responded that distance learning is being used in basic RN, RN-to-BSN, and advanced practice programs. Most of the programs are postlicensure programs, such as RN to BSN, MSN, or postmaster's certification programs. Three of the state boards of nursing (New York, Wisconsin, and Illinois) reported an entry-level RN program that offered most of its coursework through distance education, and many state boards reported that such programs were in development. Almost half (45%) of the states reported that they have programs that offer the majority of the coursework through distance education (NCSBN, 2004).

DISCUSSION POINT

Is distance education more appropriate for one educational level than another (e.g., graduate-level education more so than undergraduate education? RN to BSN more than RN entry?) Why or why not?

STUDENT NEEDS IN DISTANCE LEARNING

Historically, much of the literature on distance learning has been directed at preparing faculty members to teach online or looking at special needs that faculty teaching distance courses might have. More recently, however, there has been greater awareness that distance students also have unique needs.

Palloff and Pratt (2003) proposed that what the virtual student needs is very clear: communication and feedback, interactivity and a sense of community, and adequate direction and empowerment to carry out the tasks required of the course. The NCES (2005) reported, however, that it might be more complex than that, because online learners range in age from late adolescence to late adulthood. To meet student needs, distance education faculty are challenged to move beyond traditional pedagogical teaching strategies that work well in a classroom setting. As characteristics of nursing students change—that is, they are older and have more life experience—the need to emphasize adult learning theory becomes more important to present courses that are technologically effective and meaningful from the virtual learner's standpoint (Rounds & Rappaport, 2008).

In addition, distance students frequently need clarification regarding how they are to engage with the instructor, the material, or one another. Unlike the traditional classroom, where a student often has a choice of whether to participate in a discussion, online learners generally do not have this option. For this reason, online learning needs to be learner centered and learner focused (Palloff & Pratt, 2003).

Palloff and Pratt (2003) suggested that the virtual student:

- Needs to have access to a computer and modem or high-speed connection and the skills to use them

- Must be open-minded about sharing personal details about his or her life, work, or other educational experiences

- Cannot be hindered by the absence of visual cues in the communication process

- Should be willing to commit a significant amount of time to his or her studies weekly and should not see the course as the "softer, easier way"

- Is or can be developed into a critical thinker

- Has the critical ability to reflect

- Most important, holds a belief that high-quality learning can happen anywhere and anytime

Meeting these student needs does not mean that all students will be satisfied with their distance education experience. Some students report dissatisfaction with online courses related to the technology in use, course content, and breakdown in communication. Indeed, Huston, Shovein, Damazo, and Fox (2001) suggested that a student's computer skill levels are often predictive of his or her satisfaction with distance learning. Other students express frustration with not being given the independence and freedom they need to complete online course requirements. Most students who choose distance education as a learning modality are self-motivated and disciplined, and certainly these two characteristics should be predictive of success.

DISCUSSION POINT

What technology hardware and skills are typically needed by the distance learner to be successful in completing distance education courses?

CONTROVERSIES REGARDING DISTANCE EDUCATION IN NURSING

Can Nursing Be Taught Online?

Using distance education to teach nurses is not without controversy. When first introduced, there were concerns, which are still voiced today, that Internet education for a practice- and competency-based profession such as nursing would fail to produce individuals who were equally competent to those from traditional programs.

Common questions about the appropriateness of distance education for nurses include whether there is adequate clinical experience and adequate opportunity to develop necessary skills such as professional socialization and critical thought. The inherent nature of nursing as a clinical profession requires that all students have the opportunity to develop professional practices through collaboration with faculty, peers, mentors, and experts. Clinical practice experiences are essential to the socialization and development of this professional role. Nursing is a practice- and competency-based profession, which makes the opportunity for clinical experience an issue of great concern.

Accrediting bodies require that all distance education courses in nursing have the same clinical requirements as those in the traditional setting. For example, schools providing distance programs must deem clinical sites and preceptors competent and the various accrediting bodies, including the Joint Commission and state departments of health service, must document that established standards are met at the facilities. Establishing quality clinical preceptorships for students in remote settings can be a challenge but is essential to ensuring that distance students receive the same level and quality of clinical practicum experiences as students in more traditional programs.

DISCUSSION POINT

Should faculty be required to make on-site visits for students completing preceptorships in distance education programs?

Can Distance Education Nursing Students Be Socialized to the Professional Nursing Role?

Professional socialization has long been identified as a crucial aspect of nursing students' development. One's first response to distance education might be that such socialization is likely to be very difficult without the face-to-face interaction of traditional education. However, the literature actually suggests that both socialization and student interactions can be enhanced by using distance education technologies.

One study (Huston et al., 2001) suggested greater-than-expected increases in role and campus socialization, as well as in computer literacy, as a result of a primarily distance learning RN-to-BSN bridge course. Of note, students quickly created support groups online to discuss common challenges and issues associated with their return to school. The study concluded that an RN-to-BSN bridge course can be used successfully to ease the transition of students re-entering the academic environment and may be the link that allows RN-to-BSN students effectively to face the concurrent challenges of

role socialization and computer literacy while mastering course content and course objectives (Huston et al.). Similarly, research by Billings, Skiba, and Connors (2005) noted that distance nursing students reported being generally satisfied with how Web-based courses socialized them to the profession.

This socialization may, in fact, be enhanced by what many experts consider to be increased communication and connection between and among students in distance education teaching modalities such as online chats, discussion boards, and "webinars." Distance education students are frequently found to communicate openly with each other and with their faculty and to form close bonds. More reflection before interaction often leads to more logical and coherent viewpoints than those expressed by classroom-based students. Indeed, many faculty members say that they get to know students better in online programs than in face-to-face classes because students are typically required to participate actively in every class and/or feel more comfortable expressing themselves from a distance.

In addition, it is more difficult for one or two learners to dominate the conversation, a complaint often heard in traditional classrooms. The shy student has an equal chance of being heard in the online learning community. Furthermore, because it is a faceless environment, distance learners often feel freer to share personal information, thoughts, and feelings and may take more risks, although new research by Voss (2008) disputes this (see Research Study Fuels the Controversy on page 40). In addition, because online students have more opportunities to develop their communication skills, an increased focus on these opportunities may support essential 8 of the new *Essentials* document, which recognizes that collaboration and communication among health care professionals is critical to delivering high-quality and safe patient care (AACN, 2008). The better the communication skills of the nurse, the better equipped is she or he to communicate and collaborate effectively with other nursing professionals and other professionals on the health care team.

Furthermore, a recent study (Kubsch, Hansen, & Huyser-Eatwell, 2008) determined that professional values—those standards for action accepted by the practitioner and professional group—were emphasized in RN-to-BSN completion programs. The flexibility of these programs to teach outside the medical high-tech model resulted in higher mean scores on perceived

Research Study Fuels the Controversy: Variations in Student Learning Success

This study focused on incorporating online learning into a traditional face-to-face postgraduate forensic entomology unit with a heavy emphasis on problem-based learning activities. Students were surveyed to evaluate their perceptions of the online component and its value as a learning tool.

STUDY FINDINGS

Online learning was positively received by students, who considered it a valuable supplement to traditional teaching delivery. Students demonstrated a preference for online activities over paper versions and felt that online activities increased their understanding of the lab and assignment exercises. Students also liked the convenience, flexibility of access to information, communication options, quiz feedback, and interaction activities offered as part of the online component. Of particular note, 84% of students believed that the online material helped them to learn the subject matter quickly. When asked to what extent the online material assisted them in mastering the course content, 16% responded that it was essential and 84% said that it was helpful. In addition, only 11% of students felt that online modes of discussion with teachers and peers were more comfortable than face-to-face engagement. Rather, the increased communication observed was likely related to online advantages such as the flexibility offered in terms of access hours and locations.

Voss, S. (2008). *Resurrecting the dead: Use of online learning in forensic science*. Centre for Forensic Science, University of Western Australia, Teaching and Learning Forum. Available at: http://lsn.curtin.edu.au/tlf/tlf2008/refereed/voss.html. Accessed September 30, 2008.

professional values among the subjects pursuing their BSN degree.

Because so many online programs are directed at BSN completion, this curricular emphasis on professional values provides an opportunity to develop the strong professionalism and professional values recognized as fundamental to the profession (see essential 8 of the new *Essentials* document). In addition, because each nurse's professional values influence how her or his roles are enacted, the development of strong values will influence the nurse's role as leader, a trait emphasized in essential 2, Basic Organizational and Systems Leadership for Quality Care.

Can Students in Distance Learning Programs Achieve Desired Learning Outcomes?

Although outcomes achieved with traditional classroom learning have been viewed as the gold standard of quality education, many experts suggest that online education is as effective as classroom learning. Perhaps this is because the learner-centered environment compensates for the lack of face-to-face interaction.

Numerous experts and studies (Armstrong, Gessner, & Cooper, 2000; Buckley, 2003; Zucker & Asselin, 2003; Billings, 2007; University of Florida, 2008) suggest little difference in student learning outcomes between students who learn via distance education and those in traditional pedagogy formats, such as classroom lectures, conferences, or seminars. For example, a study by Harrington and Walker (2004) of a staff development program determined that the computer-based group consistently gave more-positive ratings and increased their knowledge scores significantly more than the instructor-led group, although there were differences between groups in long-term knowledge gains. Their study also showed that, at least in the large continuing education program, the scores of the computer-based group were significantly higher than those of the instructor-led groups on all six measures of satisfaction with the learning experience.

Indeed, there are a number of studies that suggest that distance education learners may have better outcomes than traditional learners. For example, Maring, Costello, and Plack (2008) found that distance students enrolled in a pathophysiology course performed significantly better on test questions than students in a traditional classroom ($t = 5.16, P < .001$); however, students continued to express a strong preference for the traditional classroom format. The researchers also found that increases in exam scores for the distance students were inversely correlated to cumulative grade point averages. Therefore they concluded that students with less academic ability may benefit from the self-paced learning and Internet resources to master coursework requiring factual recall of information.

Some studies suggested that the learning outcomes of distance students benefit most when the role of faculty changes to facilitator or guide rather than provider of information, and they proposed that critical thought is developed more quickly for the distance student in response, partly, to the asynchronous and collaborative nature of the experience. The ability of online education to foster thoughtful discussion—through e-mail, chat rooms, and discussion boards—may be the technology's greatest strength.

In addition, students in online courses can be directed to use evidence-based practice sources. The development of this skill—to easily navigate and discover these resources—will make empirical data more easily available for use in practice. Distance learning, then, allows students to develop skills such as critical thought and retrieval of empirical evidence, which are both required outcomes for the nursing graduate. These findings suggest that essential 3, Scholarship for Evidenced-Based Practice, may be easily met as online students reference current evidence-based studies found on evaluated Web resources. In addition, online learning is a good example of how nurses can learn the effect of one kind of technology on their practice and on their delivery of patient care. Enhanced capability to learn and teach online will also assist in meeting essential 4, Information/Patient Care Technology.

How Do Faculty Roles Differ in Distance Education from Traditional Settings?

As technology becomes more integrated into distance education and the role of the student evolves, so too must the role of the distance faculty educator. According to Watts (2003), distance education faculty need to use the new technologies along *with* students in an exploration and analysis of the world and its meaning.

In addition to preparing and posting materials, faculty must be able to respond to students' e-mail and review online activity in chat rooms in a timely manner. Bonnel (2008) concurred, arguing that although faculty who teach in online courses often express concern about

the time required to provide feedback in distance courses, such feedback is critical to the learning experience. Indeed, Bonnel argued that a purposeful approach to feedback in course design is what often brings about new learning opportunities and that a lack of feedback can lead to student procrastination and even course failure.

The transition from the traditional classroom to the online classroom, however, is not easy. Mancuso-Murphy (2007) suggested that

if the move is done in a systematic and orderly way, with the incorporation of a theory of learning, teaching strategies that address multiple learning styles, use of technology with multiple capabilities, and a focus on creating an interactive, collaborative community of learners, course redesign for the Web can result in a high-quality educational experience with pleasing results for both faculty and students (p. 259).

CONSIDER
The transition from a traditional classroom to online learning and emancipatory teaching often requires faculty to transition to new teaching and learning paradigms, and intrapersonal conflict is likely during the transition (Shovein, Huston, Fox, & Damazo, 2005).

Because of the uniqueness of distance faculty and student interactions, students would be wise to evaluate certain characteristics of their instructor. Distance learning can be disquieting for faculty as they lose familiar landmarks such as visual cues and body language. This is because the distance faculty must not only have content expertise, they must be able to nurture and support students through what is often a new learning experience for students, who are often re-entry learners.

Students then can evaluate several key characteristics that increase the likelihood that an instructor will be successful in facilitating an online course:

■ Flexibility

■ A willingness to learn from one's students

■ A willingness to give up control to the learners in both course design and the learning process

■ A willingness to collaborate

■ A willingness to move away from the traditional faculty role (Palloff & Pratt, 2002)

DISCUSSION POINT

Given that there are inadequate numbers of nursing faculty to teach the nurses that will be needed to solve the current nursing shortage—and that nursing faculty are even "grayer" than nurses in general—does distance education offer new opportunities for retired faculty to re-enter the workforce and teach part-time without the commitment of being on-site?

How Can Quality in Distance Education Programs Be Assured?

The number of distance education programs in nursing has increased dramatically, and this increase can be expected to continue. Yet, it is not always easy to discern the quality of these programs. Thus, in addition to identifying one's ability to be successful with teaching online, each distance education program itself must be evaluated.

Graham, Caglitary, Lim, Craner, and Duffy (2001) in their classic article applied Chickering and Gamson's (1987) "Seven Principles of Good Practice" (the gold standard for traditional undergraduate education) to online education (Box 3.2), along with corresponding lessons for online instruction. Using these principles, faculty can accomplish learner-focused online education to meet the needs and wants of the virtual student (Palloff & Pratt, 2003).

Despite the research already presented on distance learner outcomes, questions continue regarding the quality of distance education curricula, clinical standards, accreditation, and jurisdiction issues. Scientifically based knowledge about outcomes, what teaching and learning practices contribute to positive outcomes, what support needs to be in place for students and faculty, or how Web technology and its tools contribute to teaching and learning are still being discovered through research.

BOX 3.2 | **CHICKERING AND GAMSON'S CLASSIC SEVEN PRINCIPLES OF BEST PRACTICE AND CORRESPONDING LESSONS FOR ONLINE EDUCATION**

Principle 1. Good practice encourages student–faculty contact.
Lesson for online instruction: Instructors should provide clear guidelines for interaction with students.
Principle 2. Good practice encourages cooperation among students.
Lesson for online instruction: Well-designed discussion assignments facilitate meaningful cooperation among students.
Principle 3. Good practice encourages use of active learning techniques.
Lesson for online instruction: Students should present course projects.
Principle 4. Good practice gives prompt feedback.
Lesson for online instruction: Instructors need to provide two types of feedback—information feedback and acknowledgment feedback.
Principle 5. Good practice emphasizes time on task.
Lesson for online instruction: Online courses need deadlines.
Principle 6. Good practice communicates high expectations.
Lesson for online instruction: Challenging tasks, sample cases, and praise for quality work communicate high expectations.
Principle 7. Good practice respects diverse talents and ways of learning.
Lesson for online instruction: Allowing students to choose project topics allows diverse views to emerge.

Source: Graham, C., Caglitay, K., Lim, B.-R., Craner, J., & Duffy, T. M. (2001). Seven principles of effective teaching: A practical lens for evaluating online courses. The Technology Source. SUNY Network. Available at: **http://technologysource.org/article/seven_principles_of_effective_teaching/**. Accessed September 26, 2008.

BOX 3.3 | STANDARDS FOR DISTANCE EDUCATION NURSING PROGRAMS

1. Student outcomes are consistent with the stated mission, goals, and objectives of the program.

2. The institution assumes the responsibility for establishing a means to assess student outcomes, including both program and specific course outcomes, and that results are used for continuous program improvement.

3. Mechanisms for ongoing faculty development and involvement in the area of distance learning and the use of technology in the teaching–learning process are established.

4. Appropriate technical support for faculty and students is provided.

5. The program provides learning opportunities that facilitate development of students' clinical competence and professional role socialization and measures these student outcomes.

6. The program provides or makes available resources for the student's successful attainment of all program objectives.

7. Each accreditation and program review entity incorporates the review of distance education programs as a component of site visitor/evaluator training.

Source: American Association of Colleges of Nursing (2005). *Alliance for nursing accreditation statement on distance education policies.* Available at: **http://www.aacn.nche.edu/Education/disstate.htm.** Accessed September 26, 2008.

The continuing question of quality outcomes in distance learning programs for nursing has, however, been addressed by various professional nursing organizations. These identified standards should be used in assessing any distance program for nursing. For students who choose to pursue distance education, it is imperative that they choose a program approved by a regional accrediting body, the professional association of a specific field of study, and/or a state agency. For example, through its Council of Regional Accrediting Commissions, in 2000 the eight regional accrediting commissions developed a statement of commitment and best practices for electronically offered degree and certificate programs (Western Interstate Commission for Higher Education [WICHE], 2001a, 2001b).

In addition, the Alliance for Nursing Accreditation, composed of 14 national and specialty nursing organizations and accrediting/certification bodies, developed a statement on distance education policies (AACN, 2005) to assure the public that nursing education programs maintain a high standard of quality. This statement directed that distance learning programs must meet the same academic program and support standards and accreditation criteria as programs provided in face-to-face formats. Other standards for distance education nursing programs (AACN, 2005) identified by the Alliance for Nursing Accreditation are shown in Box 3.3.

More recently, the National League for Nursing Accrediting Commission (NLNAC) released its 2008 standards and criteria for multiple levels of nursing education programs, including clinical doctorate degree programs in nursing. Additional criteria have been applied for nursing education units engaged in distance education (NLNAC, 2008). These are shown in Box 3.4.

DISTANCE LEARNING AND SPECIFIC STUDENT POPULATIONS

RN-to-BSN Students

In 1996, the National Advisory Council on Nurse Education and Practice recommended that a federal policy be adopted to achieve a basic nurse workforce in which at least two thirds hold baccalaureate or higher degrees in nursing by the year 2010. Currently only 47.2% of the RN workforce possesses baccalaureate, master's, or doctoral degrees (Health Resources and Services Administration, 2004).

The benchmark study by Aiken, Clarke, Cheung, Sloane, and Silber (2003) has been a motivating factor for facilities and government to increase opportunities, funding, and compensation for those wanting to attain a BSN or advanced degree. This study showed a strong

BOX 3.4

NLNAC 2008 ADDITIONAL STANDARDS AND CRITERIA FOR DISTANCE EDUCATION: CLINICAL DOCTORATE DEGREE PROGRAMS IN NURSING

For nursing education units engaged in distance education, the following additional criteria are applicable:

1. Distance education, as defined by the nursing education unit, is congruent with the mission of the governing organization and the mission/philosophy of the nursing education unit.

2. Faculty engages in ongoing development and receives support in distance education modalities, including instructional methods and evaluation.

3. Information related to technology requirements and policies specific to distance education is clear, accurate, consistent, and accessible.

4. Learning activities, instructional materials, and evaluation methods are appropriate for the delivery format and consistent with student learning outcomes.

5. Fiscal, physical, technological, and learning resources are sufficient to meet the needs of faculty and students and ensure that students achieve learning outcomes.

6. The systematic plan for evaluation encompasses students enrolled in distance education and includes evidence that student learning and program outcomes are comparable for all students.

Source: National League for Nursing Accrediting Commission (2008). *NLAC 2008 standards and criteria. Clinical doctorate degree programs in nursing.* Available at: http://www.nlnac.org/manuals/SC2008_DOCTORATE.htm. Accessed 9/29/08.

correlation between RN education level and patient outcomes. The study's key finding was at least 1,700 preventable deaths could have been realized in Pennsylvania hospitals alone if the nursing staff had been comprised of 60% BSN-prepared nurses and the nurse-to-patient ratio had been 1:4.

A second study (Aiken, Clarke, Sloane, Lake, & Cheney, 2008) confirmed the previous findings that every 10% increase in the proportion of baccalaureate nurses on the hospital staff was associated with a 4% decrease in the risk of death. Dr. Kathleen Ann Long, past president of the AACN, stated, "Dr. Aiken's research clearly shows that baccalaureate nursing education has a direct impact on patient outcomes and on saving lives" (AACN, 2003, para 2). Perhaps these data can be used to encourage more nurses with associate degrees to complete their education with a BSN. Only 16% of associate-degree–prepared nurses go on to obtain post-RN nursing or nursing-related degrees (AACN, 2003). The accessibility and flexibility of distance RN-to-BSN programs could clearly meet the needs of a workforce that desperately needs to respond to such compelling findings.

One finding from the Aiken et al. (2003) study that was not so publicized was that a nurse's years of experience had no effect on mortality or failure-to-rescue rates. This is important information when considering that the nurse workforce is aging. It is contrary to the long-held belief that the nurse expert can compensate for advanced education with experience. Presented correctly, these data could stimulate the experienced nurse to obtain a baccalaureate degree and stimulate a career that has, perhaps, become less fulfilling. If this goal becomes easier to achieve through a distance RN-to-BSN program, the chances that a nurse would pursue this route may increase.

DISCUSSION POINT

Euripides (484–406 BCE) said, "There is in the worst of fortune, the best of chances for a happy change." Could the global nursing shortage facilitate the best chance to change our approach to distance education within the nursing profession?

Refresher Course Students

Approximately 500,000 nurses in the United States are not actively employed in nursing. Nurses not presently employed in nursing may be enticed back into the workforce because of distance education refresher courses. Traditionally, refresher courses have been provided by schools of nursing or hospital-based continuing education departments and are generally offered in the traditional approach of classroom didactic followed by clinical practice. The cost of such programs and their dependence on class size to be cost-efficient require them to pull from a large geographic area, resulting in the need for these students, in many instances, to commute long distances.

Refresher courses in nursing are vital bridges for inactive nurses returning to nursing (Hammer & Craig, 2008). Inactive nurses can be returned to the workforce if they update their knowledge and skills (Huggins, 2005). Deterrents to their return include a lack of availability or accessibility of refresher courses. Reasons for inactive nurses to complete a refresher course include their desire to return to nursing, their having older children, and a change in marital status that presumably affected their financial status (Hawley & Foley, 2004).

CONSIDER
Nurses who participate in refresher courses may experience uncertainty and lack of confidence in their abilities to cope with new information and practice and may experience a life crisis.

Educational issues have been identified as online refresher courses have evolved. Issues identified, for example, in the evaluation of a refresher course at Kennesaw State University in Georgia included technical support, including computer availability and competence, testing issues related to participants not needing a course grade or to sit for the state licensing examination, and the need for additional faculty development before teaching (White et al., 2003).

CONCLUSIONS

Is distance learning appropriate for nursing education? Can it produce nurses competent in the social, behavioral, and clinical skills needed for the humanistic, practice-oriented discipline of nursing? Those in favor of distance education say that there is no excuse for not using new and available tools. They believe that the intelligent use of technology will extend both reach and results (Watts, 2003).

Yet, despite numerous research studies suggesting that distance education is an effective method of providing education to nurses, controversy continues, and "quiet concerns" about quality perpetuate. For those unsure that distance education methods can produce desired learner outcomes, regulatory bodies are in place to evaluate these programs, and the current standards emphasize the same academic rigor as those used in evaluating on-campus programs.

Each student must determine whether distance learning is right for him or her. Similarly, each teacher will need to determine individually if he or she wants to use distance education technologies to connect with students.

The contributions of distance education to the nursing shortage could not have come at a better time. The nursing profession needs distance education to attract nurses who cannot access traditional school settings. Distance education can also help to retain and attract nurses to practice by providing advanced degrees, which correspond with higher levels of job satisfaction.

In addition, given the aging of nursing educators, the incentives of distance education may be significant to faculty retention and recruitment. Working from a "virtual classroom" in one's home might be tempting to faculty, especially those thinking of retirement. Master's-prepared nurses also could pursue careers in education more easily via online doctoral courses while remaining in the workforce.

Despite the quality safeguards and the obvious benefits of increasing the number of entry modes into nursing education, there are skeptics who will be slow to embrace any nontraditional learning method.

Brian Hutchinson, the first editor for *The Journal of Continuing Education in Nursing*, stated:

> *The decision [for using distance education] is ours—either lift the anchor or maintain the status quo. If you decide to take the plunge . . . study all alternative methods. Chart your course, but don't expect smooth sailing. Batten down the hatches. Use all relevant navigational guides. Steady at the helm . . . Damn the torpedoes . . . And full speed ahead. (Armstrong et al., 2000, p. 68)*

Perhaps the most noteworthy thing about this statement is that it was made in 1976. More than three decades later, it still holds true. The bottom line is that distance education in nursing is here to stay and is, in fact, gaining momentum. The increasing number of quality distance education programs will only assist in advancing nursing education and alleviating the nursing shortage.

Shovein et al. (2005) stated:

> The reaction to computer technology will probably follow patterns of the past, which consist of those who fearlessly embrace it, those who are prudently cautious, and those who will fight it to the end. Eventually, it will come down to the balance and the way in which the technology is applied and the purpose for which it is used. The formidable task remains what it has always been for a nursing educator, to design learning paradigms that awaken the awareness of another to a nursing consciousness.

FOR ADDITIONAL DISCUSSION

1. Can online learning using an interactive, community-based approach be used effectively across disciplines—specifically, nursing?

2. Using the standards identified in this chapter, how would one go about evaluating the quality of a distance education program in nursing?

3. Should national standards be set for distance education courses in nursing?

4. Can students learn to relate well in a multidisciplinary environment when their dominant educational experiences have been technology based?

5. How can faculty effectively oversee and assess clinical competence in distance modalities, particularly in prelicensure programs?

6. What noncurricular supports are necessary for students enrolled in distance education programs?

7. What are the findings of the research on the effectiveness of distance education? Are they valid? Are there gaps in the research that require further investigation?

8. How can online programs for nursing education provide specific content and experiences to meet the new *Essentials of Baccalaureate Education for Professional Nursing Practice*?

REFERENCES

Aiken, L., Clarke, S., Cheung, R. B., Sloane, D., & Silber, J. H. (2003). Educational levels of hospital nurse and surgical patient mortality. *Journal of the American Medical Association, 290*(12), 1617–1623.

Aiken, L., Clarke, S., Sloane, D., Lake, E., & Cheney, T. (2008). Effects of hospital care environment on patient mortality and nurse outcomes. *Journal of Nursing Administration, 35*(5), 223–229.

American Association of Colleges of Nursing (AACN) (2005). *Alliance for Nursing Accreditation statement on distance education policies.* Available at: http://www.aacn.nche.edu/Education/disstate.htm. Accessed September 26, 2008.

American Association of Colleges of Nursing (AACN) (2003). *AACN applauds new study that confirms link between nursing education and patient mortality.* Available at: http://www.aacn.nche.edu/Media/News Releases/Archives/2003/2003AikenStudy.htm. Accessed September 26, 2008.

American Association of Colleges of Nursing (AACN) (2008). *The essentials of baccalaureate education for professional nursing practice.* Available at: http://www.aacn.nche.edu/Education/bacessn.htm. Accessed September 21, 2008.

Armstrong, M., Gessner, B., & Cooper, S. (2000). POTS, PANS, and PEARLS: The nursing profession's rich history with distance education for a new century of nursing. *The Journal of Continuing Education in Nursing, 31*(2), 63–70.

Billings, D. (2007). Optimizing distance education in nursing. *Journal of Nursing Education, 46*(6), 247–248.

Billings, D. M., Skiba, D. J., & Connors, H. R. (2005). Best practices in Web-based courses: Generational differences across undergraduate and graduate nursing students. *Journal of Professional Nursing, 21*, 126–133.

Bonnel, W. (2008). Improving feedback to students in online courses. *Nursing Education Perspectives, 29*(5), 290–294.

Buckley, K. (2003). Evaluation of classroom-based, Web-enhanced, and Web-based distance learning nutrition courses for undergraduate nursing. *Journal of Nursing Education, 42*(8), 367–370.

Chickering, A. W., & Gamson, Z. F. (1987). Seven principles for good practice in undergraduate education. *American Association of Higher Education Bulletin, 1987*, 3–7.

Graham, C., Caglitay, K., Lim, B.-R., Craner, J., & Duffy, T. M. (2001). Seven principles of effective teaching: A practical lens for evaluating online courses. The Technology Source. SUNY Network. Available at: http://technologysource.org/article/seven_ principles_of_effective_teaching/. Accessed September 26, 2008.

Hammer, V., & Craig, G. (2008). The experiences of inactive nurses returned to nursing after completing a refresher course. *The Journal of Continuing Education in Nursing, 39*(8), 358–367.

Harrington, S., & Walker, B. (2004). The effects of computer based training on immediate and residual learning of facility staff. *The Journal of Continuing Education in Nursing, 35*(4), 156–163.

Hawley, J., & Foley, B. (2004). Being refreshed: Evaluation of a nurse refresher course. *The Journal of Continuing Education in Nursing, 35*(2), 84–88.

Health Resources and Services Administration. (2004). *National sample survey of registered nurses.* Available at: http://bhpr.hrsa.gov/healthworkforce/rnsurvey04/. Accessed September 21, 2008.

Huggins, M. E. (2005). Registered nurse refresher course as an adjunct in nurse recruitment. *The Journal of Continuing Education in Nursing, 36*(5), 213–217.

Huston, C., Shovein, J., Damazo, B., & Fox, S. (2001). The RN-BSN bridge course: Transitioning the re-entry learner. *The Journal of Continuing Education in Nursing, 32*(6), 250–253.

Institute for Higher Education (1999). *Policy: What's the difference? A review of contemporary research of the effectiveness of distance learning in higher education.* Available at: http://www.ihep.org/assets/files/ publications/s-z/WhatDifference.pdf. Accessed September 26, 2008.

Instructional Technology Council (2008). *2007 Distance education survey results.* Available at: http://www. presidiumlearning.com/downloads/ITCAnnual SurveyMarch2008.pdf. Accessed September 29, 2008.

Kubsch, S., Hansen, G., & Huyser-Eatwell, V. (2008). Professional values: The case for the RN–BSN Completion Education. *The Journal of Continuing Education in Nursing, 39*(8), 375–384.

Mancuso-Murphy, J. (2007). Distance education in nursing: An integrated review of online nursing students' experiences with technology-delivered instruction. *Journal of Nursing Education, 46*(6), 252–260.

Maring, J., Costello, E., & Plack, M. (2008). Student outcomes in a pathophysiology course based on mode of delivery: Distance versus traditional classroom learning. *Journal of Physical Therapy Education, 22*(1), 24–32.

National Council for Education Statistics (NCES). (2005). *Digest of educational statistics, 2005.* Available at: http://nces.ed.gov/programs/digest/d05/. Accessed September 24, 2008.

National Council of State Boards of Nursing (NCSBN) (2004). *2002–2003 NCSBN distance learning survey results.* Available at: https://www.ncsbn.org/873.htm. Accessed December 23, 2008.

National Council of State Boards of Nursing (NCSBN) (2008). *Distance learning/Web definitions: A resource for the model education rules.* Available at: https://www. ncsbn.org/836.htm. Accessed September 29, 2008.

National League for Nursing Accrediting Commission (2008). *NLAC 2008 standards and criteria. Clinical doctorate degree programs in nursing.* Available at: http:// www.nlnac.org/manuals/SC2008_DOCTORATE. htm. Accessed September 29, 2008.

Palloff, R., & Pratt, K. (2002). Beyond the looking glass: What faculty and students need to be successful online. In K. E. Rudestam & J. Schoenholtz-Read (Eds.), *Handbook of Online Learning* (pp. 171–184). Thousand Oaks, CA: Sage.

Palloff, R., & Pratt, K. (2003). *The Virtual Student: A Profile and Guide to Working with Online Learners.* San Francisco: Wiley.

Rounds, L. R., & Rappaport, B. A. (2008). The successful use of problem-based learning in an online nurse practitioner course. *Nursing Education Perspectives, 29*(1), 12–16.

Shovein, J., Huston, C., Fox, S., & Damazo, B. (2005). Challenging traditional teaching and learning paradigms: Online learning and emancipatory teaching. *Nursing Education Perspectives, 26*(6), 340–343.

Sloan Consortium (2006). *Making the grade: Online education in the United States, 2006.* Available at: http://www.sloan-c.org/publications/survey/pdf/making_the_grade.pdf. Accessed September 24, 2008.

Stokowski, L. (2004). Trends in nursing: 2004 and beyond. *Topics in Advanced Practice Nursing eJournal, 4*(1). Available at: http://medscape.com/viewarticle/466711. Accessed September 26, 2008.

University of Florida (2008). *Distance learning at the University of Florida. The distance education experience.* Available at: http://www.distancelearning.ufl.edu/students/characteristics.aspx. Accessed September 29, 2008.

Voss, S. (2008). *Resurrecting the dead: Use of online learning in forensic science.* Centre for Forensic Science, University of Western Australia, Teaching and Learning Forum. Available at: http://lsn.curtin.edu.au/tlf/tlf2008/refereed/voss.html. Accessed September 30, 2008.

Watts, M. (2003). *Technology: Taking the Distance out of learning.* San Francisco: Jossey-Bass.

Western Interstate Commission for Higher Education (WICHE) (2001a). *Best practices for electronically offered degree and certificate programs.* Available at: http://www.ncahlc.org/download/Best_Pract_DEd.pdf. Accessed December 23, 2008.

Western Interstate Commission for Higher Education (WICHE) (2001b). *Statement of commitment by the regional accrediting commissions for the evaluation of electronically offered degree and certificate programs.* Available at: http://www.ncahlc.org/download/CRAC_Statement_DEd.pdf. Accessed December 23, 2008.

White, A., Roberts, V., & Brannan, J. (2003). Returning nursing to the workforce: Developing an online refresher course. *The Journal of Continuing Education in Nursing, 34*(2), 59–63.

Zucker, D., & Asselin, M. (2003). Migrating to the Web: The transformation of a traditional RN to BS program. *The Journal of Continuing Education in Nursing, 34*(2), 86–89.

BIBLIOGRAPHY

Benjamin, R., & Ostrow, L. (2008). Technology in nursing education. *International Journal for Human Caring, 12*(2), 57–64.

Croix, W. (2006). *Down with the 50% rule: Up with online education.* Available at: http://www.worldwidelearn.com/education-advisor/indepth/down-with-the-50-percent-rule-up-with-online-education.php. Accessed December 23, 2008.

DeNeui, D., & Dodge, T. (2006). Asynchronous learning networks and student outcomes: The utility of online learning components in hybrid courses. *Journal of Instructional Psychology, 33*(4), 256–259.

Hall, C., & Fabayo, A. (2006). Nursing students' adjustment to a new phenomenon. *Journal of National Black Nurses' Association, 17*(2), 24–29.

Hurley, J. (2008). The necessity, barriers and ways forward to meet user-based needs for emotionally intelligent nurses. *Journal of Psychiatric & Mental Health Nursing, 15*(5), 379–385.

Lahaie, U. (2007). Web-based instruction: Getting faculty onboard. *Journal of Professional Nursing, 23*(6), 335–342.

Lewis, P., & Price, S. (2007). Distance education and the integration of E-learning in a graduate program. *The Journal of Continuing Education in Nursing, 38*(3), 139–143.

Martin, P. (2008). *Reviewing the AACN baccalaureate essentials: A journey in transformation.* Available at: http://www.aacn.nche.edu/Education/pdf/teleconf08. pdf. Accessed September 22, 2008.

Parker, E., & Howland, L. (2006). Strategies to manage the time demands of online teaching. *Nurse Educator, 31*(6), 270–274.

Robbins, L. K., & Hoke, M. M. (2008). Using objective structured clinical examinations to meet clinical competence evaluation challenges with distance education students. *Perspectives in Psychiatric Care, 44*(2), 81–88.

Welliver, M.D., Groom, J., Pabalate, J., Kalynych, N., McDonough, J. P., & Loriz, L. (2008). Tips for using video teleconferencing for distance education. *Nurse Educator, 33*(4), 149–150.

WEB RESOURCES

American Association of Colleges of Nursing (AACN)	http://www.aacn.nche.edu/
American Association for Higher Education (AAHE)	http://www.aahea.org/
American Nurses Association	http://www.nursingworld.org
Institute for Higher Education Policy	http://www.ihep.org/
Multimedia Educational Resource for Learning and Online Teaching (MERLOT)—free membership site with links to online learning materials along with annotations and peer reviews	www.merlot.org
National Council of State Boards of Nursing (NCSBN)	http://www.ncsbn.org
Honor Society of Nursing, Sigma Theta Tau International (STTI)	http://www.nursingsociety.org/default.aspx
University of Chicago Student Counseling and Resource Service	http://counseling.uchicago.edu/
Western Cooperative for Educational Telecommunications (WCET)	http://www.wcet.info
Western Interstate Commission for Higher Education (WICHE)	http://www.wiche.edu

CHAPTER 4

Using Simulation to Teach Nurses

• SHERRY D. FOX AND REBEKAH DAMAZO •

Learning Objectives

The learner will be able to:

1. Describe the evolution of simulation technology used in teaching nurses from the late 1990s to the present.
2. Analyze the potential impact of simulation technology on nursing education's ability to produce increased numbers of graduates in light of the current nursing shortage, inadequate numbers of nursing faculty, and inadequate clinical placement sites for nursing students.
3. Explore how the use of simulation as an adjunct to clinical nursing education can mitigate or reduce provider errors and improve patient outcomes.
4. Identify how strategies such as debriefing and guided reflection can be used to stimulate collaborative dialogue and problem solving in simulated learning experiences.
5. Explore common challenges associated with using simulation to teach nurses, including cost, time constraints, a lack of realism, and inadequately prepared educators to supervise the simulated learning experiences.
6. Review and summarize the current literature regarding the effect of simulated learning on the achievement of desired learner outcomes.
7. Consider the strengths and limitations of high-fidelity patient simulators as a replacement for traditional acute care clinical experience in nursing education.
8. Explore the likelihood that certifying and licensing boards will look to simulation as one way to validate the initial and ongoing competency of health care professionals.
9. Identify factors that should be considered and steps that should be taken before educational and health care facilities acquire simulation technology as a teaching tool.
10. Consider whether simulation could have been used more effectively as a supplement to his or her basic nursing education or ongoing continuing education as a health care professional.

Nurses the world over are familiar with the use of simulation in training. Most nursing students begin their exposure to clinical nursing cloistered in a skills lab, with static mannequins on which they can practice positioning, turning, dressings, and insertion of various tubes. The skill of injections is often practiced first on oranges, gel pads, or even classmates before the student approaches the real patient. Hypothetical patient interactions may be carried out in role-play.

Despite such rehearsals, the approach to the patient is often fraught with uncertainty, anxiety, and exposure to multiple contextual elements for which the skills lab has not prepared the student, and the practice of nurs-

ing turns out to be precisely "*practice.*" Many a wary patient has watched as a novice anxiously "practiced" some skill or assessment in the real world with varying degrees of success. The student is usually totally focused on the skill, barely able to interact with the patient or the environment.

Beyond the necessary psychomotor skills are the skills of clinical reasoning and decision making—picking up appropriate cues, making necessary assessments, and coming to appropriate conclusions about what the patient needs in a dynamic, fast-paced setting.

The skills needed to meet real-world demands cannot be easily rehearsed in traditional skills labs, with static mannequins such as the ubiquitous "Mrs. Chase." Nurse educators have tried to expand the scope of isolated skills lab practice by introducing computer vignettes, case studies, role playing, and other modalities, with positive results, but these teaching methods invariably lack many aspects of reality and interactivity for the student. Conversely, the real clinical setting lacks aspects of predictability and control in terms of the environment for learning. The instructor cannot ensure that each student attains the same, or even similar, experiences, resulting in highly variable learning outcomes.

These unmet needs were the impetus for the proliferation of high-fidelity patient simulators in the late 1990s and first decade of the 21st century. This chapter describes the emergence of sophisticated simulators as a tool for teaching nurses, provides the rationale for their use, and outlines the challenges inherent in determining how to incorporate simulation into nursing education. In addition, it presents preliminary outcomes of simulation use, as well as examples of emerging applications for staff training and competency assessment and regulatory trends. Components needed to develop a simulation center are summarized.

THE EMERGENCE OF HIGH-FIDELITY PATIENT SIMULATORS

Within the last decade, the proliferation of high-fidelity patient simulators has set the stage for a revolution in how students are taught and even in how practicing nurses are taught and their competencies assessed. Patient simulators are full-sized, computerized mannequins that can be programmed to respond in realistic ways. They can provide dynamic assessment data in real time, display programmed signs and symptoms, and respond to nursing actions.

These sophisticated mannequins evolved from low-technology mannequins and task trainers (such as Resusci Annie and intravenous [IV] arms) as computer technology advanced. In the 1980s, sophisticated simulators were in use for the training of anesthesiologists and military personnel (Hovancsek, 2007); nurse anesthetist programs also benefited. However, the costs for such early versions of patient simulators were prohibitive for most schools of nursing. As the industry has grown and the array of products has expanded, patient simulators are now within affordable ranges for many nursing schools and hospital systems and are poised to

become an important technological adjunct for nursing education in the 21st century.

One of the major providers of human patient simulators claims that more than 2,500 of its simulators are in institutions worldwide, with exponential growth (Medical Education Technologies Incorporated, 2008). A recent study reported on baccalaureate nursing schools and the use of simulators (Katz, 2007). Of responding baccalaureate schools of nursing accredited by the National League for Nursing Accrediting Commission (NLNAC), 78.9% ($n = 78$) had patient simulators. Of the schools that did not have simulators, 68.6% planned to purchase them within the next 2 years.

DEMANDS ON NURSING EDUCATION

This proliferation of patient simulators is fueled by multiple demands on nursing education. At the forefront of these challenges is a critical nursing shortage, which is projected to worsen as baby boomers age and leave the workforce, affecting the need for health care services (American Association of Colleges of Nursing [AACN], 2008). Many of these retiring boomers are part of the nursing workforce, further compounding nursing shortages. Schools of nursing are under pressure to expand enrollments and to produce competent graduates quickly. Despite steady increases in nursing enrollments, growth is not fast enough to meet the expected demand for nurses over the next decade. The capacity of the educational system is severely challenged by the lack of nursing faculty and the scarcity of clinical placements for students to apply their theoretical knowledge.

> ### CONSIDER
> With an expected 2% to 3% yearly increase in demand for nurses, the nursing shortage could grow to 500,000 by the year 2025. A 2008 report by health care leaders estimated that we should be producing 30,000 more nurses every year (AACN, 2008).

Even when clinical placements are adequate for students to meet learning objectives, the practice setting never provides a uniform set of experiences for all students. Critical events that occur infrequently are experienced by a very limited number of students. For example, most students have no opportunity to experience a code, yet they are expected to perform competently on their first encounter with one, with the balance of life and death hanging on cardiopulmonary resuscitation (CPR) skills that have been practiced only briefly, periodically with CPR recertification. More important, the rapid assessment of patient deterioration and the advanced decision making needed to prevent the actual cardiac arrest are expert skills that need ongoing rehearsal and reinforcement, which students and novice nurses usually do not receive. On-the-job training is not the ideal place to develop such critical competencies.

DISCUSSION POINT
Think of a clinical occurrence in which you felt unprepared to handle the situation. What type of practice or rehearsal could have prepared you better?

SIMULATION AND HEALTH CARE QUALITY

Nursing educators in academia, as well as in staff development, face challenges on many fronts in preparing and maintaining a well-educated, competent nursing workforce that is adequate in numbers and in appropriate skills to meet today's health care demands. Above all, the consumer of health care wants assurances that today's nurses are competent and that the care provided is safe and free from errors and omissions that can lead to prolonged illness or death.

The landmark Institute of Medicine (IOM) report *To Err Is Human* promoted simulation training as one way to prevent and mitigate errors (Kohn, Corrigan, & Donaldson, 2000): In simulation for modeling crisis management, "small groups that work together—whether in the operating room, intensive care unit, or emergency department—learn to respond to a crisis in an efficient, effective, and coordinated manner" (pp. 176–177). The report proposed the development of simulation technology, although it cautioned that simulation "that will allow full, interdisciplinary teams to practice interpersonal and technical skills in a non-jeopardy environment where they can receive meaningful feedback and reinforcement" (p. 177) would be a great challenge. Since this report, simulation technology and its implementation have made great strides in the area of simulation training for the professions and for interprofessional teams.

CONSIDER
The Agency for Healthcare Research and Quality (AHRQ) supports simulation research through its patient safety program, funding 19 grant projects totaling $5 million in 2006, to evaluate the role of simulation in improving the safety of health care. The agency asserted that "Simulation in health care creates a safe learning environment that allows researchers and practitioners to test new clinical processes and to enhance individual and team skills before encountering patients" (AHRQ, 2008).

Practicing nurses must keep up with changes in technology and the effect on patient care, at the same time dealing with nursing staff shortages, rapid turnover, the use of traveling nurses, and the necessity for mentoring students and new nurses. New nurses are often hired directly into settings demanding high-level competencies, without the luxury of practice experience in lower-acuity settings. Acuity levels in today's hospitals and other clinical settings do not allow for quiet reflection for decision making. The pace is fast, and the nurse who is not well practiced is at risk to make serious errors in omission and commission.

Even with the best efforts of nursing academia to produce competent graduates, nursing educators know that a new graduate, at best, is a novice nurse, lacking confidence and competence in many areas. Del Bueno (2005), using a competency assessment tool, estimated that only 35% of new graduate registered nurses (RNs) meet expectations for entry-level clinical judgment. She attributed this deficiency to the tendency of nursing programs to focus on content rather than application. Students need consistent experience, in simulation and in real settings. A recent ranking of 36 new nurse graduate competencies by front-line nurse leaders in service settings (3,500 nurse managers, directors, educators, and charge nurses) revealed consistent agreements on new graduate deficiencies (Advisory Board Company, 2008). All six "Management of Responsibilities" competencies—appropriate follow-up, ability to take initiative, completion of tasks within the expected time frame, ability to track multiple responsibilities, ability to prioritize, and delegation of tasks—were in the lower one third of new-graduate proficiencies. Several critical thinking competencies (recognition of changes in patient status, interpretation of assessment data, and ability to anticipate risk) were also in the bottom one third of competencies. Only 10% to 19% of nurse leaders agreed that new graduates exhibited these competencies. Nursing educators, as well as nurses responsible for orienting new nurses, are faced with the challenge of developing the competency levels of new nurses.

USING SIMULATION FOR NURSING EDUCATION AND STAFF DEVELOPMENT

Fortunately, the "perfect storm" of health care chaos and increased demands on nursing educators is crossing paths with the recent revolution in technology producing lifelike, interactive human mannequins—high-technology patient simulators. Simultaneously, as production and market competition grow, these simulators are becoming priced at levels that make them more affordable. The planned integration of patient simulators in nursing, for academic education as well as for staff development, is one major avenue to producing higher levels of competency and safe practice for nursing.

Durham and Alden (2008, p. 1), in a handbook for nurses produced by the federal Agency for Healthcare Research and Quality (AHRQ), proposed that the "use of simulation as a teaching strategy can contribute to patient safety and optimize outcomes of care, providing learners with opportunities to experience scenarios and intervene in clinical situations within a safe, supervised setting without posing a risk to a patient." Similarly, Salas, Wilson, Burke, and Priest (2005) supported simulation as effective in improving patient safety, based on initial data regarding its effectiveness. Reducing medical errors is one area where the health care community can and should benefit from using simulation-based training to assure patient safety. However, it is important to note that simulation is only effective if it is designed and delivered appropriately.

CAPABILITIES OF PATIENT SIMULATORS

Human patient simulators are categorized as "high-fidelity" simulation, compared with the "lower fidelity" of task trainers (mannequins that have limited capabilities, designed for specific tasks, such as pelvic models and IV arms) and static mannequins such as the Mrs. Chase

"dummy." Fidelity refers to the degree of realism. High-fidelity mannequins can be programmed to display selected signs and symptoms and to respond to the actions of the learner. The student can listen to preprogrammed heart, lung, and bowel sounds, can assess pulses at anatomically correct sites, can visualize respirations and pupil responses, and can observe displays of physiologic parameters such as the electrocardiogram (ECG), blood pressure, pulse oximetry, and temperature on a simulated patient monitor. These parameters can all change in a planned trajectory or under the control of a skilled operator. The simulators can be preprogrammed to speak or to respond through operator voices. Three major companies produce a variety of simulators (infant, child, adult, birthing) (Medical Education Technologies Incorporated [METI], Laerdal, and Gaumard), with more companies and products emerging rapidly. A range of sophisticated features is available, with the more complex models used for anesthesiology and military training.

Simulation is an educational strategy that allows realistic reproduction of aspects of real health care settings and patient events, which are designed by or under the control of the instructor. Students participate in the simulation scenario just as they would in the actual setting. Students interact with the mannequin, make physical assessments, monitor physiologic parameters, and observe the programmed trajectory of an episode. The student's interventions can affect the trajectory, for better or worse. All of the student's actions can be recorded for later reflection and debriefing and may be observed by peers to stimulate collaborative dialogue and problem solving. Possibly the most powerful component of simulations is the *debriefing*, which is a requisite at the completion of a scenario (Henneman, Cunningham, Roche, & Curnin, 2007). Debriefing, guided by a skilled educator, can produce insightful reflection on the events, help students to analyze and explain the reasoning behind actions, and facilitate the exploration of alternative approaches.

Decker (2007b) described the process of *guided reflection*, which she equated with the art of nursing. Decker hypothesized that "if simulated learning experiences are based on the principles of experiential learning, and guided reflection is embedded into the simulated learning experience, then the experience should promote the insight needed for the development of clinical judgment that promotes quality patient care" (p. 76). Research is needed to support this hypothesis, one of many challenges posed for nurse educators using simulation teaching strategies.

Rising to this challenge, Kuiper, Heinrich, Matthias, Graham, and Bell-Kotwall (2008) tested debriefing with a clinical reasoning model, comparing scores on a clinical reasoning tool for the same students in real clinical situations versus simulation. There was no significant difference between the clinical reasoning scores in the real and simulated experiences. The authors concluded that simulated experiences allow practice with clinical reasoning skills, promoting similar thinking as in authentic clinical experiences.

DISCUSSION POINT
Following a critical patient incident, what type of discussion ensues in your clinical setting? Who provides input? What type of record is available to trace the actions that occurred (or were omitted)? (One example might be a debriefing session following a "code.")

BENEFITS OF SIMULATION

Unlike real clinical practica, in which an instructor's vigilance is spread over many students and many patients, with simulation the instructor can observe every step the student makes, allowing for many teachable moments and the possibility of coaching to correct fallacies of judgment and erroneous actions. Simulations can expose students to rare events that they do not commonly see in practice in which competent performance is critical but rarely possible without practice opportunities. Faculty can ensure that all students have exposure to specific critical learning experiences.

Unlike the real world of student clinical experience, faculty observing simulated learning experiences may choose not to rescue the "patient" by preventing student mistakes. Students may be allowed to experience the full consequences of their decisions, even to the point of the "death" of their "patients," which can profoundly affect the students' learning and retention of what they have learned.

Simulations can be designed for team practice, enhancing collaboration and improving team communication skills. Simulations that provide for interdisciplinary training, including the full array of roles in a patient care scenario, are becoming an important part of staff development. Health care professionals are pre-dominantly trained in their individual disciplines, yet they must be able to come together as teams, with little or no interdisciplinary training. Therefore, simulation can provide the common ground for health care teams to learn how to function as teams (Miller, Riley, Davis, & Hansen, 2008). Patient safety requires highly organized systems of care, yet the training of the individuals who comprise the teams has been neglected. The IOM report *To Err Is Human* emphasized the need for team training using simulation (Kohn et al., 2000).

In addition, the level of difficulty in simulation can be adapted for the student level. Simulators are differentiated according to the complexity needed for specific objectives. For example, anesthesiology training and advanced military training for casualty management involve highly complex simulators with advanced capabilities. However, the standard mannequins in use in most schools of nursing can be programmed for simple to advanced scenarios by manipulating one or more parameters to the level of difficulty. A novice student may have to respond to a simple declining blood pressure, whereas an advanced student may be dealing with a plummeting oxygen saturation, apparent respiratory distress, tachycardia, pharmacological effects, and distressed family members.

Beyond uses in teaching assessment and providing realistic skills practice, scenarios can be developed and validated to provide for the development of critical thinking and clinical decision making and can be used for competency evaluation (Decker, Sportsman, Puetz, & Billings, 2008). The ability for nurse educators to be able to observe a complete set of actions, question a student's line of thinking, and provide guidance when the student fails to notice or incorporate important cues is a powerful teaching adjunct, allowing for many more of the precious "teachable moments" valued by faculty.

Depending on how the learning environment is managed, students generally respond very positively to the learning opportunities in simulation, reporting increased self-confidence and lower anxiety levels (Hovancsek, 2007, p. 5; Jeffries and Rizzolo, 2006). They also express value in learning from each other when a collaborative approach is used in which classmates observe and contribute to each other's scenarios (Lasater, 2007b).

Experiential learning (including simulation) "is especially adaptable to adult learners; [it gives] opportunity to see real consequences of one's actions, to feel the exhilaration of success and the frustration of failure" (Gilley, 1990,

p. 261). Because nursing schools have many nontraditional learners, it is important to recognize the value added with simulation. High-fidelity simulation is a learning strategy that helps to keep students fully engaged and requires them to address complex patient problems and events.

Gassert (2006) asserted that the use of simulation could reduce the number of clinical hours required for students, providing a wider range of patient illnesses and events. Expanded clinical capacity provided by simulation could support the admission of increased numbers of students.

DISADVANTAGES OF SIMULATION

The use of patient simulators may not be a total panacea for educators. Initial costs for the acquisition of the simulators are prohibitive for many programs. Beyond the initial investment, ongoing considerations of space, technician support, and faculty training mandate continuing expenses. One program estimated the ongoing costs at $1,000 per hour of instruction (National Council of State Boards of Nursing [NCSBN], 2005). A basic high-fidelity simulator costs $30,000 to $40,000 and has an expected shelf life of around 3 years. Models that sense and respond to medications and have other sophisticated features necessary for anesthesiology or military training can cost as much as $250,000. Institutions must augment their traditional equipment budgets to accommodate this emerging technology.

In addition, the number of students who can work with the simulators at one time is limited, and students require intensive faculty involvement, which is often more time consuming than regular clinical supervision for a group of students. Traditional student-to-faculty ratios may need to be evaluated as simulation users become more knowledgeable about the most effective use of simulation time schedules. Faculty may need to rethink the "8-hour" student shift and replace it with shorter, more frequent training days.

Students may also feel put on the spot and experience anxiety, especially when being observed by faculty and peers. However, in her research analyzing the use of simulation to develop clinical judgment, Lasater (2007b) reported that, despite the fact students may report that simulations were "anxiety producing" or made them "feel like an idiot," the group participants consistently verbalized that they did learn through the scenarios. These findings corroborate other researchers who support the heightened learning achieved when students experience simulation (Jeffries and Rizzolo, 2006; Radhakrishnan, Roche, & Cunningham, 2007; Beyea, von Reyn, & Slattery, 2007; Jarzemsky & McGrath, 2008).

Another disadvantage is that students might not function as if the scenario was real, perceiving an artificiality to the setting (NCSBN, 2005). Most educators acknowledge where realism is lacking when discussing cases with students. It is important for the faculty designing the case scenario to understand the degree of realism required to accomplish the stated learning objectives.

Simulators continue to evolve. There are now simulators that bleed, cry, and speak in as many languages as are available for programming. Moulage techniques are being used to create everything from gaping wounds, to pressure sores, to rashes. Simulation centers are also incorporating standardized patients of various ages and ethnicities (such as actors trained to portray a specific set of patient problems), which provide added realism. Many students in simulations begin to interact with the "patient" as if it were real. Students who are "unable to suspend disbelief" may accomplish as much as those who become immersed in the simulation script (Lasater, 2007b).

Although recognizing the promise of simulation, the NCSBN (2005) offered the caution that students "must practice in authentic situations." Although recognized as a complement to actual clinical practice, simulation should not replace it. Where simulation is done well it does not replace clinical practice but rather provides experience and skill that will enhance practice. Finding the optimum balance, however, between clinical practice and simulation is not easy and will require ongoing research. (See Research Study Fuels the Controversy on page 57.)

Although it is important to note the cautionary views on simulation, it is noteworthy that those who are using and evaluating simulation are passionate champions of this rapidly advancing field. Today's simulation is not focused on isolated skill building. It builds on a skills foundation and requires students to acquire cognitive and affective skills and to develop clinical judgment (Lasater, 2007b). In many areas students are required or encouraged to practice in a team of health professionals, building competencies essential for working within teams. One area of concern, however, relates to the student who becomes confident in simulation and may take on tasks beyond his or her level of expertise. It is essential that faculty provide simulations that are within the scope of practice, geared to the student's level.

Research Study Fuels the Controversy: Can Simulation Develop Nursing Expertise?

Day (2007) expressed concerns about the ability of nurses/students truly to develop expertise as described by Benner's model of "Novice to Expert" through simulation. Noting that expertise is developed within the complex context of practice settings, she asserted that the development of expertise in nursing requires experience and the "right kind of engagement with practice situations" (p. 507). She cautioned that simulations are removed from the context of the patient, requiring different assumptions and roles than those experienced by students in simulation. Acknowledging the promise of high-fidelity simulation, she expressed the belief that simulation will likely not speed the acquisition of skills for new graduates if clinical time with real patients is replaced.

In an alternative view, Beeman (2008) developed a tiered critical care education program based on Benner's model of "Novice to Expert." Simulations were developed to teach and assess levels of critical care expertise, from the advanced beginner to expert. Carefully designed scenarios for each level were used to foster clinical advancement and to provide for performance evaluation. The ultimate goal for this ambitious program is to demonstrate optimized patient outcomes and patient safety as a result of achieving clinical excellence (p. 50).

Both authors valued simulation, but Day saw the potential as much more limited than did Beeman. Beeman's approaches are used with practicing nurses, so the question of replacing clinical time is not an issue, as it might be with student nurses. However, Beeman evidenced confidence that the clinical reasoning needed to develop true expertise can be nurtured and evaluated through well-designed, complex scenarios with skilled faculty not necessarily requiring the context of the real patient encounter.

DISCUSSION POINT

1. Which position (Day or Beeman) do you find most compelling? (Consider the education of student nurses vs. ongoing proficiency development for practicing nurses.)
2. As a practicing nurse, would you consider ongoing training and evaluation with simulation as a requirement to advance your career as an opportunity or a threat?

Day, L. (2007). Simulation and the teaching and learning of practice in critical care units. *American Journal of Critical Care, 16,* 504–507.
Beeman, L. (2008). Basing a clinician's career on simulation: Development of a critical care expert into a clinical simulation expert (pp. 31–51). In R. Kyle & W. Murray (Eds.), *Clinical Simulation: Operations, Engineering and Management.* New York: Elsevier.

Perhaps the most significant barrier to the use of simulation is the need for well-trained faculty who can devise the best uses of simulation within specific curricula. All too often, expensive simulators are purchased but not effectively used, lacking a champion who can bring about the extensive curricular planning and faculty training needed. It is not uncommon for expensive mannequins to lie dormant in their shipping crates long after their arrival. Seasoned educators may find the technology interface daunting (Starkweather & Kardong-Edgren, 2008). Despite the availability of predeveloped scenarios for nursing education, nursing faculty will have their own priorities and will desire modifications that must be programmed into the computer. The availability of skilled technicians who can assist with the computer interface removes one of the major faculty hurdles but poses additional costs.

Effective simulations also require expert debriefing. Debriefing is a skilled function, bringing to bear the faculty member's clinical expertise, as well as his or her educational savvy. One approach to preparing faculty for the challenges is attendance at teaching conferences that focus on simulation; another approach is individual training sessions for groups of faculty. For example, California State University, Chico, integrates simulation training in the preparation of all nursing education master's students, preparing future educators with the skills needed to incorporate simulation into nursing education.

SIMULATION FOR PRACTICE SETTINGS

Patient simulators are not and will not be relegated only to academic settings for the initial training of nursing students. Beyea (2004) promoted human patient simulation for its potential to increase patient safety by teaching technical and professional skills or by testing new processes and procedures in a controlled, predictable environment with no threat to patient safety. She described several applications at Dartmouth-Hitchcock Medical Center, including the following:

- Developing skill and competency related to pediatric and moderate sedation.
- Team training related to emergency cesarean sections, helping team members to develop synergy.
- Developing competencies of new graduates for high-risk clinical situations such as laryngospasm, pulmonary embolus, heart failure, and acute coronary syndrome, incorporating assessment, priority setting, intervention, and outcomes evaluation.

Many others have extolled the benefits of simulation for developing proficiency in critical care settings. Beyea et al. (2007) developed a nurse residency program using human patient simulation to address issues related to the orientation time required for new graduates to become competent and to feel confident. A 12-week program was developed, with didactic courses, weekly simulation experiences, and clinical time with a preceptor. At the end of the residency, the nurses were evaluated with simulations designed to assess competence. The program resulted in a markedly reduced time for orientation, with the program participants able to take full patient assignments. Participants were better prepared for skills. The simulation experiences allowed early identification of areas in which participants needed remediation or more guidance. The residents improved in self-rated confidence, competence, and readiness for independent practice. An overwhelming majority of the participants were positive about the simulation experiences. Similarly, Ackermann, Kenny, and Walker (2007) described the development of a simulator program to aid in the transition of new graduate nurses, promoting critical thinking, decision-making, and clinical confidence.

Morris et al. (2007) also incorporated the patient simulator as part of an overall critical care institute for orienting new graduates and inexperienced RNs into critical care units. The simulator facilitated the development of critical thinking skills and provided educators with ongoing assessment of the orientee's ability to apply knowledge.

Beeman (2008) described a tiered approach to nursing staff development, using simulation technology for three different levels of clinical expertise (based on Benner's model of Novice to Expert). An elaborate simulation center provides academic training, as well as staff development training, for medical residents, nurses,

nurse technicians, respiratory therapists, pharmacists, and paramedics. Evaluation components are incorporated into the simulations and are used as part of performance evaluation for clinical advancement.

Rauen (2004) described the use of simulation for orientation in cardiac surgery, as well as in step-down and critical care nursing orientations. She noted that the skill levels and abilities of nurses varied, but their evaluations of simulation training were universally positive. She concluded,

Critical care nursing is fast paced and requires a high level of attention to details, quick assessment skills, and critical thinking. These skills are difficult to teach and are best learned through experience and practice. Simulation allows the opportunity to learn and practice critical care skills in a controlled and safe environment (p. 51).

Anderson and Leflore (2008) described the benefits of simulation for operating room team training as a tool that can increase effective communication and overall team effectiveness.

Wolf (2008) described the use of simulation to teach assessment and intervention skills for emergency nurses, using a "paradigm case" model described by Benner. Following 4 hours of classroom instruction, six nurses completed three to five simulation scenarios representing different diagnoses and indications for triage. The scenarios revealed gaps in the nurses' assessment and triage processes and indicated areas for refining training. All of the nurses felt that the combination of training methods was helpful and improved triage skills. Follow-up with chart reviews showed great improvement in triage accuracy, particularly for the least experienced nurses. Wolf concluded that simulation training can improve triage accuracy, leading to better patient care.

Simulation is also promoted as a strategy for retooling nurses. Burns et al. (2006) promoted the use of simulation as a re-entry mechanism for nurses who have been out of the workforce. RNs responded positively, claiming that simulation greatly reduced their anxiety. In addition, the training program was effective as a recruiting tool for the hospital.

Yaeger and Arafeh (2008) described the value of simulation training for obstetric and neonatal care providers to obtain hands-on training of neonatal resuscitation. Studies have indicated that the ability to adequately perform neonatal resuscitation may not be achieved by traditional training methods. Simulation training is seen as an important enhancement to former models of neonatal resuscitation training.

Miller et al. (2008) described the use of "in situ" training in which human patient simulators are brought into the practice unit where the health care team normally functions to provide team training to enhance perinatal safety. This ambitious pilot study provided 35 simulations in six hospitals, with more than 700 participants. Extensive debriefing following the simulations allowed participants to develop insight into communication lapses, team failures, and latent conditions. The authors emphasized the value of team versus individual training as a means to improve processes and safety.

In situ training has also been used for ambulatory care (Maynes, 2008) to provide emergency training to clinic staff. Maynes pointed out that in situ training allows staff to find and use equipment and supplies in their own units, often resulting in changes in the type of equipment as inadequacies became apparent during simulations. Similar results have been found in other in situ simulations, such as finding out that the anesthesiologist could not reach the crash cart in an operating room simulation or that emergency room staff could not locate an IV fluid warmer to deal with a near-infant drowning victim with hypothermia.

Acute care and ambulatory settings are finding patient simulators extremely valuable for ongoing staff development, as well as for interdisciplinary team training. Patient simulators are likely to be in every nurse's future to maintain practice competence and to develop new skills.

RESEARCH ON SIMULATION OUTCOMES

Agencies that have instituted simulation training are usually very positive about their outcomes. However, research on simulation outcomes for nursing is in its infancy. Much of the literature is of a developmental nature, describing programs and processes but not evaluating outcomes. Is there evidence that these expensive programs lead to better learning than traditional teaching strategies? Schools of medicine, training in anesthesiology, and the military have been using sophisticated patient simulators for a long time and have performed studies on the effect on learning.

Issenberg, McGaghie, Petrusa, Gordon, and Scalese (2005) performed an extensive review of outcomes research on simulation in medical education conducted between the years 1969 and 2003. They focused on 109 studies that used a simulator as an educational assessment or intervention with quantitative measures, using experimental or quasi-experimental methodology.

From this review they concluded, "While research in this field needs improvement in terms of rigor and quality, high-fidelity medical simulations are educationally effective and simulation-based education complements medical education in patient care settings" (Issenberg et al., p. 10). Their recommendations for effective learning with simulators are listed in Box 4.1.

| BOX 4.1 | TIPS FOR EFFECTIVE TEACHING THROUGH SIMULATION |

- Provide feedback during the learning experience with the simulator.
- Ensure that learners repetitively practice skills on the simulator.
- Integrate simulators into the overall curriculum.
- Ensure that learners practice with increasing levels of difficulty (if available).
- Adapt the simulator to complement multiple learning strategies.
- Ensure that the simulator provides for clinical variation.
- Ensure that learning on the simulator occurs in a controlled environment.
- Provide individualized (in addition to team) learning on the simulator.
- Clearly define outcomes and benchmarks for the learners to achieve by using the simulator.
- Ensure that the simulator is a valid learning tool.

Source: Issenberg, S., McGaghie, W., Petrusa, E., Gordon, D., & Scalese, R. (2005). Features and uses of high-fidelity medical simulations that lead to effective learning: A BEME systematic review. *Medical Teacher, 27*, 10–28.

Although the research reviewed by Issenberg et al. was based on medical students, it is reasonable to believe that these findings and recommendations apply to nursing education as well. Ravert (2002) reviewed nine quantitative studies that measured outcomes of computer-based simulation; 75% showed positive effects. She noted that more research is needed, but simulation posed enormous potential as an educational strategy.

Perceived Satisfaction, Decreased Anxiety, and Increased Confidence

Most of the studies performed in nursing have focused on how acceptable this mode of learning is to students and their satisfaction levels. In general, this mode of learning is very well received by students (Robertson, 2006; Schoening, Sittner, & Todd, 2006; Bantz, Dancer, Hodson-Carlton, & Van Hove, 2007; Jeffries, 2008).

Feingold, Calaluce, and Kallen (2004) surveyed baccalaureate nursing students ($n = 65$) and faculty ($n = 4$) after two semesters of clinical simulation activities. The survey tool measured perceptions of realism, value of the experience, and ability to transfer skills to the real world. An overwhelming majority of the students and faculty thought that the simulations were realistic; they perceived value in the simulations, believing that they "tested clinical skills and decision making, reinforced clinical skills and enhanced learning" (p. 161). Faculty unanimously agreed that the simulation learning experiences would transfer to real clinical settings, whereas only half of the students perceived this, a curious finding that merits further study. The authors suggested simulation as a cost-effective adjunct to clinical experiences, preparing students for the care of acutely ill patients and complex technology and enhancing safety for patients.

Bremner, Aduddell, and Amason (2008) compared two groups of first-year nursing students to examine the effects of using the human patient simulator prior to the first clinical experience. One group ($n = 71$) worked with the simulator one week prior to the clinical experience; the other group ($n = 78$) experienced the traditional skills lab. The authors concluded that the intervention group experienced less anxiety and greater comfort in their first clinical experience. The simulator group believed that the experience gave them confidence in their assessment skills, helped to relieve stress on the first clinical day, and should be a component of the nursing curriculum.

In addition, outcomes research on simulation extends beyond the United States; simulation is in use worldwide. Kiat, Mei, Nagammal, and Jonnie (2007) surveyed 260 second-year nursing students in Singapore 6 months after initiation of simulation in the curriculum. The students each experienced 20 hours in simulation training. The questionnaire asked about perceived benefits, the actual experience with the simulation, factors related to the effectiveness of the training, and whether they would choose to attend simulation training. Students were overwhelmingly positive about the experience, perceiving simulation as an enjoyable way to learn, allowing them to think on their feet, to identify areas for improvement, to make mistakes without causing harm, and to increase confidence. More than 95% of the students would choose to participate in more simulation training. The authors concluded that appropriately used simulation has the potential to revolutionize learning in nursing, bridging theory and practice.

Attitudes of Practicing Nurses toward Simulation

Simulation training is still in its infancy and not yet understood or well accepted by practicing nurses, most of whom did not experience this form of learning in their initial training. However, hospital systems are beginning to realize the value of simulation centers for ongoing training of nursing and other health professional staff. For nurses who were not exposed to simulation in their educational programs, simulation can be a new, possibly daunting experience.

DeCarlo, Collingridge, Grant, and Ventre (2008) surveyed 523 practicing nurses in a university hospital to determine their prior simulation exposure, perceived barriers to participation in simulation, and priorities for education. Nurses who had prior experience with simulation perceived the lack of reality as one barrier to simulation; those with no prior experience perceived unfamiliarity with the equipment as a barrier; and those who worked in nonacute areas perceived simulation as a stressful, intimidating environment. However, the value of simulation for learning to manage rare events was recognized as a priority by less-experienced nurses and those practicing in acute care areas. This research demonstrates that practicing nurses may need well-designed simulations carried out in a supportive, nonthreatening manner to minimize barriers to their participation.

Learning Outcomes with Simulation

Perhaps more relevant to educators is the degree to which simulation experiences actually contribute to learning outcomes. The research literature is sparse in this area but is growing rapidly. Radhakrishnan et al. (2007) performed a pilot study on a small group ($n = 12$) of senior nursing students to identify performance areas sensitive to improvement following practice with a patient simulator. Half of the students were assigned to a control group, who completed their regular senior clinical rotation; half of the students completed two 1-hour simulations with two complex patients, in addition to their regular clinical rotation. At the end of the rotations, all students participated in a two-patient simulation and were evaluated on achievement of objectives related to safety, basic assessment, prioritization, problem-focused assessment, interventions, delegation, and communication. Simulation students scored significantly higher on two scales—Safety and Basic Assessment—with no difference seen in the other measures. The safety scale involved patient identification, with more of the intervention group checking the patient identification, which is critical for safe administration of medications and other treatments. The intervention group also performed better in assessing and reassessing basic vital signs, which is critical for monitoring emergent patient conditions.

Lasater (2007a, 2007b) reported on students' experience with the development of clinical judgment through high-fidelity patient simulation. The first portion of the study (Lasater, 2007a) involved the development and pilot testing of a rubric to assess levels of performance in clinical judgment. The developed rubric provided clear expectations for student learning and a standard for providing feedback, serving as a guide for students' development of clinical judgment.

In the second portion of the study (Lasater, 2007b), focus groups were conducted with 8 volunteer students, part of the larger population of 48 students who participated in weekly simulation scenarios in lieu of a clinical day per week. Five major codes were condensed from 13 primary themes—the strengths and limitations of high-fidelity simulation; the paradox of feeling anxiety and feeling stupid while experiencing increased learning and awareness; the desire for more direct feedback about performance; the value of students' connections with others; and general recommendations for better facilitation and learning. A major strength perceived by students was that simulation integrated theoretical learning with psychomotor skills and clinical practice learning, requiring them to critically think about what to do. A second strength was the breadth of experiences, allowing students to see conditions they were rarely exposed to in their clinical rotations.

Although perceived as extreme situations, the scenarios forced students to anticipate events that could happen, which is useful in the development of clinical judgment, for example, observing the rapid onset of anaphylactic shock following administration of an antibiotic. Limitations of the simulator were also noted, such as the lack of facial expressions and other visual cues. Learning from each other's experiences, collaborating as teams, and hearing others' stories were important sources of learning.

These findings emphasized the critical nature of the debriefing period and the reflective thinking that can occur. Lasater also recommended engaging students who served in the role of observer, in that the quality of perceived learning was not as great for student observers as for the actively engaged students.

Extending Lasater's work on the importance of the debriefing, Kuiper et al. (2008) reported on the use of a specific model—the *Outcome Present State-Test* (OPT)—as a rating tool for clinical reasoning. The OPT tool has been in use since 2003, with good interrater reliability (87%). Use of the OPT model encourages the use of "cognitive critical thinking strategies of organization, comparison, classification, evaluation, summarization, and analysis" (Kuiper et al., 2008, p. 3). Students in the study completed OPT worksheets as part of their regular clinical experiences and also used the OPT as part of simulation debriefing. Students worked together as a group to complete the OPT worksheets following the simulation. Scores on the OPT rating scale were compared for OPT worksheets completed during regular clinical experience and the simulation OPT worksheets. No significant differences were found between the scores. The authors concluded that the simulation experiences provided students practice with the expected clinical reasoning skills, similar to actual clinical experiences. The authors recommended the use of simulation in coordination with didactic experiences and for remediation, concluding, "Simulation allows for errors in decisions and judgments without jeopardizing patient safety, yet enhances clinical reasoning competence" (Kuiper et al., 2008, p. 12).

Nehring, Ellis, and Lashley (2001) reviewed existing studies on the use of patient simulators. Nine studies testing the effectiveness of patient simulation in medicine, anesthesiology, and nursing found that students rated simulator experiences as positive. The authors reported on their experience with a convenience group of 42 senior nursing students on completion of specific advanced medical-surgical modules (airway obstruction, congestive heart failure, pulseless electrical activity, and hypovolemic shock). The students were given a lecture on these topics, followed by a pretest. The students then worked with the patient simulator in groups of five or six, where they worked with three case scenarios related to the topics. Following the simulations, the students completed a post test, with significant improvement in their scores. The post tests were repeated 5 to 7 days later, with no change in scores, indicating retention of learning.

These findings are similar to those of Johnson, Flagg, and Dremsa (2007) (see Research Study Fuels the Controversy). In this study, posttest analyses showed no dif-

ference between group learning skills using a CD-ROM application and patient simulators on lower-level cognitive skills; however, the simulator group had significantly higher scores on cognitive and critical thinking skills.

Wayne et al. (2006) also used simulation-based education methods to train 38 medicine residents in advanced cardiac life support (ACLS). Following standard ACLS instruction, the residents participated in 8 hours of training using a patient simulator. Residents with the simulator training had a 38% increase in ACLS skills compared with residents who had not yet experienced the simulator training. Long-term follow-up of the residents indicated that their ACLS skills did not deteriorate over a 14-month period, without any further ACLS training. Previous studies have shown rapid decay of ACLS skills; a comparable group of residents without simulation training demonstrated a 17% skills decline at the end of their residency, despite two ACLS courses. The authors believed programs using simulation as an adjunct to ACLS training could be useful to help develop and maintain ACLS skills. Although this study

Research Study Fuels the Controversy: Simulation Most Effective in Developing Higher-Level Critical Thinking

Johnson, Flagg, and Dremsa (2007) designed a prospective, randomized study to compare cognition and critical thinking outcomes using a patient simulator versus interactive CD-ROM in training for the care of combat casualties exposed to chemical agents. The study involved 99 volunteer health professionals from active duty or reserve military units. Following a carefully designed, valid, and reliable pretest on the care of casualties exposed to chemical agents, subjects were randomly assigned to a control group, a patient simulator group, or an interactive

CD-ROM group. The two experimental groups completed instruction in the assigned modalities; the control group received no instruction. The patient simulator group interacted with three patient scenarios; the CD-ROM group was exposed to the same three scenarios, with the ability to make choices and receive computerized feedback on treatment choices. One month following the interventions, subjects were retested. The instrument contained items that measured lower-level cognition skills, as well as higher-level cognition and critical thinking skills.

STUDY FINDINGS
The baseline pretest showed no differences among groups on any of the cognitive levels. The posttest analyses showed no difference between the CD-ROM group and the patient simulator group on the lower-level cognitive skills. However, the simulator group had significantly higher scores on cognitive and critical thinking skills. The authors postulated that the teaching

strategies used with the patient simulator allowed the participants the ability to see the actual effectiveness of interventions related to the use of atropine and fluid resuscitation in a simulated realistic situation. Because critical thinking is postulated to occur within the context of the situation, the authors concluded that the simulation training was the most effective in achieving higher-level critical thinking skills.

Johnson, D., Flagg, A., & Dremsa, T. (2007). Effects of using a Human Patient Simulator (HPS™) versus a CD-ROM on cognition and critical thinking. *Medical Education Online, 13*(1). Available at: http://www.med-ed-online.org/pdf/T0000118.pdf. Accessed July 29, 2008.

related to medical residents, it is likely that the findings would transfer to practicing critical care nurses, who take the same ACLS courses periodically.

In addition, a major study by Draycott et al. (2008) demonstrated the excellent potential for simulation training to affect health care outcomes. A retrospective, observational study compared the management and neonatal outcomes of births complicated by shoulder dystocia. All maternity staff was trained on birth training mannequins at a mandatory multiprofessional, 1-day training course at a British hospital. Birth records (15,908) for the 3 years before the training were compared with 13,117 births 3 years after the training. Clinical management improved after the training on several parameters. There was a significant reduction in neonatal injury. All of the outcomes could be attributed to several factors—the mandatory training of 100 percent of the staff, the teaching of simplified methods, and the use of a high-fidelity trainer. Further research would be needed to sort out the contribution of each, but presumably the training's effectiveness was enhanced by the use of simulation practice.

REGULATORY TRENDS RECOGNIZE THE VALUE OF SIMULATIONS

It is likely that many certifying and licensing boards will look to simulation as one way to validate the initial and ongoing competency of health professionals. There will be reluctance to embrace this new technology unless the validity and reliability of assessment methods can be assured, but as more research emerges, simulation will become an accepted tool for competency assessment in many areas. The American Academy of Pediatrics (AAP) steering committee on Neonatal Resuscitation Programs (NRP) announced its commitment to base newborn resuscitation on the best evidence-based science available. With that in mind, AAP incorporates practice on an infant simulator as part of its Neonatal Resuscitation Program. This announcement prompted the Laerdal Corporation to collaborate with the AAP to develop an infant simulator specifically designed for NRP training (American Academy of Pediatrics, 2007).

As part of heightened emergency preparedness efforts, the U.S. Department of Health and Human Services (DHHS), together with the Joint Commission on the Accreditation of Healthcare Organizations and

other agencies, is preparing to extend disaster training to the inpatient bedside environment. High-fidelity human patient simulators will be used for training in disaster and terrorism response and treatment, as well as in patient safety and other issues raised in the IOM report *To Err Is Human* (Ramirez, 2008).

The American Board of Physician Specialties (ABPS) and METI have teamed up to develop a new certification examination for disaster medicine incorporating simulation (ABPS, 2006).

SIMULATION AND PATIENT SAFETY

Simulation is poised to become an essential component of efforts to meet quality and safety initiatives. Administrators are becoming more cognizant of the important role simulation could play in increasing the safety and quality of health care and the concomitant reduction in financial risk. Risk managers of health care systems are beginning to recognize the value of simulation training for containing the costs of legal suits. Harvard University Medical Center examined the high cost of malpractice in the 1990s for their anesthesiologists and pursued simulation as an anesthesia risk control strategy. Because of success both in controlling costs and malpractice litigation, the risk control strategy was extended to obstetrical providers. The program was successful in developing, implementing, and evaluating an obstetric simulation-based team training course grounded in *crisis resource management* (CRM) principles. The results were highly satisfied participants who reported using the CRM principles taught with patient simulation. Participants still valued their participation 1 year after completing the course, and, as an added benefit, received a 10 percent reduction in annual obstetrical malpractice premiums. This study supported the idea that simulation-based CRM training can serve as a strategy for mitigating adverse perinatal events and has the added benefit of reducing the cost of malpractice insurance (Gardner, Walzer, Simon, & Raemer, 2008).

SIMULATION IN CONTINUING EDUCATION FOR NURSES

All licensed professions require ongoing education to maintain and expand the competency needed in a dynamic health care system. Yet, traditional methods of continuing education are under scrutiny. An interdisciplinary conference on continuing education for the health professions acknowledged that professional continuing education is in disarray, with too little emphasis on improving clinical performance to provide high-quality care and the preponderance of continuing education offered in the form of lectures (Hager, Russell, & Fletcher, 2008).

In addition, there is little evidence that lectures endured for continuing education requirements actually improve practice (see Chapter 18). Among many recommendations to improve the effectiveness of continuing education, the value of simulations was acknowledged: "Interactive scenarios and simulations are promising approaches to CE, particularly for skills development, whether the skill is a highly technical procedure, history taking or a physical examination technique" (Hager et al., 2008, p. 19).

Simulation centers are on the threshold of fulfilling this potential. An international survey of 40 nursing schools and simulation centers revealed that nine of the programs offered continuing education using patient simulators in such areas as airway management, nurse anesthesia updates, critical care certification, ACLS, and RN refresher courses (Nehring & Lashley, 2004). Simulation centers in rural settings offer the opportunity for the latest technology and procedures to be introduced, making available trainings usually confined to academic medical centers, where there are many opportunities to encounter complex and high-risk patients. The rural professionals on the front line, who often provide early triage and care to stabilize patients for transport to medical centers, can benefit greatly from team training simulations to improve outcomes for uncommon critical events.

National and international trends ensure that students, nurse educators, and practicing nurses will encounter high-fidelity human patient simulators in their career pathways. However, not every setting has embarked on the process of establishing such learning centers. The first step may be starting a center. Nurses in practice or in education settings may have to become the champions who instigate the establishment of simulation centers, as well as be involved in the initial planning stages.

DEVELOPING A SIMULATION CENTER

Beginning on the pathway to developing a simulation center for an academic or service setting is a daunting task, with a steep learning curve. Despite the proliferation of such centers, many have been developed by serendipitous approaches rather than careful business plans. Few "how-to" resources were available for early adopters. More resources will be available for the next generation of centers, including work described by Seropian, Brown, Gavilanes, and Driggers (2004), Spunt (2007), and Kyle and Murray (2008). Most important, development of an effective simulation program requires much more than the purchase of a mannequin.

The American Hospital Association Committee on Health Professions (2007) delineated steps that should be taken before hospitals consider the acquisition of simulators. The first step should be an assessment of the simulators currently available within the institution and the region. Next, a clear purpose and specific objectives should be outlined to ensure regular use. Hospitals need to consider how the simulators will be used and by whom. Given the initial cost of developing a simulation center and maintaining it, a multiyear business plan is essential.

Human resources should also be assessed, such as potential champions, potential faculty, potential staffing, and the administrative structure for oversight. Space will need to be allocated in accordance with the types of trainings anticipated, with enough space to accommodate team trainings and observers. A budget plan that covers capital expenses, as well as maintenance, repair, and replacement is essential, including ongoing software upgrades. Plans for revenue generation should be considered. However, the Committee cautioned that early centers have found that simulation is a "cost of doing business," not likely to bring a positive return on investment. Savings may result from risk reduction, but will be hard to quantify.

Seropian et al. (2004) described a comprehensive approach to simulation program development, including vision development, a business plan, getting buy-in from potential funding sources, deciding on the type of equipment to purchase, where to house it, and technical adjuncts needed such as audiovisual equipment. Early in the process, training must occur for the faculty. Curriculum development is crucial—the faculty who determine the curriculum must make decisions on how simulation will be integrated. Seropian et al. concluded that the development of a simulation program "involves organization, curricular thought, simulation skill, and a whole new view of health care education and clinical experience" (p. 174). It is likely that many academic and practice settings will realize that simulation is a valued adjunct to educating nurses and nursing staff to maintain cutting edge competencies.

Given the high cost of simulation centers and the need to keep such centers fully functioning, partnerships in which several agencies collaborate and share financial sponsorship provide mutual benefits. Partnerships among academic centers and hospitals allow for ongoing maximal use of the center when the schools are out of session, as well as allow for expanded use covering more than one hospital shift (Metcalfe, Hall, & Carpenter, 2007). In addition to partnerships, use of nonfaculty nurses and retired nurses, either as volunteer or paid staff, can help to extend the faculty in labor-intensive simulations in a cost-effective manner (Foster, Sheriff, & Cheney, 2008).

Along with plans for developing the center, a plan for training of the faculty who will work with the students is essential. Teaching with simulation is not business as usual. Many faculty find the technology involved daunting. Even with skilled technicians to soften the technical interface, nursing faculty must deliberate on the best ways to integrate simulation into the curriculum. Clear learning outcomes must be delineated, along with specific objectives for each simulation. The degree of realism required to meet the learning objectives must be determined and incorporated. To achieve economical use of faculty and precious time with the simulators, faculty must develop strategies to engage groups of students so that more than one student can benefit from the learning in the scenario. The reflective learning that occurs after a scenario is completed requires skilled faculty (Bremner, Aduddell, Bennett, & VanGeest, 2006; Lasater, 2008a). Fortunately, many faculty are rising to the challenge. Most national nursing conferences now include sessions on the use of simulation, curriculum design, and ongoing research. Indeed, Decker (2007a) posed the question as to whether it is even ethical to train nurses without using simulation in an era in which these resources are readily available and when outcomes research suggests such positive outcomes (see Research Study Fuels the Controversy).

Research Study Fuels the Controversy: Is It Ethical to Train Nurses *without* the Use of Simulation?

Given new simulation technology, which allows for much greater demonstration of competency before entering the real patient care setting, is it ethical to continue to educate students *without* simulation? Decker (2007a) discussed the educational ethics related to the use of patient simulators as a means to provide realistic training for students without endangering patients versus traditional clinical learning experiences in which patients are subject to the ministrations of inexperienced students.

STUDY FINDINGS

Discussing ethical principles of justice, autonomy, beneficence, nonmaleficence, veracity, and compassion, Decker presented examples of how simulation training might lead to more ethical care for patients. For example, Decker asked, "Are nurse educators and other healthcare professionals demonstrating compassion when they allow students to perform procedures for the first time on clients instead of first providing students with simulated experiences?" (p. 16). Decker raised questions for nursing faculty to consider regarding their obligation to assure nursing student competencies prior to engaging in patient care, in light of the looming opportunities presented by patient simulators. She posed a need for a change in the culture of nursing education, related to use of simulation.

QUESTIONS FOR DISCUSSION

1. When a student approaches a patient procedure, is it ethical to ask for the patient's consent without fully disclosing the student's qualifications to perform the procedure?
2. In comparing traditional models of nursing education—skills labs followed by clinical practice—with simulation prior to clinical practice:
   a. Which model provides for greater patient safety?
   b. Which model provides for the greatest security for the patient?
   c. Which model provides for the greatest confidence building for students?

Decker, S. (2007). Simulations: Education and ethics. In P. Jeffries (Ed.), *Simulation in Nursing Education: From Conceptualization to Evaluation* (pp. 11–19). New York: National League for Nursing.

CONCLUSIONS

The advance of technology in health care is relentless; simulation brings significant technological change to nursing education as well. Regardless of how nurses were initially educated, all nurses can anticipate exposure to simulation technology, whether as students, new graduates, or orientees, when transitioning to new specialties, for demonstrating ongoing competency, and even for continuing education. Nurses in staff development or responsible for training nurses for specialty settings will need to consider simulation as a teaching and competency assessment strategy. In a profession that requires lifelong learning, the question of how best to learn new competencies is partially answered by the promise of simulation.

FOR ADDITIONAL DISCUSSION

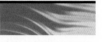

1. Consider your first skill applied to a real patient, such as giving an injection or starting an intravenous line. How confident were you of your skill? How anxious were you? How much of your anxiety was transmitted to the patient? Would simulation practice have improved your confidence and decreased your anxiety?

2. Reflect on a crisis situation in patient care that you had to solve quickly on your own. Would prior simulation practice have helped you in your ability to anticipate and critically analyze the situation? Why or why not?

3. Consider a clinical situation in which you experienced profound learning, something you will never forget. Is there a way to replicate that situation through simulation so that others could experience the same learning? Why or why not?

4. Simulation has been faulted for not being totally realistic. Which factors in patient care can readily be incorporated into simulation? Which cannot?

5. Consider the anxiety experienced by students in a simulation who are being observed by faculty and peers. In the clinical setting, is there more or less anxiety when you are uncertain of your actions and are being observed by patients, family, nurses, physicians, and others?

REFERENCES

Ackermann, A., Kenny, G., & Walker, C. (2007). Simulator programs for new nurses' orientation: A retention strategy. *Journal for Nursing in Staff Development, 23*(3), 136–139.

Advisory Board Company (2008). Capturing the academic and industry perspectives. Available at: http:www.advisoryboardcompany.com/offerings.html. Accessed August 14, 2008.

Agency for Healthcare Research and Quality (2008). *Improving patient safety through simulation research.* Available at: http://www.ahrq.gov/qual/simulproj.htm. Accessed August 30, 2008.

American Academy of Pediatrics (2007). *NRP Instructor Update, 16*(2), 1–12.

American Association of Colleges of Nursing (2008). *Nursing shortage fact sheet.* Available at: http://www.aacn.nche.edu/media/factsheets/nursingshortage.htm. Accessed July 28, 2008.

American Board of Physician Specialties (2006). METI and ABPS team up to develop world's first American Board of Disaster Medicine Certification Examination. Available at: http://www.abpsga.org/events/past_news.html?story=42. Accessed July 30, 2008.

American Hospital Association Committee on Health Professions (2007). *Clinical simulators: Considerations for hospitals.* Available at: http://www.hret.org/hret/programs/content/simulatorsreport.pdf. Accessed July 27, 2008.

Anderson, M., & Leflore, J. (2008). Playing it safe: Simulated team training in the OR. *AORN Journal, 87*(4), 772–779.

Bantz, D., Dancer, M., Hodson-Carlton, K., & Van Hove, S. (2007). A daylong clinical laboratory: From gaming to high-fidelity simulators. *Nurse Educator, 32*(6), 274–277.

Beeman, L. (2008). Basing a clinician's career on simulation: Development of a critical care expert into a clinical simulation expert. In R. Kyle & W. Murray (Eds.), *Clinical Simulation: Operations, Engineering and Management* (pp. 31–51). New York: Elsevier.

Beyea, S. (2004). Human patient simulation: A teaching strategy. *AORN Journal.* Available at: http://findarticles.com/p/articles/mi_mOFSL/is_4_80/ai_n6274052/print?tag=artBody;coll. Accessed July 30, 2008.

Beyea, S. C., von Reyn, L., & Slattery, M. (2007). A nurse residency program for competency development using human patient simulation. *Journal for Nurses in Staff Development, 23*(7), 77–82.

Bremner, M., Aduddell, K., & Amason, J. (2008). Evidence-based practices related to the human patient simulator and first year baccalaureate nursing students' anxiety. *Online Journal of Nursing Informatics, 12*(1), 1–10.

Bremner, M., Aduddell, K., Bennett, D., & VanGeest, J. (2006). The use of human patient simulators: Best practices with novice nursing students. *Nurse Educator, 31*(4), 170–174.

Burns, H., Sakraida, T., Englert, N., Hoffman, R., Tuite, P., & Foley, S. (2006). Returning nurses to the workforce: Developing a fast track back program. *Nursing Forum, 41*(3), 125–132.

Day, L. (2007). Simulation and the teaching and learning of practice in critical care units. *American Journal of Critical Care, 16*, 504–507.

DeCarlo, D., Collingridge, D., Grant, C., & Ventre, K. (2008). Factors influencing nurses' attitudes toward simulation-based education. *Simulation in Healthcare: The Journal of the Society for Simulation in Healthcare, 3*(2), 90–96.

Decker, S. (2007a). Simulations: Education and ethics. In P. Jeffries (Ed.), *Simulation in Nursing Education: From Conceptualization to Evaluation* (pp. 11–19). New York: National League for Nursing.

Decker, S. (2007b). Integrating guided reflection into simulated learning. In P. Jeffries (Ed.), *Simulation in Nursing Education: From Conceptualization to Evaluation* (pp. 73–85). New York: National League for Nursing.

Decker, S., Sportsman, S., Puetz, L., & Billings, L. (2008). The evolution of simulation and its contribution to competency. *The Journal of Continuing Education in Nursing, 39*(2), 74–80.

Del Bueno, D. (2005). A crisis in critical thinking. *Nursing Education Perspectives, 26*, 278–282.

Draycott, T., Crofts, J., Ash, J., Wilson, L. V., Yard, E., Sibanda, T., & Whitelaw, A. (2008). Improving neonatal outcome through practical shoulder dystocia training. *Obstetrics & Gynecology, 112*(1), 1–7.

Durham, C., & Alden, K. (2008). Enhancing patient safety in nursing education through patient simulation. In R. G. Huges (Ed.), *Patient Safety and Quality: An Evidence-Based Handbook for Nurses* (AHRQ Publication No. 09-0043). Rockville, MD: Agency for Healthcare Research and Quality. Available at: http://www.ahrq.gov/qual/nurseshdbk/docs/durhamc_epsne.pdf. Accessed July 24, 2008.

Feingold, C., Calaluce, M., & Kallen, M. (2004). Computerized patient model and simulated clinical experiences: Evaluation with baccalaureate nursing students. *Journal of Nursing Education, 43*, 156–163.

Foster, J., Sheriff, S., & Cheney, S. (2008). Using nonfaculty registered nurses to facilitate high-fidelity human patient simulation activities. *Nurse Educator, 33*(3), 137–141.

Gardner, R., Walzer, T. B., Simon, R., & Raemer, D. B. (2008). Obstetric simulation as a risk control strategy: Course design and evaluation. *Journal of the Society for Simulation in Healthcare, 3*(2), 119–127.

Gassert, C. (2006). Impact of technology and simulated learning on nursing shortages. *Nursing Outlook, 54*(3), 166–167.

Gilley, J. W. (1990). Demonstration and simulation. In M. W. Galbraith (Ed.), *Adult Learning Methods: A Guide for Effective Instruction* (pp. 261–281). Malabar, FL: Krieger.

Hager, M, Russell, S., & Fletcher, S. (Eds.) (2008). *Continuing Education in the Health Professions: Improving Healthcare through Lifelong Learning.* New York: Josiah Macy, Jr. Foundation.

Henneman, E., Cunningham, H., Roche, J., & Curnin, M. (2007). Human patient simulation: Teaching students to provide safe care. *Nurse Educator, 32*(5), 212–217.

Hovancsek, M. (2007). Using simulation in nursing education. In P. Jeffries (Ed.), *Simulation in Nursing*

Education: From Conceptualization to Evaluation (pp. 1–9). New York: National League for Nursing.

Issenberg, S., McGaghie, W., Petrusa, E., Gordon, D., & Scalese, R. (2005). Features and uses of high-fidelity medical simulations that lead to effective learning: A BEME systematic review. *Medical Teacher, 27*, 10–28.

Jarzemsky, P., & McGrath, J. (2008). Look before you leap: Lessons learned when introducing clinical simulation. *Nurse Educator, 33*(2), 90–95.

Jeffries, P., and Rizzolo, M. (2006). Designing and implementing models for the innovative use of simulation to teach nursing care of ill adults and children: A national, multi-site, multi-method of study. In P. Jeffries (Ed.), *Simulation in Nursing Education: From Conceptualization to Evaluation* (pp. 147–159). New York: National League for Nursing.

Jeffries, P. (2008). Designing simulations for nursing education. *Annual Review Nursing Education, 6*, 161–177.

Johnson, D., Flagg, A., & Dremsa, T. (2007). Effects of using a human patient simulator (HPS™) versus a CD-ROM on cognition and critical thinking. *Medical Education Online, 13*(1). Available at: http://www.med-ed-online.org/pdf/T0000118.pdf. Accessed July 29, 2008.

Kardong-Edgren, S., Starkweather, A., & Ward, L. (2008). The integration of simulation into a clinical foundations of nursing course: Student and faculty perspectives. *International Journal of Nursing Education Scholarship, 5*(1), Article 26. Available at: http://www.bepress.com/ijnes/vol5/iss1/art26/. Accessed December 30, 2008.

Katz, G. (2007). *Simulation use in BSN programs.* Unpublished doctoral study. California State University, Chico, School of Nursing.

Kiat, T., Mei, T., Nagammal, S., & Jonnie, A. (2007). A review of learners' experience with simulation based training in nursing. *Singapore Nursing Journal, 34*(4), 37–43.

Kohn, L., Corrigan, J., & Donaldson, M. (Eds.) (2000). *To Err Is Human: Building a Safer Health System.* Washington, DC: National Academy Press.

Kuiper, R., Heinrich, C., Matthias, A., Graham, M., & Bell-Kotwall, L. (2008). Debriefing with the OPT model of clinical reasoning during high fidelity patient simulation. *International Journal of Nursing Education Scholarship, 5*(1), Article 17. Available at: http://www.bepress.com/ijnes/vol5/iss1/art17. Accessed December 30, 2008.

Kyle, R., & Murray, W. (Eds.) (2008). *Clinical Simulation: Operations, Engineering and Management.* New York: Elsevier.

Lasater, K. (2007a). Clinical judgment development: Using simulation to create an assessment rubric. *Journal of Nursing Education, 46*, 496–503.

Lasater, K. (2007b). High-fidelity simulation and the development of clinical judgment: Students' experiences. *Journal of Nursing Education, 46*, 269–276.

Maynes, R. (2008). Human patient simulation in ambulatory care nursing. *AAACN Viewpoint, 30*(1), 11–14.

Medical Education Technologies Incorporated (2008). Available at: http://www.METI.com. Accessed August 12, 2008.

Metcalfe, S., Hall, V., & Carpenter, A. (2007). Promoting collaboration in nursing education: The development of a regional simulation laboratory. *Journal of Professional Nursing, 23*(3), 180–183.

Miller, K., Riley, W., Davis, S., & Hansen, H. (2008). In situ simulation. *Journal of Perinatal & Neonatal Nursing, 22*(2), 105–113.

Morris, L., Pfeifer, P., Catalano, R., Fortney, R., Hilton, E. L., McLaughlin, J., Nelson, G., Palamone, J., Rabito, R., Wetzel, R., & Goldstein, L. (2007). Designing a comprehensive model for critical care orientation. *Critical Care Nurse, 27*(6), 37–61.

National Council of State Boards of Nursing (NCSBN) (2005). Clinical instruction in prelicensure nursing programs. Available at: http://www.ncsbn.org/Final_Clinical_Instr_Pre_Nsg_programs.pdf. Accessed July 21, 2008.

Nehring, W., & Lashley, F. (2004). Current use and opinions regarding Human Patient Simulators in nursing education: An international survey. *Nursing Education Perspectives, 25*(5), 244–248.

Nehring, W., Ellis, W., & Lashley, F. (2001). Human patient simulators in nursing education: An overview. *Simulation & Gaming, 32*, 194–199.

Radhakrishnan, K., Roche, J., & Cunningham, H. (2007). Measuring clinical practice parameters with human patient simulation: A pilot study. *International Journal of Nursing Education Scholarship, 4*(1), Article 8. Available at: http://www.bepress.com/ijnes/vol4/iss1/art8/. Accessed December 30, 2008.

Ramirez, M. (2008). Implications of NIMS integration plan for hospitals and healthcare. Available at:

http://ezinearticles.com/?Implications-of-NIMS-Integration-Plan-For-Hospitals-and-Healthcare&id=672536. Accessed August 2, 2008.

Rauen, C. (2004). Simulation as a teaching strategy for nursing education and orientation in cardiac surgery. *Critical Care Nurse, 24*(3), 46–51.

Ravert, P. (2002). An integrated review of computer-based simulation in the education process. *CIN: Computers, Informatics, Nursing, 20*(5), 203–206.

Robertson, B. (2006). An obstetric simulation experience in an undergraduate nursing curriculum. *Nurse Educator, 31*(2), 74–78.

Salas, E., Wilson K. A., Burke, C. S., & Priest, H. A. (2005). Using simulation-based training to improve patient safety: What does it take? *Journal on Quality and Patient Safety, 31*(7), 363–371.

Schoening, A., Sittner, B., & Todd, M. (2006). Simulated clinical experience: Nursing students' perceptions and the educators' role. *Nurse Educator, 31*(6), 253–258.

Seropian, M., Brown, K., Gavilanes, J., & Driggers, B. (2004). An approach to simulation program development. *Journal of Nursing Education, 43*(4), 170–174.

Spunt, D. (2007). Setting up a simulation laboratory. In P. Jeffries (Ed.), *Simulation in Nursing Education: From Conceptualization to Evaluation* (pp. 105–122). New York: National League for Nursing.

Starkweather, R., & Kardong-Edgren, S. (2008). Diffusion of innovation: Embedding simulation into nursing curricula. *International Journal of Nursing Education Scholarship, 5*(1), Article 13. Available at: http://www.bepress.com/ijnes/vol5/iss1/art13/. Accessed December 30, 2008.

Wayne, D., Siddall, V., Butter, J., Fudala, M. J., Wade, L. D., Feinglass, J., & McGaghie, W. C. (2006). A longitudinal study of internal medicine residents' retention of advanced cardiac life support skills. *Academic Medicine, 81*(10 Suppl), s9–s12.

Wolf, L. (2008). The use of human patient simulation in ED triage training can improve nursing confidence and patient outcomes. *Journal of Emergency Nursing, 34*(2), 169–171.

Yaeger, K., & Arafeh, J. (2008). Making the move: From traditional neonatal education to simulation-based training. *Journal of Perinatal & Neonatal Nursing, 22*(2), 154–158.

BIBLIOGRAPHY

Diefenbeck, C., Plowfield, L., & Herrman, J. (2006). Clinical immersion: A residency model for nursing education. *Nursing Education Perspectives, 27*(2), 72–79.

Jeffries, P. (2005). A framework for designing, implementing and evaluating simulations used as teaching strategies in nursing. *Nursing Education Perspectives, 26*(2), 96–103.

Jeffries, P. (Ed.) (2006). *Simulation in Nursing Education: From Conceptualization to Evaluation.* New York: National League for Nursing.

Jeffries, P. (2008). Getting in S.T.E.P. with simulations: Simulations take educator preparation. *Nursing Education Perspectives, 29*(3), 70–73.

King, C., Moseley, S., Hindenlang, B., & Kuritz, P. (2008). Limited use of the human patient simulator by nurse faculty: An intervention program designed to increase use. *International Journal of Nursing Education Scholarship, 5*(1), Article 12. Available at: http://www.bepress.com/ijnes/vol5/iss1/art12/. Accessed December 30, 2008.

Kyle, R., & Murray, W. (Eds.) (2008). *Clinical Simulation: Operations, Engineering and Management.* New York: Elsevier.

Waldner, M., & Olson, J. (2007). Taking the patient to the classroom: Applying theoretical frameworks to simulation in nursing education. *International Journal of Nursing Education Scholarship, 4*(1), Article 18. Available at: http://www.bepress.com/ijnes/vol4/iss1/art18/. Accessed December 30, 2008.

WEB RESOURCES

Advanced Initiatives in Medical Simulation (AIMS)	http://www.medsim.org/
Bay Area Simulation Collaborative (BASC)	http://www.bayareanrc.org/
Center for Immersive and Simulation-Based Learning	http://cisl.stanford.edu/
Center for Advanced Pediatric and Perinatal Education (CAPE)	http://cape.lpch.org/
Gaumard Scientific Co.	www.gaumard.com
Harvard Center for Medical Simulation	http://harvardmedsim.org/cms/
International Nursing Association for Clinical Simulations and Learning	http://www.inacsl.org/
Laerdal Patient Simulators	http://www.laerdal.com
Laerdal Simulation User Network	http://simulation.laerdal.com/
Medical Education Technologies (METI)	http://www.meti.com
Simulation Innovation Resource Center	http://sirc.nln.org/
Society for Simulation in Healthcare (SSH)	http://www.ssih.org

JOURNALS

Clinical Simulation in Nursing. Elsevier, Inc.
Simulation in Healthcare. Lippincott, Williams, & Wilkins.
CIN: Computers, Informatics, Nursing. Lippincott, Williams, & Wilkins.

CHAPTER 5

The Current Nursing Shortage: Causes, Consequences, and Solutions

• CAROL J. HUSTON •

Learning Objectives

The learner will be able to:

1. Explore factors affecting the current supply of registered nurses (RNs) in the United States as well as the current and projected demand through 2020.
2. Compare regional differences in the supply and demand for registered nurses in the United States.
3. Discuss consequences of the current shortage on quality of health care, current working conditions for RNs, and RN retention rates.
4. Analyze the relationship between recruitment and retention in resolving a nursing shortage.
5. Identify the relationship between nursing shortages and the state of the national economy.
6. Explore the impact of non-monetary factors such as working conditions, empowerment, and shared decision making on retention rates of registered nurses.
7. Analyze the impact of salary as an incentive for resolving nursing shortages.

8. Address the educational challenges inherent in solving the nursing shortage given unfilled faculty positions, resignations, projected retirements, low faculty pay schedules, and the shortage of students being prepared for the faculty role.
9. Identify specific strategies being used to recruit and retain older nurses in the workforce.
10. Differentiate between and provide examples of both short term and long term solutions to nursing shortages.
11. Identify benchmark research findings that examine the relationship between nurse staffing levels and clinical outcomes of patients.
12. Outline strategies directed at both supply and demand factors that have been proposed in an effort to reduce the current nursing shortage and analyze the efficacy of each.
13. Reflect upon his/her personal commitment to a career in professional nursing.

As government and private insurer reimbursement declined in the 1990s and managed care costs soared, many health care organizations, and hospitals in particular, began downsizing to achieve cost containment by eliminating registered nursing jobs or by replacing registered nurses (RNs) with unlicensed assistive personnel. Even hospitals that did not downsize during this period often did little to recruit qualified RNs.

This downsizing and shortsightedness regarding recruitment and retention contributed to the beginning of an acute shortage of RNs in many health care settings by the late 1990s. Peter Buerhaus, an expert on health care

workforce needs, suggested that the health care quality and safety movement also exacerbated the shortage in the late 1990s as research emerged to demonstrate the relationship between nurse staffing and patient outcomes and the public became aware of how important an adequately sized workforce was to patient safety (Roman, 2008).

Unlike earlier nursing shortages, which typically lasted only a few years, the current shortage has lasted longer and been more severe than any nursing shortage experienced thus far. In fact, Herbst (2007, para 1) stated that hospital administrators and nurses' advocates consider the current shortage to be a "staffing crisis."

The nursing shortage is also widespread geographically (indeed, worldwide). Hinshaw (2008) and Aiken (2007) suggested that there are shortages in both developing and developed countries, with the shortage in developed countries exacerbating the shortages in developing countries as a result of nurse migration (see Chapter 6). The shortage also exists in all practice settings, although it is greatest in acute care hospitals. Rural areas have greater shortages than urban areas (Cramer, Nienaber, Helget, & Agrawal, 2006). In addition, the causes of the current shortage are numerous and multifaceted, which makes resolution even more difficult.

How significant is the shortage? Projections made early in the 21st century suggested a national shortfall of at least 760,000 nurses by 2020. Recent research by Buerhaus and colleagues, however, has revised the projected shortage to 340,000 as a result of more people entering the profession in their late 20s and early 30s (Roman, 2008). Projections by Dr. Linda Aiken, Professor of Nursing and Sociology and Director of the Center for Health Outcomes and Policy Research at the University of Pennsylvania, are similar (Smalarz, Corbett, & Doonan, 2007).

These revised projections do not mean, however, that the crisis has passed. Indeed, Buerhaus, in an interview with *RN* editor Linda Roman, stated

We have reduced the magnitude of the future shortage hurricane from a Category Five, on a huge amount of steroids, down to a Category Three. But that can still kill you. It would cause unprecedented damage if it were to fully develop—It would shut down most of the system and cause care to be rationed.

To assess more accurately the depth or significance of the current nursing shortage, data must be examined regarding both the demand for RNs and the supply. Assessing the demand for RNs is, in many ways, more complicated than assessing the supply. However, from an economic perspective, this shortage is being driven more by the supply side of the supply/demand equation than the demand side. This makes the problem even more difficult to solve because it will require more than the short-term, quick-fix solutions that have worked in the past.

> CONSIDER
> This nursing shortage is not likely to be fixed by the same short-term, quick-fix solutions that worked in the past.

In addition, solving the current nursing shortage will be expensive. Buerhaus suggested that "The U.S. needs to spend at least $1 billion to make any inroads into the nursing shortage. . . If we're lucky, we'll get $50 or $60 million" ($1 Billion Needed to Address, 2003/2004).

This chapter will explore the current nursing shortage, including the current and projected demand for RNs, as well as the supply. In addition, consequences of the shortage will be examined, together with strategies that have been proposed in an effort to confront what is likely one of the greatest current threats to quality health care.

> CONSIDER
> The current nursing shortage is a global public health crisis.

THE DEMAND

"*Demand*" is defined by the *Merriam Online Dictionary* (2008a) as the quantity of a commodity or service wanted at a specified price and time. In the case of nursing, demand would be the amount of a good or service (in this case, an RN) that consumers (in this case, an employer) would be willing to acquire at a given price. A shortage occurs when employers want more employees at the current market wages than they can get. Demand then is derived from the health status of a population and the use of health services.

The demand for professional nurses in both the short- and long-term future continues to increase. In fact, employment of registered nurses is expected to grow much faster than average for all occupations through 2014, and, according to the November 2007 projections from the U.S. Bureau of Labor Statistics, more than 587,000 new nursing positions will be created through 2016 (a 23.5% increase), making nursing the nation's top profession in terms of projected job growth (Dohm & Shniper, 2007).

Buerhaus, Staiger, and Auerbach (2009) concurred, predicting an increase in demand for registered nurses that will continue to grow 2% to 3% per year. Indeed, Buerhaus et al. suggested that the deficit of full-time nurses will reach 500,000 by 2025. This is less than the 2006 projections by the U.S. Health Resources and Services Administration (HRSA), which suggested that 1 million new nurses would be needed by 2020 and that all 50 states in the United States would experience a nursing shortage of some degree by 2015, but it is just as unattainable (American Association of Colleges of Nursing [AACN], 2006a).

Hinshaw's (2008) demand projections are also daunting, suggesting that the 6% RN shortage at the beginning of the 21st century will swell to 29% by 2020 if the issue is not addressed, but Hinshaw noted that part of this shortage will come from the projected 40% increase in demand, compared to the projected 6% growth in the supply of nurses. These figures are in line with recent data from the Massachusetts Nursing Association, which show that the state vacancy rate for nursing faculty, which was at 5 percent in 2006, surged to 14 percent by June 2008 (Jordan, 2008). Finally, the American Hospital Association notes that there were 126,000 unfilled positions for RNs in U.S. hospitals as of January 2006 but suggested that this was just the "calm before the storm," given current shortage projections (Clarke & Cheung, 2008).

Causes of Increased Demand

There are multiple demand factors driving the current shortage, including a growing population, medical advances that increase the need for adequately educated nurses, and the increased acuity of hospitalized patients. Other factors driving demand are the technological advances in patient care and an increasing emphasis on health care prevention.

In addition, a growing elderly population with extended longevity will require more nursing care. The Institute for the Future of Aging Services (2007) suggested that between now and 2015, the population aged 85 years and older will increase by 40%. As life expectancy in the United States increases, more nurses are needed to assist the individuals who are surviving serious illnesses and living longer with chronic diseases.

Heinz (2004) agreed, stating that the demand for health care will continue to grow at a staggering rate as the baby-boom generation enters the later stages of their lives. The increased needs of these individuals will require intense health care services, as well as greater hospital bed occupancy and highly skilled nursing care. This is at least part of the reason that nursing home bed occupancy was 84% in 2006 (U.S. Department of Health and Human Services, 2007). As a result, the demand for health care is expected to steadily increase, and the numbers of nurses to care for these patients will lag behind.

Geographical Maldistribution of Nurses

Besides shortages of nurses in acute care settings, the nursing workforce is poorly distributed geographically. As the 21st century began, the greatest concentration of employed nurses was in New England and the lowest concentration was in the Pacific region. Indeed in 2006, the number of RNs per 100,000 population varied from a low of 588 in California to a high of 2,093 in the District of Columbia (The New York Center for Health Workforce Studies, 2006). The mean for the United States was 802 per 100,000 population.

The reality, however, is that virtually all states have been affected by the current shortage. The situation in some states, however, is especially dire. Seguritan (2007, para 8) suggested that "states in the West and Southwest have a disproportionate number of nursing vacancies because of rapid population growth, which exacerbates a widening gap in the number of facilities and staff compared to patients that need care." Indeed, the California Board of Registered Nursing reported that "the nursing shortage in California is worse now than it was in 2000 in terms of the number of working RNs per capita," declining from 544 full-time equivalent RNs per 100,000 population in 2000 to 539 in 2005 (National Council State Boards of Nursing [NCBSN], 2008a, para 2).

Similarly, using publicly accessible databases, Lin, Lijun, Turek, Jurascjek, and John (2008) reported that all regions in California exhibit growing shortages, with shortfalls ranging from 3% to 600% by 2020. Based on a modified version of the grading rubric of the California Regional Registered Nurse Workforce Report Card, only two regions will receive a grade above "C" in 2020, and the number of "F" grades will grow to nine.

THE SUPPLY

"*Supply*" refers to the quantity of goods or services that are ready for use or purchase (*Merriam Webster Online Dictionary*, 2008b). To evaluate the supply of RNs in the United States, it is necessary to look at both RNs who are currently working and those who are eligible to work but do not. In addition, the current and potential student pool must be part of the supply discussion. The bottom line is that the supply of registered nurses is expected to grow little in the coming decade or two, but large numbers of nurses are expected to retire. Indeed, Buerhaus suggested that the full effect of the shortage will not be felt until between 2015 and 2020, when demand for nurses is expected to grow well beyond the number of RNs available (Roman, 2008).

The United States has about 2.9 million registered nurses (RNs) filling about 2.4 million jobs (U.S. Department of Health and Human Services, 2006). This is not enough. The U.S. Department of Labor reported more than 126,000 RN job vacancies in 2006 (Seguritan, 2007). "Indeed, it is estimated that 8.5% of the nursing positions in the U.S. are unfilled—and some expect that number to triple by 2020 as 80 million baby boomers retire and expand the ranks of those needing care" (Herbst, 2007, para 1).

These figures are similar to those released in July 2007 by the American Hospital Association (AHA), which suggested that U.S. hospitals had approximately 116,000 vacancies at the end of 2006, translating into a national RN vacancy rate of 8.1% (AHA, 2007). Similarly, the National Commission on Nursing Workforce for Long-Term Care (2005) revealed that nearly 100,000 vacant nursing positions existed in long-term care facilities on any given day, and the nurse turnover rate in that setting exceeded 50%.

DISCUSSION POINT

What factors cause turnover to be so high in long-term care facilities? Is the shortage of licensed health care professionals in long-term care more heavily influenced by supply or demand?

Enrollment in Nursing Schools

The number of students enrolled or projected to enroll in nursing programs is also an important factor in determining RN supply. Unfortunately, some schools of nursing have chosen to close nursing programs due to funding cuts or to reduce program size. Still others have been forced to turn away potential students because of a lack of faculty. Despite this, enrollment in nursing schools has steadily increased every year for almost a decade (see Table 5.1). Unfortunately, however, these increases are not adequate to replace those nurses who will be lost to retirement in the coming decade.

In fact, the Council on Physician and Nurse Supply has determined that 30,000 additional nurses must be graduated annually to meet the nation's health care needs, an expansion of 30% over the current number of annual nurse graduates (AACN, 2008b). The HRSA's predictions are even direr, suggesting that nursing schools must increase the number of graduates by 90% to adequately address the nursing shortage (AACN, 2007). With preliminary data showing a 7.4% increase in graduations from baccalaureate nursing programs in 2007, one can see that schools are falling far short of meeting this target.

Unfortunately, enrollment increases are not possible without a significant boost in federal and state funding to prepare new faculty, enhance teaching resources, and upgrade nursing school infrastructure. More money is needed in the form of nursing scholarships and loans to encourage young people to enter nursing. In addition, individual nurses and professional organizations must support legislation to improve financial access to nursing education. The Tri-Council for Nursing (comprising the American Association of Colleges of Nursing,

---

| TABLE 5.1 | Number of Candidates Taking the National Council Licensure Examination for Registered Nurses (NCLEX-RN): First-Time, U.S.-Educated Candidates Only |

Program	2001	2002	2003	2004	2005	2006	2007
Diploma	2,310	2,424	2,565	3,162	3,540	3,810	3,688
Baccalaureate	24,832	25,806	26,630	30,648	35,496	41,349	45,781
Associate	41,567	42,310	47,423	53,275	60,053	65,390	69,890
Total	68,579	70,604	76,727	87,177	99,187	110,713	119,579

Source: National Council State Boards of Nursing (2008). *NCLEX examination pass rates.* Available at: https://www.ncsbn.org/1237.htm. Accessed May 24, 2008.

the American Nurses Association, the American Organization of Nurse Executives, and the National League for Nursing) has also urged nurses to advocate for increased nursing education funding under Title VIII of the Public Health Service Act, as well as other publicly funded initiatives, so that there will be the necessary capacity and resources to educate future nurses.

There have been increases in federal money for nursing education over the last decade. The passage of legislation such as the 2002 Nurse Reinvestment Act encouraged more students to choose nursing as a career and helped students financially to complete their education. It also encouraged graduate students to complete their studies and assume teaching positions in nursing schools. In addition, many states introduced or passed legislation designed to improve working conditions and attract more nurses.

Many hospitals have joined forces with local schools of nursing to offer scholarships in exchange for a student's willingness to work in that institution after graduation (Henderson & Hassmiller, 2007). Hospitals are also lending master's and doctorally prepared advanced nurses such as nurse practitioners, clinical nurse specialists, and clinical nurse leaders to supplement faculty positions.

Private foundations have also stepped up to offer funding for nursing education. In 2008, the Robert Wood Johnson Foundation (RWJF) joined with the American Association of Colleges of Nursing (AACN) to create the Robert Wood Johnson Foundation New Careers in Nursing (RWJF, 2008). Through grants to schools of nursing, the program funds up to 500 scholarships of $10,000 each annually to schools that offer accelerated baccalaureate and master's nursing programs.

In 2006, the RWJF announced a 5-year, $10 million initiative called Partners Investing in Nursing's Future. "In collaboration with the Northwest Health Foundation, RWJF funded local foundations to make significant investments in the nursing challenges in their communities" (Henderson & Hassmiller, 2007, p. 96).

Ironically, recruitment efforts into the nursing profession the last decade were very successful, and the problem is no longer a lack of nursing school applicants. Indeed, enrollment in nursing programs of education has increased steadily since 2001. The problem is that there are inadequate resources to provide nursing education to those interested in pursuing nursing as a career, including an insufficient number of clinical sites, classroom space, nursing faculty, and clinical preceptors.

Indeed, Bolt (2008) suggested that it often costs colleges more to educate nurses than they collect in tuition and state funding. For example, Lane Community College in Eugene, Oregon, suggested that a nursing education costs $5,000 more per student each year than what it brings in through student tuition, state and local taxes, and other support, including donations. As a result, they turn away qualified applicants, despite the critical shortage of nurses (Bolt).

DISCUSSION POINT

Should the increased cost of nursing education be passed on to students? Would students enrolled in public universities be willing to pay more for their education than students in other majors?

Indeed, the AACN (2007) reported that 30,709 qualified applicants were turned away from baccalaureate nursing programs in 2007. More than 38,000 were turned away in 2006, and more than 37,000 were turned away in 2005, so the problem is not new (AACN, 2007). The number turned away in 2007 rises to 40,285 qualified applicants when both baccalaureate and graduate nursing programs are included (AACN, 2008a).

Although program costs are a major deterrent to increasing nursing school enrollment, the greatest problem is an inadequate number of nursing faculty to teach students interested in pursuing nursing as a career. By 2007, 71.4% of nursing schools cited faculty shortages as the major reason they had denied qualified students admission (AACN, 2008a), and a 2006 report by the National League for Nursing (NLN) identified a 7.9% vacancy rate for full-time faculty in baccalaureate and higher degree programs (Issues in Nursing, 2008). According to a 2006 survey by the AACN, there were 637 faculty vacancies at 329 nursing schools with baccalaureate and/or graduate programs across the country, and an additional 55 faculty positions were needed just to accommodate student demand (AACN, 2006c). This translates into approximately 1.9 faculty vacancies per school.

The situation was even worse in a more recent study (AACN, 2008a), which showed a total of 767 faculty vacancies at 344 nursing schools with baccalaureate and/or graduate programs across the country. The national nurse faculty vacancy rate was identified as 8.8%, which translates into approximately 2.2 faculty vacancies per school. Most of the vacancies (86.2%) were faculty positions requiring or preferring a doctoral degree (AACN).

Mary Ann Peters, the Director of Graduate Nursing Programs at La Salle University in Philadelphia, went so far as to suggest that nurse educators might be considered as candidates for the endangered species list (Issues in Nursing, 2008). She suggested that this is because there simply are not enough nurses with the educational credentials needed for the faculty role and because academic institutions do not provide a high enough salary to draw new individuals to it. She concluded that the profession and society must develop a strategic plan and support it with adequate funding because excellent education is essential to the future of a vital evolving profession and superior patient care.

The RWJF agreed, suggesting that the time it takes to earn the degree typically required for full faculty status, the reluctance to give up practice opportunities, and the low pay incentive sharply curtailed interest in academic careers in nursing (RWJF, 2007). The RWJF recommended granting funding stipends to those willing to teach nursing, raising academic salaries, engaging health care providers to pay a greater share of the cost of workforce training, and developing new degree programs to better prepare nurse educators and speed their entry into the faculty role. The RWJF also suggested that leaders in academia, government, the health care industry, and professional associations must collaborate across sectors to put these policies into place.

Increasing the number of nursing students in the pipeline as a strategy for addressing the current nursing shortage clearly depends on having enough qualified faculty to teach them. The AACN (2008a) warns that if not addressed, the shortage of nurse educators will continue to halt further progress in reversing the national nursing shortage. Clearly, the same energy that was directed at recruiting young people for nursing must now be directed at recruiting nursing faculty.

In response, Nurses for a Healthier Tomorrow (NHT) launched a national advertising campaign entitled "Nursing education . . . pass it on" in February 2004 (NHT, n.d.). The seven faculty recruitment print ads depicted nurse educators expressing the personal satisfaction and rewards that they receive from their job. The campaign also included four colorful ads depicting nurse educators who encourage teaching careers, an outreach campaign to nursing journals and the mass media, ready-to-run articles in a special edition of the NHT newsletter, and a new career profile on the nurse educator posted on the NHT Web site.

In addition, many federal and private sources of funding have been created for students considering graduate nursing education. The 2002 Nurse Reinvestment Act includes a student loan repayment program for nurses willing to serve in faculty roles after graduation (NHT, n.d.). Similar programs are also available through the National Health Service Corps and the Bureau of Health Professions. In addition, the Nurse Faculty Education Act of 2005 provided $12 million to help recruit new nursing faculty and doctoral students, given that more than half of doctoral degree holders are expected to enter faculty roles (Nursing Doctorate Programs, 2006).

As a result, survey data by the AACN (2005) showed a 13.7% increase in enrollment in master's degree programs in nursing and a 7.3% increase in research-focused doctoral programs. In addition, nurses now have more opportunities to earn doctoral degrees as a result of the emergence and rapid growth of new Doctor of Nursing Practice (DNP) degree programs: "Twenty-four universities and colleges including early adopters Purdue University, Columbia University, the University of Kentucky and the University of Tennessee Memphis have launched DNP programs, and nearly 200 more are looking to do so" (Nursing Doctorate Programs, 2006, para 2). Other long-term strategies for addressing the nursing faculty shortage are shown in Box 5.1.

CONSIDER

Unfilled faculty positions, resignations, and projected retirements continue to pose a threat to the nursing education workforce.

Part-Time and Unemployed Nurses: An Untapped Pool?

Some experts have suggested that too much emphasis has been placed on recruiting young people to solve the nursing shortage, and that supply could more easily be increased by bringing unemployed or part-time nurses back to nursing full-time.

The reality is, however, that the percentage of RNs who are not employed in nursing has dropped significantly since 1977, from more than one in four RNs to one in six (Buerhaus et al., 2009). In addition, the number of RNs working full-time increased from 68% in 1977 to just greater than 70% in 2004, and the number of hours during a given week worked by both full- and part-time RNs combined increased by approximately 6.5% between 1983

BOX 5.1   **LONG-TERM STRATEGIES FOR ADDRESSING THE NURSING FACULTY SHORTAGE**

---

1. Recruitment
   - Provide a position image/role model for advanced education in nursing education.
   - Recruit young people from middle and high schools to become nursing faculty.
   - Streamline the education track to higher academics.
   - Provide financial support or tuition forgiveness in exchange for teaching service.
   - Develop mentoring/support programs for new academics.
2. Retention
   - Provide better salaries and benefits for nursing faculty.
   - Create positive work environments and reasonable teaching assignments.
   - Reward teaching excellence.
   - Create faculty development and mentorship programs.
3. Collaboration
   - Develop relationships with state legislators for support and funding.
   - Partner with high schools, colleges, health care institutions, and governmental agencies to create support for higher education in nursing.

Source: Adapted from Allen, L. (2008). The nursing shortage continues as faculty shortage grows. *Nursing Economics, 26*(1), 35–40.

---

and 2006 (Buerhaus et al., 2009). Thus, the pool of part-time and unemployed nurses has already been tapped.

Research conducted by McIntosh, Val Palumbo, and Rambur (2006) agreed, and suggested that a viable *shadow workforce* (those who are no longer working in the profession but possess the necessary training and experience to do so) does not exist. They also disputed the notion that large numbers of nurses left the profession due to workplace dissatisfaction and are now available to return. Instead, they found that only 12% of those who left for retirement would consider returning (see Research Study Fuels the Controversy on page 78).

In addition, the literature on re-entry of RNs into the workplace is often pessimistic, suggesting that such programs take a great deal of effort for the results they provide. Nonetheless, research by Williams, Stotts, and Jacob (2006) suggested that a major portion (27.6%) of nurses who leave nursing do so because of a conflict between parenting duties and scheduling requirements (13.5%) at work. This suggests that these nurses might return to nursing if given the opportunity to work part-time and if shifts were flexible and shorter.

In fact, Buerhaus et al. (2009) suggested that the current shortage has been lessened, at least in part, by the

re-entry of older RNs into employment. This was especially true earlier in this decade when the U.S. economy first began to stall. In fact, the "employment growth of older RNs (over the age of 50) has increased every year since 2000 for an astounding net gain of more than 257,000 full time equivalent (FTE) RNs" (Buerhaus et al., 2009, p. 119). In contrast, the total net employment growth of RNs aged 21 to 34 years was only roughly 36,000, which was effectively negated by a similar net decrease in employment (roughly 40,000 FTE RNs) by RNs aged 35 to 59 years. Buerhaus et al. warned, however, that the increased demand by boomers and the aging workforce will make the re-entry of older RNs only a brief reprieve in a shortage that is far from over (Despite Americans' High Regard, 2008).

Using Foreign-Born Nurses to Relieve the Shortage

The shortage has also been alleviated at least in part by the importation of RNs from foreign markets. Buerhaus et al. (2009) suggested that the number of foreign-born RNs in the U.S. workforce between 1994 and 2001 averaged 6.0% each year. By 2002, it doubled to 12.5%. After

Research Study Fuels the Controversy: Does a "Shadow Workforce" of Inactive Nurses Exist?

The researchers in this study surveyed the entire list of Vermont nurses with inactive or lapsed licenses in January 2004 (*n* = 3,682), using a tool developed by M. T. Shore in 1990 entitled Identification of Factors Which Would Attract Inactive Registered Nurses Back to the Hospital Setting.

STUDY FINDINGS

The researchers found that a shadow workforce of inactive nurses did not exist in the Vermont area. In addition, the research suggested that retirement and family responsibility were the primary personal reasons for leaving nursing, although 21% of respondents indicated that non-nursing job opportunities were an explanation for leaving. Stressful work environments, the physical nature of the job, excessive paperwork, and work hours/scheduling were also factors contributing to withdrawal from the profession. The factors considered most important in consideration of re-entering the workforce were accessibility of re-entry programs, flexible work schedules, free or affordable re-entry programs, and an orientation program. The study concluded that greater attention should be directed at helping nurses to identify with the profession and being encouraged to remain active through creative postretirement employment alternatives.

McIntosh, B., Val Palumbo, M., & Rambur, B. (2006). Does a 'shadow workforce' of inactive nurses exist? *Nursing Economics, 24*(5), 231–238.

a temporary decline in 2005, likely related to the expiration of work visas, the employment of foreign-born nurses surged forward again in 2006, outstripping the growth in employment among nurses born in the United States: "Overall, the rapid growth in employment of foreign-born RNs accounts for more than one-third (37%) of the total growth of total RN employment in the United States since 2002" (Buerhaus et al., 2009, p. 118).

Widespread, transnational nursing migration is likely to continue for some time, given the success hospitals have had with foreign recruitment and the time required to strengthen the domestic nurse supply pipeline. Such practice, however, could potentially have negative implications in terms of the domestic job market and health care quality. In addition, using foreign-born labor has complex international implications, creating a drain on some countries' health care systems while shoring up the economies of countries that purposefully export their workers. Because the importation of nurses has such complex ramifications, a separate chapter is devoted to its discussion (see Chapter 6).

ROOTS OF THE SHORTAGE

Many factors contribute to the current nursing shortage in acute care settings, including an aging workforce, increased employment of nurses in outpatient or ambulatory care settings, high turnover due to worker dissatisfaction, inadequate long-term pay incentives, and an increasing recognition by nurses that they can make more money and act more autonomously as free agents than as full-time employees of a health care organization. These factors and others (Box 5.2) will be discussed in this section.

Nursing as a "Graying" Population

Nursing is a graying population—even more so than the population at large. This means that the nursing workforce is retiring at a rate faster than it can be replaced. The most recent national RN survey (*2004 National Sample Survey of Registered Nurses*), released in March 2006, indicates that the average age of the registered nurse in the United States is 46.8 years, more than 1 year older than the estimated average age of 45.2 years in the 2000 survey (Hart, 2006).

Indeed, the average age of the working nurse has been increasing for some time. Only 26.6 percent of the RN population in the survey was younger than 40 years, just 16.6 percent was younger than 30 years, and the largest group of RNs was aged 45 to 49 years (Hart, 2006). This rising average age reflects a two- to three-decade-long trend toward older students entering nursing education programs, as well as a general decline in interest in nursing as a career among younger people. In

BOX 5.2 | CAUSES OF THE CURRENT NURSING SHORTAGE

- Increasing elderly population (more individuals who are chronically ill).
- Increased acuity in acute care settings, requiring higher-level nursing skills.
- Downsizing and restructuring of the late 1990s, which eliminated many RN positions.
- A relatively healthy economy in the late 1990s and early 2000, which encouraged some nurses to change from full time employment to part-time or to quit.
- Aging RN workforce.
- Workplace dissatisfaction.
- Women choosing fields other than nursing for a career.
- Aging faculty for RN programs.
- Inadequate nursing programs to accommodate interested applicants.
- Low ceiling on wages for RNs without advanced degrees.
- Future educator pool for RNs more limited than demand.

addition, "the average age becomes even starker when confronted with the average of RN retirement, which is approximately 52 years" (Hinshaw, 2008, p. 56).

A 2007 study, however, suggests that this trend might be reversing. Auerbach, Buerhaus, and Staiger (2007) found that although the number of people entering nursing in their early to mid-20s remains at its lowest point in 40 years, greater numbers of individuals in their late 20s and 30s are entering the field, which should serve to decrease the age of the average nurse. In addition, the study showed that people born in the 1970s are now almost as likely to become nurses as people born during the 1950s, when interest in nursing careers was at its height. The researchers suggested that this projected increase in nursing will mitigate the severity of the nursing shortage in 2020.

Yet, retirement projections for the profession are grim. The *Nursing Management Aging Workforce Survey*, released in July 2006, reported that 55% of surveyed nurses planned to retire between 2011 and 2020, and, by and large, employers were taking little action to retain aging workers (Orlovsky, 2006). These retirement numbers are consistent with those reported by the Massachusetts Nursing Association in 2008 that more than 50% of the state's 132,841 licensed nurses are in their 50s and will be leaving the work force within 10 years (Jordan, 2008).

Another survey, by AMN Healthcare, suggested that 35% of baby-boomer nurses said that they "plan to retire, change profession, work part-time, switch to a less demanding role, or work as travel nurses" in the next 1 to 3 years (Baby-Boomer Nurses Are on Their Way Out, 2008, para 1). The most common reason given for their intent to change their current work situation was burnout and declining satisfaction with the work.

Orsolini-Hain and Malone (2007) suggested that the loss of so many experienced nurses in such a short time will actually result in a "brain drain" or gap in clinical nursing expertise. This could result in "increased medical errors and concomitant negative health outcomes for millions of Americans who need an expert and highly educated workforce to deliver care" (p. 167). Orsolini-Hain and Malone went on to suggest that the current nursing shortage should not be addressed merely by increasing the number of RNs. Instead, policy initiatives are needed to address the "expertise gap" as well.

DISCUSSION POINT

Why is there so little discussion about the "expertise gap" that will occur as a result of impending nursing retirements?

Similarly, Letvak (2008) stated that we cannot afford to lose the experience of so many older nurses. He pointed out that older workers typically have higher job satisfaction and lower turnover. In addition, "they are more dedicated to their jobs, take pride in a job well done, have good listening skills, are not intimidated by difficult personalities, and demonstrate maturity" (p. 22).

DISCUSSION POINT
What factors have led to the "graying" of the
nursing workforce? Does there appear to be any
short-term resolution of these factors?

The Nursing Faculty Are Grayer Yet

To further confound the nursing shortage and efforts to
address it, the average age of nursing faculty members
continues to increase, narrowing the number of productive years nurse educators can teach. With the average age of Ph.D.-prepared nurse educators being almost
54 years and the average retirement age for nursing faculty being 62.5 years (La Rocco, 2006), one must question where the faculty will come from to teach the new
nurses needed to solve the current shortage. In addition,
with only 13% of nurses holding master's or doctoral
degrees (U.S. Department of Health and Human Services, 2006) and the lag time required to educate master's- or doctorally-prepared faculty, the faculty shortage may end up being the greatest obstacle to solving
the current nursing shortage.

> **CONSIDER**
> Even if enough students can be recruited to
> become nurses, there will not be enough faculty
> to teach them.

The Exodus to Nonacute Care Settings

Another factor compounding the nursing shortage in
acute care hospitals is the number of nurses leaving the
acute care hospital for employment in community
health settings. About two thirds of nurses receive their
paychecks from hospitals, whether from working in the
hospital itself or in a clinic or home care practice associated with a hospital (Sounart, 2008). Connie Curran,
editor of *Nursing Economics*, suggested, however, that
working overtime has become standard practice in
acute care hospitals, that pay raises are difficult to come
by as a result of decreasing reimbursement, and that although hospitals traditionally have been generous with
health care benefits, pensions are hard to come by. Curran argued that these factors will drive nurses away
from hospitals and into other settings (Sounart). Indeed, Curran stated that "the estimate is now that there

are about 200,000 nurses moving into retail 'minute
clinics,' insurance companies, and other outside organizations" (Sounart, 2008, para 7).

The Free Agent Nurse

An increase in the number of free agent nurses is another aspect that must be examined in assessing supply
and demand factors of the current nursing shortage.
Full-time employment of nurses is decreasing. Instead,
nurses are increasingly assuming the role of *free agent*, a
term more common to Generation X than their older
counterparts, and this contributes to a shortage in acute
care agencies. A free agent nurse is often an independent contractor who sells his or her services to an employer, with the condition that he or she maintains control over the number of hours they are willing to work
and working conditions.

Per-diem and *traveling nurses* are two types of free
agents. The relationship between the free agent and his
or her employing organization is based on a free and
open exchange, more of a partnership than an unequal
dependency relationship. Typically, the free agent nurse
makes a higher hourly wage than other full-time or
part-time employees in a health care organization in exchange for not receiving health care and retirement
benefits. Such nurses also have greater control over if
and when they want to work.

Historically, health care organizations have sought
to employ full-time workers (employees) so that they
could better control the availability of needed human
resources. However, the free agent model of nursing is
gaining momentum in health care organizations as they
recognize that they need to supplement their full-time
employee pool with these skilled workers and that significant benefit costs can be accrued from using free
agent or temporary workers.

Critics of the increased use of free agent nurses, particularly traveling nurses, suggest that this practice may
negatively affect the quality of care related to inconsis-
tency of caretakers and a reduced ability to determine
the competencies of the specific free agent nurse. In an
effort to address these quality concerns, Aiken, Xue,
Clarke, and Sloane (2007) compared outcomes and adverse events between supplemental nurses working in
hospitals and permanent staff. This study found that a
high proportion of supplemental nurses work in critical

care units, where the needs for nurses with specialized skills is high. Analyses, however, suggested that supplemental nurses were no less qualified than permanent staff nurses and that, in fact, the supplemental nurses were more likely to hold baccalaureate and higher degrees. The study concluded that having more supplemental nurses might in some cases have a positive effect on patient outcomes. More research is needed, however, on the effect of the free agent nurse on the current nursing shortage.

Workplace Dissatisfaction

Perhaps one of the most significant yet least addressed factors leading to the current RN shortage is workplace dissatisfaction, resulting in high turnover levels and nurses leaving the profession. Long shifts, low autonomy, mandatory overtime, and being forced to work weekends, nights, and holidays prompts many nurses to look for other jobs.

In a recent study, Hayes et al. (2006) found that turnover is driven by a number of organizational factors, including experienced workload, stress and burnout, management and leadership style, degree of workplace empowerment, promotional opportunities, work schedules, and other economic and market factors.

A study by Ward-Smith et al. (2007) also reinforced the physical demands of the job as a factor influencing job satisfaction. Nurses in this study indicated that workplace physical demands (specifically the 12-hour shift) were the most challenging aspect of their job. When this response was separated out by age groups, older nurses felt the physical demands were greatest, whereas younger nurses reported that both physical and mental challenges were equally demanding.

In addition, research by Buerhaus, Donelan, Ulrich, DesRoches, and Dittus (2007) found that the most common reasons for the current nursing shortage as identified by staff nurses providing direct care were salary and benefits, lack of adequate career options for women, faculty shortages, and having to work undesirable hours. Fifty-six percent of respondents in this study also reported that there was inadequate time for direct patient care, including hands-on care, patient/family teaching, and discharge planning. Buerhaus et al. concluded that improving the hospital workplace continues

to be among the most pressing challenges confronting the nurse workforce.

Hospital administrators appear to think the same. A 2008 survey showed that staff retention was the number one concern identified by top-level hospital executives for the next 12 months (van der Pool, 2008). Retention was ranked even higher than the economy and Medicaid/Medicare reimbursement cuts.

> ### CONSIDER
> The nursing shortage cannot be resolved until we address the underlying issues of worker dissatisfaction that caused it in the first place.

Is Pay an Issue?

Salaries also provide mixed incentives for young people to become nurses and for nurse retention. The economy at the end of the 20th century was fairly strong, with low unemployment and rising consumer confidence. This resulted in some RNs, who were often the second breadwinner in the family unit, reducing their work hours or leaving the workplace entirely. Many of these same RNs, however, returned to work after the September 11, 2001, attack on the World Trade Center in New York City, as a result of declining stock market values and lower levels of consumer confidence.

Wages for registered nurses have increased with rising demand and progression of the shortage. The average hourly wage for nurses in the United States in 2008 ranged from $21.49 for a nurse with less than 1 year of experience to $29.60 for a nurse with 20 years of experience or more (Pay Scale, 2008). This equates to a median annual salary ranging from $45,017 to $58,088. Nursing salaries also vary by state, with the median hourly rate in North Carolina being $23.98, as compared to $32.87 in California (Pay Scale, 2008). Figures compiled by O'Brien (2008) are similar, with the national average nurse salary being $56,785, and with nurses in California having the highest average salary and nurses in Tennessee making the least.

Sounart (2008) suggested that whereas many U.S. health care facilities opted to increase nursing salaries in response to the current nursing shortage, recent surveys show that nursing salaries might be leveling out. Herbst (2007) agreed, suggesting that wages for registered nurses rose just 1.34% from 2006 to 2007, well below than the inflation rate. He suggested that this was due to declining insurance reimbursement to health care organizations, as well as global nurse migration, with nearly one third of the RNs joining the U.S. workforce coming from outside the United States.

In fact, a 2008 salary survey of 7,500 nurses from across the United States suggested that nursing salaries are actually declining. The ADVANCES Salary Survey 2008 reported average nursing salaries in 2007 of $59,650 per year, nearly $3,000 higher than the 2008 average of $56,785 (Sounart, 2008). These numbers are still up, however, from the 2006 averages reported by the U.S. Bureau of Labor Statistics in 2006 of $53,240, with an average hourly rate of $25.60 (Sounart).

> **DISCUSSION POINT**
> Historically, nursing is considered to be an altruistic profession. How critical do you think pay is as a motivator for people to want to become nurses?

In contrast to the mixed findings for staff nurses, salary is clearly a deterrent for nursing faculty: "Not only are academic salaries lower than they are for clinical practice, and administrative positions of advanced practice nurses, but the cost of securing advanced academic degrees is costly" (Allen, 2008, p. 37). Indeed, many graduate students who may have become educators in the past are now opting instead for better-paying positions in clinical and private practice. The average salary of a nurse practitioner in 2007 was $81,397, an 8.8% increase between 2005 and 2007, and an impressive 55% increase over the last decade (Rollet & Lebo, 2008). In contrast, the AACN (2008a) reported that full-time associate professor nurse faculty with a master's degree earned an annual average salary of $66,588.

One reason that nursing faculty salaries are so poor comparatively is that nursing education has never had the same federal funding support as medical education. Roberson (2007) reported that "hospitals receive significant federal funding for medical education, but they are not similarly subsidized for training nurses." In addition, "nursing education programs can lose money for colleges, limiting colleges' willingness to expand their programs and raise faculty salaries" (Roberson, 2007, para 20–23). Clearly, increasing faculty salaries and providing tuition support for graduate students considering a career as a nursing faculty will be an essential part of addressing the increasing faculty shortage.

> **DISCUSSION POINT**
> What incentives should be offered to nurses who earn master's or doctoral degrees to become nursing faculty members rather than advanced practice nurses engaged in clinical practice?

Retention: An Undervalued Strategy

An often ignored or at least undervalued aspect of nursing shortages is that highly trained, employable nurses are *voluntarily* leaving the profession because they are dissatisfied with their work. A study by Kovner, Brewer, Fairchild, Poornima, and Kim (2007) found that 13% of newly licensed RNs had changed principal jobs after 1 year, and 37% reported that they felt ready to change jobs. A report released by the PricewaterhouseCoopers Health Research Institute (2007) also found that although the average nurse turnover rate in hospitals was 8.4%, the average voluntary turnover for first-year nurses was 27.1%.

This high level of turnover is disruptive to organizational functioning and threatens the quality of patient care. It is also expensive. The costs associated with replacing a registered nurse range from $10,000 to $60,000 per RN, depending on the specialty (Hayes et al., 2006). Figures cited by Letvak (2008) are similar, suggesting that the total cost to replace one RN is estimated to be between $62,100 and $67,100. Jones (2008) suggested even greater variability in turnover cost, estimating costs between $22,000 and $64,000 per nurse turnover, primarily because some studies capture the less obvious costs such as productivity losses.

Not all health care organizations, however, have high turnover rates. Research by Rondeau, Williams, and Wagar (2008) suggested that organizations perceived to be employers-of-choice, such as magnet hospitals, retain their employees and are more capable of replacing losses than less-sought-after employers. Therefore, having a healthy work environment provides an advantage in the competition for scarce nursing resources.

In addition, Rondeau et al. (2008) found that external labor market forces, including local job markets, have the potential to negate even the most ardent recruitment and retention campaign. Given that these external forces are often beyond the control of the employer, the researchers concluded that employers are better off trying to create positive work environments to be employers-of-choice than trying to control a labor market that is often beyond their control. Clearly, organizations that pay attention to the employee market and understand what people are looking for in the work environment have a better chance to recruit and retain top talent.

CONSIDER

Retention of precious nurse resources must be a very real part of the solution to the nursing shortage; health care institutions must make a commitment to improving working conditions for nurses.

THE CONSEQUENCES OF THE SHORTAGE

What are the consequences of a nursing shortage? To answer this question, it is critical first to recognize that patient outcomes are sensitive to nursing interventions and that, as a result, nurse staffing (total hours of care, as well as staffing mix) affects patient outcomes. This supposition is certainly supported by a review of the literature, which increasingly suggests that RN staffing affects patient outcomes such as inpatient mortality and other measures of quality of hospital care.

The benchmark 2006 report *Nurse Staffing and Quality of Patient Care* by the Agency for Healthcare Research and Quality suggested that inadequate staffing and heavy workloads threaten patient safety and health care quality (Kane, Shamliyan, Mueller, Duval, & Wilt, 2007). Indeed, numerous studies have been conducted to describe the relationship between nurse staffing levels and clinical outcomes of patients at both the hospital and unit levels (see Chapter 10). Unruh (2008) found that more than 45 U.S studies and 20 international studies explored the relationship between hospital nurse staffing and patient outcomes, and most studies concluded that there are statistically significant relationships between staffing and patient outcomes. However, researchers agree that additional research is necessary.

As study findings are released, collective bargaining agents, the government, policy makers, and special interest groups are taking note and increasingly calling for regulatory oversight of nurse staffing issues. It seems that the public is listening. According to a 2002 poll by Vanderbilt University Medical Center's School of Nursing and Center for Health Services Research, most

Americans are worried about how the nursing shortage will affect their ability to receive proper medical care (Honor Society of Nursing, Sigma Theta Tau International, n.d.-a). The study showed that:

- Eighty-one percent of Americans recognize that there is a nursing shortage; 65% believe that it is either a major problem or a crisis.

- Ninety-three percent agree (and 80% strongly agree) that the nursing shortage jeopardizes the quality of health care in the United States.

- Seniors, age 55 years and older, are particularly sensitive to the shortage's effect on the quality of the health care system.

ADDITIONAL STRATEGIES FOR SOLVING THE SHORTAGE

Just as the issues that caused the current shortage are complex, so too must be the solutions to the problem. Only some of the solutions that have been presented to address the current nursing shortage are included here, including redesigning the workplace, increasing the number of nursing students in the pipeline, importing foreign nurses, improving nursing's image, increasing the faculty pool, and moving toward a self-service approach to patient care. In addition, Box 5.3 includes a list of 11 strategies created by the Honor Society of Nursing, Sigma Theta Tau International (n.d.-b) for reducing the current shortage.

Redesigning the Workplace for an Older Workforce

The age of the current nursing workforce is an important factor in the current nursing shortage because nursing can be both physically and mentally taxing, even to the young. Some experts have suggested that more attention should be given to retaining older workers or bringing retired nurses back into the workforce.

Research by Hart (2007) and the RWJF (2006) seminar study *Wisdom at Work: The Importance of the Older and Experienced Nurse in the Workplace* support the idea that health care organizations can and should actively employ strategies to retain older workers. The RWJF research identified many reasons that older nurses leave the hospital, including heavy patient loads and inadequate

| BOX 5.3 | STRATEGIES FOR ADDRESSING THE SHORTAGE |

■ Demonstrate to health care leaders that nurses are the critical difference in America's health care system.

■ Reposition nursing as a highly versatile profession in which young people can learn science and technology, customer service, critical thinking, and decision-making skills.

■ Construct practice environments that are interdisciplinary and build on relationships among nurses, physicians, other health care professionals, patients, and communities.

■ Create patient care models that encourage professional nurse autonomy and clinical decision making.

■ Develop additional evaluation systems that measure the relationship of timely nursing interventions to patient outcomes.

■ Establish additional standards and mechanisms for recognition of professional practice environments.

■ Develop career enhancement incentives for nurses to pursue professional practice.

■ Evaluate the effects of the nursing shortage on the preparation of the next generation of nurse educators, nurse administrators, and nurse researchers and take strategic action.

■ Implement and sustain a marketing effort that addresses the image of nursing and the recruitment of qualified students into nursing as a career.

■ Promote higher education to nurses of all educational levels.

■ Develop and implement strategies to promote the retention of RNs and nurse educators in the workforce.

Source: Honor Society of Nursing, Sigma Theta Tau International (n.d.-b). *Facts on the nursing shortage in North America*. Available at: **http://www.nursingsociety.org/Media/Pages/shortage.aspx**. Accessed September 1, 2008. Reprinted with permission.

nurse staffing. In addition, the work is considered physically demanding and emotionally challenging, which can lead to injuries and burnout (Larkin, 2007). Strategies suggested in the RWJF study to address these concerns include ergonomics, health promotion, education and career enhancement, and policies and procedures.

The Bernard Hodes Group (2007) agreed, suggesting that employers must be able to accommodate aging workers with technology aimed at reducing physical strain, such as electrically operated beds, bariatric equipment, and mechanical lift devices. Other strategies suggested for retaining aging nurses include flexible scheduling and benefits, and continuing education aid and wellness programs (Bernard Hodes Group). Keefe (2007) further agreed, suggesting that flexibility in scheduling and the ability to maintain benefits while working fewer hours are key issues in retaining experienced older nurses.

In addition, RNs must be made to feel valued, and physician–nurse relationships reflecting collegiality and collaboration should be fostered. In addition, environments of shared governance should be created in which nurses actively participate in all decision making related

to patient care. Staff nurses should feel empowered, and autonomy should be encouraged. In a survey of 1,440 nurses age 55 to 65 years, those who stated their intent to continue working in their current position felt that they had job security and were valued. They also felt that they had opportunities for independent thought and action on the job (Keefe, 2007).

Federwish (2008) described such a program in his description of the Center for Third Age Nurses at Holy Names University in Oakland, California. This center assists nurses age 45 years or older to look at the possibilities for staying engaged in nursing. Instead of talking about retirement, the center encourages the nurses to consider new career pathways and options such as shorter shifts. The program also encourages these experienced nurses to become mentors and to renew their commitment to nursing well into the future. More programs like these will offer older RNs the opportunity to continue to be involved in their professions for many years after they reach the age at which they would be eligible for retirement. Additional strategies for retaining older workers are shown in Box 5.4.

BOX 5.4 | **STRATEGIES FOR RETAINING OLDER WORKERS**

- Flexible shift options of 4, 6, and 8 hours, as well as job-sharing.
- Clustering patient assignments and keeping supplies and equipment in central locations to avoid extensive walking.
- Using lift teams, special beds, and equipment to curtail work-related injuries and strain.
- Review and adapt benefits package to accommodate different needs.
- Use older nurses for nonphysical work such as patient admissions and discharges.
- Move older nurses and other allied health professionals into areas and positions that maximize the use of their expertise while being less physically taxing.
- Use older staff as mentors and preceptors.

Source: Hart, K. A. (2006). *The aging workforce. Implications for recruiters.* Available at: **http://www.hodes.com/publications/talentmatters/archives/hcmatters_jul06.asp.** Accessed December 12, 2006.

Changing Nursing's Image

In addition, more efforts must be made to improve the public's image of nursing. Again, this will not be an easy task, given the historical roots of nursing stereotypes and the profession's long history of being unable to effectively change public perceptions regarding professional nursing roles and behaviors (see Chapter 20). It is also clear that despite the public's long-standing esteem for registered nurses, as documented in public opinion polls, that this has not translated into an adequate number of individuals wanting to be nurses (Donelan, Buerhaus, Des Roches, Dittus, & Dutwin, 2008).

There are initiatives underway, however, that seek to promote not only a more positive image of nursing, but also recruitment to the profession. For example, Johnson & Johnson, in conjunction with several professional nursing organizations, including the Honor Society of Nursing, Sigma Theta Tau International, launched a multiyear, $30 million national campaign during the Winter Olympics in 2003 to attract more people to the nursing profession. This "Campaign for Nursing's Future," which is the largest private sector initiative in decades, and perhaps ever, to address the nursing shortage, includes a Web site that describes the benefits of a career in nursing and provides links to nursing schools and scholarship programs. It also profiles nurses in a variety of nursing careers. The campaign also includes a scholarship fund for undergraduate students and nursing faculty.

A Self-Service Approach to Patient Care

One must also at least consider some fairly radical approaches to the nursing shortage that do not include increasing the number of nurses available. The best known of these is the *self-service model*. This model suggests that family members can be used as caregivers to supplement RNs by providing most bedside care during the immediate and post–acute hospital periods. Indeed, self-service nursing is the preferred model of care in many countries. Sapountzi-Krepia et al. (2008) described such a model as "*informal care*" and suggested that it is a common phenomenon in Greece as a result of the nursing shortage. Patients' relatives stay by their bedside for long hours and assist with care. This care often reflects specific nursing duties.

Critics of the self-service approach to care suggest that hospitalized patients are far too ill and their needs are too complex to be cared for by a layperson. They also argue that care is too sophisticated, and the technology routinely used for care is not known to individuals outside of health care. Sapountzi-Krepia et al. (2008) agreed, suggesting that it is disquieting to have hospital staff suggest to relatives that there is a need to stay at the patient's bedside or to hire a private paid patient's helper. Instead, they suggest that hospitals should introduce specific staffing policies to reduce this burden on families.

Bern-Klug and Forbes-Thompson (2008, p. 43), however, in their qualitative study of family members of nursing home residents, found that "family members often hold themselves responsible for overseeing the care of their loved one, representing the resident's perspective and history, and keeping the family connections." They concluded that these role expectations are important to family members but called on nursing staff to "maximize constructive family involvement and minimize the stress families may experience if they are not able to fulfill their role expectations" (p. 43).

CONCLUSIONS

Many factors have led to the significant professional nursing shortage of the early 21st century. Health care providers, the public, and legislators are beginning to recognize that both the problem and the potential consequences are severe. One would be hard-pressed to find a Congressperson or Senator who would not identify the current nursing shortage as one of the most serious issues affecting health care today.

Smalarz et al. (2007) agreed, suggesting that the current nursing shortage may dramatically reduce access to care and adversely affect the health care delivery system: "Shortages of human capital within the clinical workforce could erode patient care and outcomes, overwhelm many health care facilities, and further strain the clinical workforce left to grapple with the demand for services" (p. 1).

Yet, efforts to address the shortage have been too few and far between. Short-term solutions to the shortage have been attempted, including importing foreign nurses and increasing federal money for nursing education. The passage of legislation such as the Nurse Reinvestment Act has encouraged more students to choose nursing as a career and has helped students financially to complete their education. It has also encouraged graduate students to complete their studies and assume teaching positions in nursing schools.

In addition, many states have introduced or passed legislation designed to improve working conditions or attract more nurses. For example, New York introduced a series of bills in 2008 that provide recruitment incentives for nursing programs and loan reimbursements for students in nursing programs across the state (Wargas, 2008): "One of the bills calls for the preservation of nursing students' rights to claim unemployment insurance benefits while they are studying to become a registered nurse. Another creates a nursing assistance program within the state Department of Health to provide loans for prospective nursing students" (Wargas, 2008, para 3). Another bill would establish the Empire State Professional Nursing Scholarship Program for nursing students, whereas similar legislation would reimburse nursing students for loans if they work at hospitals or other health care facilities in New York after graduation (Wargas).

Long-term planning and aggressive intervention, however, will be needed for some time at the national and regional levels to ensure that an adequate, highly qualified nursing workforce will be available in the future to meet health care needs in the United States.

More must be done to address the current, increasingly severe nursing shortage, and it is increasingly obvious that multiple solutions to the shortage will be needed. These solutions will require the best thinking of experts and will likely reshape fundamental core underpinnings that have been a part of the nursing work world for decades, if not centuries.

FOR ADDITIONAL DISCUSSION

1. In what ways do other professions do a better job of attracting younger workers—both men and women?

2. Are salaries a significant driver in the current nursing shortage? At what level would salaries not be a factor?

3. How would increasing the educational level for entry into practice affect the current nursing shortage?

4. Will the demand for RNs in the future be affected by growing technological developments?

5. Why has the nursing workforce historically suffered some degree of a shortage every 10 to 15 years?

6. If magnet hospital criteria were to become the baseline for organizational structure and performance, would nursing shortages exist?

7. Why are starting salaries for nurses with master's and doctoral degrees in academia so low?

8. Why do many health care organizations choose to expend more money on recruitment than on retention strategies? Which is more effective in the short term? In the long term?

9. Is implementation of mandatory minimum staffing ratios in acute care hospitals likely to reduce the nursing shortage in California?

REFERENCES

$1 billion needed to address U.S. shortage of nurses (2003/2004). *Australian Nursing Journal, 11*(6), 21.

Aiken, L. H. (2007). U.S. labor market dynamics are key to global nurse sufficiency. *Health Services Research, 42*(3), 1299–1320.

Aiken, L. H., Xue, Y., Clarke, S. P., & Sloane, D. M. (2007). Supplemental nurse staffing in hospitals and quality of care. *Journal of Nursing Administration, 37*(7/8), 335–342.

Allen, L. (2008). The nursing shortage continues as faculty shortage grows. *Nursing Economics, 26*(1), 35–40.

American Association of Colleges of Nursing (2005). *New data confirms the shortage of nursing school faculty hinders efforts to address the nation's nursing shortage.* Available at: http://www.aacn.nche.edu/Media/News-Releases/2005/Enrollments05.htm. Accessed April 10, 2005,

American Association of Colleges of Nursing (2006a). *Nursing shortage.* Available at: http://www.aacn.nche.edu/Media/FactSheets/NursingShortage.htm. Accessed January 11, 2007.

American Association of Colleges of Nursing (2006b). *Student enrollment rises in U.S. nursing colleges and universities for the 6th consecutive year.* Available at: http://www.aacn.nche.edu/Media/NewsReleases/06Survey.htm. Accessed January 11, 2007.

American Association of Colleges of Nursing (2006c). *Nursing faculty shortage.* Available at: http://www.aacn.nche.edu/Media/FactSheets/FacultyShortage.htm. Accessed January 11, 2007.

American Association of Colleges of Nursing (AACN) (2007). *Press release. Enrollment growth slows at U.S. nursing colleges and universities in 2007 despite calls for more registered nurses.* Available at: http://www.

aacn.nche.edu/Media/NewsReleases/2007/enrl.htm. Accessed May 26, 2008.

American Association of Colleges of Nursing (AACN) (2008a). *Fact sheet. Nursing faculty shortage.* Available at: http://www.aacn.nche.edu/Media/factsheets/FacultyShortage.htm. Accessed May 26, 2008.

American Association of Colleges of Nursing (AACN) (2008b). *Fact sheet. Nursing shortage.* Available at: http://www.aacn.nche.edu/Media/FactSheets/NursingShortage.htm. Accessed May 26, 2008.

American Hospital Association (AHA) (2006). *The state of America's hospitals—Taking the pulse.* Available at: http://www.aha.org/aha/content/2006/PowerPoint/StateHospitalsChartPack2006.PPT. Accessed January 11, 2007.

American Hospital Association (AHA) (2007). *The 2007 state of America's hospitals—Taking the pulse.* Available at: www.aha.org/aha/content/2007/PowerPoint/StateofHospitalsChartPack2007.ppt. Accessed May 26, 2008.

Auerbach, D. I., Buerhaus, P. I., & Staiger, D. O. (2007). Better late than never: Workforce supply implications of later entry into nursing. *Health Affairs, 26*(1), 178–185.

Baby-boomer nurses are on their way out. Clinical rounds (2008). *Nursing, 38*(6), 25.

Bern-Klug, M., Forbes-Thompson, S. (2008). Family members' responsibilities to nursing home residents. "She is the only mother I got." *Journal of Gerontological Nursing, 34*(2), 43–52.

Bernard Hodes Group (2007). *The aging workforce: Implications for recruiters.* Available at: http://www.hodes.com/publications/talentmatters/archives/hcmatters_jul06.asp. Accessed September 1, 2008.

Bolt, G. (2008). Costly prescription: A cure for Oregon's nursing shortage won't come cheap—Who will pay the bill? *The Register Guard.* Available at: http://www.registerguard.com/csp/cms/sites/dt.cms.support.viewStory.cls?cid=103327&sid=1&fid=1. Accessed May 28, 2008.

Buerhaus, P. I., Donelan, K., Ulrich, B. T., DesRoches, C., & Dittus, R. (2007). Trends in the experiences of hospital-employed registered nurses: Results from three national surveys. *Nursing Economics, 25*(2), 69–80.

Buerhaus, P. I., Staiger, D. O., & Auerbach, D. I. (2009). *The Future of the Nursing Workforce in the United States. Data, Trends, and Implications.* Boston: Jones & Bartlett.

Clarke, S. P, & Cheung, R. B. (2008). The nurse shortage: Where we stand and where we're headed. *Nursing Management, 39*(3), 23–28.

Cramer, M., Nienaber, J., Helget, P., & Agrawal, S. (2006). Comparative analysis of urban and rural nursing workforce shortages in Nebraska hospitals. *Policy, Politics & Nursing Practice, 7*(4), 248–260.

Despite Americans' high regard, nursing shortage still looms (2008). *Nursing Economics, 26*(3), 219.

Dohm, A., & Shniper, L. (2007). Employment outlook: 2006–16. Occupational employment projections to 2016. *Monthly Labor Review,* pp. 86–125. Available at: http://www.bls.gov/opub/mlr/2007/11/art5full.pdf. Accessed January 2, 2009.

Donelan, K., Buerhaus, P., Des Roches, C., Dittus, R., & Dutwin, D. (2008). Public perceptions of nursing careers: The influence of the media and nursing shortages. *Nursing Economics, 26*(3), 143–150.

Federwish, A. (2008). Reinventing, not retiring. *Nurse-Week (California Edition), 21*(11), 14–15.

Hart, K. A. (2006). *The aging workforce. Implications for recruiters.* Available at: http://www.hodes.com/publications/talentmatters/archives/hcmatters_jul06.asp. Accessed December 12, 2006.

Hart, K. A. (2007). The aging workforce: Implications for health care organizations. *Nursing Economics, 25*(2), 101–102.

Hayes, L. J., O'Brien-Pallas, L., Duffield, C., Shamian, J., Buchan, J., Hughes, F., Spence Laschinger, H. K., North, N., & Stone, P. W. (2006). Nurse turnover: A literature review. *International Journal of Nursing Studies, 43,* 237–263.

Heinz, D. (2004). Hospital nurse staffing and patient outcomes. *Dimensions of Critical Care Nursing, 23*(1), 44–51.

Henderson, T. M., & Hassmiller, S. B. (2007). Hospitals and philanthropy as partners in funding nursing education. *Nursing Economics, 25*(2), 95–99.

Herbst, M. (2007). *A critical shortage of nurses.* Available at: http://www.businessweek.com/bwdaily/dnflash/content/aug2007/db20070828_104375.htm?chan=search. Accessed May 25, 2008.

Hinshaw, A. S. (2008). Navigating the perfect storm: Balancing a culture of safety with workforce challenges. *Nursing Research (Supplement), 57*(15), S4–S10.

Honor Society of Nursing, Sigma Theta Tau International (n.d.-a). *National poll shows most Americans worried about nursing shortage.* Available at: http://www.nursingsociety.org/Career/CareerMap/Pages/cmap_article7.aspx. Accessed August 29, 2008.

Honor Society of Nursing, Sigma Theta Tau International (n.d.-b). *Facts on the nursing shortage in North America.* Available at: http://www.nursingsociety.org/Media/Pages/shortage.aspx. Accessed September 1, 2008.

Institute for the Future of Aging Services (2007). *The long term care workforce: Can the crisis be fixed?* Available at: http://www.futureofaging.org/publications/pub_documents/LTCCommissionReport2007.pdf. Accessed May 26, 2008.

Issues in nursing. How do we tackle the nurse faculty shortage? (2008). *Nursing 2008, 38*(2), 44–45.

Jones, C. B. (2008). Revisiting nurse turnover costs. *Journal of Nursing Administration, 38*(1), 11–18.

Jordan, K. (2008). *No easy Rx for nursing crisis. Students turned away due to faculty exodus.* BostonHerald.com. News and Opinion. Available at: http://news.bostonherald.com/news/regional/general/view/2008_06_29_No_easy_Rx_for_nursing_crisis:_Students_turned_away_due_to_faculty_exodus/srvc=home&position=also. Accessed June 30, 2008.

Kane, R. L., Shamliyan, T., Mueller, C., Duval, S., & Wilt, T. J. (2007). *Nurse staffing and quality of patient care* (Evidence Report/Technology Assessment, Number 151). Rockville, MD: Agency for Healthcare Research and Quality. Available at: http://www.ahrq.gov/downloads/pub/evidence/pdf/nursestaff/nursestaff.pdf. Accessed June 30, 2008.

Keefe, S. (2007). Retaining experienced older nurses. *Advance for Nurses (Northern California and Northern Nevada), 4*(28), 19–20.

Kovner, C. T., Brewer, C. S., Fairchild, S., Poornima, S., & Kim, H. (2007). Newly licensed RNs' characteristics, work attitudes, and intentions to work. *American Journal of Nursing, 107*(9), 58–70.

La Rocco, S. A. (2006). Who will teach the nurses? *Academe.* Available at: http://www.aaup.org/publications/Academe/2006/06mj/06mjlaro.htm. Accessed January 16, 2007.

Larkin, M. (2007). Professional issues. Shortage strategies. Retaining the experienced nurse. *Journal of Nursing Administration, 37*(4), 162–163.

Letvak, S. (2008). Retirement or rehirement? *Advance for Nurses (Northern California and Northern Nevada), 5*(15), 21–23.

Lin, V., Lijun, J., Turek, X., Juraschek, D., & John, S. (2008). California regional registered nurse workforce forecast. *Nursing Economics, 26*(2), 85–105.

McIntosh, B., Val Palumbo, M., & Rambur, B. (2006). Does a 'shadow workforce' of inactive nurses exist? *Nursing Economics, 24*(5), 231–238.

Merriam Webster's Online Dictionary (2008a). *Demand.* Available at: http://www.merriam-webster.com/dictionary/demand. Accessed May 25, 2008.

Merriam Webster's Online Dictionary (2008b). *Supply.* Available at: http://www.merriam-webster.com/dictionary/supply. Accessed May 25, 2008.

National Commission on Nursing Workforce for Long-Term Care (2005). *Act now for your tomorrow. Final report of the National Commission on Nursing Workforce for Long-Term Care.* Available at: http://www.ahca.org/research/workforce_rpt_050519.pdf. Accessed May 26, 2008.

National Council State Boards of Nursing [NCBSN] (2008a). *State updates on nursing shortage issues and activities. California.* Available at: https://www.ncsbn.org/763.htm.Accessed May 26, 2008.

National Council of State Boards of Nursing (2008b). *NCLEX examination pass rates.* Available at: https://www.ncsbn.org/1237.htm. Accessed May 24, 2008.

Nursing doctorate programs changing the face of healthcare, US. (2006). Available at: http://www.medicalnewstoday.com/articles/55298.php. Accessed May 26, 2008.

Nurses for a Healthier Tomorrow (n.d.). *Campaign news.* Available at: http://www.nursesource.org/campaign_news.html. Accessed May 30, 2008.

O'Brien, A. (2008). Salary survey 2008. *Advance for Nurses (Northern California and Northern Nevada), 5*(4), 9–14.

Orlovsky, C. (2006). *Mass nurse retirement expected in 2011. Survey.* Available at: http://www.amnhealthcare.com/News.aspx?id=15444. Accessed December 6, 2006.

Orsolini-Hain, L., & Malone, R. E. (2007). Examining the impending gap in clinical nursing expertise. *Policy, Politics & Nursing Practice, 8*(3), 158–169.

PayScale (2008). *Hourly rate survey report for job: Registered Nurse (RN).* Available at: http://www.payscale.com/research/US/Job=Registered_Nurse_(RN)/Hourly_Rate. Accessed May 26, 2008.

PricewaterhouseCoopers' Health Research Institute (2007). *What works: Healing the healthcare staffing shortage.* Available at: http://www.pwc.com/extweb/pwcpublications.nsf/docid/674D1E79A678A042852 5730D006B74A9. Accessed June 30, 2008.

Roberson, J. (July 10, 2007). *Healthcare crisis is growing.* Available at: http://www.dallasnews.com/shared content/dws/classifieds/news/jobcenter/healthcare/stories/DN-HEALTHWORKERS_10bus.ART0.State.Edition1.36da38a.html. Accessed May 25, 2008.

Robert Wood Johnson Foundation (RWJF) (2006).*Wisdom at Work: The Importance of the Older and Experienced Nurse in the Workplace.* Princeton, NJ: Author.

Robert Wood Johnson Foundation (RWJF) (2007). *The nursing faculty shortage: Public and private partnerships address a growing need. Charting Nursing's Future.* Available at: http://www.rwjf.org/files/publications/other/nursingfuture4.pdf. Accessed June 30, 2008.

Robert Wood Johnson Foundation (RWJF) (2008). *New careers in nursing scholarship program.* Available at: http://www.newcareersinnursing.org/. Accessed May 25, 2008.

Rollet, J., & Lebo, S (2008). 2007 salary survey results: A decade of growth. *Advance for Nurse Pracitioners.* Available at: http://nurse-practitioners.advanceweb.com/editorial/content/editorial.aspx?cc=105177. Accessed May 26, 2008.

Roman, L. (2008). Nursing shortage: Looking to the future. *RN, 71*(3), 34–36, 38–41.

Rondeau, K. V., Williams, E. S., & Wagar, T. H. (2008). Turnover and vacancy rates for registered nurses: Do local labor market forces matter? *Health Care Management Review, 33*(1), 69–78.

Sapountzi-Krepia, D., Raftopoulos, V., Psychogiou, M., Sakellari, E., Toris, A., Vrettos, A., & Arsenos, P. (2008). Dimensions of informal care in Greece: The family's contribution to the care of patients hospitalized in an oncology hospital. *Journal of Clinical Nursing, 17*(10), 1287–1294.

Seguritan, R. S. (2007). *US immigration updates.* Available at: http://www.bastapinoy.com/immigration_RS_070322.htm. Accessed May 25, 2008.

Smalarz, A., Corbettt, G., & Doonan, M. (2007). *Policy brief. The health care workforce: Facing peril or opportunity.* Accessible at: http://www.physiciannursesupply.com/Articles/princeton-14-policy-brief.pdf. Accessed May 25, 2008.

Sounart, A. (2008). *Have nursing salaries reached their limit?* AMN Healthcare Inc. Available at: http://www.nursezone.com/nursing-news-events/more-news.aspx?ID=17587. Accessed May 27, 2008.

The New York Center for Health Workforce Studies (2006). *The United States health workforce profile* (p.135). Available at: http://www.albany.edu/news/pdf_files/U.S._Health_Workforce_Profile_October2006_11-09.pdf. Accessed May 25, 2008.

Unruh, L. (2008). Nurse staffing and patient, nurse, and financial outcomes. *American Journal of Nursing, 108*(1), 62–71.

U.S. Department of Health and Human Services (2006). *What is behind HRSA's projected supply, demand, and shortage of registered nurses?* Available at: http://bhpr.hrsa.gov/healthworkforce/reports/behindrnprojections/index.htm. Accessed January 11, 2007.

U.S. Department of Health and Human Services (2007). *Health, United States, 2007.* Centers for Disease Control and Prevention, National Center for Health Statistics. Available at: http://www.cdc.gov/nchs/data/hus/hus07acc.pdf. Accessed May 26, 2008.

U.S. Department of Health and Human Services, Health Resources and Services Administration (USDHHS-HRSA) (2002). *Projected supply, demand and shortages of registered nurses, 2000–2020.* Available at: http://bhpr.hrsa.gov/healthworkforce/reports/rnproject/report.htm. Accessed May 18, 2004.

van der Pool, L. (2008). Staff retention tops hospital exec concerns. *Boston Business Journal.* Available at: http://www.bizjournals.com/boston/stories/2008/08/18/daily7.html. Accessed August 29, 2008.

Ward-Smith, P., Hunt, C., Smith, J. B., Teasley, S. L., Carroll, C. A., & Sexton, K. (2007). Issues and opportunities for retaining experienced nurses at the bedside. *Journal of Nursing Administration, 37*(11), 485–487.

Wargas, R. (2008). Nursing shortage prompts bill package in state leg. *Suffolk Life Newspapers.* Available at: http://www.zwire.com/site/news.cfm?newsid=19725669&BRD=1776&PAG=461&dept_id=6365&rfi=6. Accessed May 28, 2008.

Williams, K. A., Stotts, R. C., Jacob, S., Stegbauer, C. C., Roussel, L., & Carter, D. (2006). Inactive nurses: A source for alleviating the nursing shortage? *Journal of Nursing Administration, 36*(4), 205–210.

BIBLIOGRAPHY

AAN: Technology may to be blame for nursing shortage. (2008). *Healthcare Benchmarks & Quality Improvement, 15*(2), 17–19.

Alberta's action plan for nurse recruitment and retention. (2008). *Canadian Nurse, 104*(2), 7.

Clark, S. P., & Cheung, R. B. (2008). The nurse shortage: Where we stand and where we're headed. *Nursing Management, 39*(3), 22–28.

Davis, D. A., & Napier, M. D. (2008). Strategically addressing the nursing shortage: A closer look at the nurse funders collaborative. *Health Affairs, 27*(3), 876–881.

Evans, M. (2008). Men could fill nursing's gaps. *Modern Healthcare, 38*(19), 14.

Mangan, K. (2007). Shortage of doctors and nurses predicted. *Chronicle of Higher Education, 53*(47), 30.

Matrone, J. A. (2007). Small state, big problem. Rhode Island nurse leaders take a second look at the state's shortage. *Journal of Nursing Administration, 37*(3), 119–121.

Ober, S., & Craven, G. (2008). New center to champion nursing in America established to avert nurse shortage. *Journal of Infusion Nursing, 31*(2), 67–68.

Politicians hold the key to solving nursing shortage (2008) *Healthcare Traveler, 15*(9), 6.

Shipman, D., & Hooten, J. (2008). Without enough nurse educators there will be a continual decline in RNs and the quality of nursing care: Contending with the faculty shortage. *Nurse Education Today, 28*(5), 521–523.

Titus, R. (2008). Low pay drives nursing shortage. *NurseWeek (Southwest), 9*(4), 11.

Wallace, N. (2008). Coming to the aid of nurses. *Chronicle of Philanthropy, 20*(9), 2.

Westendorf, J. (2007). The nursing shortage. *Plastic Surgical Nursing, 27*(2), 93–97.

WEB RESOURCES

AACN–Media Relations Nursing Shortage Fact Sheet (2004)	http://www.aacn.nche.edu/Media/Backgrounders/shortagefacts.htm
American Association of Colleges of Nursing	http://www.aacn.nche.edu
American Hospital Association	http://www.aha.org/aha/about/index.html
American Nurses Association	http://www.ana.org
Bureau of Labor Statistics	http://www.bls.gov/
Discover Nursing campaign. Johnson & Johnson Healthcare Systems, Inc.	http://www.discovernursing.com
National Council of State Boards of Nursing	http://www.ncsbn.org
National League for Nursing	http://www.nln.org
National Student Nurses Association	http://www.nsna.org
Nurses for a Healthier Tomorrow. Nurse Educator Recruitment Campaign	http://www.nursesource.org/campaign_news.html

CHAPTER 6

Importing Foreign Nurses

• CAROL J. HUSTON •

Learning Objectives

The learner will be able to:

1. Examine how the scope of global nurse migration has changed over the last decade.
2. Analyze "push" and "pull" factors that encourage nurses to migrate internationally.
3. Identify primary donor and recipient countries of migrating nurses.
4. Explore potential negative effects of international migration, including "brain drain" from "supplier" countries.
5. Apply the ethical principles of autonomy, utility, and justice in arguing for or against global nurse recruitment and migration.
6. Consider whether embedded *ethos* or *straight thinking* concepts provide an appropriate philosophical foundation for exploring the ethical dimensions of nurse migration.
7. Outline common key components of position statements on nurse migration adopted by professional associations such as the International Council of Nurses (ICN), the International Centre on Nurse Migration,

AcademyHealth, and the World Health Organization.

8. Explore national and international efforts to develop best practices or regulatory oversight of international nurse recruitment and migration.
9. Differentiate between the types of work visas foreign nurses use to gain entry for employment in the United States.
10. Outline the certification process required by the Commission on Graduates of Foreign Nursing Schools for migratory nurses to receive an occupational or permanent visa in the United States.
11. Discuss the need for ongoing cultural, professional, and psychological support for foreign nurses after their arrival in their importer country to assist them in successful socialization.
12. Reflect on personal beliefs and values regarding the use of widespread international recruitment and nurse migration to address nursing shortages.

Many countries have historically had cyclical shortages of nurses, but typically they were caused by increasing demand outstripping a static or slowly growing supply of nurses. The current situation is more serious. Demand continues to grow while supply decreases as a result of an aging workforce, a projected dramatic increase in nursing retirements in the coming decade, and an inadequate number of new graduates from nursing education programs. Indeed, almost all of the developed countries in the world are reporting nursing shortages.

One increasingly common means of alleviating the current nursing shortage has been to recruit foreign nurses. In fact, the number of international migrants has doubled since 1970, and nurses are increasingly a part of that migratory stream (Kingma, 2007).

International recruitment and *nurse migration*—moving from one country to another in search of employment—has been viewed as a relatively inexpensive, "quick-fix" solution to rapidly increasing health care worker shortages. The current situation, however, is different from those in the past, when nurse migration was mostly based on individual motivation. Now there is active planning of large-scale international nurse recruitment, often from developing countries. In fact, research completed by AcademyHealth reported that there were 267 U.S. based international nurse recruitment firms as of 2007, representing a 10-fold increase from the late 1990s (Pittman, Folsom, Bass, & Leonhardy, 2007). In addition, recruiter Web sites reported operations in 74 countries. Brush (2008, p. 20) suggested that nurse migration used to be a one-way exchange among a few developed and developing countries, but now it is a "more complicated and circuitous stream of global health workers flowing in new directions and patterns."

This recruiting onslaught affects the ability of developing countries to develop sustainable health care systems and provide appropriate care to their citizens. Indeed, Brush and Sochalski (2007) suggested that few donor nations are prepared to manage the loss of their nurse workforce to such widespread migration. Other health care leaders have gone so far as to suggest that the active recruitment of health care professionals from low-income countries with limited health care resources is a crime (Benetar, 2007; Mills et al., 2008).

Kuehn (2007) also pointed out that, ironically, when developing nations educate their health care workers only to have them leave for developed countries, they are in effect subsidizing wealthier nations. The International Organization for Migration estimated that developing nations spend $500 million each year to educate health care workers who then migrate to North America, Western Europe, and South Asia (Kuehn).

CONSIDER
Nurse migration flows vary in direction and magnitude over time in response to socioeconomic factors present in donor and destination countries (Kingma, 2007).

In addition, developing countries recruit from each other, even within the same geographical region. For example, "approximately 80 percent of nurses immigrating to the United States are from developing countries, however close to 60,000 nurses residing in the U.S. come from Canada, the United Kingdom, Ireland and other developed countries also facing nursing shortages" (Sanvik, 2005, para 2). Table 6.1 summarizes the current dynamic nature of nurse migration in select countries around the world.

GLOBAL MIGRATION OF NURSES: "PUSH" AND "PULL" FACTORS

To understand what is driving the global migration of nurses, it is first necessary to examine what are known as the "push" and "pull" factors of nursing migration. *Push factors* are those factors that push or drive nurses to want to leave their countries to go to another. Low pay, inadequate opportunities for career advancement or continuing education, sociopolitical instability, and unsafe workplaces are examples of push factors. Other factors that act as push factors in some countries include the effect of human immunodeficiency virus and acquired immunodeficiency disease on health system workers, concerns about personal security in areas of conflict, and economic instability.

Pull factors are those factors that draw the nurse toward a different country. Pull factors typically include higher pay, more-developed career structures, opportunities for further education and professional development, and, in some cases, safety from the threat of violence (more prevalent in less developed countries). Other pull factors, such as the opportunity to travel or to participate in foreign aid work, also influence some nurses. A summary of push and pull factors for nurse migration is given in Table 6.2.

CONSIDER
Nurse migration is often a symptom of deep-seated problems in a country's nursing labor markets relating to long-term relative underinvestment in the profession and its career structure (Buchan, 2006).

It is important to remember that developed countries, such as Australia, the United Kingdom, and the United States, are the primary destinations of most migrant nurses, and developing nations are primarily the donors. For example, about 8% of U.S. registered nurses (approximately 219,000) are estimated to be foreign educated, but 80% of those who do migrate to the United States are from lower-income countries (Aiken, 2007). In London alone, 25% of the nursing workforce is internationally recruited (Denton, 2006). In fact, in some poor or transitional countries such as Ghana, Malawi, Swaizland, and the Philippines, more than half of the registered nurses have migrated (Gostin, 2008). In fact,

TABLE 6.1	Effect of Push–Pull Migration on Select Countries
Africa	Clemens and Pettersson (2008) reported that approximately 70,000 African-born professional nurses were working overseas in a developed country in the year 2000. This represents about 1/10 of African-born professional nurses, although the fraction of health professionals abroad varies enormously across African countries, from 1% to greater than 70%, depending on the occupation and the country.
Australia	Australia has called for a national workforce plan but does have a shortage of nurses, primarily in rural areas. Australia is identified as both a primary donor and a recipient country for migrant nurses and primarily recruits from the United Kingdom and New Zealand.
China	Fang (2007) stated that as a result of lack of limited job opportunities, low salary, and low job satisfaction, many Chinese nurses intend to migrate. Commercial recruiters have expressed a strong interest in recruiting Chinese nurses, but there are limited examples of successful ventures. It is likely that China will become an important source of nurses for developed nations in the coming years.
Canada	Canada is both a source and a destination country for international nurse migration, with an estimated net loss of nurses. The United States is the major beneficiary of Canadian nurse emigration, resulting from the reduction of full-time jobs for nurses in Canada due to health system reforms. Canada faces a significant projected shortage of nurses (Little, 2007).
India	Khadria (2007) stated that despite the extremely low nurse-to-population ratio in India, hospital managers in India are not concerned about the growing exodus of nurses to other countries. In fact, they are actively joining forces with profitable commercial ventures that operate as both training and recruiting agencies.
Ireland	As little as 25 years ago, Ireland had an abundant pool of nurses. Humphries, Brugha, and McGee (2008) suggested, however, that Ireland began actively recruiting nurses from overseas in 2000 and has recruited almost 10,000 nurses, primarily from India and the Philippines, since that time. Thus, Ireland has moved from being a traditional exporter of nurses to an importer.
Israel	Ehrenfeld, Itzhaki, and Michal (2007) suggested that Israel has welcomed large numbers of nurse immigrants but that the nation's expenditures for health care and nursing education have, at times, had to take a back seat to the government's efforts to house new immigrants, to relocate groups, and to defend the nation against politically motivated violence and attacks. All of this has been in the context of regional conflicts and international debates.
Lebanon	El-Jardali, Nuhad, Diana, and Mouro (2008) suggested that Lebanon is facing a problem of excessive nurse migration to countries of the Persian Gulf, North America, and Europe. An estimated one in five nurses who receive a bachelor's of science in nursing migrates out of Lebanon within 1 or 2 years of graduation, with the majority of nurses migrating to countries of the Gulf. The main reasons for migration include shift work, high patient/nurse ratios, lack of autonomy in decision making, lack of a supportive environment, and poor commitment to excellent nursing care (El-Jardali et al.).
New Zealand	New Zealand is both a source and destination country. North (2007) reported that the international movement of nurses in New Zealand was minimal during the 1990s but jumped sharply in 2001 and has remained high since that time. North also reported that movement of New Zealand RNs to Australia is expedited by the Trans-Tasman Agreement, whereas the entry of foreign RNs to New Zealand is facilitated by nursing being an identified Priority Occupation.

(continued)

TABLE 6.1	Effect of Push–Pull Migration on Select Countries *(Continued)*
Philippines	Lorenzo, Galvez-Tan, Icamina, and Javier (2007) suggested that the Philippines is a job-scarce environment, and even for those with jobs in the health care sector, poor working conditions often motivate nurses to seek employment overseas. The country is dependent on labor migration to ease a tight domestic labor market. National opinion has generally focused on the improved quality of life for individual migrants and their families and on the benefits of remittances to the nation; however, a shortage of highly skilled nurses and the massive retraining of physicians to become nurses elsewhere has created severe problems for the Filipino health system, including the closure of many hospitals.
Saudi Arabia	Saudi Arabia now gets most of its nurses from the Philippines—the same place where most countries, including the United States, are doing the majority of their recruiting.
United Kingdom	Buchan (2007) suggested there has been rapid growth in inflow of nurses to the United Kingdom from other countries. In contrast to the 10% of foreign nurses in the United Kingdom in the early 1990s, 40% to 50% of more recent nurse registrants in the United Kingdom have come from other countries, principally the Philippines, Australia, India, and South Africa. Outflow has been at a lower level, mainly to other English-speaking developed countries—Australia, the United States, New Zealand, Ireland, and Canada. The United Kingdom is a net importer of nurses.
United States	Aiken (2007) suggested that about 8 percent of U.S. registered nurses, numbering around 219,000, are foreign educated. Eighty percent are from lower-income countries. The Philippines is the major source country, accounting for more than 30% of foreign-educated U.S. nurses. Nurse immigration to the United States has tripled since 1994, to close to 15,000 entrants annually. Foreign-educated nurses are located primarily in urban areas, most likely to be employed by hospitals, and somewhat more likely to have a baccalaureate degree than native-born nurses.

TABLE 6.2	Push and Pull Factors for Nurse Migration

Push Factors	Pull Factors
Low pay (absolute and/or relative)	Higher pay (and opportunities for remittances)
Poor working conditions	Better working conditions
Lack of resources to work effectively	Better-resourced health systems
Limited career opportunities	Career opportunities
Limited educational opportunities	Provision of post basic education
Impact of human immunodeficiency virus (HIV) and acquired immunodeficiency disease (AIDS)	Political stability
Unstable/dangerous work environment	Travel opportunities
Economic instability	Aid work

Source: Buchan, J. (2006). The impact of global nursing migration on health services delivery. *Policy, Politics, & Nursing Practice (Supplement), 7*(3), 16S–25S.

Research Study Fuels the Controversy: Why Do Nurses Emigrate?

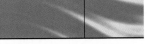

This study of 139 nursing students in Uganda assessed their views on practice options and their intentions to migrate.

STUDY FINDINGS

Seventy percent of participants reported wanting to work outside Uganda and said it was likely that within 5 years they would be working in the United States (59%) or the United Kingdom (49%). About one fourth (27%) said they could be working in another African country. Survey respondents reported that financial remuneration was the greatest push factor encouraging them to migrate. Those wanting to work in urban, private, or U.K./U.S. practices were less likely to express a sense of professional obligation and/or loyalty to their native country. Those who lived in rural areas were less likely to report wanting to migrate. Students with a desire to work in urban areas or private practice were more likely to report an intent to migrate for financial reasons or in pursuit of a country with stability, whereas students wanting to work in rural areas or public practice were less likely to want to migrate overall.

Nguyen, L., Ropers, S., Nderitu, E., Zuyderduin, A., Luboga, S., & Hagopian, A. (2008). Intent to migrate among nursing students in Uganda: Measures of the brain drain in the next generation of health professionals. *Human Resources for Health, 6*(1), 5.

Buchan (2006) suggested that for English-speaking nurses with an internationally recognized qualification, "the world is their oyster, and they can move wherever they want to practice" (p. 175).

Destination countries are able to recruit nurses as a result of a large number of pull factors. Many internationally recruited nurses suggest they would have preferred to remain in their home country with family and friends and in a familiar culture and environment, but push and pull factors overwhelmingly influenced their decision to migrate. Such was the case in research done by Nguyen et al. (2008), which suggested that financial remuneration was the greatest push factor encouraging Ugandan student nurses to migrate (see Research Study Fuels the Controversy).

> ### CONSIDER
> A nurse's motivation to migrate is multifactorial, not limited to financial incentives, and barriers exist that discourage or slow the migration process (Kingma, 2007).

THE EFFECT OF GLOBAL MIGRATION ON DEVELOPING COUNTRIES

A review of the literature suggests that different countries have experienced different effects as a result of the push–pull of international nurse migration. In some cases, aggressive recruitment, by which large numbers of recruits are sought, may significantly deplete a single health facility or contract an important number of newly graduated nurses from a single educational institute. This has significant local and regional implications.

Some national governments and government agencies have, however, actually encouraged the outflow of nurses from their country, including Fiji, Jamaica, India, Mauritius, and the Philippines. For many years, the Philippines government actively endorsed and facilitated initiatives aimed at educating, recruiting, training, and placing nurses around the world. This was likely the result of a financial imperative, to encourage the generation of remittance income. Remittances of overseas Filipinos were expected to reach US $14.7 billion in 2007, up $1.9 billion from 2006 (International Centre on Nurse Migration, 2007). This represents 10% of the gross domestic product (GDP) for the Philippines (Kingma, 2007).

> ### CONSIDER
> Migrating nurses provide value to source countries, in that health care workers often send remittances back home to support their families and bolster the economy; they may form clinical or educational partnerships between countries; and, after a time, some workers return home with enhanced skills and experience (Gostin, 2008).

The mass export of nurses from the Philippines is also a response to a labor market oversupply. The Philippines currently produces 100,000 to 150,000 nurses every year, and less than 5% of them are employed in the Philippines, either by the government or the private sector (Gamolo, 2008). The Philippine Overseas Employment Administration deployed a total of 13,525 licensed nurses around the world in 2006 (James, 2008), and, according to the Trade Union Congress of the Philippines, more than 21,000 new Filipino nurses sought U.S. jobs in 2007 (Gamolo). The Trade Union continues to encourage the deployment of surplus nurses and other highly skilled workers rather than unskilled workers, whose skills are more easily replaceable.

China, with the second-largest nursing workforce in the world (2.2 million nurses), is another country actively seeking to export nurses. Xu (2004) suggested that push factors for the migration of Chinese nurses include a significant surplus of nurses, especially those prepared at the secondary school level; a declining socioeconomic status of nurses; and the underdevelopment of nursing as a profession. In fact, Xu predicted that China will replace the Philippines as the country exporting the largest number of nurses to the United States in the foreseeable future.

In contrast, Fang (2007) suggested that there is actually a severe shortage of nurses in China, with only 1 nurse per 1,000 population, yet there is a very high level of unemployment and underemployment of nurses. Therefore, there is a surplus of nurses who can and do want to migrate. Fang suggested that even if the Chinese government were to increase the nursing jobs available and improve working conditions, some surplus would still exist. He concluded that China will likely become an important source of nurses for developed nations in the coming years.

India is also gaining ground as one of the world's leading nurse exporters. In 2004, for example, India surpassed the Philippines in terms of the number of nurses admitted to the U.K. Registrar for the first time (Brush, 2008).

Nonetheless, recent reports from South Africa, Ghana, China, the Caribbean, and even the Philippines highlight that such a significant outflow of nurses has had negative effects, including reductions in the level and quality of services and the loss of specialist skills. Indeed, Bayron (2006) reported that more than 100,000 nurses have left the Philippines since 1994, causing public health experts in that country to suggest that their health care system is on the brink of collapse. Similarly, African ministers of health have repeatedly brought resolutions to the World Health Assembly stating that health care worker migration is crippling their health care systems (Kuehn, 2007). Taiwan too has expressed concerns about the brain drain that has occurred as a result of the migration of nurses from there (Brush, 2008).

It is this brain drain that is one of the most critical negative consequences of widespread nursing migration from developing countries. Brain drain refers to the loss of skilled personnel and the loss of investment in education that is experienced when those human resources migrate elsewhere. The Federation for American Immigration Reform [FAIR] (n.d.) defines brain drain as the flow of skilled professionals from less developed countries to more developed countries and suggests that this practice results in developing countries losing the individuals they can least afford to lose because they are the ones "who are skilled and educated, who perform crucial services contributing to the health and economy of the country, and who create new jobs for others" (para 1).

Complaints of brain drain are heard from donor countries such as India, the Philippines, South Africa, and Zimbabwe. These nations argue that their human health care resources are being extracted at a time when they are needed most. Although these negative effects of international migration on "supplier" countries have been more openly recognized and addressed the last few years, concerted efforts to address the problem continue to be limited.

In addition, many of the countries that are exporting nurses are also experiencing a nursing shortage. For example, Africa has the countries with the lowest number of nurses in the world in absolute terms and in terms of nurses to care for the population—often 100-fold less than the United States (Buchan, 2006). This leaves Africa "struggling very, very hard, at the moment, to deliver even minimum health care" (Buchan, p. 195).

CONSIDER

The majority of countries importing foreign nurses are primarily white, and donor nations typically export nurses of color. The issue of race and the global economics of nursing should be examined in terms of effect on both supplier and donor countries.

CONSIDER

The positive global economic/social/professional development associated with international migration must be weighed against the substantial brain and skills drain experienced by donor countries.

It should be noted, however, that brain drain is not just occurring in nursing. Despite Europe's efforts to stop its scientific brain drain, more and more of the continent's brightest young researchers are choosing to pursue careers abroad. In Germany, for example, record numbers of highly qualified individuals are choosing to work abroad, marking the biggest mass exodus in 60 years (Paterson, 2008). Countries in Eastern Europe, including Poland, Latvia, and Lithuania, are reporting the same, creating a marked brain drain in that region (Eastern Europe Fears Brain Drain, 2006).

In addition, CSR Europe (2008) suggested that 30% of professionals from African countries work abroad, requiring African countries to invest $4 billion annually to replace them. In addition, 20,000 skilled professionals, scientists, academics, and researchers leave the African continent annually, "depriving many African countries of the human and intellectual capital they need to develop" (CSR Europe, para 1).

Just because the brain drain that occurs in nursing resources also occurs in other disciplines does not make it acceptable. It does, however, suggest that the individual's right to choose cannot be easily negated simply because the donor country does not want to lose its intellectual resources.

Finally, one must consider whether recruiting foreign nurses to solve acute staffing shortages is simply a poorly thought out quick fix to a much greater problem and whether, in doing so, not only are donor nations harmed, the issues that led to the shortage in the first place are never addressed. Certainly, one must at least question whether wholesale foreign nurse recruitment would even be necessary if importer nations made a more concerted effort to improve the working conditions, salaries, empowerment, and recognition of the home-born nurses they already employ. Indeed, one must question whether importation occurs in an effort to avoid the costs of doing so. Clearly, many nursing organizations and nursing leaders have begun to recognize the negative effects of international migration on "supplier" countries, but efforts to address the problem have been inadequate.

> ### CONSIDER
> Importing foreign nurses to solve the nursing shortage only puts a Band-Aid on the problem. The factors that led to the nursing shortage in the first place still need to be resolved.

> ### DISCUSSION POINT
> If the money that is being spent on recruitment and immigration of foreign nurses was instead spent on resolving the domestic nursing issues that led to a shortage in the first place, would international nurse recruitment even be necessary?

GLOBAL NURSE RECRUITMENT AND MIGRATION AS AN ETHICAL ISSUE

Controversy regarding the ethics of international recruitment of nurses is not new. Whenever resources are limited, ethical issues regarding their allocation are likely to arise. In the case of global nurse recruitment and migration, the ethical principles of autonomy, utility, and justice seem most relevant. Certainly, there must be some sort of a balance between the right of individual nurses to choose to migrate (autonomy), particularly when push factors are overwhelming, and the more utilitarian concern for the donor nations' health as a result of losing scarce nursing resources.

Gostin (2008) agreed, suggesting that health care workers should not be deprived of their human rights and be tied to an impoverished life at home with grim prospects. In addition, international law guarantees an individual the right to freedom of movement and residence [as established in the Universal Declaration of Human Rights (United Nations General Assembly, 1948) and the International Covenant on Civil and Political Rights (Office of the United Nations High Commissioner for Human Rights, 1976). The individual's right to migrate is central to self-determination.

> ### DISCUSSION POINT
> Should the right for the individual nurse to migrate (autonomy and self-determination) override what might be best for the donor nation (utilitarianism)?

Justice, or fairness, is another ethical principle that seems appropriate to this discussion because it examines how social and material goods are distributed to or withheld from members of a group or society, particularly in relation to fairness. Drevdahl and Shannon (2008) suggested that the relative ease with which health care professionals are able to get specialized visas to work is in direct contrast with immigrants employed in low-wage positions. They suggested that this in itself is a violation of basic human rights and global expectations of justice.

McElmurry, Solheim, Kishi, Coffia, and Janepanish (2006) suggested another ethical principle violation in their assertion that the unmanaged flow of nurse migration violates the ethical principles underlying the concept of "health for all." Gostin (2008) agreed, suggesting that nurse migration often disadvantages societies that are already the poorest and least healthy and that, because nursing shortages are associated with poor outcomes, not only is critical intellectual capital taken away from the developing country, but also the donor country's health outcomes are likely to worsen.

McElmurry et al. (2006) also suggested that nurse migrants are often placed in vulnerable, inequitable work roles and that employers in donor countries often fail to address the basic causes of their own underlying nurse shortage. They argued that ethical foreign nurse recruitment can occur only if donor countries (1) leave developing countries enhanced rather than depleted, (2) contribute to national health outcomes consistent with essential care for all people, (3) are based on community participation, (4) address common nursing labor issues, and (5) involve equitable and clear financial arrangements (McElmurry et al.).

The following question then must be asked: Does global recruitment violate the principle of justice, particularly if such migration does not solve the underlying shortage and when such retention is done at the expense of the donor country? Kingma (2007) expressed the same concern in her assertion that injecting migrant nurses into dysfunctional health systems—ones that are not capable of attracting and retaining staff domestically—will not solve the nursing shortage.

Milton (2007) suggested that the ethics of nurse migration become even more complex when nurse leaders must consider whether the issue should be viewed using philosophical frameworks that contain embedded *ethos* or *straight thinking* concepts. She concluded that there are ethical considerations for having an ethos or straight thinking for doing what is right and good for the discipline of nursing and the community, and she argued that the discipline of nursing must focus on creating health policies that value humans and health, as well as human dignity.

Clearly, donor countries have an ethical obligation to do what they can to provide their nurses with a safe, satisfying, and economically rewarding work environment. Importer countries have an ethical obligation to do what is necessary to be more self-reliant in meeting their professional workforce needs and to avoid recruiting nurses from those countries that can least afford to experience brain drain. Finally, professional health care associations must lead the way in addressing how best to respond to these ethical concerns.

PROFESSIONAL ORGANIZATIONS RESPOND

Given the current extent of nurse migration and the multiplicity of ethical dilemmas associated with it, many professional organizations, representing nurses from around the world, have weighed in on the issue. Some have provided formal position statements to guide both donor and importer countries. Others have attempted to provide guidance to the individual nurse considering global migration.

The International Council of Nurses

One international agency, the International Council of Nurses (ICN), has issued several position statements arguing for ethics and good employment practices in international recruitment (Box 6.1). The ICN, a federation of more than 128 national nurses' associations, represents millions of nurses worldwide (ICN, 2008). The *ICN Position Statement: Nurse Retention, Transfer, and Migration* confirms the right of nurses to migrate, as well as the potential beneficial outcomes of multicultural practice and learning opportunities supported by migration, but acknowledges potential adverse effects on the quality of health care in donor countries (ICN, 1999).

The ICN (1999) position statement also condemns the practice of recruiting nurses to countries where authorities have failed to implement sound human resource planning and to seriously address problems that cause nurses to leave the profession and discourage them from returning to nursing. The position statement also denounces unethical recruitment practices that exploit nurses or mislead them into accepting job responsibilities and working conditions that are incompatible with their qualifications, skills, and experience. The ICN and its member national nurses' associations call for a regulated recruitment process, based on ethical principles that guide informed decision making and reinforce sound employment policies on the part of governments, employers, and nurses, thereby supporting fair and cost-effective recruitment and retention practices.

| BOX 6.1 | ICN POSITION STATEMENT ON NURSE RETENTION, TRANSFER, AND MIGRATION (1999) |

ICN and its member associations firmly believe that quality health care is directly dependent on an adequate supply of qualified nursing personnel.

ICN recognizes the right of individual nurses to migrate, while acknowledging the possible adverse effect that international migration may have on health care quality.

ICN condemns the practice of recruiting nurses to countries where authorities have failed to address human resource planning and problems that cause nurses to leave the profession and discourage them from returning to nursing.

In support of the above, ICN:

■ Disseminates information on nursing personnel needs and resources and on the development of fulfilling nursing career structures.

■ Provides training opportunities in negotiation and socioeconomic welfare-related issues.

■ Disseminates data on nursing employment worldwide.

■ Takes action to help reduce the serious effects of any shortage, maldistribution, and misutilization of nursing personnel.

■ Advocates adherence nationally to international labor standards.

■ Condemns the recruitment of nurses as a strike-breaking mechanism.

■ Advocates for open and transparent migration systems (recognizing that some appropriate screening is necessary to ensure public safety).

■ Supports a transcultural approach to nursing practice.

■ Promotes the introduction of transferable benefits, e.g., pension.

National nurses' associations are urged to:

■ Encourage relevant authorities to ensure sound human resources planning for nursing.

■ Participate in the development of sound national policies on immigration and emigration of nurses.

■ Promote the revision of nursing curriculum for basic and post basic education in nursing and administration to emphasize effective nursing leadership.

■ Disseminate information on the working conditions of nurses.

■ Discourage nurses from working in other countries where salaries and conditions are not acceptable to nurses and professional associations in those countries.

■ Ensure that foreign nurses have conditions of employment equal to those of local nurses in posts requiring the same level of competency and involving the same duties and responsibilities.

■ Ensure that there are no distinctions made among foreign nurses from different countries.

■ Monitor the activities of recruiting agencies.

■ Provide an advisory service to help nurses interpret contracts and assist foreign nurses with personal and work-related problems, such as institutional racism, violence, and sexual harassment.

■ Provide orientation for foreign nurses on the local cultural, social, and political values and on the health system and national language.

■ Alert nurses to the fact that some diplomas, qualifications, or degrees earned in one country may not be recognized in another.

■ Assist nurses with their problems related to international migration and repatriation.

Source: International Council of Nurses (1999). *Position statement: Nurse retention, transfer, and migration.* Available at: **http://www.icn.ch/psretention.htm.** Accessed June 25, 2008.

BOX 6.2 | ICN PRINCIPLES OF ETHICAL NURSE RECRUITMENT

1. Effective planning and development strategies must be introduced, regularly reviewed, and maintained to ensure a balance between supply and demand of nurse human resources.

2. Nursing legislation must authorize regulatory bodies to determine nurses' standards of education, competencies, and standards of practice and to ensure that only individuals meeting these standards are allowed to practice as a nurse.

3. Because the provision of quality care relies on the availability of nurses to meet staffing demand, nurses in a recruiting region/country and seeking employment should be made aware of job opportunities.

4. Nurses should have the right to migrate if they comply with the recruiting country's immigration/work policies (e.g., work permit) and meet obligations in their home country (e.g., bonding responsibilities, tax payment).

5. Nurses have the right to expect fair treatment (e.g., working conditions, promotion, and continuing education).

6. Nurses and employers are to be protected from false information, withholding of relevant information, misleading claims, and exploitation (e.g., accurate job descriptions, benefits/allocations/bonuses specified in writing, authentic educational records).

7. There should be no discrimination between occupations/professions with the same level of responsibility, educational qualification, work experience, skill requirement, and hardship (e.g., pay, grading).

8. When nurses' or employers' contracted or acquired rights or benefits are threatened or violated, suitable machinery must be in place to hear grievances in a timely manner and at reasonable cost.

9. Nurses must be protected from occupational injury and health hazards, including violence (e.g., sexual harassment), and made aware of existing workplace hazards.

10. The provision of quality care in the highly complex and often stressful health care environment depends on a supportive formal and informal supervisory infrastructure.

11. Employment contracts must specify a trial period when the signing parties are free to express dissatisfaction and cancel the contract with no penalty. In the case of international migration, the responsibility for covering the cost of repatriation needs to be clearly stated.

12. Nurses have the right to affiliate to and be represented by a professional association and/or union to safeguard their rights as health professionals and workers.

13. Recruitment agencies (public and private) should be regulated, and effective monitoring mechanisms, such as cost-effectiveness, volume, success rate over time, retention rates, equalities criteria, and client satisfaction, should be introduced.

Source: Adapted from International Council of Nurses (2007). *Position statement: Ethical nurse recruitment.* Available at: http://www.icn.ch/psrecruit01.htm. Accessed June 25, 2008.

In addition, the ICN adopted a position paper on ethical nurse recruitment in 2001 that was revised and reaffirmed in 2007 (ICN, 2007). This document identifies 13 principles (see Box 6.2) necessary to create a foundation for ethical recruitment, whether international or intranational contexts are being considered. The ICN suggests that all health sector stakeholders—patients, governments, employers, and nurses—will benefit if this ethical recruitment framework is systematically applied. In addition, policy questions and subsidiary research questions related to international nurse recruitment are shown in Box 6.3.

The International Centre on Nurse Migration

Another organization, the International Centre on Nurse Migration (ICNM), established in 2005, represents a collaborative project launched by the ICN and the Commission on Graduates of Foreign Nursing Schools (CGFNS). The ICNM is an international resource for the development, promotion, and dissemination of research, policy, and information on nurse migration, with an ultimate goal being to "establish dynamic, effective global and national migration policy and practice that facilitate safe

| BOX 6.3 | INTERNATIONAL NURSE MOBILITY: QUESTIONS ON POLICY AND SUBSIDIARY RESEARCH |

Source Countries

Policy

- Should outflow be supported or encouraged? (to stimulate remittance income or to end oversupply)
- Should outflow be constrained or reduced? (e.g., to reduce "brain drain"; if so, how?—what is effective and ethical?)
- Should recruitment agencies be regulated?

Research

- What are the destination countries for outflow?
- How much of outflow is permanent or temporary? (short or long term?)
- How much of outflow is going to health sector–related employment/education in other countries and what proportion to non–health-related destinations?
- What is the size of outflow to other countries compared to the outflow to other sectors within the country?
- What is the effect of outflow?
- Why are nurses leaving?
- How should flows be monitored?

Destination Countries

Policy

- Is inflow sustainable?
- Is inflow a cost-effective way of solving skills shortages?
- Is inflow ethically justifiable?
- Should recruitment agencies be regulated?

Research

- What are the source countries for inflow?
- How much of inflow is permanent or temporary?
- How much of inflow is going to health sector–related employment/education in the country and what proportion to non–health-related destinations?
- Is inflow effectively managed?
- Why are nurses coming?
- How should flows be monitored?

International Agencies

- How should international flows of nurses be monitored?
- In the context of the working relationship with the country's government, what is the appropriate role/response of the agency to the issue of international nurse mobility?
- Should the international agency intervene in the process (e.g., developing ethical framework, supporting government-to-government contracts, introducing regulatory compliance)?

Source: Buchan, J., Parkin, T., & Sochalski, J. (2003). *International nurse mobility: Trends and policy implications.* Available at: **http://www.icn.ch/Int_Nurse_mobility%20final.pdf.** Accessed February 10, 2004. Reprinted with permission.

patient care and positive practice environments for nurse migrants" (ICNM, 2008, para 1).

One priority of the ICNM will be to address gaps in policy, research, and information with regard to the migrant nurse workforce, including screening and workforce integration (CGFNS, 2005). In addition, the Centre's Web site is intended to act as a portal for policy, research studies, and other information regarding migration trends and statistics. According to Judith Oulton, Chief Executive Officer of the ICN, "The Centre provides an important asset in understanding and acting on the needs of migrating nurses, employers and policy makers throughout the global community" (CGFNS, 2005, para 4).

The AcademyHealth Project: Achieving Consensus on Ethical Standards of Practice for International Nurse Recruitment

AcademyHealth, a professional society of 4,000 individuals and 125 affiliated organizations throughout the United States and abroad, has also taken an active role in working to assure the ethical recruitment of international nurses (AcademyHealth, 2008). Funded through a grant from the John D. and Catherine T. MacArthur Foundation in collaboration with the O'Neill Institute for National and Global Health Law at Georgetown University, AcademyHealth convened a task force of recruiters, hospitals, and foreign-educated nurses to develop draft standards of practice about global nurse recruitment, as well as recommendations on how to institutionalize these standards. In late 2007, AcademyHealth released a report on year 1 of its 2-year project—the International Recruitment of Nurses to the United States: Toward a Consensus on Ethical Standards of Practice (Pittman et al., 2007).

In September 2008, AcademyHealth celebrated the formal release of its new Voluntary Code of Ethical Conduct for the Recruitment of Foreign Educated Nurses to the United States. The Code is designed to increase transparency and accountability throughout the process of international recruitment and ensure adequate orientation for foreign-educated nurses. It also provides guidance on ways to ensure recruitment is not harmful to source countries.

The World Health Organization

Another international organization involved in establishing guidelines for nurse migration is the World Health Organization (WHO). In an effort to balance the right of workers to migrate with a need to assure that global health care needs are met, the WHO launched the Health Worker Migration Policy Initiative in 2007. The initiative brings together professional organizations and other groups to "develop a roadmap and code of practice for health worker migration" (Kuehn, 2007, p. 1854). Simultaneously, individual organizations have launched their own efforts to encourage ethical recruitment of health workers and to spread the benefits of health worker migration more equitably among developed and developing nations (Kuehn).

The proposed code, as called for by a resolution of the World Health Assembly in 2004, will promote ethical recruitment, protect migrant health workers' rights, and encourage governments in both developed and developing nations to actively address the push and pull factors that promote nurse migration (WHO, 2007). The Code of Practice will be the first of its kind on a global scale for migration.

In addition, 2004 WHO Resolution 57.19 urges member states to mitigate the adverse effects of health care worker migration by forming country and regional agreements such as the South Africa/United Kingdom Memorandum of Understanding, the Pacific Code, and the Caribbean Community agreement (Gostin, 2008).

THE MISTREATMENT OF FOREIGN NURSES

Despite the costs and investment of time and energy that goes into recruiting foreign nurses, some health care organizations treat imported nurses poorly once they arrive. These nurses may receive substandard jobs or wages or be subjected to illegal practices by their employers. For example, Pittman et al. (2007) report that 18% of recruiting firms charge foreign nurses an up-front fee, a practice that has been found illegal in connection with the recruitment of temporary farm workers in the United States and that is prohibited in the U.K. Code of Practice for the International Recruitment of Health Care Professionals. In addition, most recruiters charge migrant nurses a "buyout" or breach fee

BOX 6.4 | QUESTIONABLE PRACTICES REPORTED BY INTERNATIONAL NURSES

- Denying nurses the right to obtain a copy of the contract at the time of signing.
- Altering contracts both before nurses' departure from their home country and on arrival in the sponsor country without their consent.
- Imposing excessive demands to work overtime, in some cases with no differential pay, combined with threats that nurses will be reported to immigration authorities if they refuse to comply.
- Retention of green cards by employers, delays in processing Social Security numbers and RN permits, and payment of nurses at lower rates until documentation is complete.
- Delaying payments and paying for fewer hours than actually worked.
- Paying wages below direct-hire counterparts and in some cases other per-diem nurses.
- Providing substandard housing.
- Offering insufficient clinical orientation.
- Requiring excessively high breach fees and refusing to allow nurses to pay buy-outs in installments.

Source: Pittman, P., Folsom, A., Bass, E., & Leonhardy, K. (2007). *U.S. based international nurse recruitment: Structure and processes of a burgeoning industry. Report on year I of the Project International Recruitment of Nurses to the United States: Toward a consensus on ethical standards of practice.* Available at: **http://www.intlnursemigration.org/download/Report-on-Year-I.pdf.** Accessed June 25, 2008.

of up to $50,000 for resigning prior to the end of their employment contract.

There are also reports that overzealous recruiters have made false promises to foreign nurses regarding job opportunities and wages and virtually forced the newly migrated registered nurses to work long hours in substandard working conditions. Part of the reason for this is that private for-profit agencies have increasingly become involved in the search for nursing personnel, and there is generally no designated body that regulates or monitors the content of contracts offered. Internationally recruited nurses may be particularly at risk of exploitation or abuse due to the difficulty of verifying the terms of employment as a result of distance, language barriers, cost, and naiveté.

Indeed, a 1-year study by AcademyHealth suggested that international nurses experience a number of questionable hiring or employment practices, primarily with regard to employment in nursing homes. These are shown in Box 6.4. The study concluded that although it is likely that "only a small group of recruiters and nursing homes engage in abusive practices, the very existence of such practices is indicative of oversight problems" (Pittman et al., 2007, p. 27).

Jeans (2006) went further in her assertion that the recruitment process of foreign nurses is completely corrupt and that recruiters need to be regulated. She ar-

gued that recruiters should not be allowed to "misrepresent reality, lure people with false promises, and collect huge fees for doing so" (p. 59S).

CONSIDER

Due to the lack of regulatory oversight of global nurse migration contracting, foreign nurses are at increased risk for employment under false pretenses and may be misled as to the conditions of work, remuneration, and benefits.

Pittman et al. (2007) suggested that placement agencies also add to the corruption, in that they often charge health care organizations a standard fee of $15,000 to $25,000, depending on the state and the nurse's experience, to bring in a foreign nurse. Staffing agencies, which also provide foreign nurses, are typically paid on an hourly basis for the nurses they provide, and this rate may be four times greater than the average RN hourly wage in an effort to recover their investment costs (Pittman et al.).

DISCUSSION POINT
Should there be greater regulatory oversight of foreign nurse recruitment? If so, who should be charged with this responsibility?

THE INTERNATIONAL COMMUNITY ADDRESSES THE PROBLEM

The nursing shortage and resulting global migration issues have led several national governments to intervene, and, as a result, some countries have made progress in tackling the ethical issues associated with global recruitment and migration of nurses.

Some Governments Respond

Within the last few years, many countries, including the United States, have published national nursing strategies for dealing with staff shortages. Norway has issued a policy statement on the ethics of international recruitment. The Netherlands, Ireland, and the Scandinavian countries also have good-practice guidelines on international recruitment or are looking at developing guidelines. The United Kingdom went even further when in August 2006 it began limiting nurse recruitment to the European Union (EU) countries and only granting work permits to nurses from non-EU countries if National Health Services institutions showed that jobs could not be filled by U.K. or EU applications (Depausil, W.B., as cited in Brush, 2008).

Other countries have initiated or examined various policy responses to reduce outflow, such as requiring nurses to work in their home countries for a certain amount of time after education completion or by charging the nurse a fee to migrate to another country. For example, the Nurses Association of Jamaica has demanded that the Jamaican government raise salaries in an effort to get nurses to stay (Brush, 2008).

Another response has been to recognize that outflow cannot be halted if principles of individual freedom are to be upheld, but that the outflow that does occur must be managed and moderated. The "managed migration" initiative being undertaken in the Caribbean, which has provided regional support for addressing the nursing shortage crisis and developed initiatives such as training for export and temporary migration, is one example of a coordinated intervention to minimize the negative effects of outflow while realizing at least some benefit from the process (Salmon, Yan, Hewitt, & Guisinger, 2007).

U.S. Immigration Policy

Like most national governments, the U.S. government continues to play a pivotal role in the nurse migration issue by virtue of its ability to issue travel visas. The reality is that there is a finite number of visas available as a result of tougher post-9/11 immigration standards and caps on how many green cards are issued (Coates, 2006). Clearly, commercial recruiters and employers continue to apply pressure to ease restrictions on nurse migration in an effort to mitigate the U.S. nursing shortage (Aiken, 2007), but labor certification laws and rules regarding the issuance of visas are complex.

Labor certification laws in the United States state that under normal circumstances, the Department of Labor is required by law to certify to the Department of State and the Immigration and Naturalization Service (INS) when an alien is hired that (1) no U.S. citizens and permanent residents are available or qualified for a given job and (2) the employment of an alien will not adversely affect the wages of the concerned profession (U.S. Department of Homeland Security, 2005).

The main purpose of this legal provision has been to protect the domestic labor market; however, the immigration laws have provided preferential provisions for members of certain professions in the national interest of the United States, and, as a result, the government has created a list of occupations and professions, including nursing, that do not require labor certification. Because nursing has been classified as one of the shortage areas in the U.S. economy, a so-called *blanket waiver* of the labor certification is in place.

In addition, from 1962 to 1989, foreign nurses were regarded as "professionals" under U.S. immigration laws and could therefore seek an H-1 temporary work visa in the United States. In 1989, the Immigration Nursing Relief Act (INRA) created a 5-year pilot program. The INRA stipulated that only health care facilities with "attestations" approved by the Department of Health could obtain H-1A occupation visas to employ nurses on a temporary basis. Consequently, other occupations that formerly fell into the H-1 category became part of the new H-1B category. In addition, in 1990, Congress passed the Immigration and Nationality Act, which is the legal foundation for current immigration policies. In this act, nursing continued to be listed as a shortage area.

In 1999, the Nursing Relief for Disadvantaged Areas Act created H-1C occupational visas, which were perceived largely as an effort to renew the INRA of 1989 but with more restrictions. These temporary visas were created for foreign nurse graduates seeking employment in designated U.S. facilities (serving primarily poor patients in inner cities and some rural areas). Rules published in the *Federal Register* mandated that the total number of H-1C visas be limited to 500 each year, be valid for up to 3 years, and be capped at 25 nurses in states with a population of fewer than 9 million and 50 nurses in states with a population of more than 9 million (Murthy, 2004). Once the limitation is reached, visas are generally capped for the year. Accordingly, the wait to enter the United States from countries like the Philippines, China, and India had ballooned to 3 years by 2006 (Coates, 2006).

In addition, some foreign nurses apply for work in the United States via the H-1B visa. This nonimmigrant visa status allows recruiting of shortage professionals into jobs that require a 4-year university degree. Of particular interest is the fact that RNs do not qualify for the H-1B visa: A Fifth Circuit Court ruling in February 2000 stated that RN hospital jobs do not currently require a bachelor's degree in nursing, regardless of recruiter requirements. Some nurses can still apply for the H-1B status, however, if they have a specialized skill, particularly in intensive care, management, and specialty nursing areas or if U.S. employers can convince immigration officials that specific jobs do meet the H-1B requirement on a case-by-case basis.

Another way nurses get work visas in the United States has been under the immigrant E3 to I-140 status ("green card" or permanent resident). In this case, RNs can be brought into the country and become permanent residents through petition to the INS. A problem with this visa status is that it does not require labor certification, so the Department of Labor does not have to certify that the wage offered to the nurse is the prevailing wage. However, the law does state that foreign nurses entering under I-140 cannot have a negative effect on domestic wages.

DISCUSSION POINT

Does the increased importation of foreign nurses directly or indirectly affect the prevailing wages of domestic RNs?

Still other foreign nurses have sought employment in the United States in accordance with the North American Free-Trade Agreement (NAFTA), enacted in December 1993. NAFTA established a reciprocal trading relationship between the United States, Canada, and Mexico and allowed for a nonimmigrant class of admission exclusively for business and service trade individuals entering the United States.

To complicate the matter further, on July 26, 2003, the U.S. Bureau of Citizenship and Immigration Services ruled that foreign-educated health care professionals, including nurses who are seeking temporary or permanent occupational visas, as well as those who are seeking NAFTA status, must successfully complete a screening program before receiving an occupational visa or permanent (green card) visa. This screening, completed by the CGFNS, includes an assessment of an applicant's education to ensure that it is comparable to that of a nursing graduate in the United States, verification that licenses are valid and unencumbered, successful completion of an English-language proficiency examination, and verification that the nurse has either earned certification by the CGFNS or passed the National Council Licensure Examination for Registered Nurses (NCLEX-RN).

Nurses who entered the United States after the ruling on July 26, 2003, had 1 year from entry to produce a visa certificate from a U.S. Department of Homeland Security (DHS)–approved agency such as the CGFNS. Nurses in the United States before July 26, 2003, had until July 26, 2004, to produce the certificate (Steefel, 2004). The National Council of State Boards of Nursing (NCSBN) and the Organization of Nurse Executives (AONE), however, asked the DHS to delay implementation of certification rules for certain health care workers, including nurses, for at least 18 months, suggesting that 10,000 to 15,000 nurses might not be able to continue to work if they could not obtain certification (Steefel).

The American Nurses Association (ANA), however, opposed such a delay, noting that the new rules were originally passed in 1996 and suggesting that the 1-year transition period should have been adequate for foreign nurses to start the certification process (Steefel, 2004). Yet, on July 19, 2004, the U.S. Citizenship and Immigration Services (USCIS) announced that Canadian and Mexican health care workers who entered the United States on a TN (Trade NAFTA) visa and were employed in the United States and held a valid U.S. license before September 23, 2003, would continue to be exempt from the prescreening requirements for 1 additional year (USCIS Extends Deadline, 2004).

DISCUSSION POINT

Should implementation of the new certification rules have been delayed? When do manpower issues take precedence over concerns regarding patient safety?

In addition, the CGFNS (2005) reported that a Supplemental Appropriations Bill in 2005 provided for the recapture of 50,000 immigrant visas that had gone unused between 2001 and 2005. These Employment-Based 3rd Preference (EB-3) visas were reserved for Schedule A: Registered Nurses, Physical Therapists, and Performing Artists of Exceptional Ability.

Then, in 2007, a bill known as the Nursing Relief Act of 2007 (H.R. 1358) was introduced to create a new nonimmigrant visa category for professional nurses known as the W-1:

> *The bill proposed a numerical cap of 50,000 W-1 visas per year, but allowed the limit to rise based on the demand for foreign nurses. The W-1 was to be good for three (3) years at a time, with not more than six (6) years maximum allowable. The nurses, however, could apply for a 7th year extension to protect them from lengthy green card processing times (Seguritan, 2007, para 1).*

Sponsoring employers of nurses who entered with a W-1 visa had to agree to pay migrant nurses at the wage level paid to similarly situated employees or the prevailing wage for the occupational classification, whichever was greater. In addition, the employment of foreign nurses could not adversely affect the working conditions of nurses employed at the worksite (Seguritan, 2007). This bill was referred to the House Committee on the Judiciary in March 2007 but was not voted on.

Instead, Bill 1348 was introduced into the Senate proposing the Comprehensive Immigration Reform Act of 2007. This bill, among other things, established a temporary guest worker program through H-2C visas, which provided for 3-year stays, with one additional 3-year extension (GovTrack.us, 2008). This bill was still under consideration at the time of this writing.

ENSURING COMPETENCY OF FOREIGN NURSES: COMMISSION ON GRADUATES OF FOREIGN NURSING SCHOOLS AND THE NCLEX-RN EXAMINATION

Nursing is one of the most highly regulated health professions in the United States, and a license is required to practice in all 50 states and U.S. territories. Before 1977, endorsement and taking the State Board Test Pool Ex-amination (SBTPE) were the two ways for foreign nurses to obtain a license. The SBTPE tested the foreign graduate's English-language proficiency and knowledge of U.S. nursing practice, but, alarmingly, only a small percentage (15% to 20%) of foreign RNs typically passed the NCLEX-RN.

As a result of this high failure rate and a concern for patient safety, the ANA and the NLN, with collaboration from the Department of Labor and the INS, established the CGFNS in 1977 as an independent, nonprofit organization. The mission of CGFNS was to protect foreign nurse graduates and the U.S. public "by assuring the integrity of health professional credentials in the context of global migration and by fostering the equitable treatment of healthcare professionals as they expand their horizons" (CGFNS, 2008a).

The strategies CGFNS identified to accomplish this mission were to evaluate and test foreign graduates via a certification program before they left their home countries to ensure that there was a reasonable chance for them to pass the NCLEX-RN in the United States. Through a contract with the NLN, which had designed the NCLEX-RN, a CGFNS qualifying examination was developed. The examination consists of two parts to test the applicant's knowledge of nursing and the English language (both written and oral). In addition, a credentials review is required to earn the CGFNS Certificate. Passage of the certification exam meets one of the immigration requirements for securing an occupational visa to work in the United States (CGFNS, 2008b). Today, the CGFNS qualifying examination is offered in 50 cities around the world (CGFNS, 2008b).

A study released in April 2008 suggested that the CGFNS Certification Program Qualifying Exam has been and continues to be a strong predictor of performance on the NCLEX-RN examination:

> *The April 2006 through March 2007 Validity Study revealed that foreign-educated nurses who passed the CGFNS Qualifying Exam on the first attempt had a 92.4% chance of passing NCLEX on the first attempt. The findings of the current study include an overall pass rate on the NCLEX-RN examination for CGFNS Certificate Holders of 90.8% versus 40.7% for non-Certificate Holders (CGFNS, 2008c).*

The CGFNS examination, however, should not be mistaken as substitute for the state board licensing examination. Indeed, most states in the United States require foreign nurses to pass the CGFNS certification before they are allowed to take the NCLEX-RN.

The NCSBN has also taken steps to make it easier for foreign RNs to take the NCLEX-RN. Until 2005, the NCLEX-RN was offered only in the United States and its territories. In fact, prior to 2005, the only option foreign nurses had was to earn the CGFNS certificate, secure a job offer from a U.S. employer, and take the NCLEX-RN only after they arrived in the United States with their green cards (NCLEX RN Now Given Outside U.S., n.d.). Now the exam is offered at 18 international locations, including Manila, Philippines; London, England; Seoul, South Korea; Hong Kong; Sydney, Australia; Toronto, Montreal, and Vancouver, Canada; Frankfurt, Germany; Mumbai, New Delhi, Hyderabad, Bangalore, and Chennai, India; Mexico City, Mexico; Taipei, Taiwan; and Chiyodaku and Yokohama, Japan (NCSBN, 2008).

Gamolo (2008) reported that the Philippines readily topped the list of countries with the most foreign nurses taking the NCLEX for the first time in 2007, with 21,499. India came in second, with 5,370 examinees; followed by South Korea, with 1,906; Canada, with 888; and Cuba, with 673.

ASSIMILATING THE FOREIGN NURSE THROUGH SOCIALIZATION

The ethical obligation to the foreign nurse does not end with his or her arrival in a new country. The sponsoring country must do whatever it can to see that the migrant nurse is assimilated into the new work environment, as well as the new culture. Coates (2006) suggested that this process is not easy and that it is time consuming.

For example, language skills are often a significant issue for foreign nurses. This was obvious in a story shared by St. Rose Dominican Hospitals about their experience in recruiting five Korean nurses in 2005 (Mower, 2007). Although the recruitment agency assured the hospital that the nurses' language skills would be addressed and improved in the time it took to have visas issued, it quickly became apparent that the nurses' verbal skills were inadequate for the job. After spending between $15,000 and $17,000 to recruit and train each of the five nurses, the hospital had to enroll the nurses in English courses at the University of Nevada, Las Vegas.

Cheryl Peterson, a senior policy analyst with the American Nurse's Association, suggested, however, that language is just the tip of the iceberg. She suggested that the nursing profession has conducted little research into how to properly acclimate foreign nurses into the field (Mower, 2007). In addition, she added that hospitals rarely follow other, possibly more successful, transitional programs, instead choosing their own home-grown methods to socialize migrant nurses.

Ryan (2003) suggested that socialization to the professional nursing role is one of four basic needs that must be addressed if foreign nurses are to adapt successfully to U.S. workplaces. Ryan suggested that initially foreign nurses must be introduced to U.S. jargon and variations in nursing practice delivery so that language will not be a significant barrier. Then many must be supported through a period of cultural, professional, and psychological dissonance that is associated with anxiety, homesickness, and isolation. Finally, these nurses must be integrated within the institution so that they develop a sense of community life on the nursing unit.

The importance of appropriate professional and cultural socialization for foreign nurses cannot be overestimated. Aboderin (2007), in an exploratory qualitative investigation, found that Nigerian nurses who had migrated to the United Kingdom in an effort to improve their economic status actually experienced a loss of professional and social status in their host country. This is because the Nigerian nurses come from a national perspective by which "nurses belong not to the poor 'masses' but to a relatively privileged population segment—by virtue of their position as educated professionals. This privilege, (as well as their specific choice of profession), makes their global migration possible" (Aboderin, p. 2244). However, Nigerian nurses who migrate often experience values conflicts in terms of what constitutes a good life: to live well (in due material comfort), among one's people "at home." This supports the idea of a decidedly "local" normative perspective and suggests that country-specific strategies are needed to improve the employment satisfaction and retention of foreign nurses.

Bola, Driggers, Dunlap, and Ebersole (2003) stated that international nurses also frequently experience culture shock regarding nonverbal communication, which may interfere with their assimilation: "Patients or staff with limited cultural competence may interpret nonverbal communication, such as eye contact or smiling, as disrespectful" (Bola et al., p. 41).

Ryan (2003) suggested that using a cultural diversity enhancement group (CDEG) and a "buddy program" might help to socialize these international nurses. A CDEG includes staff nurses and management personnel from varied ethnic backgrounds who agree to "buddy" with the international nurses to make them feel welcomed in the organizational culture and to assist them regarding basic services, places, or necessary items they need to know about or have. Bola et al. (2003) concurred, suggesting that without a support system, international nurses might question their ability to solve problems and function successfully because the values and behaviors helpful in solving problems in their home country may not be helpful elsewhere.

Many migrant nurses are afraid to express dissatisfaction or to ask for help for fear they will no longer have a job or because they fear being sent home. In addition, many of the families left behind in donor countries count on the migrant RN sending money home to improve their living standard. All of these factors place migrated nurses at increased risk for abuse and failure to assimilate.

CONSIDER

Recruiting internationally may be a quick-fix solution, but it is far from clear that it is a cost-effective solution.

CONCLUSIONS

Nurse migration and its associated ethical dilemmas are among the most serious issues facing the nursing profession. Buchan (2006) suggested that the growing trend of nurse migration during the last 5 to 10 years will continue. In addition, there will be increased competition among countries for qualified registered nurses, although "the United States is likely to be at the top of the table in terms of opportunities and what it pays nurses" (Buchan, p. 229).

Clearly, developed countries have an advantage in terms of pull factors to recruit migrant nurses from less developed countries, and less developed countries are the ones most likely to suffer the devastating effects of brain drain. One must ask, however, whether this quick-fix solution to the nursing shortage has become too commonplace and too easy. Does it keep recruiter countries from dealing with the issues that led to their shortage in the first place? Does it negatively affect prevailing domestic wages and artificially alter what should be normal supply/demand curves in the health care marketplace? Of even greater concern is the lack of regulatory oversight of contracting with foreign nurses, placing them at risk for unethical, if not illegal, employment practices in their host country.

Some countries and professional nursing organizations are beginning to address these issues. So, too, are national governments and regulatory agencies in an effort to protect both the migrant nurses and the public those nurses will serve. Yet, in the meantime, what may be hundreds of thousands of nurses are migrating internationally, and the potentially negative effects of this increasing trend on both the migrant nurse and the donor nation are becoming ever more apparent. Chopra, Munro, and Lavis (2008) suggested that despite pronounced international concern, little research and few solutions exist regarding the problem. Brush (2008, p. 23) agreed, suggesting that "despite ongoing debate about how best to manage nurses' international mobility, nurse migration remains relatively unchecked, uncoordinated, and individualized, such that some countries suffer from its effects while others benefit."

FOR ADDITIONAL DISCUSSION

1. Are the requirements for foreign nurses to get visas in the United States adequate?

2. Does achieving CGFNS certification and passing the NCLEX-RN examination in the United States assure competency of the foreign nurse graduate?

3. As long as international nurse recruitment is a viable option, will the problems that have led to a nursing shortage in the first place be addressed?

4. Should donor countries develop nurse migration policy efforts that limit human resource exports?

5. How can government and professional nursing organizations work together to ensure that recruitment practices of foreign nurses are both ethical and appropriate?

6. How does the ethical principle of veracity (truth telling) apply to the zealous recruiting efforts seen, particularly in developing countries?

7. Is government regulatory oversight of foreign nurse recruitment efforts in conflict with U.S. values of capitalistic free enterprise?

REFERENCES

Aboderin, I. (2007). Contexts, motives and experiences of Nigerian overseas nurses: Understanding links to globalization. *Journal of Clinical Nursing, 16*(12), 2237–2245.

AcademyHealth (2008). *About us.* Available at: http://www.academyhealth.org/about/index.htm. Accessed June 25, 2008.

Aiken, L. H. (2007). U.S. nurse labor market dynamics are key to global nurse sufficiency. *Health Services Research, 42*(3p2), 1299–1320.

Bayron, H. (2006). *Philippine medical brain drain leaves public health system in crisis.* NewsVOAcom. Available at: http://www.voanews.com/english/archive/2006-05/2006-05-03-voa38.cfm. Accessed June 25, 2008.

Benetar, S. R. (2007). An examination of ethical aspects of migration and recruitment of health care professionals from developing countries. *Clinical Ethics, 2*(1), 1–6.

Bola, T. V., Driggers, K., Dunlap, C., & Ebersole, M. (2003). Foreign-educated nurses. Strangers in a strange land. *Nursing Management, 34*(7), 39–42.

Brush, B. L. (2008). Global nurse migration today. *Journal of Nursing Scholarship, 40*(1), 20–25.

Brush, B. L., & Sochalski, J. (2007). International nurse migration: Lessons from the Philippines. *Policy, Politics, & Nursing Practice, 8*(1), 37–46.

Buchan, J. (2006). The impact of global nursing migration on health services delivery. *Policy, Politics, & Nursing Practice (Supplement), 7*(3), 16S–25S.

Buchan, J. (2007). International recruitment of nurses: Policy and practice in the United Kingdom. *Health Services Research, 42*(3p2), 1321–1335.

Buchan, J., Parkin, T., & Sochalski, J. (2003). *International nurse mobility: Trends and policy implications.* Available at: http://www.icn.ch/Int_Nurse_mobility%20final.pdf. Accessed February 10, 2004.

Chopra, M., Munro, S., & Lavis, J. N. (2008). Effects of policy options for human resources for health: An analysis of systematic reviews. *Lancet, 371*(9613), 668–674.

Clemens, M., & Pettersson, G. (2008). New data on African health professionals abroad. *Human Resources for Health, 6*, 1. Available at: http://www.human-resources-health.com/content/6/1/1. Accessed January 5, 2009.

Coates, C. (2006). *Local initiative: Despite shortage, hospitals avoid foreign nurses. Goliath: Business Knowledge on Demand.* Available at: http://goliath.ecnext.com/coms2/gi_0199-5944858/Local-initiative-despite-shortage-hospitals.html. Accessed June 25, 2008.

Commission on Graduates of Foreign Nursing Schools (CGFNS) (2005). *CGFNS and ICN launch new 'International Centre on Nurse Migration.'* Available at: http://www.cgfns.org/files/pdf/hs/2005/hs_summer_05.pdf. Accessed June 26, 2008.

Commission on Graduates of Foreign Nursing Schools (CGFNS) (2008a). *Mission and history.* Available at: http://www.cgfns.org/sections/about/hist.shtml. Accessed June 25, 2008.

Commission on Graduates of Foreign Nursing Schools (CGFNS) (2008b). *CGFNS certification program.* Available at: http://www.cgfns.org/sections/programs/cp/. Accessed June 25, 2008.

Commission on Graduates of Foreign Nursing Schools (CGFNS) (2008c). *CGFNS international's certification program qualifying exam for foreign educated nurses predicts success for passing NCLEX-RN examination.* Available at: http://www.cgfns.org/sections/announcements/news/default.shtml. Accessed June 25, 2008.

CSR Europe (2008). *Alleviating brain drain.* Available at: http://www.csreurope.org/solutions.php?action=

show_solution&solution_id=512.Accessed June 25, 2008.

Denton, S. (2006). Nation-to-nation challenges to addressing the effects of emerging global nurse migration on health care delivery. *Policy, Politics, & Nursing Practice (Supplement), 7*(3), 76S–80S.

Drevdahl, D., & Shannon, D. K. (2008). Exclusive inclusion: The violation of human rights and US immigration policy. *Advances in Nursing Science (ANS), 30*(4), 290–302.

Eastern Europe fears brain drain (2006). SIAWorkPermit.com. Available at: http://www.workpermit.com/news/2006_02_20/europe/eastern_europe_fears_brain_drain.htm. Accessed June 25, 2008.

Ehrenfeld, M., Itzhaki, S., & Michal, B. (2007). Nursing in Israel. *Nursing Science Quarterly, 20*(4), 372–375.

El-Jardali, F., Nuhad, M., Diana, J., Mouro, G. (2008). Migration of Lebanese nurses: A questionnaire survey and secondary data analysis. *International Journal of Nursing Studies.* Available at: http://www.sciencedirect.com/science?_ob=ArticleURL&_udi=B6T7T-4RR8351-1&_user=10&_coverDate=02%2F01%2F2008&_alid=758586279&_rdoc=1&_fmt=high&_orig=search&_cdi=5067&_sort=d&_docanchor=&view=c&_ct=1&_acct=C000050221&_version=1&_urlVersion=0&_userid=10&md5=c00f67455055682b21dcc17b1863e11b. Accessed January 5, 2009.

Fang, Z. Z. (2007). Potential of China in global nurse migration. *Health Services Research, 42*(3, Part 2), 1419–1428.

Federation for American Immigration Reform [FAIR] (n.d.). *Brain drain.* Available at: http://www.fairus.org/site/pageserver?pagename=iic_immigrationissuecenterse514. Accessed June 25, 2008.

Gamolo, N. O. (2008). Top stories. RP nurses seen as prime export commodity. *The Manila Times.* Available at: http://www.manilatimes.net/national/2008/mar/10/yehey/top_stories/20080310top6.html. Accessed June 25, 2008.

Gostin, L. (2008). The international migration and recruitment of nurses: Human rights and global justice. *Journal of the American Medical Association, 299*(15), 1827–1829.

GovTrack.us (2008). S. 1348: Comprehensive Immigration Reform Act of 2007. Available at: http://www.govtrack.us/congress/bill.xpd?tab=summary&bill=s110-1348. Accessed June 25, 2008.

Humphries, N., Brugha, R., & McGee, H. (2008). *Overseas nurse recruitment: Ireland as an illustration of the dynamic nature of nurse migration.* Available at: http://www.ncbi.nlm.nih.gov/sites/entrez. Accessed June 25, 2008.

International Centre on Nurse Migration (2007). *International nurse migration & remittances fact sheet 2007.* Available at: http://www.icn.ch/matters_icnm_remittances.pdf. Accessed June 25, 2008.

International Council of Nurses (ICN) (1999). *Position statement: Nurse retention, transfer, and migration.* Available at: http://www.icn.ch/psretention.htm. Accessed June 25, 2008.

International Council of Nurses (ICN) (2007). *Position statement: Ethical nurse recruitment.* Available at: http://www.icn.ch/psrecruit01.htm. Accessed June 25, 2008.

International Council of Nurses (ICN) (2008). *About ICN.* Available at: http://www.icn.ch/abouticn.htm. Accessed June 24, 2008.

James, E. (2008). *Global brain drain. Advance Perspective: Nurses.* Available at: http://community.advanceweb.com/blogs/nurses3/archive/2008/04/10/global-brain-drain.aspx. Accessed June 25, 2008.

Jeans, M. E. (2006). In-country challenges to addressing the effects of emerging global nurse migration on health care delivery. *Policy, Politics, & Nursing Practice (Supplement), 7*(3), 58S–61S.

Khadria, B. (2007). International nurse recruitment in India. *Health Services Research, 42*(3p2), 1429–1436.

Kingma, M. (2007). Nurses on the move: A global overview. *Health Services Research, 42*(3p2), 1281–1298.

Kuehn, B. M. (2007). Global shortage of health workers, brain drain stress developing countries. *Journal of the American Medical Association, 298*(16), 1853–1855.

Little, L. (2007). Nurse migration: A Canadian case study. *Health Services Research, 42*(3p2), 1336–1353.

Lorenzo, F. M. E., Galvez-Tan, J., Icamina, K., and Javier, L. (2007). Nurse migration from a source country perspective: Philippine country case study. *Health Services Research, 42*(3p2), 1406–1418.

McElmurry, B., Solheim, K., Kishi, R., Coffia, M., & Janepanish, W. (2006). Ethical concerns in nurse migration. *Journal of Professional Nursing, 22*(4), 226.

Mills, E. J., Schabas, W. A., Volmink, J., Walker, R., Ford, N., Katabira, E., Anema, A., Joffres M., Cahn, P., & Montaner, J. (2008). Should active recruitment of health workers from sub-Saharan Africa be viewed as a crime? *Lancet, 371*(9613), 685–688.

Milton, C. (2007). The ethics of nurse migration: An evolution of community change. *Nursing Science Quarterly, 20*(4), 319–322.

Mower, L. (2007). *Hospitals hire foreign nurses with care. Language, medical skills equally critical.* Reviewjournal.com. Available at: http://www.lvrj.com/news/8795217.html. Accessed June 26, 2008.

Murthy, S. (2004). *United States immigration. Overview: H1C visas for registered nurses.* Available at: http://www.murthy.com/news/UDh1covr.html. Accessed July 24, 2004.

National Council of State Boards of Nursing (2008). *NCSBN selects the Philippines as international testing site for NCLEX examinations.* Available at: https://www.ncsbn.org/1152.htm. Accessed June 26, 2008.

NCLEX-RN now given outside USA at testing centers (n.d.). Available at: http://www.mdnurse.com/NCLEXRN.html. Accessed June 25, 2008.

Nguyen, L., Ropers, S., Nderitu, E., Zuyderduin, A., Luboga, S., & Hagopian, A. (2008). Intent to migrate among nursing students in Uganda: Measures of the brain drain in the next generation of health professionals, *Human Resources for Health, 6*(1), 5.

North, N. (2007). International nurse migration: Impacts on New Zealand. *Policy, Politics, & Nursing Practice, 8*(3), 220–228.

Office of the United Nations High Commissioner for Human Rights (1976). *International Covenant on Civil and Political Rights.* Available at: http://www.unhchr.ch/html/menu3/b/a_ccpr.htm. Accessed January 5, 2009.

Paterson, T. (2008). German brain drain at highest level since 1940s. *The Independent.* Berlin. Accessible at: http://www.independent.co.uk/news/world/europe/german-brain-drain-at-highest-level-since-1940s-451250.html. Accessed June 25, 2008.

Pittman, P., Folsom, A., Bass, E., & Leonhardy, K. (2007). *U.S. based international nurse recruitment: Structure and practices of a burgeoning industry. Report on year I of the Project International Recruitment of Nurses to the United States: Toward a consensus on ethical standards of practice.* Available at: http://www.intlnursemigration.org/download/Report-on-Year-I.pdf. Accessed June 25, 2008.

Ryan, M. (2003). A buddy program for international nurses. *Journal of Nursing Administration, 33*(6), 350–352.

Salmon, M., Yan, J., Hewitt, H., & Guisinger, V. (2007). Managed migration: The Caribbean approach to addressing nursing services capacity. *Health Services Research, 42*(1), 1354–1372.

Sanvik, S. (2005). Experts on global nursing shortage provide recommendations to stem crisis. *Bio Medicine.* Available at: http://news.bio-medicine.org/medicine-news-3/Experts-on-global-nursing-shortage-provide-recommendations-to-stem-crisis-8828-1/. Accessed June 24, 2008.

Seguritan, R. S. (2007). *Nursing Relief Act of 2007. U.S. Immigration Updates.* Available at: http://www.bastapinoy.com/immigration_RS_070322.htm. Accessed June 26, 2008.

Steefel, L. (2004). Bridges or barriers. *Nurseweek (California), 2004,* 11–13.

United Nations General Assembly (1948). *The Universal Declaration of Human Rights.* Available at: http://www.un.org/Overview/rights.html. Accessed January 5, 2009.

USCIS extends deadline for prescreening requirement for some Canadian and Mexican nurses. (2004). *Nursing World.* Available at: http://www.nursing-world.org/inc/prtnewsarchive.htm. Accessed July 22, 2004.

U.S. Department of Labor (2005a). Petitions for Aliens to Perform Temporary Nonagricultural Services or Labor (H-2B); Proposed Rule. *Federal Register, 70*(17), 3984; 8 CFR 214. Available at: http://bulk.resource.org/gpo.gov/register/2005/2005_3984.pdf. Accessed January 5, 2009.

U.S. Department of Labor (2005b). ETA Proposed Rule. Post-Adjudication Audits of H-2B Petitions in All Occupations Other Than Excepted Occupations in the United States. *Federal Register, 70*(17), 3993–3997; 20 CFR 655. Available at: http://www.dol.gov/eta/regs/fedreg/proposed/2005001222.htm. Accessed January 5, 2009.

World Health Organization (WHO) (2007). *New initiative seeks practical solutions to tackle health worker migration.* Available at: http://www.who.int/mediacentre/news/notes/2007/np23/en/index.html. Accessed June 26, 2008.

Xu, Y (2004). *Are Chinese nurses a viable source to relieve the U.S. nurse shortage?* Presented at AcademyHealth Meeting, San Diego, California. Abstract 2078. Available at: http://gateway.nlm.nih.gov/MeetingAbstracts/ma?f=103625112.html.

BIBLIOGRAPHY

Arah, O. A., Obgu, U. C., & Okeke, C. E. (2008). Too poor to leave, too rich to stay: Development and global health correlates of physician migration to the United States, Canada, Australia, and the United Kingdom. *American Journal of Public Health, 98*(1), 148–154.

Biesky, T. (2007). Foreign-educated nurses: An overview of migration and credentialing issues. *Nursing Economics, 25*(1), 20–23, 34.

Cooper, R. A., & Aiken, L. H. (2006). Health services delivery: Reframing policies for global nursing migration in North America—A U.S. perspective. *Policy, Politics, & Nursing Practice (Supplement), 7*(3), 66S–70S.

Dwyer J. (2007). What's wrong with the global migration of health care professionals? Individual rights and international justice. *Hastings Center Report, 37*(5), 36–43.

Humphries, N., McGee, R., & Hannah, B. (2008). Overseas nurse recruitment: Ireland as an illustration of the dynamic nature of nurse migration. *Health Policy, 87*(2), 264–272.

Jolley, J. (2007). Now and then. Always nurses. *Paediatric Nursing, 19*(7), 12.

Keatings, M. (2006). Health services delivery: Reframing policies for global nursing migration in North America—A Canadian perspective. *Policy, Politics, & Nursing Practice (Supplement), 7*(3), 58S–61S.

Nichols, B. L. (2006). The impact of global nurse migration on health services delivery. *Policy, Politics, & Nursing Practice (Supplement), 7*(3), 6S–8S.

Perrin, M. E., Hagopian, A., Sales, A., & Huang, B. (2007). Nurse migration and its implications for Philippine hospitals. *International Nursing Review, 54*(3), 219–226.

Pittman, P., Aiken, L. H., & Buchan, J. (2007). *Health Services Research, 42*(3p2), 1275–1280.

Raghuram, P. (2007). Interrogating the language of integration: The case of internationally recruited nurses. *Journal of Clinical Nursing, 16*(12), 2246–2251.

Rosenkoetter, M., & Nardi, D. (2007). American Academy of Nursing Expert Panel on Global Nursing and Health: White paper on global nursing and health. *Journal of Transcultural Nursing, 18*(4), 305–315.

Smith, P., & Mackintosh, M. (2007). Profession, market and class: Nurse migration and the remaking of division and disadvantage. *Journal of Clinical Nursing, 16*(12), 2213–2220.

Yan, J. (2006). Health services delivery: Reframing policies for global nursing migration in North America—A Caribbean perspective. *Policy, Politics, & Nursing Practice (Supplement), 7*(3), 71S–75S.

Yearwood, E. L. (2007). The crisis of nurse migration in developing countries. *Journal of Child & Adolescent Psychiatric Nursing, 20*(3), 191–192.

WEB RESOURCES

American Organization of Nurse Executives (AONE): Policy Statement on Foreign Nurse Recruitment (Approved by the AONE Board of Directors, December 2003)	http://www.hospitalconnect.com/aone/advocacy/ps_foreign_recruitment.html
Commission on Graduates of Foreign Nursing Schools	http://www.cgfns.org/
Commonwealth Code of Practice for the International Recruitment of Health Workers	http://www.thecommonwealth.org/shared_asp_files/uploadedfiles/%7B7BDD970B-53AE-441D-81DB-1B64C37E992A%7D_CommonwealthCodeofPractice.pdf
Global Health Workforce Alliance	www.ghwa.org

International Council of Nurses: International Forum Discusses Alternatives to Nurse Migration	http://www.icn.ch/sewapr-sept03.htm#2
International Nurse Mobility Trends and Policy Implications (World Health Organization, International Council of Nurses, and Royal College of Nursing)	http://www.icn.ch/global/Issue5migration.pdf
International Labour Organization—International Labour Migration	http://www.ilo.org/public/english/protection/migrant/
The ABC's of Healthcare Immigration: Nonimmigrant Visa Options for Nurses	http://www.visalaw.com/h06jul/4hjul06.html
National Council Licensure Examination for Registered Nurses (NCLEX-RN) (providing information on the NCLEX examination)	http://www.ncsbn.org/
International Centre on Nurse Migration	http://www.intlnursemigration.org/
International Council of Nurses	http://www.icn.ch/
Sigma Theta Tau, International Honor Society of Nursing: Position Statement on International Nurse Migration	www.nursingsociety.org/aboutus/Documents/policy_migration.doc
Nurses Board of Victoria: Position Statement: Ethical Recruitment of Overseas Nurses	http://www.nbv.org.au/media/43646/position%20statement%20%20ethical%20recruitment%20of%20overseas%20nurses.pdf

CHAPTER 7

Unlicensed Assistive Personnel and the Registered Nurse

• CAROL J. HUSTON •

Learning Objectives

The learner will be able to:

1. Identify driving forces leading to the increased use of unlicensed assistive personnel (UAP) in acute care settings beginning in the early 1990s.
2. Name common job titles for UAP.
3. Differentiate between the minimum mandated educational preparation of certified nurses aides (CNAs) and UAP.
4. Analyze current research studies that explore the effect of increased UAP use on manpower (direct care and supervisory) costs.
5. Explore current benchmark research linking staffing mix with patient outcomes and summarize the state of the literature.
6. Discuss how the role of the registered nurse (RN) as delegator has changed with the increased use of UAP.
7. Examine how the role of delegator and supervisor of UAP increases the scope of liability for the RN.

8. Explore strategies for restructuring work environments and clarifying role expectations so that professional nurses spend less time on nonnursing tasks.
9. Identify safeguards that health care organizations can put in place to increase the likelihood that UAP are used both effectively and appropriately as members of the health care team.
10. Outline current state legislation seeking to address minimum UAP education and competencies.
11. Discuss factors contributing to both the current and projected shortages of UAP, particularly in long-term care settings.
12. Reflect on the personal self-confidence and skill that an RN might need in delegating to UAP.

In an effort to contain spiraling health care costs, many health care providers in the 1990s restructured their organizations by eliminating registered nurse (RN) positions and/or by replacing licensed professional nurses with unlicensed assistive personnel (UAP). UAP are "individuals trained to function in an assistive role to RNs to provide patient care as delegated by the nurse" (Steefel, 2007, para 1). The term includes, but is not limited to, nurse aides, nurse extenders, health care aides, technicians, orderlies, assistants, and attendants.

Although the acronym UAP will generally be used throughout this chapter, it is noteworthy that in 2007, the American Nurses Association (ANA) stopped using the term UAP and replaced it with NAP, suggesting that many *nursing assistive personnel* (NAP) are now licensed or for-

mally recognized in some manner (ANA, 2007). The ANA argued that use of the term "unlicensed" is inaccurate.

Regardless of nomenclature, unlicensed workers are a significant part of the health care landscape and have been for some time. By the late 1990s, hospitals began actively recruiting the RNs who had been let go just a few years before. RNs who lost their jobs, however, were slow to return to the acute care setting, despite a widespread, worsening nursing shortage. As a result, hospitals again increased their use of UAP early in the 21st century in an effort to supplement their licensed nursing staff.

Both as a result of the restructuring of the 1990s and the current serious nursing shortage, the skill mix in many hospitals includes a significant percentage of UAP. In fact, almost all RNs in acute care institutions and long-term care facilities are involved in some way with the assignment, delegation, and supervision of UAP.

Several reasons are commonly cited for the increased use of UAP. The primary argument for using UAP in acute care settings is usually cost, although the professional nursing shortage is a contributing factor (Marquis & Huston, 2009). Another widely recognized benefit of using UAP is that they can free professional nurses from tasks and assignments (specifically, nonnursing functions) that can be completed by less well-trained personnel at a lower cost.

So why has the increased use of UAP created so much controversy? The answer is that in many institutions, UAP are not supplements to, but replacements of, professional RN staff. This is of concern because empirical research exists regarding what percentage of the staffing mix can safely be represented by UAP without negatively affecting patient outcomes. In addition, minimum national educational and training requirements have not been established for UAP, and their scope of practice varies from institution to institution. All of these issues raise serious questions as to whether greater use of UAP represents an effective solution to dwindling health care resources or whether it is an economically driven, short-term response that could lead to compromised patient outcomes.

This chapter, however, does not argue for the elimination of UAP. Instead, it addresses what safeguards must be incorporated in the use of UAP so that safe, accessible, and affordable nursing care is possible.

MOTIVATION TO USE UNLICENSED ASSISTIVE PERSONNEL

The primary arguments for using UAP are maximizing human resources and cost reduction. UAP can maximize human resources because they free professional nurses from tasks and assignments that do not require independent thinking and professional judgment. This is significant because much of a typical nurse's time is spent on nonnursing tasks and functions. Nonnursing tasks and functions are those routine or standardized activities that can be done by an individual with minimal training and do not require a great deal of individual client assessment, independent thought, or decision making. Examples of nonnursing activities include making a bed, doing vital signs, feeding clients, measuring intakes and outputs, and obtaining a weight or height.

Research by Buerhaus, Donelan, Ulrich, DesRoches, and Dittus (2007) suggested that only 41% of the time in a typical RN workweek is spent on direct patient care. The remainder of the time is directed at engaging in patient care documentation (23%), locating supplies and equipment related to patient care (8%), transporting patients (5%), making patient-related telephone calls (8%), engaging in meetings or activities related to patient safety or quality improvement (7%), and engaging in shift changes or other hand-off functions (7%).

Domrose (2008) presented similarly disturbing findings in her study of 767 medical/surgical nurses in 36 hospitals across the country in 2005 and 2006. This study found that nurses spent less than 40% of their time in patient's rooms and that less than 20% of nursing time—about 1 hour and 20 minutes per shift—was spent on patient care activities. In addition, only 7% of time was spent on patient assessment and reading vital signs.

DISCUSSION POINT

Why are professional registered nurses still completing so many nonnursing tasks? Are they reluctant to delegate them to ancillary personnel, or are there inadequate support personnel to take on these tasks?

Cost savings associated with UAP use—the second argument for increased UAP use—are less clear. A meta-analysis by Thungjaroenkul, Cummings, and Embleton (2007) found that a lack of coherence in definitions and measurement tools for cost makes it difficult to conclude with certainty the results of nurse staffing on hospital costs. They concluded, however, that patient costs were generally reduced with greater RN staffing due to the higher knowledge and skill level of the RN to provide more effective nursing care and the reduction in patient resource consumption.

Likewise, a study by Needleman, Buerhaus, Stewart, Zelevinski, and Mattke (2006) found a negative relationship between the cost estimation based on length of stay (LOS) and the ratio of RNs to other nursing staff. In other words, increasing the hours provided by RNs yielded cost savings resulting from lowered death rates and reduced LOS. The study also noted that increasing nursing hours, with or without increasing the proportion of hours provided by RNs, reduced days, adverse outcomes, and patient deaths, but with a net increase in hospital costs of 1.5% or less at the staffing levels modeled.

Many experts, however, have reported that UAP use failed to produce anticipated cost savings in some hospitals. Many of these hospitals resumed reliance on RNs due to the greater flexibility associated with a larger cadre of RNs.

EDUCATIONAL REQUIREMENTS FOR UNLICENSED ASSISTIVE PERSONNEL

Some monitoring of the regulation, education, and use of UAP has been ongoing since the early 1950s; however, most of this has been for *certified nurse's aides*. The Omnibus Budget Reconciliation Act (OBRA) of 1987 established regulations for the education and certification of *nurse's aides* (minimum of 75 hours of theory and practice and successful completion of an examination in both areas). No federal or community standards have been established, however, for training the more broadly defined UAP.

Indeed, most UAP training is completed by the employing facility and occurs without formal certification. Formal training programs that do exist are completed at vocational schools and community colleges and typically focus on long-term care, providing certifications only as necessary to meet state requirements.

Still, this formal training is often inadequate. In 2002, the Office of the Inspector General of the Department of Health and Human Services issued a report on *Nurse Aide Training* (Texas Nurses Association [TNA], 2004). This report, which looked at the training of nurse aides for nursing homes, concluded that nurse aide training had not kept pace with the changes in long-term care settings and that teaching methods for nurse aides were ineffective and teaching sessions too brief to provide the didactic and hands-on experience that was necessary to achieve competence. The report urged improvement of competency evaluation program requirements for nurse aides.

Of even more concern is the fact that nurse aides are used even more widely today than in 1998 when TNA convened its first task force on the subject. Today, nurse aides are being used in many settings other than long-term care. Extended utilization and reports on the need to set specific competency-based training make it inappropriate for nurse aides to continue to be trained to deliver care only in long-term care settings (TNA, 2004). For efficiency and safety, it is clear that a standardized curriculum that addresses the skill sets needed in the many settings where nurse aides are used should be implemented. The TNA argued that because aides

support the care delivered by RNs and licensed vocational nurses, it is logical that the aides' education should be under the purview of the nursing board.

Similar to long-term care, the education and training of UAP in acute care settings is inadequate. In fact, there are no required educational standards or guidelines for the use of UAP in acute care settings. Instead, UAP educational and training requirements for acute care settings are generally facility based, and the UAP is often trained only in the skill sets needed for that particular facility (Case, 2004). This is important to remember when UAP transfer from one facility to another because no assumption should be made about UAP competency levels to perform certain tasks, despite their work experience.

CONSIDER

A high school diploma may not be required to work as UAP in acute care settings.

Some agencies argue that the work experience reported by their UAP is a substitute for formal education and training. Potter and Grant (2004) reported that experienced UAP shared stories of "knowing their patients." This level of knowing did not involve scientific principles or a detailed knowledge base such as that possessed by an RN but was a practical level of knowing that allowed them to contribute to the patient care process.

DISCUSSION POINT

Is it possible for RNs to assess individual UAP's "knowing" of patients and, if so, should this influence their task assignment to that UAP?

The increased use of UAP, called by some the "deskilling of the nursing workforce," has raised concern among consumers and legislators alike. The result has been the introduction of legislation at the state level. Some states have introduced legislation to regulate UAP practice through registration and certification. Others have proposed direct regulation of UAP by passing legislation that requires UAP to be certified by meeting education and competency requirements. Still others require the state boards of nursing or the department of health to register or certify UAP.

In 2007, the ANA suggested six actions that should be taken to create a national and/or state policy agenda about the educational preparation of UAP or NAP and

AMERICAN NURSES ASSOCIATION'S (2007) RECOMMENDATIONS FOR A NATIONAL AND/OR STATE POLICY AGENDA FOR NURSING ASSISTIVE PERSONNEL (NAP)

1. Recognize that the NAP should never be considered or used as a replacement for registered nurses or licensed practical nurses.
2. Aggressively promote the understanding that delegation is an integral part of professional nursing practice and not a supervisory act connected to acting on behalf of the employer.
3. Establish recognized competencies for the NAP that will guide the development of a core curriculum.
4. Promote national nursing initiatives to establish criteria and guidelines for the clinical training of the NAP through the use of evidence-based research, preparing the NAP to provide routine care in predictable patient functions.
5. Establish systems for training, certification, registry, and disciplinary monitoring of the NAP.
6. Support continued efforts to implement recommendations related to patient safety and quality and the nursing work environment articulated in reports generated by the Institute of Medicine such as *To Err is Human: Building a Safer Health System; Crossing the Quality Chasm: A New Health System for the 21st Century;* and *Keeping Patients Safe: Transforming the Work Environment of Nurses.*

Source: Excerpted from American Nurses Association (2007). *Position statement. Registered nurses utilization of nursing assistive personnel in all settings.* Available at: http://www.nursingworld.org/MainMenuCategories/HealthcareandPolicyIssues/ANAPositionStatements/uap/UnlicensedAssistivePersonnel.aspx. Accessed August 28, 2008.

the competencies they should have for safe practice. These are shown in Box 7.1.

DISCUSSION POINT

Why has the movement to regulate UAP education and training occurred only at the state level? Why has there been no national movement to do the same?

The need for state legislation to regulate UAP education and training should not imply, however, that all UAP are undereducated and unprepared for the roles they have been asked to fill. Indeed, UAP educational levels vary from less than that of a high school graduate to those holding advanced degrees (Case, 2004). This merely suggests that RNs, in delegating to UAP, must make no assumptions about the educational preparation or training of that UAP. Instead, the RN must carefully assess what skills and knowledge each UAP has or risk increased personal liability for the failure to do so.

UNLICENSED ASSISTIVE PERSONNEL SCOPE OF PRACTICE

In addition to existing state regulations regarding UAP education and training, as well as required competen-

cies, many professional nursing organizations have studied the use and effect of UAP and are adopting position statements regarding their use. The International Council of Nurses (ICN), in their position statement *Delegation and Supervision,* stated that UAP cannot perform tasks without supervision, and they define supervision as providing guidance and overseeing the delegated activities either through direct observation or through verbal instruction and direction (Steefel, 2007). "The bottom line is that RNs must be available for supervision and support and must evaluate tasks that UAP perform, and follow-up on the information reported" (Steefel, para 11).

In the early 1990s, the ANA took the position that the control and monitoring of assistive personnel in clinical settings should be performed through the use of existing mechanisms that regulate nursing practice. Typically, this includes the state board of nursing, institutional policies, and external agency standards.

In follow-up, many state boards of nursing issued recommendations regarding scope of practice for UAP or attempted to delineate the relationship between RNs and UAP. Few states, however, used the ANA or National Council of State Boards of Nursing (NCSBN) definitions for delegation, supervision, or assignment. Most states also report that there are no standardized curricula in place for UAP employed in acute-care hospitals. The end result, then, is that there is no universally accepted scope of practice for UAP.

Some state boards of nursing have issued task lists for UAP (lists of activities considered to be within the scope of practice for UAP). However, in creating such a list, an unofficial scope of practice is created, and this suggests that such individuals will be performing activities independently. Task lists also suggest that there is no need for delegation, in that the UAP already has a list of nursing activities that he or she may perform without waiting for the delegation process (Marquis & Huston, 2009).

DISCUSSION POINT

What happens when the condition of a patient changes? Is the training of UAP adequate to recognize changes in clients' conditions that warrant seeking intervention from the licensed nurse?

One major national effort to define the scope of practice for UAP was undertaken by the ANA in their delineation of tasks appropriate for UAP practice in the early 1990s. Multiple revisions have followed. Yet, despite the efforts by the ANA and state boards of nursing, the reality is that at the institutional level, most health care organizations interpret regulations broadly, allowing UAP a broader scope of practice than that advocated by professional nursing associations or state boards of nursing. In addition, although some institutions limit the scope of practice for UAP to nonnursing functions, many organizations allow the UAP to perform skills traditionally reserved for the licensed nurse.

CONSIDER

Given the lack of national regulatory standards regarding the scope of practice for UAP, many health care institutions allow UAP to complete tasks traditionally reserved for licensed practitioners.

In some cases, UAP known as *unlicensed medication administration personnel* (UMAP) or *medication technicians* (MT) also administer medications. In addition, *Certified Medicine Aides* (CMAs) have worked in licensed nursing home settings since the 1970s (Maryland Board of Nursing, 2008). In fact, Mitty and Flores (2007) reported that more than half of the states in the United States permit UAP or medication technicians to assist with or administer medications. Mitty and Flores suggested that this nursing activity (or task) is more likely authorized as a result of state-assisted living regulations than by support and approval of the state board of nursing. They also suggested that the terms "assistance" and "administration" are either poorly defined or used interchangeably in many of these regulations, raising concerns for most nurses in terms of delegation, liability for practice, and accountability.

CONSIDER

More than half of the states in the United States allow UAP to assist with or administer medications.

A similarly expanded scope of practice for UAP in assisted living settings was reported by Young et al. (2008), who noted that medications in most assisted living settings are managed primarily by UAP, with limited professional involvement. This is in contrast to skilled nursing facilities (SNFs), where licensed nurses are engaged in medication administration.

UAP also administer drugs in school settings. School nurses, however, are waging a battle to stop the expansion of UAP practice in terms of the drugs they are allowed to administer (e.g., currently only licensed school nurses can administer insulin). Gursky and Ryser (2007) suggested that because school nurses are often assigned multiple schools and cannot be present at all sites simultaneously, tasks must often be delegated to UAP.

It is the position of the National Association of School Nurses, however, that the use of assistive personnel may be appropriate to supplement professional school nursing services in certain situations, but they should never supplant school nurses or be permitted to practice nursing without a license (Safe Staffing for School Nurses, 2008).

Indeed, a University of Iowa study conducted by McCarthy, Kelly, and Reed (2000) reported that nearly half of the school nurses surveyed reported medication errors in their schools during the previous year. A major factor in medication errors was the use of "unlicensed assistive personnel" such as school secretaries, health aides, teachers, parents, and even students to administer medications. Only 25% of the nurses said they administered all the medication in their schools. The other 75% said that unlicensed personnel routinely dispense medications to students.

The reality, then, is that in many settings, UAP are inappropriately performing functions that are within the legal practice of nursing. This is likely a violation of the state nursing practice act and poses a threat to public safety: "This model of practice, however, is considered a viable alternative to care provided primarily by registered nurses and demand for UAP is only expected to grow" (Kleinman & Saccomano, 2006, p. 163).

CONSIDER

Many patients given direct care by UAP assume that UAP are licensed nurses. This confusion is promulgated when health care professionals do not include their credentials on their nametags or do not introduce themselves to patients according to their actual job title.

Steefel (2007) warned that certain professional responsibilities related to nursing care must never be delegated. These professional responsibilities include patient assessment, nursing diagnosis, care planning, patient teaching, and health education.

It is critical, then, that the RN never lose sight of his or her ultimate responsibility for ensuring that patients receive appropriate, high-quality care. This means that although the UAP may complete nonnursing functions such as bathing the patient, taking vital signs, and measuring and recording intake and output, it is the RN who must analyze that information using highly developed critical thinking skills and then use the nursing process to see that desired patient outcomes are achieved. Only RNs have the formal authority to practice nursing, and activities that rely on the nursing process or require specialized skill, expert knowledge, or professional judgment should never be delegated.

UNLICENSED ASSISTIVE PERSONNEL AND PATIENT OUTCOMES

The outcomes associated with the increased use of UAP are not fully known; however, considerable evidence exists that demonstrates a direct link between decreased RN staffing and declines in patient outcomes. Some of these declines in patient outcomes include an increased incidence of patient falls, nosocomial infections, increased physical restraint use, and medication errors.

In a Delphi survey of 24 experts from 10 countries, Van den Heede, Clarke, Sermeus, Vleugels, and Aiken

(2007) found that the highest consensus levels regarding sensitivity to nurse staffing were for nurse-perceived quality of care, patient satisfaction, and pain. Nursing care hours per patient day (NCHPPD) received the highest consensus score as a valid measure of the number of nursing staff. As a skill mix variable, the proportion of RNs to total nursing staff achieved the highest consensus level.

Hall, Doran, and Pink (2004), in their descriptive, correlational study of 19 teaching hospitals in Ontario, Canada, found that the lower the proportion of professional nursing staff employed on a unit, the higher was the number of medication errors and wound infections. Similarly, Dunton, Gajewski, Taunton, and Moore (2004) reported that higher fall rates were associated with fewer nursing hours per patient day and a lower percentage of registered nurses, although the relationship varied by unit type.

There are also outcome data available regarding the use of UAP to assist with and administer medications. Young et al. (2008) looked at medication administration errors in assisted living settings (where UAP administer most of the medications) in 12 sites in three states (Oregon, Washington, and New Jersey). Of their 4,866 observations, there were 1,373 errors (a 28.2% error rate). Of these, 70.8% were wrong time, 12.9% were wrong dose, 11.1% were an omitted dose, 3.5% were an extra dose, 1.5% were an unauthorized drug, and 0.2% were the wrong drug.

Canham et al. (2007) found similar problems with errors in the school setting, where school office staff members (UAP) are typically delegated this task. In that study, five school nurses developed and participated in a medication audit of 154 medications. Audit results showed a wide range of errors and discrepancies, including problems with transcription, physician orders or lack thereof, timing, documentation, and storage.

A more complete review of the literature on the relationships among nurse staffing, staffing mix, and patient outcomes is included in Chapter 5.

REGISTERED NURSE LIABILITY FOR SUPERVISION AND DELEGATION OF UNLICENSED ASSISTIVE PERSONNEL

Delegation has long been a function of registered nursing, although the scope of delegation and the tasks being delegated have changed dramatically over the last two decades. In the 1990s, some health care institutions began assigning nonnursing health care workers to nursing departments under the supervision of a nurse manager. As a result, the professional nurse (RN) role changed in many acute care institutions from one of direct care provider to one requiring delegation of patient care to others.

This role of delegator and supervisor increased the scope of legal liability for the RN. Although there is limited case law involving nursing delegation and supervision, it is generally accepted that the RN is responsible for adequate supervision of the person to whom an assignment has been delegated. Although nurses are not automatically held liable for all acts of negligence on the part of those they supervise, they may be held liable if they were negligent in the supervision of those employees at the time that those employees committed the negligent acts (Marquis & Huston, 2009).

Liability is based on a supervisor's failure to determine which patient needs could safely be assigned to a subordinate or for failing to closely monitor a subordinate who requires such supervision. Experienced nurses have traditionally been expected to work with minimal supervision. The RN who delegates care to another competent RN does not have the same legal obligation to closely supervise that person's work as when the care is delegated to UAP. In assigning tasks to UAP, then, the RN must be aware of the job description, knowledge base, and demonstrated skills of each person.

Quallich (2005) developed a guide to assist nurses in determining situations in which delegation can appro-priately be done. Although the list created by Quallich was for a urologic unit, it is an example of the type of guideline that should be available on all units when delegating to UAP. Most important, the guide gives examples of tasks that cannot be delegated. Some examples of professional responsibilities include patent assessment, care planning, patient teaching, and patient outcome evaluation and interpreting test results.

In addition, Newhouse, Steinhauser, and Berk (2007) developed a test with acceptable estimates of reliability and validity to identify UAP who could successfully perform their job in four essential knowledge-based domains (math, patient data collection, medical terminology, and reporting abnormal data) and suggested that the tool be used as a screening tool for UAP.

The ANA has also identified general principles for RNs to use in delegating to NAP. These are shown in Box 7.2.

CONSIDER

The UAP has no license to lose for "exceeding scope of practice," and nationally established standards to state what the limits should be for UAP in terms of scope of practice do not exist. It is the RN who bears the legal liability for allowing UAP to perform tasks that should be accomplished only by a licensed health care professional.

BOX 7.2 | AMERICAN NURSE ASSOCIATION (2007) RECOMMENDATIONS FOR REGISTERED NURSES WHO WORK WITH NURSING ASSISTIVE PERSONNEL (NAP)

1. Recognize and utilize the legal authority that is vested to the RN by the state nurse practice act specific to the delegation of nonprofessional tasks to an adequately trained NAP.

2. Acknowledge and understand the guidance inherent in the professional and specialty nursing scope and standards of practice with regard to the delegation of nonprofessional tasks to an adequately trained NAP.

3. Understand the relevant employer policies, procedures, and position descriptions related to utilization of NAP within the facility.

4. Utilize the right and obligation to know the set of skills that the NAP is competent to perform in order to promote safe patient care. This information should be documented and readily available to the RN.

5. Exercise decision-making authority, based on professional judgment, regarding whether or not to delegate a particular task to the NAP relevant to the patient care situation.

Excerpted from American Nurses Association (2007). *Position statement. Registered nurses utilization of nursing assistive personnel in all settings.* Available at:
http://www.nursingworld.org/MainMenuCategories/HealthcareandPolicyIssues/ANAPositionStatements/uap/UnlicensedAssistivePersonnel.aspx. Accessed August 28, 2008.

The bottom line is that delegating to UAP is similar to delegating to other types of health care workers. RNs are always accountable for the care given and must be responsible for instructing UAP as to who needs care and when. The UAP should be accountable for knowing how to properly perform their segment of assigned care and for knowing when other workers should be called in for tasks beyond the limits of their knowledge and training. As such, the UAP does bear some personal accountability for their actions, despite the legal doctrine of *respondeat superior* (the employer can be held legally liable for the conduct of employees whose actions he or she has a right to direct or control).

Case (2004) agreed, arguing that although *respondeat superior* applies only to the employer, an RN, LPN, UAP, and other employees are nonetheless responsible for their own actions. The RN then may be sued individually for delegation only if it is inappropriate according to the state's nurse practice act and the policies of the facility (Case).

DISCUSSION POINT

Do most UAP believe that they can be held legally liable and accountable for their actions if they are delegated to do something by an RN that is beyond their scope of practice or training?

Regardless of liability issues, the need for nurses to have highly developed delegation skills has never been greater than it is today. The ability to use delegation skills appropriately will help to reduce the personal liability associated with supervising and delegating to UAP. It will also ensure that clients' needs are met and their safety is not jeopardized.

CREATING A SAFE WORK ENVIRONMENT

There are things that health care organizations can do to increase the likelihood that UAP are used both effectively and appropriately as members of the health care team. First, the organization must have a clearly defined organization structure in which RNs are recognized as leaders of the health care team. This organization structure must facilitate RN evaluation of UAP job performance and encourage UAP accountability to the RN.

Job descriptions must also be developed by health care agencies that clearly define the roles and responsibilities of all categories of caregivers. These descriptions

should be consistent with that state's nurse practice legislation, as well as with community standards of care, and should reflect differences between the roles of licensed and unlicensed personnel. Policies should facilitate adequate supervision of UAP by RNs and restrict UAP to simple tasks that can be performed safely. In addition, worker credentials should be readily apparent on the nametags worn by nursing health care personnel.

Second, uniform training and orientation programs for UAP must be established to ensure that preparation is adequate to provide at least minimum standards of safe patient care. These training and orientation programs should be based on clearly defined job descriptions for UAP. In addition, organizational education programs must be developed for all personnel to learn the roles and responsibilities of different categories of caregivers. In addition, to protect their patients and their professional license, RNs must continue to seek current information regarding national efforts to standardize scope of practice for UAP and professional guidelines regarding what can be safely delegated to UAP.

In addition, there must be adequate program development in leadership and delegation skills for RNs before UAP are introduced. Delegation is a learned skill, and much can be done to better prepare RNs for this role. Educational programs that produce graduate nurses must explore the nature of the RN role, with a focus on professional nurse leadership roles, to better prepare them to meet the challenges of working in restructured health care settings. Practicing RNs should have opportunities for continuing education in the principles of delegation and supervision. This will allow them not only to recognize the limitations of UAP scope of practice, but also to gain confidence in differentiating between skills requiring licensure and those that do not. (See Research Study Fuels the Controversy on page 125.)

THE UNLICENSED ASSISTIVE PERSONNEL SHORTAGE

Finally, if all the issues related to the education, training, scope of practice, and delegation to UAP are resolved, there may be an even greater problem. There may not be enough UAP to meet the need that has been established. High turnover rates and severe shortages of direct-care workers are a problem in the health care industry.

Research Study Fuels the Controversy: Registered Nurses, Unlicensed Assistive Personnel, and Patient Care

This qualitative study used a phenomenological approach to describe nurses' experiences of delegation to UAP in a large metropolitan hospital. Seventeen in-depth interviews were conducted with acute care nurses to examine the nature and significance of delegation to UAP.

STUDY FINDINGS

The research found that nurses define delegation in a variety of ways. For some nurses, delegation is viewed explicitly, in that the UAP is asked to carry out a particular task. Other nurses view delegating to UAP as involving both explicit and implicit tasks. The authors concluded that delegation implies interdependence between the nurse and the UAP and that interventions are needed to improve the relationship and communication between them to improve the quality of care. They also suggested that ultimately the shared values of nurses and UAP must focus on achieving optimal outcomes for patients.

Standing, T. S., & Anthony, M. K. (2008). Delegation: What it means to acute care nurses. *Applied Nursing Research, 21*(1), 8–14.

There are 2.3 million UAP, comprising almost 25% of all health care workers in health care delivery settings (Rainer, 2004), and a Bureau of Labor Statistics report estimated that by 2008, the demand for nonprofessional direct care staff, such as UAP, will have increased by more than 80% from the 1998 level.

Indeed, there is a nationwide shortage of well-trained UAP in all settings, and although many states report recruitment and retention of support personnel as a major area of concern, few are actively addressing the situation. Similarly, a study in 2002 by the Center for Health Workforce Studies in New York found that more than 50% of states reported a shortage of certified nurse aides (Healthcare Workforce Shortage, n.d.)

One problem contributing to this shortage is the high turnover rate for nursing assistants. A survey by Kluger (2006) of 854 facility administrators in six states showed that the average annual staff turnover rate for certified nurse aides was 56.4%.

The reasons for this high turnover rate are varied, but low pay and the physical and emotional demands of the job are certainly a part of it. Pfefferle and Weinberg (2008) added that many direct care workers encounter negative messages from their managers, supervisors, coworkers, and sometimes residents about the meaning and value of their work. As a result, many unlicensed workers "cast themselves as the last defense for residents, as the ones doing the work that no one else will do" (Pfefferle & Weinberg, p. 959).

In addition, few employers provide UAP employer-paid benefits such as health insurance coverage, retirement benefits, or childcare. Furthermore, there are limited career paths for aides who do not want to achieve a licensed job category (e.g., LPN, RN), and they often have little direct input into organizational decision-making.

Working conditions are also often less than ideal. Because of high UAP turnover and absenteeism, those UAP who do work must often work short-handed, which leads to greater stress. A study released by the California HealthCare Foundation in December 2004 showed that only 1 in 10 of California's skilled nursing facilities fully comply with all federal care standards for minimum nursing staff requirements, and that requirement is only 3.2 hours of nursing care per patient per day (Nursing Homes Fall Short, 2004 on page 125).

> ### CONSIDER
> "The number of staff on duty [in nursing homes] varies according to the three shifts of the day, but the brunt of work falls on the certified nursing aides. They perform the hands-on tasks needed by residents for an average of less than $10 an hour, and the way those direct-care workers approach their jobs makes all the difference in the satisfaction of patients and families" (Rotstein, 2002, para 65).

Overcoming both the current and future UAP shortage will not be easy. The pool of younger women, who traditionally comprise UAP (particularly in long-term care settings), is stagnant (Rotstein, 2002). Rotstein stated this lack of manpower—or more accurately, womanpower—is already used often by the long-term care industry to defend its shortcomings. Indeed, a government study found that fewer than 1 in 10 nursing homes employs the optimum number of nurses and aides. Few facilities are ever cited for understaffing, however, because minimum government standards are set far below the levels needed to help assure high-quality care (Rotstein).

Indeed, Rainer (2004) suggested that a variance in minimum staffing levels exists across hospitals and nursing homes and, according to the *Keeping Patients Safe* report, minimum standards for staffing in nursing homes need to be updated. Federal regulations are out of date and do not reflect new knowledge on safe staffing levels. Minimum standards for RNs require only one licensed nurse in a nursing home, regardless of its size.

The bottom line, then, is that the demand for UAP is growing rapidly and the difficulty of meeting future demand is exacerbated by the fact that the population of persons who have traditionally filled these jobs is declining.

CONCLUSIONS

The increased use of UAP presents both opportunities and challenges for the American health care system. The position of the American Nurses Association (2007, p. 8) is that "the utilization of nursing assistive personnel (NAP) in the provision of specific aspects of direct and indirect patient care, as a result of delegation and direction by a registered nurse, is an appropriate, safe, and resource-efficient method of providing nursing care." Clearly, this is the case, and UAP play an increasingly integral role in care delivery. Indeed, they provide most of the paid long-term care needed in this country.

Nonetheless, the challenge continues to be to use UAP only to provide personal care needs or nursing

tasks that do not require the skill and judgment of the RN. With increasing patient loads and the current nursing shortage, many health care organizations and the RNs who work within them are tempted to allow UAP to perform tasks that should be limited to professional nursing practice. Nurses must remember, however, that the responsibility for assuring that patients are protected and that UAP do not exceed their scope of practice ultimately falls to the RN. When UAP are allowed to encroach into professional nursing care, patients are placed at risk.

As noted by Stepanek (2003, para 21),

UAP were brought into health care ostensibly to assist the RN in the provision of care: The lines defining the practice between these non-licensed "helpers" and highly-educated RNs have blurred to the point where patients no longer routinely know the qualifications of the person providing their care. Name badges that previously read, "Registered Nurse" now read "nursing services staff," leaving patients uninformed and less than confident. This "removing of the guardrails" that once ensured patients with quality nursing should be every bit as terrifying as a rocky mountain drive is to a committed acrophobic . . . if not more so.

When patients approach health care, they too assume that the guardrails are in place; however, for patients, the blurring of the lines between the practice of RNs and UAP makes it nearly impossible to make an informed decision about continuing their journey.

Certainly at some point, given the increasing complexity of health care and the increasing acuity of patient illnesses, there is a maximum representation of UAP in the staffing mix that should not be breached. Those levels have not yet been determined. Nor have states been able to reach a consensus regarding the education, training, and scope of practice needed for UAP to safely practice. Until these answers are found, the likelihood is that UAP will continue to constitute a significant portion of the nursing workforce and the boundary between UAP and RN practice will continue to be blurred.

FOR ADDITIONAL DISCUSSION

1. Is cost or the nursing shortage the greater driving force in increased UAP use in acute care hospitals today?

2. Is institutional training and certification of UAP a precursor to future initiatives for institutional licensure of registered nurses?

3. Are the cost savings associated with increased UAP use offset by the need for greater supervision by RNs and potential declines in patient outcomes?

4. Should UAP be allowed to administer medications? Perform intravenous cannulation? Change sterile dressings?

5. Do you believe that patients typically are aware whether it is the UAP or licensed nurse that is caring for them?

6. How comfortable do you believe most RNs are in the role of delegator to UAP? Do you believe most RNs feel clarity regarding role differentiation between the RN and the UAP?

7. Should the training and certification of UAP fall under the purview of state boards of registered nursing?

REFERENCES

American Nurses Association (ANA) (2007). *Position statement. Registered nurses utilization of nursing assistive personnel in all settings.* Available at: http://www.nursingworld.org/MainMenuCategories/HealthcareandPolicyIssues/ANAPositionStatements/uap/UnlicensedAssistivePersonnel.aspx. Accessed August 28, 2008.

Buerhaus, P., Donelan, K., Ulrich, B. T., DesRoches, C., & Dittus, R. (2007). Trends in the experiences of hospital-employed registered nurses: Results from three national surveys. *Nursing Economics, 25*(2), 69–80.

Canham. D. L., Bauer, L., Concepcion, M., Luong, J., Peters, J., & Wilde, C. (2007). An audit of medication administration: A glimpse into school health offices. *Journal of School Nursing, 23*(1), 21–27.

Case, B. (2004). Delegation skills. *Advance for Nurses, 1*(3), 20–26.

Domrose, C. (2008). Not enough hours. *Nurse Week (California), 2*(13), 32–33.

Dunton, N., Gajewski, B., Taunton, R. L., & Moore, J. (2004). Nurse staffing and patient falls on acute care hospital units. *Nursing Outlook, 52*(1), 53–59.

Gursky, B. S., & Ryser, B. J. (2007). A training program for unlicensed assistive personnel. *Journal of School Nursing, 23*(2), 92–97.

Hall, L. M., Doran, D., & Pink, G. H. (2004). Nurse staffing models, nursing hours, and patient safety outcomes. *Journal of Nursing Administration, 34*(1), 41–45.

Healthcare workforce shortage (n.d.). *Medical News.* Available at: http://www.hosa.org/emag/articles/medical_news_october03.pdf. Accessed August 28, 2008.

Kleinman, C. S., & Saccomano, S. J. (2006). Registered nurses and unlicensed assistive personnel: An uneasy alliance. *The Journal of Continuing Education in Nursing, 37*(4), 162–170.

Kluger, M. (2006). Staff turnover in nursing homes. *American Journal of Nursing, 106*(10), 71.

Marquis, B., & Huston, C. (2009). *Leadership Roles and Management Functions in Nursing* (6th ed.). Philadelphia: Lippincott Williams & Wilkins.

Maryland Board of Nursing. (2008). *Medicine aide versus medication technician—What is the difference?* Available at: http://www.mbon.org/main.php?v=norm&p=0&c=medtech/medaide_vs_medtech.html. Accessed June 26, 2008.

McCarthy, A., Kelly, M. W., & Reed, D. (2000). Medication administration practices of school nurses. *Journal of School Health, 70*(9), 371–376.

Mitty, E., & Flores, S. (2007). Assisted living column. Assisted living nursing practice: Medication management: Part 2 supervision and monitoring of medication administration by unlicensed assistive personnel. *Geriatric Nursing, 28*(3), 153–160.

Needleman, J., Buerhaus, P., Stewart, M., Zelevinski, K., & Mattke, S. (2006). Nurse staffing in hospitals: Is there a business case for quality? *Health Affairs, 25*(1), 204–211.

Newhouse, R. P., Steinhauser, M., & Berk, R. (2007). Development of an unlicensed assistive personnel job screening test. *Journal of Nursing Measurement, 15*(1), 36–45.

Nursing homes fall short, study finds (2004). *The Sacramento Bee,* December 1, 2004, p. A3, columns 1–3.

Pfefferle, S. G., & Weinberg, D. B. (2008). Certified nurse assistants making meaning of direct care. *Qualitative Health Research, 18*(7), 952–961.

Potter, P., & Grant, E. (2004). Understanding RN and unlicensed assistive personnel working relationships in designing care delivery strategies. *Journal of Nursing Administration, 34*(1), 19–25.

Quallich, S. A. (2005). A bond of trust: Delegation. *Urologic Nursing, 25*(9), 120–123.

Rainer, S. (2004). Nurses work environments require changes for the safety of patients. Available at: http://www.njsna.org/Rainer's%20Report/march_5_2004.htm. Accessed August 9, 2004.

Rotstein, G. (2002). No place like home: Nursing homes struggle with too few nurses, aides for growing elderly population. *Health and Science.* Available at: http://www.post-gazette.com/healthscience/20020922nursinghomes0922p1.asp. Accessed April 18, 2005.

Safe staffing for school nurses (2008). *The Nursing Voice (ANA\C), 13*(2), 1.

Standing, T. S., & Anthony, M. K. (2008). Delegation: What it means to acute care nurses. *Applied Nursing Research, 21*(1), 8–14.

Steefel, L. (2007). Learning to let go. *Nursing Spectrum/Nurse Week (New York).* Available at: http://include.nurse.com/apps/pbcs.dll/article?AID=200770405020. Accessed June 27, 2008.

Stepanek, C. (2003). Executive director's column. Removing the guardrails. *Nebraska Nurse, 36*(4), 2, 4.

Texas Nurses Association (TNA) (2004). *Nursing issues.* Available at: http://www.texasnurses.org/nursingissues/proposedres_04.htm. Accessed April 18, 2005.

Thungjaroenkul, P., Cummings, G., & Embleton, A. (2007). The impact of nurse staffing on hospital costs and patient length of stay: A systematic review. *Nursing Economics, 25*(5), 255–265.

Van den Heede, K., Clarke, S. P., Sermeus, W., Vleugels, A., & Aiken, L. H. (2007). International experts' perspectives on the state of the nurse staffing and patient outcomes literature. *Journal of Nursing Scholarship, 39*(4), 290–297.

Young, H. M., Gray, S. L., McCormick, W. C., Sikma, S. K., Reinhard, S., Johnson, T. L., Christlieb, C., & Allen, T. (2008). Types, prevalence, and potential clinical significance of medication administration errors in assisted living. *Journal of the American Geriatric Society.* Available at: http://www.blackwellsynergy.com.mantis.csuchico.edu/doi/pdf/10.1111/j.1532-5415.2008.01754.x. Accessed June 26, 2008.

BIBLIOGRAPHY

Anderson, K. A. (2008). Grief experiences of CNAs: Relationships with burnout and turnover. *Journal of Gerontological Nursing, 34*(1), 42–49.

Castle, N., Engberg, J., Men, A., & Engberg, J. (2008). Nurse aide agency staffing and quality of care in nursing homes. *Medical Care Research & Review, 65*(2), 232–252.

Center for American Nurses (2007). Registered nurse utilization of nursing assistive personnel statement for adoption. *Prairie Rose, 76*(2), 17–18.

Cherry, B., Ashcraft, A., & Owen, D. (2007). Perceptions of job satisfaction and the regulatory environment among nurse aides and charge nurses in long-term care. *Geriatric Nursing, 28*(3), 183.

Cready, C. M., Yeatts, D. E., Gosdin, M. M., & Potts, H. F. (2008). CNA empowerment: Effects on job performance and work attitudes. *Journal of Gerontological Nursing, 34*(3), 26–35.

Greenberg, M. E. (2007). Nurse entitlement: Protecting what is ours. *AAACN Viewpoint, 29*(4), 4–5.

Howe, L. (2008). Education and empowerment of the nursing assistant: Validating their important role in skin care and pressure ulcer prevention, and demonstrating productivity enhancement and cost savings. *Advances in Skin & Wound Care, 21*(6), 275–281.

Hutton, S., & Gates, D. (2008). Workplace incivility and productivity losses among direct care staff. *AAOHN Journal, 56*(4), 168–175.

Lugo, N. R. (2007). For high-quality care, team up with techs. *Nursing Spectrum (Florida Edition), 17*(10), 36–37.

Metzner, L. (2006). Medication aides: A regulatory update. *Colorado Nurse, 106*(3), 3–4.

Sanders, N. (2008). Update from the Board of Nursing. Frequently asked questions: Delegation by nurses to unlicensed assistive personnel (UAPs). *Alaska Nurse, 58*(1), 9.

Snyder, L. A., Chen, P. Y., & Vacha-Haase, T. (2007). The underreporting gap in aggressive incidents from geriatric patients against certified nursing assistants. *Violence and Victims, 22*(3), 367–379.

Steefel. L. (2007). Nurses can benefit by learning to trust UAPs. *Nursing Spectrum/Nurseweek (California).* Available at: http://include.nurse.com/apps/pbcs.dll/article?AID=2007304120013. Accessed June 27, 2008.

2007 Convention Resolution: Use of LP/VNs and Unlicensed Assistive Personnel (2007). *Journal of Practical Nursing, 57*(2), 10.

Yeatts, D. E., & Cready, C. M. (2007). Consequences of empowered CNA teams in nursing home settings: A longitudinal assessment. *Gerontologist, 47*(3), 323–339.

WEB RESOURCES

American Association of Colleges of Nursing, Tri Council for Nursing, Statement on Assistive Personnel to the Registered Nurse	http://www.aacn.nche.edu/Publications/positions/tricounc.htm
Arizona Nurses Association, Position Statement on the Use of Unlicensed Assistive Personnel When under the Direction of the Registered Nurse	http://www.aznurse.org/default.asp?PageID=10001164
Association of Women's Health, Obstetric, and Neonatal Nurses (AWOHNN), Position Statement, The Role of Unlicensed Assistive Personnel in the Nursing Care for Women and Newborns	http://www.awhonn.org/awhonn/content.do?name=05_HealthPolicyLegislation/5H_PositionStatements.htm
Commonwealth of Massachusetts, Office of Health and Human Services	http://www.mass.gov/?pageID=eohhs2subtopic&L=5&L0=Home&L1=Provider&L2=Certification,+Licensure,+and+Registration&L3=Occupational+and+Professional&L4=Nurse+Aides&sid=Eeohhs2
National Council State Board of Nursing, Delegation and Nursing Assistive Personnel Issues	https://www.ncsbn.org/314.htm
Oncology Nursing Society, Position statement on the use of assistive personnel in cancer care, Revised October 2007	http://www.ons.org/publications/positions/AssistivePersonnel.shtml
Society of Gastroenterology Nurses and Associates, Position Statement, Role Delineation of Assistive Personnel	http://www.sgna.org/Resources/statements/statement8.cfm
South Carolina Board of Nursing, Position Statement, The Practice of Nursing in a School Setting	http://www.llr.state.sc.us/POL/Nursing/index.asp?file=schoolsetting.htm
South Carolina Board of Nursing, Position Statement, Delegation of Nursing Care Tasks To Unlicensed Assistive Personnel (UAP)	http://www.llr.state.sc.us/POL/Nursing/index.asp?file=uaptasks.htm

CHAPTER 8

Socialization and Mentoring

• JEANNE MADISON •

Learning Objectives

The learner will be able to:

1. Define socialization, resocialization, and mentoring.
2. Identify common situations that increase nurses' need for socialization and resocialization.
3. Analyze the historical impact of gender socialization and feminism on the advancement of nursing as a profession.
4. Explore the relationship between professional oppression and empowerment and between oppressed-group behavior and horizontal violence.
5. Describe how Kramer's work on reality shock for new graduate nurses influenced socialization research in nursing.
6. Investigate strategies to assist new graduate nurses with socialization to the professional nursing role.
7. Describe why experienced nurses experiencing role transition often need resocialization, and identify specific strategies to promote such resocialization.
8. Provide examples of positive and negative socialization behaviors common in health care workplace settings.
9. Describe characteristics of classic mentoring relationships, as well as stages common to most mentoring relationships.
10. Compare and contrast the roles of mentor, role model, preceptor, coach, and guide in promoting professional socialization and resocialization.
11. Contrast the historical availability of mentors for men and women and determine whether these trends have changed over time.
12. Postulate reasons that mentoring was historically less available in "traditionally female" occupations as compared to the situation for women in general.
13. Examine how mentors, preceptors, role models, and guides have influenced his or her own professional development and socialization to professional nursing.

Nurses today have many entries and exits from the health care workplace. Nurses change clinical specialties with ease and leave employers for childbirth or child care, to care for elderly parents, for advanced education, or for international nursing experience. Sometimes they return to the health care workplace, often years later, as re-entry or "new" nurses. It is not uncommon for one individual to have multiple careers that are widely divergent and bear little relationship to each other.

Nurses also change from full-time to part-time employment and back again. They enter nursing for the first, second, or third time as young adults, in middle age, or as seniors, and they come from diverse ethnic, religious, and social backgrounds. Many are educated in one country but practice in several other countries. Given this individual variation, as well as diversity in practice patterns, how these nurses are socialized and resocialized in the health care workplace in the 21st century is of profound importance.

SOCIALIZATION: ROLES, SKILLS, VALUES, AND CHANGE

Socialization is the process by which a person acquires the technical skills of his or her society, the knowledge of the kinds of behavior that are understood and acceptable in that society, and the attitudes and values that make conformity with social rules personally meaningful, even gratifying. Socialization has also been called enculturation.

Resocialization occurs when individuals are forced to learn new values, skills, attitudes, and social rules as a result of changes in the type of work they do, the scope of responsibility they hold, or in the workplace setting itself (Marquis & Huston, 2009). Individuals who frequently need resocialization include experienced nurses who change work settings, either within the same organization or in a new organization, and nurses who undertake new roles. Some nurses adapt easily to resocialization, but most experience some stress with role change.

Before the 1970s, little thought was given to how socialization and resocialization occurred in the health care workplace or how new graduates experienced the transition from student to graduate nurse. It was generally believed that because nurses were educated in the hospital environment, they would not be unduly surprised or alarmed by changes in responsibility and accountability on graduation from their nursing program. Kramer's work (1974, 1981) on "reality shock" and issues associated with professional socialization led to a renaissance of this thinking, which continues today.

The latest emphasis on socialization research in nursing occurred, coincidentally, at the same time as another sweeping social phenomenon that profoundly changed nursing and the health care workplace forever: the feminist movement. Research about nursing and women's issues expanded significantly against the backdrop of feminism in the Western world.

To nurses in practice and leadership roles, the incongruencies between the subservience of the work world and the professional practice environment expected by university or college-educated, "enlightened feminist" graduates became abundantly clear. The research spotlight on the female-dominated nursing workplace revealed serious shortcomings and the consequences of maintaining the professional socialization status quo. In addition, an increase in the number of men undertaking nursing education further changed the dynamics within the profession. Clearly, change was needed to meet the expectations of the new professional nurse and to move nursing from under a medical model into an accountable and self-governing profession.

During the 1970s, significant nursing research focused on analyzing the health care workplace in an effort to understand the long-standing mechanisms that disempowered, denigrated, and marginalized nurses and the nursing profession. It was evident that the oppressive forces in place were entrenched, powerful, and advantageous to those who were in power. Reversing the trajectory of negative nurse socialization was no simple task and could be undertaken only by nurses, individually and collectively.

> ### CONSIDER
>
> The oppression of nurses has come not only from outside groups, such as medicine and health care administration, but also from within the profession.

THE HEALTH CARE WORKPLACE IN THE 21ST CENTURY

Negative and positive socialization patterns in the nursing workplace have received wide attention in the literature. The expression used for negative socialization is *horizontal violence*, and it includes manifestations such as bullying, harassment, verbal abuse, and intimidation. Positive socialization is exemplified in the various supportive behaviors associated with mentoring, preceptoring, role modeling, coaching, and guiding. Only recently has significant progress been made for nurses to understand issues associated with the nexus between professional oppression and empowerment.

Anger and Hostility

Exactly what is the experience of new nurses as they are socialized into the health care environment of the 21st century? Ironically, for many nurses it seems easier or safer to turn anger and feelings of intimidation inward or to peers rather than toward supervisors or other organized and long-standing oppressors. Hutchinson, Vickers, Jackson, and Wilkes (2006) described the level of anger and bullying ethos that can dominate behaviors in particular nursing teams. Their research found that bullying sought to "change how individuals thought about themselves, eroding their self-image, destroying their self confidence and shattering the fundamental values they held about their world and themselves" (p. 235).

Additionally and unfortunately, not all nurses are altruistic or interested in the development of other nurses and the nursing profession. Many nurses can identify colleagues in the workplace who habitually target entry-level and/or vulnerable staff to undertake responsibilities and tasks that benefit the taskmaster. Often, delegation of tasks in this manner is a pattern or habit and can involve a number of dependent, unacknowledged, and exploited staff. Fawning and groveling behavior is encouraged and expected by the taskmaster. This person can abuse his or her (perceived) authority, position, or experience and, in the guise of a pseudomentoring bond, encourage the development of an inappropriate workplace relationship. Such relationships should not be confused with mentoring and need to be exposed and named.

Registered nurses are well placed to recognize and name unacceptable workplace behaviors that they observe. Madison and Minichiello (2004) noted that remaining silent or ignoring obviously unhelpful, negative, and discriminatory action in the workplace is no longer an option. Taking action can be intimidating and frightening, but it is necessary and part of a professional's responsibility.

Oppression and Horizontal Violence

The literature is clear that horizontal violence is not unique to nursing; rather, it is found in most oppressed groups and professions. Researchers agree that negative socialization and oppressive behaviors must be eliminated before nurses can assume positive socialization strategies and empower themselves. Understanding typical oppressed-group behavior and horizontal violence is the first step to developing effective change strategies that will reduce and eliminate it.

Oppressed groups typically believe they are oppressed because they are deficient in some way, and, most important, the oppressor defines these deficiencies (Freire, 1968). As this distorted perception is internalized, the oppressed group inadvertently perpetuates the process of oppression. Unsupportive, disempowering, and controlling behaviors *within* the hierarchical nursing structure can easily be identified and demonstrated by horizontal violence. In addition, the oppressive, controlling strategies used by the medical profession and hospital administrators (usually men) are also relatively easy to identify. However, the relationship between those behaviors and the self-inflicted, dysfunctional, oppressive behaviors demonstrated within the nursing profession have been exposed and analyzed only recently.

Oppressed-group behavior includes a number of widely accepted characteristics: feelings of inferiority, powerlessness, inequality, and self-doubt that perpetuate feelings of oppression, which engender feelings of inferiority. Sometimes nurses do not recognize the language they use and the (not so) hidden message that they unintentionally convey.

CONSIDER

How often do we hear or say, "I'm just a med-surg nurse," or "Oh, you work on a medical floor," or "I just work in a nursing home," rather than hearing or saying, "I am a medical surgical specialist," or "Oh, you're a medical nursing specialist," or "I'm a specialist in caring for the elderly"?

Some nursing workplaces can have a culture of oppression and exploitation in the absence of a rational self-confidence and pride. Intentional positive reinforcement is rare or nonexistent. Historically, nurses have been exploited by the delegation of tasks that were no longer interesting or challenging to medical practitioners. Their salaries and hours of work are unlike those of any other female-dominated profession.

Just as women are marginalized in society, so nurses continue to be marginalized in the health care workplace. Predominantly male, medical practitioners empowered themselves through their dominance and abuse of power over nurses and women in the workplace. Socially and culturally, physicians have worked hard to maintain their dominance in health care and to control and restrict nurses and other health practitioners. Personal and professional violence against women and nurses from the medical and administrative staff seems to continue in many health care organizations.

The oppression of nurses still sometimes begins early in the educational program when nurses are in their most formative and vulnerable stage. Hoel, Giga, and Davidson (2007) noted how students on clinical placements described indirect bullying behaviors such as insensitivity, indifference, and humiliation. They considered the challenge for students in reconciling such workplace behavior with the "caring" strategies that attracted the students to nursing in the first instance. Early in the education of nursing students, curriculum must include strategies that cultivate empowerment and positive personal and professional growth.

Early workplace experiences must allow students to see nurses treating each other in positive and supportive ways.

Hoel et al. (2007) noted that students, who have fairly limited time in individual clinical placement, may have difficulties in finding support, strong relationships, or mentors to help them deal with inappropriate workplace behaviors. Acknowledging that new graduates are confronted with a challenging and sometimes very negative workplace is critical to progressing the discussion to positive socialization strategies and the ways in which nurses can empower one another.

DISCUSSION POINT

What and where are some of the resources nurses can access if they need advice and support when attempting to confront issues of inappropriate, unhelpful, and negative workplace behaviors?

SOCIALIZATION AND MENTORING: EMPOWERMENT

Mentoring is an intense, positive, discreet, exclusive, one-on-one relationship between an experienced professional and a less experienced novice. The contemporary literature is filled with various definitions and descriptions of mentoring. The mentor relationship is described as similar to the parent–child relationship in that it is usually charged with emotion and is a serious and mutual, nonsexual, loving relationship. The expression "inquisitive teacher" is used when discussing a mentor. From these descriptions, one can assume that mentoring is a high-level human relationship of some significance.

Descriptions of mentors include terminology such as caring, trusting, experienced, dedicated, and almost always some elusive quality frequently called "chemistry." Clearly, a mentoring relationship is different from the more superficial role model or preceptor that is also discussed in the nursing literature. Kilcullen (2007, p. 102) described the roles of a mentor to students in the clinical setting as "enhancing learning for students, through support, acting as role models, performing socialization roles, and acting as assessors." Fitzpatrick (2007, p. 61) described the role of a mentor to students as that of a storyteller who assists "future generations of nurses to move through those mazes that either hasten or slowed our own professional progress."

CONSIDER

Mentoring has been identified as one of the most powerful socialization strategies for professional and career advancement.

Perhaps most important for nurses is the research from the late 1970s and 1980s that focused on the unique nature of mentoring among women. Sargent (1977) discussed the many positive aspects of the mentor relationship as described in the literature but emphasized what she considered to be most important. The true value, beyond the teaching, sponsoring, and sharing roles, is the "blessing" in and of itself. To warrant the time and attention ("the blessing") of the mentor is the real worth to the mentee; to have someone believe in one enhances one's belief in oneself.

The business and management literature contains many references and discussions regarding the mentor–mentee phenomenon. Its value to organizational, as well as personal, development has been clearly established over the last 30 years. Schein (1978, pp. 177–178) discussed the obvious situation that exists in organizations when new employees look to more experienced personnel for advice and information. Schein developed several roles that the willing experienced "mentor" can assume to assist in the development of the new "mentee." The analysis concluded with the observation that the mentor does not necessarily have to be a recognized power figure within the organization, but that experience and willingness to share are important. Other characteristics common to mentoring are shown in Box 8.1.

Kanter (1977) was one of the earliest businesswomen to identify and use the term *sponsor* to describe the mentor relationship. According to Kanter, the very important role that sponsors play in the power struggle at all levels of the organization has three primary characteristics (pp. 181–184):

1. The ability to be often in a position to fight for a mentee. The propensity to point out superior performance at important times and promote or support a recommendation from a novice are essential ingredients of the sponsor relationship.

2. The ability to bypass the hierarchy and obtain inside information within the organization.

3. "Reflected power," or support from those with formal or informal power to accelerate the movement of the novice up the organizational ladder.

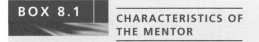

BOX 8.1 — CHARACTERISTICS OF THE MENTOR

Open: willing to see multiple perspectives.

Flexible: professionally agile and able to try different approaches.

Perceptive: insightful and knowledgeable about motives and subtitles.

Believes: someone who sees potential, "believes in" the mentee.

Vision: sees the possibilities, the big picture.

Positive: exudes energy and confidence.

Motivates: gives the mentee reason to change and stretch.

Willing: available with an "open door" policy.

Unobtrusive: steps back while pushing for growth.

Protects: able to shield the mentee from workplace danger.

Stages of the Mentoring Relationship

Schira (2007) described the phases in mentoring relationships (Box 8.2). The first phase includes finding and connecting with a more experienced person in the workplace. A mentoring relationship can be established when a "chemistry" is present that fosters reciprocal trust and openness. The second phase includes teaching, modeling, and insider knowledge that fosters a sense of competence and confidence. The intensity of the relationship can escalate to high levels during this learning, listening, and sharing phase. The third phase includes a sense of change and growth as the mentoring relationship begins to move to a conclusion. The intensity wanes as the mentee begins to move toward independence. The last stage finds both the mentee and the mentor achieving a different, independent relationship, based, it can be hoped, on positive, collegial characteristics.

Separation and redefinition are often difficult because the mentor and mentee may share different perceptions about whether it is time to separate and what their new relationship should be. It is critically important for mentees *and* mentors that they should outgrow the need for such intense coaching if the mentor has done a good job of cultivation. Unfortunately, some mentoring relationships get "stuck" and fail to move forward the development of the novice. Personal and workplace circumstances and distractions can cause mentors and protégés to reach a comfort zone that prevents positive and ongoing development of the novice.

Typical mentoring relationships are usually characterized by the participants as intense. Any intense, high-level, interpersonal human relationship that evolves and changes can become a problem and have unfortunate ramifications, particularly in the workplace. As any intense relationship comes to a close, both participants must synchronize the separation or changed relationship. The literature identifies that most mentoring relationships evolve into a warm, lifelong, collegial friendship. Occasionally, either the mentor or protégé is unprepared for the end of a mentoring relationship, or an end is foisted on the participants due to job changes; this can cause serious unhappy individual and workplace consequences.

DISCUSSION POINT
What strategies can be used when a mentee or protégé remains grateful and connected to the mentor but also begins to feel confined or restricted by a mentoring relationship?

BOX 8.2 — STAGES OF THE MENTORING RELATIONSHIP

1. Finding and connecting.
2. Learning and listening.
3. Changing and shifting.
4. Mentoring others.

Source: Schira, M. (2007). Leadership: A peak and perk of professional development. *Nephrology Nursing Journal, 34*(3), 289–294.

Mentoring Opportunities for Men and Women: Historical Differences

Before the 1970s, the business world functioned on "the good ol' boys" network, with mentoring relationships between men an expected, accepted way to progress up the ladder of opportunity and promotion. The older, more experienced males were used to seeking out the younger, newer workplace (male) colleague whom they deemed a protégé worthy of "judgment of potential." The golf course, the locker room, and after-work drinks between work colleagues all advanced exclusively male mentoring relationships and, in the meantime, excluded women from promotional opportunities. This male-to-male mentoring phenomenon spawned the famous invisible, or "glass," ceiling that reduced career advancement opportunities for women and thus affected the predominantly female nursing profession.

Historically, there were not enough mentors for all the women who wanted one. In the past, far fewer women were in the workplace, and they were usually not at the higher, more visible organizational positions. The lack of emphasis on team sports for a girl in childhood could reduce her effectiveness in later life on a business or professional "team." In addition, solitary activities such as cooking and piano lessons are more common to young girls. Although the socialization of girls has undoubtedly changed in the last 20 years, at least some of these elements continue to exist.

Boys are still traditionally encouraged to participate in football, baseball, and basketball, developing expertise to use in a team effort. Another reason is the potential sexual aspects found in a close personal, albeit business or professional, relationship. Some men may subconsciously wish to avoid the potential complications of close cross-gender work relationships. It is conceivable that many men *still* fail to perceive talent that merits attention in career women.

> ### CONSIDER
> The socialization of young girls and boys has changed in subtle and not so subtle ways over the last 20 years as research has developed new ways of understanding learning and development. The effect of these changes will gradually change the workplace in expected and sometimes unexpected ways.

In addition, a shortage of mentors for women may be a result of the low number of women in top-level business management who are both willing and available to be mentors to other women. Moreover, the emphasis on the affiliative socialization needs of women could affect the mentoring process. "Belonging" is still associated with feminine socialization; "achieving" is often the focus of socialization for men. Because the purpose of mentoring is achievement, it would seem that mentoring would be inconsistent with feminine socialization; however, the skills of cooperation and collaboration could also support and enhance mentoring.

> ### CONSIDER
> It would be the unusual employer today who does not foster women into leadership roles. Employers are now developing strategies to encourage people from diverse backgrounds (i.e., ethnic, cultural, religious) to achieve promotion and fill leadership roles.

Fortunately, mentoring opportunities for women are increasing. However, the gains are slower for women from diverse backgrounds. Women of color, very young or older women, and women with disabilities have more difficulty finding mentors than their white or more accepted counterparts. Not having an influential mentor or sponsor can slow professional growth and development, reduce opportunities for advancement, and perpetuate the typical male-dominated organizational hierarchy.

Mentoring in Nursing

The presence or absence of mentoring within the nursing profession received attention only in the 1970s when the phenomenon became an important researchable topic. So much societal emphasis had been placed on gaining access to male-dominated professions that the predominantly female service-oriented professions remained underdeveloped. The labeling of "traditional" and "female" apparently had been influential in reducing appropriate attention to the mentoring process in these "traditionally female" occupations. Clearly, mentoring was identified and highly regarded in male-dominated workplaces long before it was noted as having potential for women and, later, nurses.

> ### CONSIDER
> Mentoring opportunities for all women, and thus for nurses, have been far more limited than for their male counterparts.

Vance (1977, 1982, 2000) was one of the earliest nurse researchers to explore mentoring in nursing. The mentoring phenomenon and its many permutations are widely acclaimed and largely accepted as an effective strategy for the personal and professional development of nurses in the workplace. It is not an uncommon occurrence to find an editorial or reflective comment in scholarly nursing journals regarding the benefits and positive outcomes associated with mentoring relationships. A 2005 Internet search of "nurses" and "mentoring" via Google uncovered 852 sites. In 2008 there were a phenomenal 2,590,000 sites.

DISCUSSION POINT

What alternatives are available to nurses who are new to a workplace or feel that a professional change is on the horizon, if there do not seem to be any available mentors for advice?

Clearly, nurses must actively seek out and perpetuate mentoring relationships. There is an overwhelming number of positive consequences for nurses who find the supportive interpersonal model that fits their current professional practice and health care workplace. The highly educated professional workforce found in today's health care organizations includes many nurses in powerful positions. Nurses must accept responsibility for individual and collective action to create and maintain an environment that is rewarding and supports positive socialization strategies for themselves and their professional colleagues.

Increasing Opportunities for Mentoring

Not surprisingly, contemporary nursing literature encourages a more assertive, less passive approach to developing a mentoring relationship. Emphasis is placed on the responsibility of leading nurses to bring along, indeed seek out, newer nurses to develop within an area of expertise. Newer nurses are urged to seek out a mentor or mentors to assist them, especially at critical points in their career progress, such as in the beginning or during a change of career direction or promotion. Waiting for a mentor to find a protégé is not always an effective strategy.

As the nursing workforce ages, health care organizations need to identify new ways of valuing mature, older, and experienced nurses and other health care professionals. It is not just the novice in a mentoring relationship who benefits. The mentor also receives many advantages. The recognition as a "wise one" is evident for many coworkers to see. The gratitude, challenge, and revitalization of acting in a mentoring role are renewing and pleasurable. Participating in and watching a novice develop confidence, assertiveness, and professional skills are high-level rewards for a mentor.

CONSIDER

In some cultures, older (less productive and dependent) people were literally or figuratively pushed away to die in isolation. Today, Western cultures are changing the way older people are viewed by placing value and appreciation on the wisdom that comes with experience.

Before the current nursing shortage, research into the mentoring phenomenon was essentially limited to strategies to assist nurses to gain promotion up and away from the bedside. Encouraging nurses to stay in nursing, and particularly at the bedside, became a new and strategically important goal of mentoring and other supportive behaviors. As the shortage of bedside nurses has spiraled out of control, interest has increased in how mentoring, role modeling, and other supportive behaviors might socialize nurses and improve retention.

Value of Mentoring in Recruitment and Retention

In an effort to improve recruitment as well as retention, some organizations have initiated programs that "assign" mentors and mentees when the workplace situation does not allow for spontaneous mentoring relationships to develop. Much of the current literature identifies the importance of an organization's leaders and high visibility health professionals to demonstrate the valuing of supportive and positive behaviors. Recognizing the ever more diverse nature of the nursing and health care work environment would seem fundamental to recruitment, retention and fostering mentoring values.

Bally (2007) described the current concern for organizations—an aging, soon-to-retire workforce and the necessity to establish a workplace that is attractive to a younger, perhaps less patient workforce. A health care workplace culture of respect and empowerment would seem to be the current imperative of nursing leaders. Thupayagale-Tshweneagae and Dithole (2007) agreed and described the important strength that comes with unity and a respect for diversity among registered nurses. Experienced nurses bring diverse specialist skills to the health care workplace. Respecting and then actively acknowledging the ever-expanding nursing specialties will foster a workplace that enjoys good recruitment and retention statistics.

A culturally competent health care workplace must also understand and appreciate the contribution of racial and ethnic diversity. Bond, Gray, Baxley, Cason, and Denke (2008) explored challenges associated with the socialization of Hispanic nurses into the health care arena. Their interest was in improving the understanding of how Hispanic nurses might view nursing and nursing education differently, in hopes of addressing recruitment and retention, as well as improving health disparities among a large minority.

Mentoring and Developmental Stages

Nurses should be acquainted with adult developmental issues and life transitions as they relate to wellness and illness. Linking this information to the mentoring phenomenon and workplace socialization is important. It will be clear that establishing a mentoring relationship can be enormously important not only to the novice, but also to the mentor.

It was only in the 1970s that Gail Sheehy (1976) in *Passages* and Daniel Levinson (1978) in *The Seasons of Man's Life* connected mentoring and adult developmental theory. They emphasized that people continue to change throughout their adult life. Levinson found, among other information, that in early adulthood (ages 20 to 40 years), several distinct developmental changes occur in a certain sequence. Young people between 22 and 28 years of age enter the adult world. From 28 to 33 years of age they analyze what has occurred so far and take steps to alter or change what they feel is inappropriate. From 33 years of age to midlife, they invest in realizing their goals or, as Sheehy describes, "climbing the career ladder."

Near age 40 years, people stop to take stock of the first half of their life. The compromises that were necessary in the first half of their life and the realization or lack of realization of their goal(s) are crucial components of the infamous midlife transition. At approximately 45 years of age, a pattern is established that modifies a life structure to accommodate the midlife analysis. Both Levinson and Sheehy identified that for many people the last half of their adult life is the fullest and most satisfying. There was evidence that the same transitional periods versus stable periods continue throughout adulthood.

Both works point out clear life stages marked by internal changes not directly related to external changes,

such as divorce, death, marriage, births, and the like. Both Sheehy and Levinson refer to the period of the post-midlife review as being fulfilling, renewing, and satisfying or being full of resignation and stagnation, depending on how one has dealt with previous transitional periods. This conceptual framework is relevant and pertinent for the nurse in the 21st century.

> CONSIDER
> Research indicates that internal (life) changes occur despite external or extrinsic changes. Nurses in today's health care environment frequently encounter workplace transfers and employment changes, as well as longer and more diverse careers. The health care workforce has greater differences in age, ethnicity, and gender than ever before.

The changes and growth, or lack of growth, demonstrated in the different life stages are interconnected. There are always new heights to be climbed, but the next step is not simply another rung on the same ladder. The top of the first ladder turns out to be the bottom rung on a new ladder (Levinson, 1978, p. 154). During the final thrust toward achievement of success, individuals must devote themselves to that end at the expense of other important parts of themselves. Many believe that if they become the president of the company or the shop steward or whatever their dream might be, they will achieve happiness and contentment forever. At midlife an internal mechanism forces most adults to look at the price that has been paid for the place in which they find themselves.

Levinson and Sheehy both described the importance of recognizing the costs and gains and the necessary trade-offs that come to light during midlife analysis. The wisdom that may develop after midlife sets the stage for mentoring. At certain transitional points in life, the mentor relationship has profound and significant value to both participants. Seeing the ladder ahead, one can often see someone ahead who has been climbing.

Schein's (1978) research included the observation that the midlife analysis exposes a career spent as a leader or a key contributor or as dead wood. Levinson stated that the mentor functions primarily as a transitional figure. The mentor "is usually older than the protégé by a half-generation, roughly 8 to 15 years" and is experienced as a "responsible, admirable, older sibling" (Levinson, 1978, pp. 177–178). It would appear that the pre-midlife adult would be most susceptible to the protégé role, just as the post-midlife adult would be most susceptible to the mentoring role. Welcoming, acquainting, guiding, hosting, and counseling roles would serve both adults well.

Levinson referred to "generativity," or the sense that one feels for the continuity of life and the concern for the future generations. This can be seen at home, at work, in friendships, in government, and by many nurses. Usually, only after midlife does this sense of responsibility for the development of others take an active form. A clear understanding of adult developmental theory lends credence to the significance and importance of mentoring for the mentor as well as for the protégé.

CREATING A SUPPORTIVE ENVIRONMENT FOR SOCIALIZATION AND RESOCIALIZATION

The workplace environment is key to nurse satisfaction, retention, and patient care (Schira, 2007; Woelfle & Mc-Caffrey, 2007; Fletcher, 2006). Employers and nurse leaders have significant responsibility for creating a workplace that genuinely values supportive behaviors, such as mentoring. Many health care organizations encourage and recommend that nurses take advantage of the opportunity to mentor throughout their professional careers. The literature is replete with multiple examples of various forms of formal and informal mentoring programs.

> ### CONSIDER
> Today's nurses encounter higher workloads and sicker patients than ever before. Energy to combat demeaning and abusive behaviors from workplace colleagues is in short supply because so much energy must be directed to providing safe and competent patient care. This situation encourages workplace and professional "silence," which is an impediment to individual and professional growth.

Leadership

Highly visible organizational leader(s) must "walk the walk," not merely "talk the talk." All leaders and managers in health care facilities need to demonstrate supportive behaviors and identify and support formal and informal mentoring or other supportive programs at individual as well as departmental levels. For positive socialization, such as mentoring, to flourish and for the nursing profession to reach its greatest potential, registered nurses need to be proactive and find ways to facilitate professional and individual growth-producing workplace strategies (Box 8.3).

A workplace culture in which mutual respect is evident in all written and verbal communications is an important strategy for organizations. One of the favorite pastimes of employees everywhere is to closely observe, and then dissect, each word, behavior, and nuance of their managers, supervisors, and leaders. Appropriate acknowledgment, respectful tones, and public positive reinforcement can have long-term and lasting individual and group consequences. On the other hand, an impatient, poorly expressed personal or

---

BOX 8.3 | **TRAITS OF WORK CULTURES THAT PROMOTE POSITIVE SOCIALIZATION**

1. Mutual respect is evident in all written and verbal communications.
2. There is appropriate acknowledgment of the ideas and work of others.
3. Superior performance is sought and recognized publicly.
4. Roadblocks to goal achievement or unnecessary bureaucracy in the workplace are identified and addressed promptly.
5. Expectations are clear.
6. Criticism is constructive and given in private.

professional observation from a high-visibility person in the organization will be described and embellished throughout the organization for far longer than anyone could anticipate.

Organizational leaders can use a language that creates a positive and supportive work environment. What is included in the language is as important as what is excluded. Seeking out superior performance, knowing and using people's names, acknowledging the ideas or work of others, and identifying and reducing roadblocks or unnecessary bureaucracy in the workplace need to be everyday occurrences for leaders and managers. On the other hand, "constructive criticism" or even "suggestions" can be unhelpful and, more important, go unheeded when presented in front of others. Employing these basic interpersonal and professional communication skills is essential in a workplace that hopes to attract and retain high-quality health care professionals.

Organizations are responsible for the ongoing education and training of all employees, including leaders and managers. Poorly trained and performing leaders are the responsibility of the organization's executive and corporate level. Allowing inadequate leaders and leadership to prevail in an organization has long-term serious and negative consequences. Alternatively, an effective,

---

Research Study Fuels the Controversy: Inactive Nurses Become Active Again

A recent phenomenological research study into the experiences of nurses who have undertaken a refresher or "re-entry" program is of interest when exploring issues associated with mentoring and the health care workplace.

STUDY FINDINGS

The worldwide shortage of registered nurses has generated substantial research into the phenomenon of re-entering the workplace after a significant period of absence. This study found that mentoring was a significant factor to nine nurses who were interviewed as they were completing a refresher course. The informant nurses had been away from the clinical setting from 5 to 27 years. Their educational background varied from an Associate Degree in Nursing to a master's degree in a field other than nursing. Hammer and Craig described the informant nurses as demonstrating high levels of self-efficacy and motivation, which are important characteristics for embarking on a significant personal and career change activity.

Previous research has identified the importance of a mentor during life-changing transitions; certainly, re-entering the workplace after a significant absence rates as a significant life transition. The informant nurses experienced challenges with the expectation that they would have to organize their own clinical placements, as well as to interact with more experienced nurses. One nurse described the greeting she received from a potential employer: "You are 50 some odd years old; why are you doing this? We want younger girls to come in."

Most of the informant nurses described stressors related to peer relationships and unit politics. This research challenged the common perception that mentors are usually a generation-and-a-half older than their mentee. Mentors or guides in the new workplace can be considerably younger than their mentee.

The informant nurses were unanimous in the view that having one specified nurse colleague to answer questions, provide support, and assist them in the specific clinical setting was closely linked with ultimately positive experiences and outcomes. The early orientation period was of critical importance to these nurses. One of the expectations of these informant nurses was in keeping with widely researched and accepted adult education strategies—self-direction and involvement in educational decisions and experiences was essential.

Nurses who contemplate a way to return to "active duty" need to acquire current skills and familiarity with new procedures and equipment. Understanding how to develop and reintegrate nurses returning to the workplace after significant absences is important to nursing. Today's workplace needs to recognize that the current generation expects and organizes their lives to include multiple career phases. Integrating newly hired, older nurses in an era of multiple careers and life goals is important. Determining ways to support and foster positive long-term professional development is of significance to the international health care arena.

Hammer, V. R., & Craig, G. P. (2008). The experiences of inactive nurses returned to nursing after completing a refresher course. *Journal of Continuing Education in Nursing, 39*(8), 358–368.

persuasive role model and leader can energize and empower numerous employees and thereby promote a positive, effective workplace. This is particularly important in a health care workplace, where highly educated professionals quite clearly know what they expect from their work environment and organizational leadership.

Sponsors, Guides, Preceptors, and Role Models

Organizations can also create work environments supportive of socialization through their use of sponsors, guides, preceptors, and role models. Shapiro, Haseltine, and Rowe (1978) suggested that a continuum exists with mentors and peer pals as endpoints, and sponsors and guides as internal points on the continuum. At one end are the mentors, who have the most "intense and paternalistic" roles. Sponsors and then guides are at the two-thirds point; sponsors are less powerful in affecting their charges, whereas guides are invaluable in explaining the system. The peer pal, or today's clinical preceptor, is at the other end of the continuum from a mentor. The peer pal or preceptor encourages a relationship between peers as they help each other succeed and progress.

CONSIDER

Clinical coordinators or preceptors are commonly assigned to one or more student nurses during their clinical practice placement. Qualities found in the various supportive roles identified here may or may not be readily available to students in today's health care workplace.

A surprising level of camaraderie can develop between preceptors and students when preceptored clinical experiences are organized. Attention to the socialization of developing nurses in the real world of evening, night, and weekend shifts can be expected to promote a bond between experienced and less experienced nurses. Their experiences do not support the notion that nurses "eat their young." Smedley (2008) explored the development of successful preceptor skills as experienced nurses facilitated the learning, focus, and comfort in the health care workplace of less experienced nurses. She found and identified several characteristics important to successful preceptors; consistent with the literature presented here, three of them were positive attitudes, patience, and the desire to motivate others to learn.

Similarly, Hammer and Craig (2008) found that having one specified nurse colleague to answer questions, provide support and assist the individual nurse in the specific clinical setting was closely linked with ultimately positive experiences and outcomes. The early orientation period was of critical importance to these nurses. (See Research Study Fuels the Controversy on page 140.)

CONCLUSIONS

Understanding the socialization of novice nurses and the resocialization of nurses in transition or at the peak of their performance is critical to the nursing profession and the health of society. The realization of the full potential of nurses and the nursing profession has a direct effect on patient care and patient outcomes. The history and knowledge available through the nursing research reviewed here authenticates the importance of understanding and developing a range of strategies that enhance positive, supportive socialization among nurses. The continuing evolution toward professionalization and autonomy that sustains and enhances nurse empowerment is the most effective recruitment and retention strategy available.

Nurses comprise the largest group of health professionals, and most nurses practice nursing within an organization. Considering that hospitals are substantial business enterprises with complicated, multifaceted hierarchies and that nurses are largely responsible for significant departmental budgets, one cannot help but see that interest in and research on professional development and positive socialization, such as mentoring relationships, are important. Today's health care organizations, administrators, health care professionals, and particularly nurses have a vested interest in recognizing and supporting mentoring programs, relationships, and behaviors.

It is within the hospital organization that most nurses develop or grow as individuals and as professionals. Administrators and medical staff need to consider interdisciplinary mentoring relationships because this cross-fertilization will enhance professional relationships in the health care workplace. Altering the workplace to encourage real partnerships among all health professionals with clear appreciation and acknowledgment of the unique contribution of each discipline remains a challenge. There is much at stake and a way to travel still.

FOR ADDITIONAL DISCUSSION

1. What are some health care workplace behaviors associated with typical oppressed groups?
2. Describe strategies that might be effective in reducing typical oppressed-group behavior.
3. Who is advantaged when negative socialization occurs in the health care workplace? Why?
4. Describe five career changes or transitions that might be facilitated by a mentoring relationship.
5. In what ways does a mentoring relationship provide an advantage to the mentor?
6. What are the advantages and disadvantages to a nursing professional of having positive or negative socialization strategies?
7. Will having increasing numbers of men in nursing change the frequency or kinds of mentoring relationships that exist in nursing?
8. How can research continue to develop notions associated with positive socialization in the nursing profession?

REFERENCES

Bally, J. M. G. (2007). The role of nursing leadership in creating a mentoring culture in acute care environments. *Nursing Economics, 25*(3),143–148.

Bond, M. L., Gray, J. R., Baxley, S., Cason, C. L., & Denke, L. (2008). Voices of Hispanic students in baccalaureate nursing programs: Are we listening? *Nursing Education Perspectives, 29*(3), 136–142.

Campbell, S. L. (2003). Cultivating empowerment in nursing today for a strong profession tomorrow. *Journal of Nursing Education, 42*(9), 423–426.

Darling, L. A. (1984). What do nurses want in a mentor? *Journal of Nursing Administration, 14*(10), 42–44.

Fitzpatrick, J. J. (2007). Leaders, mentors, and storytellers. *Nursing Education Perspectives, 28*(2), 61.

Fletcher, K. (2006). Beyond dualism: Leading out of oppression. *Nursing Forum, 41*(2), 50–59.

Freire, P. (1968). *Pedagogy of the Oppressed.* New York: Seabury Press.

Hammer, V. R., & Craig, G. P. (2008) The experiences of inactive nurses returned to nursing after completing a refresher course. *Journal of Continuing Education in Nursing, 39*(8), 358-368.

Hoel, H., Giga, S. I., & Davidson, M. J. (2007). Expectations and realities of student nurses' experiences of negative behaviour and bullying in clinical placement and the influences of socialization

processes. *Health Services Management Research, 20*(4), 270–278.

Hutchinson, M., Vickers, M. H., Jackson, D., & Wilkes, L. (2006). They stand you in a corner; You are not to speak: Nurses tell of abusive introduction in work teams dominated by bullies. *Contemporary Nurse, 21*(2), 228–238.

Kanter, R. M. (1977). *Men and Women of the Corporation.* New York: Basic Books.

Kilcullen, N. M. (2007). Said another way: The impact of mentorship on clinical learning. *Nursing Forum, 42*(2), 95–104.

Kramer, M. (1974). *Reality shock: Why nurses leave nursing.* St. Louis, MO: Mosby.

Kramer, M. (1981). *Coping with Reality Shock.* Workshop presented at Jackson Memorial Hospital, Miami, Florida, January 27–28, 1981.

Levinson, D. (1978). *The Seasons of Man's Life.* New York: Alfred A. Knopf.

Madison, J., & Minichiello, V. (2004). The contextual issues associated with sexual harassment experiences reported by RNs. *Australian Journal of Advanced Nursing, 22*(2), 8–13.

Marquis, B., & Huston, C. (2009). *Leadership Roles and Management Functions* (6th ed.). Philadelphia: Lippincott Williams & Wilkins.

Sargent, A. G. (1977). *Beyond Sex Roles.* St. Paul, MN: West.

Schein, E. (1978). *Career Dynamics: Matching Individual and Organizational Needs.* Reading, MA: Addison-Wesley.

Schira, M. (2007). Leadership: A peak and perk of professional development. *Nephrology Nursing Journal, 34*(3), 289–294.

Shapiro, E. C., Haseltine, F. P., & Rowe, M. P. (1978). Moving up: Role models, mentors and the "patron system." *Sloan Management Review, 19*(3), 51–58.

Sheehy, G. (1976). *Passages: Predictable Crises of Adult Life.* New York: Bantam.

Smedley, A (2008). Becoming and being a preceptor: A phenomenological study. *Journal of Continuing Education in Nursing, 39*(4), 185–191.

Thupayagale-Tshweneagae, G., & Dithole, K. (2007). Unity among nurses: An evasive concept. *Nursing Forum, 42*(3), 143–146.

Vance, C. N. (1977). *A group profile of contemporary influentials in American nursing.* Doctoral dissertation, Teachers College, Columbia University.

Vance, C. (1982). The mentor connection. *Journal of Nursing Administration, 12*(4), 7–13.

Vance, C. (2000). Discovering the riches in mentoring connections. *Reflections on Nursing Leadership, 26*(3), 24–25.

Woelfle, C. Y., & McCaffrey, R. (2007). Nurse on nurse. *Nursing Forum, 42*(3), 123–131.

BIBLIOGRAPHY

Bradbury-Jones, C., Sambrook, S., & Irvine, F. (2007). The meaning of empowerment for nursing students: A critical incident study. *Journal of Advanced Nursing, 59*(4), 342–351.

Burnes, B., & Pope, R. (2007). Negative behaviours in the workplace: A study of two Primary Care Trusts in NHS. *International Journal of Public Sector Management, 20*(4), 285–303.

Cogin, J., & Fish, A. (2007). Managing sexual harassment more strategically: An analysis of environmental causes. *Asia Pacific Journal of Human Resources, 45*(3), 333.

Dyer, L. (2008). The continuing need for mentors in nursing. *Journal for Nurses in Staff Development, 24*(2), 86–90.

Fulton, J., Bøhler, A., Hansen, G., Kauffeldt, A., Welander, E., Santos, M., Thorarinsdottir, K., & Ziarko, E. (2007). Mentorship: An international perspective. *Nurse Education in Practice, 7*(6), 399–406.

Gross, D. (2008). A CLNC mentor helped me expand my CLNC business right from the start. *Legal Nurse Consulting Ezine, 19*(9), 7.

Heinrich, K. T. (2007). Dare to share: A unique approach to presenting and publishing. *Nurse Educator, 32*(6), 269–273.

Janes, G. (2008). Improving services through leadership development. *Nursing Times, 104*(13), 58–59.

Latham, C. L. (2008). Nurses supporting nurses: Creating a mentoring program for staff nurses to improve the workforce environment. *Nursing Administration Quarterly, 32*(1), 27.

LaSala, C. A., Connors, P. M., Taylor Pedro, J., & Phipps, M. (2007). The role of the clinical nurse specialist in promoting evidence-based practice and effecting positive patient outcomes. *Journal of Continuing Education in Nursing, 38*(6), 262–270.

Leners, D. W., Wilson, V. W., & Sitzman, K. L. (2007). Twenty-first century education: Online with a focus on nursing education. *Nursing Education Perspectives, 28*(6), 332–336.

Lyttle, D. (2007). My continuing journey through project LEAD (Leadership Enhancement and Development). *ABNF Journal, 18*(4), 104–106.

Mason, D. (2007). On our shoulders. *American Journal of Nursing, 107*(9), 11.

Melillo, K. D., & Futrell, M. (2008). Gerontological nursing and gerontology leader and mentor. *Journal of Gerontological Nursing, 34*(5), 7–9.

Mills, J. E., Francis, K., & Bonner, A. (2007). The accidental mentor: Australian rural nurses developing supportive relationships in the workplace. *Rural and Remote Health, 7*(4), 842.

Mooney, M. (2007). Professional socialization: The key to survival as a newly qualified nurse. *International Journal of Nursing Practice, 13*(2), 75–80.

Morris, A. H., & Faulk, D. (2007). Perspective transformation: Enhancing the development of professionalism in RN-to-BSN students. *Journal of Nursing Education, 46*(10), 445–450.

Nickle, P. (2007). Cognitive apprenticeship: Laying the groundwork for mentoring registered nurses in the intensive care unit. *Dynamics, 18*(4), 19–27.

NZNO nurse practitioner mentor system (2008). *Kai Tiaki: Nursing New Zealand, 14*(3), 5.

Santos, T. C. F., Lopes, G. T., Porto, F., & de Fonta, A. S. (2008). Opposition to the American leadership by Brazilian nurses (1934–1938). *Revista latino-americana de enfermagem, 16*(1), 130–135.

Schriner, C. L. (2007). The influence of culture on clinical nurses transitioning into the faculty role. *Nursing Education Perspectives, 28*(3), 145–149.

Scott, D. E. (2008). Learning to ask for help. *Vermont Nursing Connection, 2008*(February–April), 8.

Shinyashiki, G. T., Mendes, I. A. C., Trevizan, M. A., & Day, R. A. (2006). Professional socialization: Students becoming nurses. *Revista latino-americana de enfermagem, 14*(4), 601–607.

Tagliareni, E. M., & Malone, B. (2008). President's message: All we hope and dare to achieve. *Nursing Education Perspectives, 29*(3), 127.

Zurmehly, J. A. (2007). A qualitative case study review of role transition in community nursing. *Nursing Forum, 42*(4), 162–170.

WEB RESOURCES

A Guiding Hand	http://www.nurseweek.com/news/features/02-02/mentor.asp
American Association of Critical-Care Nurses, Education/Training/Mentoring References	http://www.aacn.org/AACN/ICURecog.nsf/Files/etm/$file/ETM.pdf
AORN Journal, Membership Committee Promotes Mentoring	http://www.findarticles.com/cf_dls/m0FSL/2_70/55525543/p1/article.jhtml
Media Kit 2008	http://www.helpatnursingspectrum.com/load_article.html?AID=930
Mentor Projects	http://www.arnm.asn.au/index.php?/content/view/23/54/
Mentor Programs for New Nurses	http://www.hcmarketplace.com/prod-5093.html
Mentoring in Health Care	http://www.questia.com
Nursing Management	http://nursingmanagement.rcnpublishing.co.uk/
Nurse Mentoring, Creating a Professional Legacy	https://www.nnsdo.org/dmdocuments/NurseMentoring.pdf
Reflections on Nursing Leadership	http://nursingsociety.org/RNL/3Q_2006/features/feature8.html
Manchester University School of Nursing, Midwifery and Social Work, Mentors Information	http://www.nursing.manchester.ac.uk/mentors/resources/nmcmentorstandards/
Texas Women's University, International Health Professions Nurse Mentor Program	http://www.twu.edu/nursing/international-mentor.asp
University of Virginia Health System, U.VA Nurse Mentoring Program Ensures High Quality Patient Care	http://www.healthsystem.virginia.edu/internet/news/Archives00/nurse_mentoring.cfm
U.S. Public Health Mentoring Program	http://phs-nurse.org/MentoringProgram.htm

CHAPTER 9

Diversity in the Nursing Workforce

• CAROL J. HUSTON •

Learning Objectives

The learner will be able to:

1. Examine the relationship between health disparities and a lack of diversity in the health care workforce.
2. Explore factors leading to the lack of ethnic and gender diversity in nursing.
3. Suggest individual, organizational, and professional strategies to increase ethnic and gender diversity in nursing.
4. Identify common barriers faced in both recruiting and retaining minority students in higher education.
5. Compare opportunity levels for decision making at senior levels of health care management between racial/ethnic minorities and whites and between men and women.
6. Identify at least four professional nursing associations that are directed at serving a specific racial or ethnic population.

7. Investigate stereotypes of male nurses that both hinder the recruitment and retention of men into nursing and pose socialization and acceptance challenges for them.
8. Compare economic and advancement opportunities for men and women in nursing.
9. Argue for or against the need for affirmative action to bring more men into the nursing profession.
10. Analyze research exploring generational differences in work values and preferences among registered nurses and explore the challenges inherent in having four generations cohabitate in the same profession at the same time.
11. Reflect on personal beliefs and values regarding the assertion that diversity, equity, and parity are moral imperatives.

Diversity has been defined as the differences among groups or between individuals, and it comes in many forms, including age, gender, religion, customs, sexual orientation, physical size, physical and mental capabilities, beliefs, culture, ethnicity, and skin color. Yet, despite increasing diversity (particularly ethnic and cultural) in the United States, the nursing workforce continues to be fairly homogeneous, at least in terms of ethnicity and gender, being white, female, and middle-aged. In fact, Dixon (2008) reported that blacks, Hispanics, and American Indians together comprise only 9% of the nursing workforce, despite their 25% representation in the U.S. population.

This lack of ethnic, gender, and generational diversity is a concern not only for the nursing profession, but also for its clients. Clearly, the nursing workforce should

be at least as diverse as the population it serves. Not only is a lack of diversity in the workforce linked to health disparities, but also minority health care professionals are more likely than their white peers to work in underserved communities, which, in turn, improves access among underrepresented groups (Giddens, 2008).

This finding was reinforced in a study by McGinnis, Moore, and Continelli (2006), which found that underrepresented minority nurse practitioners (NPs) in New York had different practice patterns than their non-underrepresented counterparts. Minority NPs were more likely to work in hospitals, community health centers, and schools, as well as in women's health, gerontology, or primary care. The implication of these findings is that minority NPs may be more likely than their non-underrepresented counterparts to provide basic services to underserved populations where these populations access care.

In response to these issues, there has been a rising clamor for greater diversity in the profession, and this is readily apparent in a review of the literature. S. K. Banschbach (2008, p. 1067), president of the American Organization of Operating Nurses (AORN), suggested that although some might "marvel at how far we have come in terms of accepting racial and gender differences," a mixture of professionals with different attributes and skills playing various roles is absolutely essential to an effective organization. Indeed, the Sullivan Commission on Diversity in the Healthcare Workforce went so far as to say that "a disproportionately white healthcare workforce cannot adequately serve a population that is increasingly non-white" (Dixon, 2008, para 6). De Leon Siantz (2008) agreed, suggesting that the elimination of health disparities in the 21st century depends on having nurse leaders who reflect the ethnic and racial diversity of the communities in which they live. Similarly, the Joint Commission (2008) recently released a report entitled *One Size Does Not Fit All: Meeting the Health Care Needs of Diverse Populations*. This report calls on health care organizations to meet the unique cultural and language needs of a diverse population and provides a tool for organizations to use that promotes patient safety and health care quality for all patients.

DISCUSSION POINT

For nursing care to be culturally and ethnically sensitive, must it be provided by a culturally and ethnically diverse nursing population?

Historically, despite this stated need for and appreciation of the benefits of a diverse health care workforce, efforts to increase the number of minority professionals have not been as successful as hoped. The reasons barriers remain are numerous, but the roots can certainly be found in racism, discrimination, and a lack of commitment to changing the situation.

CONSIDER

Barriers to increasing the number of minority health care professionals include, but are not limited to, racism, discrimination, and a lack of commitment to changing the situation.

This chapter focuses primarily on three aspects of diversity in the nursing workforce: ethnicity, gender, and age (generational factors). Factors leading to the lack of ethnic and gender diversity in nursing are explored, as are individual and organizational strategies to address the problem. (The importation of foreign nurses as a factor in workforce diversity is discussed in Chapter 6.) In addition, the efforts of current professional nursing organizations to increase diversity in the profession are examined. Finally, the effect of generational diversity on workers and workplace functioning is presented.

ETHNIC DIVERSITY

Ethnic Diversity in the United States

Demographic data from the U.S. Census Bureau continues to show increased diversification of the U.S. population, a trend that began almost 35 years ago. As of 2006, about 1 in every 3 U.S. residents was part of a group other than single-race non-Hispanic white (U.S. Census Bureau, 2007), and the 2007 U.S. census put the nation's minority population total at 102.5 million, or 34% of the U.S. population (American Association of Colleges of Nursing [AACN], 2008a).

Hispanics continue to be the largest minority group at 42.7 million and are the fastest-growing population group (U.S. Census Bureau, 2007). Blacks are the second-largest minority group (39.7 million), followed by Asians (14.4 million), American Indians and Alaska natives (4.5 million), and native Hawaiians and other Pacific islanders (990,000). The population of non-Hispanic whites who indicated no other race totaled 198.4 million in 2005 (U.S. Census Bureau, 2007).

Ethnic Diversity in Nursing

There are significant differences between the ethnic and gender demographics of the U.S. population and those of the nursing workforce in the United States (Table 9.1). Whereas the number of nurses from minority backgrounds continues to rise in the United States, it is considerably lower than the minority representation in the general population.

According to the latest National Sample Survey of Registered Nurses (NSSRN) from 2004, nurses from minority backgrounds represent just 10.7% of the registered nurse (RN) workforce. Indeed, the RN population comprises 4.2% African American, 1.7% Hispanic,

TABLE 9.1	Comparison of U.S. Population and Registered Nurse Workforce in Terms of Ethnicity and Gender	
Characteristic	**Year 2007 U.S. Census Data (% representation)**	**Year 2004 Registered Nurse Workforce (% representation)**
Gender: male	49	5.8
Gender: female	51	94.2
White (non-Hispanic)	77.1	89.3
Black/African American	12.9	4.2
Asian/Native Hawaiian	4.5	3.1
American Indian/Alaskan native	1.5	0.3
Hispanic/Latino	14.8	1.6
Two or more races	1.3	1.4

Source: AACN (2008a); United States. Population and demographics (2008); U.S. Census Bureau (2007).

3.1% Asian/Native Hawaiian, 0.3% American Indian/Alaskan Native, and 1.4% multiracial nurses.

Although the Hispanic population (at 44.3 million) is the nation's largest minority group, Bond, Gray, Baxley, Cason, and Denke (2008) suggested that Hispanics are the "missing persons" in the health professions, representing only 2% of the nursing workforce. Asians, who make up just over 4% of the U.S. population and are represented at that rate or higher in most health care segments—particularly physicians and surgeons (16.1%)—they are underrepresented as licensed practical and vocational nurses (3.6%) (Dixon, 2008).

Creating a nursing workforce that mirrors the degree of diversity in the general population will not be easy. As Dixon (2008) pointed out, "an increase of more than 20,000 minority nurses is needed to increase their proportion of the nursing workforce by just 1 percent" (para 10).

Clearly, though, increasing diversity in the nursing profession must begin with the aggressive recruitment and retention of minority students. The AACN's 2007/2008 report *Enrollment and Graduations in Baccalaureate and Graduate Programs in Nursing* is encouraging, suggesting that 26.0% of nursing students in entry-level baccalaureate programs are from minority backgrounds (AACN, 2008a). About 23.4% of master's students and 21.0% of students in research-focused doctoral programs are also from minority backgrounds. In addition, the National League for Nursing, in their *Annual Nursing Data Review for Academic Year 2005–2006*, reported "a marked increase in the percentage of graduating pre-licensure students who are members of racial or ethnic minority groups, with the increase distributed across all racial and ethnic categories: Asians, African Americans, Hispanics, and American Indians" (A Call to Action, 2008, para 1). Still more must be done to reach equal representation.

It is also important to note that according to the 2004 NSSRN, registered nurses from minority backgrounds are more likely than their white counterparts to pursue baccalaureate and higher degrees in nursing (AACN, 2008a). Only 46.5% of white nurses complete nursing degrees beyond the associate degree, in contrast to 52% of African Americans, 46.4% of Hispanics, and 72.6% of Asian nurses: "RNs from minority backgrounds clearly recognize the need to pursue higher levels of nursing education beyond the entry-level" (AACN, 2008a, para 5).

> **DISCUSSION POINT**
> Why are RNs from minority backgrounds more likely than their white counterparts to pursue higher education beyond their entry level? What factors might be contributing to this trend?

Recruiting Minority Students into Nursing

De Leon Siantz (2008) suggested that the key to recruiting more minority students into nursing is the creation of a corporate environment in schools of nursing that integrates diversity and cultural competence across academic programs, research, practice, and public policy to eliminate health disparities in partnership with faculty, students, staff, the university infrastructure, and the community at large. Sequist (2007) concurred, suggesting that financial constraints, as well as a lack of appropriate mentorship, are root causes of the low enrollment of Native American students in medical school and other health-related degree tracks. Sequist suggested that academic institutions can play a vital role in reaching out to provide the appropriate experiences and resources that will engage Native American students and help them take the next step toward a career in health care, but cautioned that these programs should always be accompanied by an appropriate evaluation structure that ensures continued improvement and facilitation of particular student needs.

Oscos-Sanchez, Oscos-Flores, and Burge (2008) outlined a different strategy for promoting the recruitment of underrepresented students in health careers in their description of a Teen Medical Academy (TMA) designed to increase career interest in medicine for underrepresented ethnic minority students from economically disadvantaged backgrounds. Students participating in the TMA reported greater interest in medical and allied health careers; confidence in the ability to achieve a health career, to learn surgical skills, and to learn other health career–related technical skills; a sense of belongingness in a health career and among doctors; and commitment to achieve a health career and meaningful work. Higher grade point average and greater involvement in extracurricular health career programs were also reported.

Unfortunately, such positive and nurturing environments for students from underrepresented backgrounds are limited in number, and the end result is that many such students either are never presented the opportunity to pursue nursing as a career or fail to receive the necessary support to successfully complete their nursing education.

In addition, many experts suggest that recruitment and retention rates are low with underrepresented groups because such groups are at greater risk of being economically disadvantaged and this, in turn, places them at greater risk of having received an inferior preparatory education. Students who complete their secondary education in economically disadvantaged communities or institutions may have inadequately developed reading, writing, and critical thinking skills and often lack access to advanced preparation in the natural and physical sciences. This makes them less viable as candidates for admission to a nursing program.

CONSIDER

Recruitment and retention of minority nursing students could improve if these students were given solid secondary academic preparation and if the environments in which they are educated were more accepting of and hospitable to students from diverse backgrounds.

Retaining Minority Students in Nursing

Despite the challenges inherent in recruiting minority students, recruiting them is still often easier than retaining them. The literature overwhelmingly suggests that minority students face more barriers than their white counterparts in completing their nursing education. Some of these barriers are shown in Box 9.1.

For some minority students, it is an inferior secondary education preparation that predisposes them to course and even program failure. In addition, because many minority students are the first in their families to attend college, it might be difficult for family members to understand and be supportive of the challenges of higher education and the rigor of academic coursework. Finances are also often a barrier to minority students, many of whom must work at least part time to subsidize the cost of their college education.

BOX 9.1

COMMON BARRIERS FOR MINORITY STUDENTS IN ACADEMIC NURSING PROGRAMS

1. Inferior academic preparation.
2. Financial problems.
3. Inadequate social support.
4. A lack of mentoring opportunities.
5. Inconsistent faculty and institutional support.
6. Inadequate numbers of minority faculty role models.

DISCUSSION POINT

Should more resources (time, energy, money) be devoted to the recruitment of or retention of minority students? Is a two-pronged approach (emphasizing both recruitment and retention) necessary? Why or why not?

Minority students also tend to experience more difficulty with social adjustment in the college environment, particularly when they are attending a predominantly white institution. Nugent, Childs, Jones, and Cook (2004) suggested that to improve the retention and graduation rates of minority students in nursing, an educational environment supporting the needs of all students, regardless of cultural, ethnic, or gender background, must exist. This environment must include academic support, financial support, self-development and professional/leadership development, faculty mentoring, and institutional awareness.

CONSIDER

Nugent et al. (2004) suggested that although much emphasis has traditionally been placed on recruitment strategies targeting minority students, it is the retention and graduation of minority students that will begin to change the cultural face of nursing.

Similarly, in their focus group interviews of 14 Mexican American nursing students from two liberal arts universities, Bond et al. (2008) found that finances, emotional and moral support, professional socialization, mentoring, academic advising, and technical support were important factors contributing to minority student's successful completion of the nursing program requirements. In addition, students identified personal determination as an important component, and the researchers concluded that faculty can play an important role in helping students capitalize on this personal determination.

Giddens (2008) also suggested that traditional curricular and pedagogical practices used in nursing programs do not accommodate the needs of diverse learners. She suggested that "attaining diversity within the nursing profession begins with attracting various student populations into nursing programs and then providing a learning environment in which all students can thrive" (p. 82).

Perhaps one of the most articulate and well-organized documents for helping culturally diverse students be successful, regardless of their educational level is the 2004 Report of the Sullivan Commission on Diversity in the Healthcare Workforce for Increasing Diversity in Nursing Education Programs. Strategies included in the document are shown in Box 9.2.

The AACN (2005) published *Effective Strategies for Increasing Diversity in Nursing Programs*. This document

BOX 9.2 | STRATEGIES IDENTIFIED BY THE SULLIVAN COMMISSION ON DIVERSITY IN THE HEALTHCARE WORKFORCE FOR INCREASING DIVERSITY IN NURSING EDUCATION PROGRAMS

1. Diversity program managers should be hired by health profession schools to develop plans to ensure institutional diversity.
2. Colleges and universities should provide an array of support services to minority students, including mentoring, test-taking skills, and application counseling.
3. Schools granting baccalaureate nursing degrees should provide "bridging programs" that help graduates of 2-year programs transition to 4-year institutions.
4. Associate nursing graduates should be encouraged to enroll in baccalaureate programs.
5. Professional organizations should work with schools to promote enhanced admissions policies, cultural competence training and minority student recruitment.
6. Organizations should provide scholarships, loan forgiveness, and tuition reimbursement programs to remove financial barriers to nursing education.

Source: Dixon, M. E. (2008). Diversity in nursing. *Advance for Nurses*. Available at: http://nursing.advanceweb.com/editorial/content/editorial.aspx?cc=57273. Accessed July 26, 2008.

highlights numerous successful campaigns undertaken by nursing schools to increase diversity in their nursing programs.

In addition, the U.S. Health Resources and Services Administration (HRSA) is addressing the need for financial support for individuals from disadvantaged backgrounds by offering the Nursing Workforce Diversity (NWD) program, which was established n 1998 to provide "grants or contracts to projects that incorporate retention programs, pre-entry preparation programs, and supports student scholarships and/or stipend programs" (HRSA, 2008, para 2). The goals of the NWD program are to improve the diversity of the nursing workforce in an effort to provide for culturally sensitive and quality health care, to create a racially and ethnically diverse nursing workforce, and to contribute to the basic preparation of disadvantaged and minority nurses for leadership positions within the nursing profession and the health care community (HRSA).

To be eligible for an NWD grant, students must come from an educationally or economically disadvantaged background (including students who belong to racial/ethnic minorities underrepresented among nurses) and express an interest in becoming a registered nurse (Rural Assistance Center, 2008). More than $302,000 was budgeted for NWD grants in 2008, and more than $318,000 was actually funded (HRSA, 2008). Unfortunately, the budgeted amount for 2009 dropped to just more than $66,000, more than $252,000 less than current funding (HRSA).

Ethnic Diversity in Education and Health Care Administration

The exact number of minority nurses in leadership positions has not been determined; however, clearly, minority nurses are underrepresented in such positions in both the academic and service sectors.

Minority Nurse Educators

Current data suggest that only 10.8% of all full-time instructional faculty members in baccalaureate and graduate programs are members of racial/ethnic minority groups, and only 5.7% are male (AACN, 2008a). The sad fact is that far too few nurses from racial/ethnic minority groups with advanced nursing degrees pursue faculty careers.

In an effort to increase the number of minority nurse scholars, the American Association of Colleges of Nursing and the Johnson and Johnson Campaign for Nursing's Future launched a national scholarship program in 2007 to increase the number of nursing faculty from ethnic minority backgrounds (AACN, 2008b). This scholarship program supports full-time nursing students in doctoral or master's degree programs, with a preference given to those completing a doctorate. Scholarship recipients must agree to teach in a U.S. school of nursing after completing their advanced degree. The first five scholarship recipients were selected for the 2008–2009 academic year, with each receiving an $18,000 scholarship. This initiative was modeled after the successful California Endowment-AACN Minority Nurse Faculty Scholarship that was successfully launched in spring 2006 to address the shortage of minority faculty in California (Program Helps Minority Nurse Scholars, 2007).

Minority Nurse Administrators

The number of minority nurses holding leadership positions in the service sector is less clear. Although there is little disagreement that minorities are underrepresented, perceptions differ as to the degree. Survey data from Witt-Kieffer, an executive search firm for health care leaders, suggested that 20% of minorities believe that minorities are well represented in health care management as compared to 41% of whites (Moon, 2007). In fact, Moon openly questioned whether any progress has been made since the early 1990s, when an industry study found that just 1% of top hospital management positions were held by minorities, despite the fact that minorities held nearly 20% of the employee positions.

Similarly, M. Evans (2007) reported that a 2002 survey by the American College of Health Executives (ACHE) found that despite the nation's increasing diversity, far fewer blacks, Hispanics, Native Americans, and Asians reported top-tier management jobs than whites, and a 2007 survey reported that only 6% of ACHE members are black, 3% are Hispanic, 3% are Asian or Pacific Islander, and fewer than 1% are American Indian or Alaskan.

Similarly, Sloane (2006, para 4) suggested that although the number of minorities in executive health care positions may have increased slightly in the last few years, many still find "they bounce off a Teflon ceiling leading to the executive suite." He argued that mentoring is key to addressing the problem so that minorities can experience the same hand up that whites often report. Only then, he suggests, can blacks and Hispanics succeed in the largely white world of the executive suite and the boardroom.

Witt-Kieffer (2008) also bemoaned the lack of minorities and women in health care leadership positions and shared research findings that the majority of CEOs report not having enough time to mentor women or minorities for such roles. Minorities fare worse than women, however, with 68% of respondents believing the health care providers fail to effectively develop minority leaders for future CEO roles, whereas only 48% believing that the same is true for women executives.

Even the means through which women and minorities are developed for leadership roles in health care differ. Fifty-five percent of CEOs reported developing future female leaders by exposure to health care provider boards/board members and board committee work, as opposed to 41% who develop minorities in the same manner (Witt-Kieffer, 2008). In addition, nearly three fourths (73%) of respondents said women leaders are developed by enabling them to attend educational conferences, as opposed to 60% who said the same of minorities.

CONSIDER

Increasing the number of ethnic minorities in executive health care positions will require an intentional commitment to do so and a well-planned development program that includes the same type of mentoring activities that white men have long enjoyed and benefited from.

Linda Hill, a professor of business administration at Harvard Business School, suggested in a 2008 interview with *Harvard Business Review* that cadres of globally savvy executives do not currently exist (Hemp, 2008). She suggested that this occurs in part because many organizations fail to view talented people as potential leaders. This may occur because "'demographic invisibles'—people who, because of their gender, ethnicity, nationality, or even age, don't have access to the tools—the social networks, the fast-track training courses, the stretch assignments—that can prepare them for positions of authority and influence" (p. 125).

Hill also suggested that other potential leaders are missed since they are viewed as "'stylistic invisibles'—individuals who don't fit the conventional image of a leader, since they don't exhibit take charge, direction setting behavior" (Hemp, 2008, p. 125). This also may represent cultural differences more than leadership ability. Clearly, then, nursing education programs and health care organizations must be more open-minded about who the profession's future leaders might be and begin to prepare nurses to be effective leaders. This will require the formal education and training that are a part of most management development programs, as well as a development of appropriate attitudes through social learning (Marquis and Huston, 2009).

One organization that has made a concerted effort to recognize and develop minority leaders is Catholic Healthcare West. In an organization with 44,000 employees and 40 hospitals, more than 50% of executives with system-wide responsibilities are women or minorities, and the organization's hiring policy calls for at least 10% of all senior management vacancies to be filled by minority candidates (Voges & Burda, 2006).

Another organization that made that commitment and established such a development program is the Hospital Corporation of America (HCA). The HCA reported that 13% of the system's chief executive officer (CEO) leadership positions were held by minorities in 2007, as compared to 5% in 2003 (Moon, 2007). This increase is a direct reflection of HCA's implementation of a program directed at cultivating minority leaders that began in 2001.

Such programs will be absolutely essential to significantly increase the number of minorities and women in health care leadership positions. Greer and Virick (2008, p. 353) concurred, suggesting that "the future of many organizations is likely to depend on their mastery of diverse succession planning given that building bench strength among women and minorities will be critical in the competitive war for talent." They went on to say that direct involvement and commitment by organization leaders are essential threshold requirements for diverse succession planning.

Greer and Virick (2008) also suggested there is a great deal that organizations can do to encourage and support diversity in the workplace, including removing career advancement barriers for women and minorities and actively planning for diverse leadership succession. Although they bemoaned the need for

Research Study Fuels the Controversy: Diversity and Succession Planning

Based on semistructured interviews with 27 Human Resource (HR) professionals from 25 organizations (24 in the United States and 1 in Canada), the authors examined both barriers to and strategies for diverse succession planning.

STUDY FINDINGS

Interviewees suggested a need to "reach deeper into the organization" and to identify potential talent earlier in filling executive positions, although at least one interviewee stressed the importance of focusing on developing high potential rather than just promulgating diversity. Another individual, however, emphasized the importance of setting diversity goals in recognition of the changing racial composition of the United States. Most interviewees agreed that developing a culture of inclusiveness is important because diverse employees often look upward in the hierarchy to see if anyone looks like them and wonder whether the environment is accepting of them.

In addition, another interviewee "stressed the importance of objective standards of potential and readiness for promotion to offset unconscious biases against women" (p. 358). Indeed, one interviewee suggested that women sometimes face so many problems in gaining acceptance that they simply decide not to pursue a particular career goal. Coaching and mentoring were identified as effective strategies for both the promotion of and retention of women and minorities in the workforce.

Greer, C. R., & Virick, M. (2008). Diverse succession planning: Lessons from the industry leaders. *Human Resource Management, 47*(2), 351–367.

special developmental programs for women and minorities, they suggested that they continue to appear to be needed for progress. Wooten (2008, p. 192), agreed, arguing there is a need to further "identify trigger points for shattering the glass ceiling, removing silos, and erasing boundaries in organizations" before we can move the inclusion journey forward. (See Research Study Fuels the Controversy.)

Ethnic Professional Associations in Nursing

There is a professional association for almost every ethnic group in nursing, including the National Black Nurses Association, established in 1971; the National Association of Hispanic Nurses, founded in 1975; the Philippine Nurses Association of America, formed in 1979; and the National Alaska Native American Indian Nurses Association. See Box 9.3 for more information on these groups.

DISCUSSION POINT

If our goal is to better appreciate and merge cultural and ethnic diversity in nursing, why do culturally and ethnically diverse nurses separate themselves with their own professional nursing organizations?

GENDER DIVERSITY

Gender Diversity in Nursing

Diversity goals in nursing are not just directed at ethnicity—they also frequently include increasing the number of men in nursing. Although men have worked as nurses for centuries, just 5.8% of the nation's 2.9 million nurses are men, a percentage that has climbed fairly steadily since the NNSRN was first conducted in 1980 (AACN, 2008a). Indeed, the number of male nurses has surged from 45,060 nurses in 1980 to 168,181 nurses in 2004, an increase of 273.2% in this time period (AACN).

Yet, despite a call to increase the number of men in nursing, progress in this regard has been slow for many reasons. Stereotypes of male nurses as being different or effeminate due to their close working relationship with women persist. In addition, most of the public would describe nursing as a female occupation, and young men often report they never even considered a career as a nurse.

The media also perpetuates the image of the nurse as female. Many media sources, and even nursing textbooks at times, refer to the comforting caregiver nurse as "she" and make no mention of men, except as sickly,

| BOX 9.3 | ETHNIC PROFESSIONAL ASSOCIATIONS IN NURSING |

Support groups and professional associations abound among nurses in the United States. Some of the groups formed to address specific issues related to ethnic diversity in nursing include the following:

National Black Nurses Association

The National Black Nurses Association (NBNA), founded in 1971, represents approximately 150,000 black nurses from the United States (with 76 chartered chapters nationwide), the Eastern Caribbean nations, and Africa (NBNA, n.d.). The mission of the NBNA is to provide a forum for collective action by black nurses to "investigate, define and determine what the health care needs of African Americans are and to implement change to make health care available to African Americans and other minorities that is commensurate with that [health care] of the larger society" (NBNA, para 4).

National Association of Hispanic Nurses

The National Association of Hispanic Nurses (NAHN) was founded in 1975 by Ildaura Murillo-Rohde and evolved out of the Ad Hoc Committee of the Spanish-Speaking/Spanish Surname Nurses' Caucus, which was formed during the American Nurses Association convention in San Francisco in 1974 (NAHN, n.d.). The NAHN strives to serve the nursing and health care delivery needs of the Hispanic community and the professional needs of Hispanic nurses. In addition, it is committed to improving the quality of health and nursing care for Hispanic consumers and to providing equal access to educational, professional, and economic opportunities for Hispanic nurses.

Philippine Nurses Association of America

The Philippine Nurses Association of America (PNAA) was formed in 1979 in an effort to address the issues and concerns of Filipino nurses in the United States. Its mission is to uphold and foster the positive image and welfare of its constituent members. In addition, the PNAA seeks to promote professional excellence and contribute to significant outcomes to health care and society (PNAA, 2006).

National Alaska Native American Indian Nurses Association

The National Alaska Native American Indian Nurses Association (NANAINA) was founded on its predecessor organization, the American Indian Nurses Association, and, later, the American Indian Alaska Native Nurses Association. The NANAINA is dedicated to supporting Alaska Native and American Indian students, nurses, and allied health professionals through the development of leadership skills and continuing education. It also advocates for the improvement of health care provided to American Indian and Alaska Native consumers and culturally competent health care (NANAINA, n.d.). Similar goals exist for the Asian and Pacific Islander population as described by the Asian and Pacific Islander Nurses Association.

demanding patients. The difficulty of male nurses socializing into what has long been perceived as a woman's occupation is depicted in Figure 9.1.

The stereotype of the male nurse as homosexual is also prevalent. Harding's (2007) study of New Zealand male nurses found that despite participants' beliefs that most male nurses are heterosexual, many male nurses are exposed to homophobia in the workplace. The heterosexual men reported employing strategies to avoid a presumption of homosexuality, including avoiding contact with gay colleagues and overt expression of their heterosexuality. Research by Snyder and Green (2008) suggested that male nurses might also seek employment in areas of nursing they perceive to be "more masculine" in an effort to dispel questions about their sexuality.

> CONSIDER
>
> Heterosexual male nurses report employing strategies to avoid a presumption of homosexuality, including avoiding contact with gay colleagues and overt expression of their heterosexuality. They also tend to seek employment in areas of nursing they perceive to be "more masculine" in an effort to dispel questions about their sexuality.

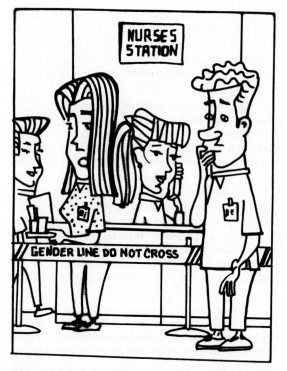

Figure 9.1. Challenges faced by men in nursing. Copyright 2002, MedZilla, Inc. http://www.medzilla.com. Reprinted with permission.

Harding (2007) concluded that a paradox exists between the public call for more men to engage in caring professions such as nursing and the repercussions they often experience as a result of the stereotype of male nurses as gay or sexually predatory. He suggested that these stigmatizing discourses deter men's entry into the profession and likely affect their retention. Nelson and Belcher (2006) agreed, suggesting that homophobia and a perception that nursing is an occupation only for women are key reasons that many men avoid choosing nursing as a profession.

Equally troubling are the research findings of Harding, North, and Perkins (2008) that whereas touch is important in nursing care, it is problematic for male nurses because women's use of touch is viewed as a caring behavior and men's touch is often viewed sexually. Male nurses in this study described their vulnerability, how they protected themselves from risk, and the resulting stress. The researchers concluded that a paradox emerges whereby the very measures employed to protect both patients and men as nurses exacerbate the perceived risk posed by men carrying out intimate care.

> ### CONSIDER
> Caregiving is not just a feminine trait.

Clearly, stereotypes that suggest that male nurses are less capable of therapeutic caring, compassion, and nurturing than female nurses hurt the profession, as well as society in general. At least partly as a result of these stereotypes, some patients have gender preferences (more commonly female) for their caregivers. This seems to be particularly true for nurses employed in labor and delivery settings.

Dorman (2008) suggested that maternal-newborn nursing is often viewed as women's domain with the exception of physicians and husbands, and went on to say that the barriers to men working in this setting are multifaceted. Many male nursing students worry that their care could be interpreted as inappropriately sexual or unprofessional. In some settings, men must still have a woman present when examining patients, and some male students feel comfortable in the labor and delivery setting only when male physicians are present.

Court cases have confused the issue further. In some cases, the courts have ruled that female gender is a legitimate qualification for labor and delivery nurses, yet other courts have found these qualifications to be discriminatory. The Association of Women's Health, Obstetric and Neonatal Nurses (AWHONN) argued that although all clients and families have the right to clinically competent, professional care, that the gender of the nurse should not be a factor (Dorman, 2008).

The issue was confused even further in a presentation at the October 2007 conference of the American Assembly for Men in Nursing, in which Josephine Devito and Scott Saccomano suggested that often it is the nursing faculty who have concerns about male students in obstetrics, not the patients and their partners (S. Evans, 2007). They encouraged nursing faculty to be sensitive to the needs of both the male student and the female patient by "creating an atmosphere of trust and professionalism as well as providing mentoring and guidance to enhance the learning experience" (Evans, p. 42). Dorman (2008) agreed, suggesting that removing barriers for male students in this setting begins with the nursing faculty, who can do much to minimize the isolation of male nursing students and reduce their stress.

Despite all these public misperceptions and barriers to practice, Susan LaRocca reported at that same conference that interviews with male nurses who joined the profession during the 1940s to 1960s, at a time when it was even more unusual for men to become nurses than today, revealed most of the men experienced tremendous satisfaction from their work (S. Evans, 2007). In addition, most felt that they could inspire young men considering nursing as a career option.

Is There a Male Advantage in Nursing?

Despite the barriers that male nurses face, Kleinman (2004) suggested their minority status also gives male nurses advantages, including those associated with hiring and promotion, that help rather than hinder their careers, unlike women in male-dominated professions. In addition, although sex role stereotyping may limit recruitment of men into nursing, Kleinman suggested that these obstacles to entry into practice are superseded by a quest for personal and professional power among men that facilitates professional career advancement in nursing. Kleinman suggested that this occurs because traditional health care organizations were organized and managed along the lines of patriarchal family structures that favor male dominance.

Tzeng and Chen (2008), in their study of male Taiwanese nurses, also found that male nurses reported gender advantages in terms of professional development. They termed this sense of superiority "the male advantage."

Men in nursing also appear to have an economic advantage. The 2008 Advance Salary Survey showed that male nurses continue to out-earn their female counterparts, with an average salary of $53,792 versus $50,615 for female nurses (O'Brien, 2008).

Similarly, research by Baldwin and Schneller (2008) found that the mean salary for female operating room managers was 93% of the mean salary for men. Male and female nurses in their study had similar education and experience, but men tended to manage more operating rooms, with a higher case volume. In addition, men supervised 50% more personnel than their female counterparts on average, had double the annual budget, and were more likely to work in teaching hospitals. Baldwin and Schneller concluded that there was evidence to suggest gender discrimination in salaries paid

to male/female operating room managers, although the unexplained differential was relatively small. In addition, they found evidence of job segregation within this narrowly defined occupation that could not be explained by differences in the average qualifications of male and female nurses.

Some experts have suggested that the more rapid career trajectory and relative higher pay for male nurses likely reflects the historical trend that more men are employed full time in their career paths whereas women tend to have career gaps related to childbearing or rearing families and often work fewer hours. This was the situation reported by O'Lynn (2008) in his community, where most male RNs worked full time and most female RNs worked 0.8 position or less.

A 2008 study, however, disputed this assumption at least in part, arguing that less than 8% of professional women born since 1956 have left the workforce for 1 year or more during their prime childbearing years (Study Disputes Opt Out Trend, 2008). In fact, the number of professional women working more than 50 hours each week increased from less than 10% for women born before 1935 to 15% for women born after 1956, and the percentage of mothers with young children working full time rose from 6% of women born from 1926 to 1935 to 38% for women born from 1966 to 1975. Although the researchers argued that the "opt-out revolution" is merely hype, they did concede that Generation X and late Baby Boomer women worked less than their male counterparts, although they worked more than previous cohorts (Study Disputes Opt Out Trend).

CONSIDER

Many experts suggest that the power of the profession would be elevated if more men were to become nurses. Yet, men in nursing hold a disproportionately large share of the high-income jobs and have higher salaries than their female counterparts.

Why Are Men Leaving Nursing?

McMillian, Morgan, and Arment (2006) suggested that whereas increased numbers of men were joining the nursing profession, disproportionate numbers of male nurses were leaving compared to female nurses. In fact, new male nurses leave the profession within 4 years of graduation at a rate almost twice that of female nurse graduates. McMillian et al. suggested that a lack of social approval, acceptance, and adequate role models beginning in nursing school are to blame. Similarly, a round-table discussion at the close of the aforementioned October 2007 conference on men in nursing concluded that the "fundamental barrier to gender equality in the field was a lack of positive, visible, and accurate male role models in nursing—both in the classroom and in clinical practice" (S. Evans, 2007, p. 42).

In studying acceptance as a factor for male nurse retention, McMillian et al. (2006) found that the most influential condition on acceptance of male nurses by their female counterparts was length of time worked with a male nurse. In addition, the researchers found that lingering nonacceptance of male nurses continued among some female nurses, and that these attitudes were likely the result of early role socialization. They concluded that nursing education could do much to eliminate sexism and discrimination by eliminating any policies that reinforce social- and gender-related segregation, by promoting nursing as a gender-neutral occupation, and by the active recruitment of male nursing instructors.

In addition, although the literature has been mixed, the majority of nursing studies that examined gender and job dissatisfaction suggested that male nurses are more dissatisfied than their female counterparts. Some experts argue that more men than women leave nursing because nursing still lacks status and therefore nurses are often demeaned by other health professionals. Male nurses may be less willing to tolerate this kind of treatment. S. Evans (2007) suggested that the climate was slowly changing for men entering the nursing profession. She suggested, however, that improving support and understanding in both the classroom and practice settings could go far in enhancing the ability to recruit, educate, and retain men in the nursing profession.

CONSIDER

Recent graduates of the nation's nursing schools are leaving the profession more quickly than their predecessors, with male nurses leaving at a much higher rate than their female counterparts.

Recruiting Men into Nursing: Is Affirmative Action Required?

There are efforts underway to increase the number of men in nursing. Some nursing schools are participating in both national and local campaigns to increase gender diversity in the profession, and the results are encouraging. In 2007 to 2008, men comprised 10.5% of students in baccalaureate programs, 8.9% of master's students, and 6.9% of students in research-focused doctoral programs, figures higher than in the current RN workforce (AACN, 2008a).

For example, the School of Nursing at Monterey Peninsula College established a men-only study group and implemented a monthly "Men in Nursing" discussion group to reduce possible feelings of isolation for male students (O'Lynn, 2008). They believed that male students should have a safe setting to share concerns that might interfere with their academic success and obtain guidance from other men who understood their situations. The school then applied for and received a grant from the Regional Health Occupations Resource Center of the Chancellor's Office of the California Community Colleges in 2007 for the purpose of recruiting and retaining men in an academic nursing program and to host a 2008 statewide conference on men in nursing (O'Lynn).

Other efforts to increase the representation of men in nursing have resulted from corporate partnerships with professional associations. For example, the American Assembly of Men in Nursing received funding from the American Association of Nurse Anesthetists, Kaiser Permanente, the Johnson & Johnson Campaign for Nursing's Future, the Nurses Service Organization, and the Nursing 2006 Foundation to promote a 30-minute film documentary called "Career Encounters: Men in Nursing" (A New Recruitment Film, 2007). The documentary features male nurses, including students, advanced practice nurses, nurse educators, and staff nurses, in a number of settings, as well as the use of a state-of-the-art simulator to train nurse anesthetists.

Some suggest that such recruitment campaigns are not enough and that affirmative action, similar to the efforts used to increase the number of women in medicine and engineering, will be required before there will be any significant increase in the number of male nurses. O'Lynn (2008) agreed, suggesting that despite a growing recognition in the professional literature that men face unique challenges in nursing school, as well as in transition to professional practice, the response from the profession as a whole has simply been a tacit acknowledgment of the topic. He suggested the need for a national initiative that would enhance the professional climate for men in nursing or promote the large-scale recruitment of men into nursing.

Many experts feel, however, that simply getting more male bodies into classroom seats is not enough. Nursing programs, they argue, must also make significant changes in their curricula and teaching styles to create a more positive and nondiscriminatory learning environment for nursing students who happen to be men.

DISCUSSION POINT

Affirmative action has been used successfully to increase the presence of some underrepresented minorities in health care. Should the same be done to increase the number of men in nursing?

GENERATIONAL DIVERSITY IN NURSING

Age has become a diversity issue during the last decade. The problem is not that the nursing workforce lacks generational diversity, but that typically four generations have not cohabitated together at the same time in a profession. This climate offers challenges and opportunities for leaders and also provides opportunities to further diversify a workforce to more closely resemble the clients they serve and to identify the best thinking of so many perspectives.

According to the 2004 NSSRN, the average age of an RN in the United States climbed to 46.8 years in 2004, the highest average age since the first comparable report was published in 1980 (Nursing Workforce Expands, 2007). In addition, only 8% of RNs were younger than the age of 30 years in 2004, compared to 25% in 1980. Given the current nursing shortage and the need to both retain and recruit older nurses and to bring new, young nurses into the field, generational issues must be examined further.

Defining the Generations

The research increasingly suggests that the different generations represented in nursing today may have different value systems, which greatly impacts the settings in which they work. Patterson (2007, p. 17), agreed, arguing that although members of a particular generational group might exhibit differences, many who grew up in the same time period have a strong identification with their own "time in history" and may act in similar ways based on the influences of that time.

For example, most experts identify four generational groups in today's workforce; the "veteran generation" (also called the "silent generation"), the "Baby Boomers," Generation X, and Generation Y (also called the "Millennials").

The *veteran generation* is typically recognized as those nurses born between 1925 and 1942. Currently, about 9% of employed nurses belong to this age group (Boivin, 2008). Having lived through several international military conflicts (World War II, the Korean War, and the Vietnam War) and the Great Depression, they are often risk averse (particularly in regard to personal finances), respectful of authority, supportive of hierarchy, and disciplined (Patterson, 2007). They are also called the *silent generation* because they tend to support the status quo rather than protest or push for rapid change. As a result, these nurses are less likely to question organizational practices and more likely to seek employment in structured settings (Marquis & Huston, 2009). Their work values are traditional, and they are often recognized for their loyalty to their employers.

The "boom generation" (born 1943 to 1960) also displays traditional work values; however, they tend to be more materialistic and thus are willing to work long hours at their jobs in an effort to get ahead. Indeed, this generation is more apt than any other to be called "workaholics," and their general inclination is to live for the present rather than the future (Patterson, 2007). Forty-seven percent of currently employed nurses and 46% of nurses working in hospitals belong to this generation (Boivin, 2008).

In addition, this generation of workers is often recognized as being more individualistic as a result of the "permissive parenting" many of them experienced growing up, constantly being told that their future contained limitless opportunities for achievement (Patterson, 2007). This individualism often results in greater creativity and thus nurses born in this generation may be best suited for work that requires flexibility, independent thinking, and creativity. Yet, it also encourages this generation to challenge rules.

In contrast, "Generation Xers" (born between 1961 and 1981), a much smaller cohort than the Baby Boomers who preceded them or the Generation Yers who follow them, may lack the interest in lifetime employment at one place that prior generations have valued, instead valuing greater work-hour flexibility and opportunities for time off. This likely reflects the fact that many individuals born in this generation had both parents working outside their home as they were growing up and they want to put more emphasis on family and leisure time in their own family units. Thus, this generation may be less economically driven than prior generations and may define success differently than the veteran generation or the Baby Boomers. They are, however, pragmatic, self-reliant, and amenable to change (Patterson, 2008). Forty-two percent of the RN workforce belongs to this generational cohort (Boivin, 2008).

"Generation Y" (born 1978 to 1986) represents the first cohort of truly global citizens. They are known for their optimism, self-confidence, relationship orientation, volunteer-mindedness, and social consciousness. They are also highly sophisticated in their use of technology, which allows them to view the world as a "smaller, diverse, highly-networked environment in which to work and live" (Patterson, 2007, p. 20). This is why some people call this generation "*digital natives.*" Generation Y currently represents only 2% of the nursing workforce, but this number will increase rapidly over the coming decade (Boivin, 2008).

Generation Y does, however, demand a different type of organizational culture to meet their needs (Piper, 2008). In fact, Generation Y nurses may test the patience of their Baby Boomer leaders: "They come to work in flip-flops listening to their iPods and are brash and ready to hit the ground running" (What Does It Take, 2008, para 2). They also "often come with a sense of entitlement that can be an affront to older workers. They want to do something meaningful today" and they "don't want to spend days at a desk listening to orientation lectures" (What Does It Take, para 6).

Mensik (2007) suggested that although generational diversity poses new management challenges, it also provides a variety of perspectives and outlooks that enhance workplace balance and productivity. She suggested that the literature often focuses on differences and negative attributes between the generations, particularly for Generations X and Y, and that a balanced view is needed.

For example, the literature repeatedly suggests that Generations X and Y may have less loyalty to their employers than the generations who preceded them, but Mensik cited current research that suggests that their commitment to employment longevity is actually greater than that of the Boomers who preceded them. Mensik concluded that instead of focusing on generational differences, nurses should instead move forward and put their energies into seeking collaboration between the generations. In addition, patients should benefit from the optimal outcomes that should occur when all generations of the workforce can work together as a higher-performing team.

Boivin (2008, para 14) also suggested that the people who benefit the most from such differences and strengths are the patients. She argued that such diversity allows patients to "have nurses caring for them who have 20 or 30 years experience under their belts, who are able to use the latest technology to prevent errors, and who are willing to challenge authority and act as patient advocates."

PROFESSIONAL ORGANIZATIONS SPEAK OUT

In the last decade many professional nursing organizations have issued position statements or recommendations on diversity. In 1997, the AACN, the national voice for baccalaureate and higher-degree education programs, drafted a position statement that suggests that diversity and inclusion have emerged as central issues for organizations and institutions and that leadership in nursing must respond to these issues by finding ways to accelerate the inclusion of groups, cultures, and ideas that traditionally have been underrepresented in higher education. Moreover, the position statement argues that health care providers and the nursing profession should reflect and value the diversity of the populations and communities they serve.

The ANA issued a position statement on discrimination and racism in health care in 1998 and stated its commitment to working toward the eradication of discrimination and racism in the profession of nursing, in the education of nurses, in the practice of nursing, and in the organizations in which nurses work. The *ANA Code of Ethics for Nurses* advocates diversity in its assertion that the nurse, in all professional relationships, practices with compassion and respect for the inherent dignity, worth, and uniqueness of every individual, unrestricted by considerations of social or economic status, personal attributes, or the nature of health problems.

The American Organization of Nurse Executives also developed a diversity statement in 2005. This statement suggests that the success of nursing leadership as a profession depends on reflecting the diversity of the communities it serves and that diversity is one of the essential building blocks of a healthful practice/work environment.

In contrast, the International Council of Nurses does not have a diversity statement, but rather has embedded *diversity* in its policy and practice. For example, the organization promotes the principles of equal opportunity employment, pay equity, and occupational desegregation.

Some professional organizations have gone beyond simply arguing the need for diversity and have instead given funds to advance the cause. Despite the backlash in the late 1990s over the practice of affirmative action in helping racial and ethnic minorities enter the health professions, the Bureau of Health Professions within the HRSA, U.S. Department of Health and Human Services, has held steadfast to its goal of ensuring representation of underrepresented minorities in the health professions by prioritizing this goal in funding opportunities.

CONCLUSIONS

Projections suggest that current ethnic minorities are likely, in the not too distant future, to become the majority of the U.S. population. This diversity, however, is not reflected in the nursing workforce or in schools of nursing. Similarly, men are underrepresented in nursing, and efforts to increase the number of men in the nursing profession are even fewer than those directed at increasing ethnic diversity. Finally, generational diversity is occurring in all health care organizations; however, few organizations have directly confronted the implications of how to deal with this diversity or examined the impact it has on the quality of care provided.

Diversity, equity, and parity are business imperatives but should also be moral imperatives. Using "change by drift" strategies to address the lack of ethnic and gender diversity in nursing has been ineffective. In addition, Chavez and Weisinger (2008) argued that contemporary organizations have likely spent millions of dollars on diversity training that has either failed or resulted in less than desired outcomes. Instead, they argued, organizations must create a "culture of diversity" that requires a longer-term, relational approach that emphasizes attitudinal and cultural transformation. Thus, energy is not directed at "managing *diversity*"; instead it is directed toward "managing for *diversity*" to capitalize on the unique perspectives of a diverse workforce. It is clear that proactive, well-thought-out strategies at multiple levels and by multiple parties will be needed before diversity in the nursing profession will mirror that of the public it serves.

FOR ADDITIONAL DISCUSSION

1. What are the strongest driving and restraining forces for increasing ethnic diversity in nursing? For increasing gender diversity in nursing? For having a multigenerational nursing workforce?

2. Should funding for diversity initiatives come from federal or state governments? From corporate partnerships?

3. Should the institutions that reap the benefits of a diverse workforce share the costs to make that happen?

4. Should there be different nursing school entry requirements for minority students than for their white counterparts?

5. Is an affirmative action approach needed to increase the number of both men and minorities in the nursing profession?

6. Will having more men in nursing raise the status of the profession?

7. What are the potential barriers to having more men in the nursing profession?

8. Why have women been better able to further their numbers in medicine than men have in nursing?

9. How does the use of mentors assist in both the recruitment and the retention of minority (ethnic and gender) nurses?

10. Does a multigenerational nursing workforce improve patient care? If so, how?

11. Which health disparities do you think would be more positively impacted if the nursing workforce was more diverse?

REFERENCES

A call to action. Strategies for dealing with the nursing shortage (2008). Cambridge College. Accessible at: http://researchlinda.blogspot.com/. Accessed July 25, 2008.

A new recruitment film for men: nurses and nurse educators in action (2007). *Nursing Education Perspectives, 28*(4), 226.

American Association of Colleges of Nursing (AACN) (2005). *Effective strategies for increasing diversity in nursing programs.* Available at: http://www.aacn. nche.edu/Publications/Issues/dec01.htm. Accessed July 26, 2008.

American Association of Colleges of Nursing (AACN) (2008a). *Fact sheet: Enhancing diversity in the nursing workforce.* Available at: http://www.aacn.nche.edu/ Media/pdf/diversityFS.pdf. Accessed July 22, 2008.

American Association of College of Nursing (AACN) (2008b). First group of minority nurse faculty scholars selected by the Johnson & Johnson Campaign for Nursing's Future and AACN. Available at: http:// www.aacn.nche.edu/Media/NewsReleases/2008/ J&JScholars.htm. Accessed July 26, 2008.

Baldwin, M. L., & Schneller, E. S. (2008). *Gender discrimination and the salaries of operating room managers.* The Fuqua School of Business, Duke University. Workforce issues. Available at: http://ashe2008. abstractbook.org/presentations/228/. Accessed July 25, 2008.

Banschbach, S. K. (2008). Diversity equals organizational strength. *AORN Journal, 87*(6), 1067–1069.

Boivin, J. (2008). Opinion. Nursing enters a new era. Four generations healing under one hospital roof. *Nursing Spectrum. NurseWeek.* Available at: http:// include.nurse.com/apps/pbcs.dll/article?AID=/ 20080811/FL02/308110018. Accessed August 11, 2008.

Bond, M. L., Gray, J. R., Baxley, S., Cason, C. L., & Denke, L. (2008). Voices of Hispanic students in baccalaureate nursing programs: Are we listening? *Nursing Education Perspectives, 29*(3), 136–142.

Chavez, C. I., & Weisinger, J. Y. (2008). Beyond diversity training: A social infusion for cultural inclusion. *Human Resource Management, 47*(2), 331–350.

de Leon Siantz, M. L. (2008). Leading change in diversity and cultural competence. *Journal of Professional Nursing, 24*(3), 167–171.

Dixon, M. E. (2008). Diversity in nursing. *Advance for Nurses.* Available at: http://nursing.advanceweb.com/ editorial/content/editorial.aspx?cc=57273. Accessed July 21, 2008.

Dorman, T. (2008). Guys in LDRP. *Advance for Nurses (Northern California and Northern Nevada), 5*(9), 19.

Evans, M. (2007). Minority execs form groups. *Modern Healthcare, 37*(33), 16.

Evans, S. (2007). Enhancing an image. *Advance for Nurses, Northern California and Northern Nevada, 9*(26), 42. Available at http://www.nursing.advance. web.com/editorial/content/editorial.aspx?cc=137532. Accessed January 30, 2009.

Giddens, J. (2008). Achieving diversity in nursing through multicontextual learning environments. *Nursing Outlook, 56*(2), 78–83.

Greer, C. R., & Virick, M. (2008). Diverse succession planning: Lessons from the industry leaders. *Human Resource Management, 47*(2), 351–367.

Harding, T. (2007). The construction of men who are nurses as gay. *Journal of Advanced Nursing, 60*(6), 636–644.

Harding, T., North, N., & Perkins, R. (2008). Sexualizing men's touch: Male nurses and the use of intimate touch in clinical practice. *Research and Theory for Nursing Practice, 22*(2), 88–102.

Health Resources and Services Administration (HRSA) (2008). *FY 2009 budget justification.* Available at: http://www.hrsa.gov/about/budgetjustification09/ healthprofessionoverview.htm. Accessed July 22, 2008.

Hemp, P. (2008). Where will we find tomorrow's leaders? A conversation with Linda A. Hill by Paul Hemp. *Harvard Business Review.* Available at: http:// harvardbusinessonline.hbsp.harvard.edu/hbsp/hbr/ articles/article.jsp?ml_subscriber=true&ml_ action=get-article&ml_issueid=BR0801&articleID= R0801J&pageNumber=1. Accessed January 16, 2009.

Joint Commission (2008). *Patient safety pulse. Joint Commission releases report on health care and diversity.* Available at: https://aphid.csuchico.edu/illiad/ illiad.dll?SessionID=O065311247Y&Action=10& Form=75&Value=88871. Accessed August 11, 2008.

Kleinman, C. S. (2004). Understanding and capitalizing on men's advantages in nursing. *Journal of Nursing Administration, 34*(2), 78–82.

Marquis, B., & Huston, C. (2009). *Leadership roles and management functions in nursing* (6th ed.). Philadelphia: Lippincott Williams & Wilkins.

McGinnis, S., Moore, J., & Continelli, T. (2006). Practice patterns of underrepresented minority nurse practitioners in New York State, 2000. *Policy, Politics & Nursing Practice, 7*(1), 35–44.

McMillian, J. Morgan, S. A., & Arment, P. (2006). Acceptance of male registered nurses by female registered nurses. *Journal of Nursing Scholarship, 38*(1), 100–106.

Mensik, J. S. (2007). A view on generational differences from a generation X leader. *Journal of Nursing Administration, 37*(11), 483–484.

Moon, S. (2007). Slow progress seen in promoting nurse executives. *Hospitals & Health Networks, 81*(4), 15–16.

National Alaska Native American Indian Nurses Association (n.d.). *About NANAINA.* Available at: http://www.nanainanurses.org/About/index.php. Accessed July 26, 2008.

National Association of Hispanic Nurses (n.d.). *About us.* Available at: http://thehispanicnurses.org/about-us/index.php?Itemid=236. Accessed July 26, 2008.

National Black Nurses Association (n.d.). *About NBA.* Available at: http://www.nbna.org/whoarewe.htm. Accessed July 26, 2008.

Nelson, R., & Belcher, D. (2006). Men in nursing: Still too few: Discrimination and stereotypes still keep many from joining nursing ranks. *American Journal of Nursing, 106*(2), 25–26.

Nugent, K. E., Childs, G., Jones, R., & Cook, P. (2004). A mentorship model for the retention of minority students. *Nursing Outlook, 52*(2), 89–94.

Nursing workforce expands as average age of RNs increases, HRSA survey finds (2007). *HRSA News.* Available at: http://newsroom.hrsa.gov/releases/2007/nursing-survey.htm. Accessed July 24, 2008.

O'Brien, A. (2008). 2008 Advance Salary Survey. *Advance for Nurses.* Available at: http://nursing.advanceweb.com/Article/ADVANCE-Salary-Survey-2008.aspx. Accessed July 26, 2008.

O'Lynn, C. (2008). Monterey Peninsula college receives grant to retain male nursing students. *Interaction— Official Publication of the American Assembly of Men in Nursing, 26*(1), 1.

Oscos-Sanchez, M. A., Oscos-Flores, L. D., & and Burge, S. K. (2008). The Teen Medical Academy: Using academic enhancement and instructional enrichment to address ethnic disparities in the American health-care workforce. *Journal of Adolescent Health 42*(3), 284–293.

Patterson, C. K. (2007). The impact of generational diversity in the workplace. *Diversity Factor, 15*(3), 17–22.

Philippine Nurses Association of America (2006). *Nursing: Caring for a stronger foundation today for the next generation.* Available at: http://www.philippinenursesaa.org/mission.htm. Accessed July 26, 2008.

Piper, L. E. (2008). The Generation-Y workforce in health care: The new challenge for leadership. *Health Care Manager, 27*(2), 98–103.

Program Helps Minority Nurse Scholars (2007). Available at: http://www.minoritynurse.com/vitalsigns/sept07_1.html. Accessed July 26, 2008.

Rural Assistance Center (2008). *Nursing workforce diversity grants.* Available at: http://www.raconline.org/funding/funding_details.php?funding_id=246. Accessed July 22, 2008.

Sequist, T. D. (2007). Health careers for Native American students: Challenges and opportunities for enrichment program design. *Journal of Interprofessional Care, 21*(Supplement 2), 20–30.

Sloane, T. (2006). Through the Teflon ceiling. *Modern Healthcare, 36*(15), 18.

Snyder, K. A., & Green, A. I. (2008). Revisiting the glass escalator: The case of gender segregation in a female dominated occupation. *Social Problems, 55*(2), 271–299.

Study disputes opt out trend for women (2008). *Workforce Management.* Available at: http://www.workforce.com/section/00/article/25/64/20.php.Accessed July 23, 2008.

Tzeng, Y., & Chen, C. (2008). The lived experience of male nursing in clinical nursing practice. *Journal of Evidence-Based Nursing, 4*(1), 61–70.

United States. Population and demographics (2008). Available at: http://www.intute.ac.uk/sciences/worldguide/html/1054_people.html. Accessed July 21, 2008.

U.S. Census Bureau (2007). *Nation's population: One-third minority.* Available at http://www.census.gov/Press-Release/www/releases/archives/population/006808.html. Accessed July 21, 2008.

Voges, N., & Burda, D. (2006). Diversity in the executive suite. *Modern Healthcare, 36*(15), 6–14.

What does it take to build bridges among the different generations? (2008). *OR Manager, 24*(4), 10.

Witt-Kieffer Executive Search Firm (2008). *Preparing future leaders in health care.* Available at: http://www.wittkieffer.com/cmfiles/reports/FutureLeaders.pdf. Accessed July 27, 2008.

Wooten, L. P. (2008). Guest editor's note: Breaking barriers in organizations for the purpose of inclusiveness. *Human Resource Management, 47*(2), 191–197.

BIBLIOGRAPHY

Baby-boomer nurses are on their way out (June 2008). *Nursing, 38*(6), 25.

Brousseau, S., Alderson, M., & Cara, C. (2008). A caring environment to foster male nurses' quality of working life in community settings. *International Journal for Human Caring, 12*(1), 33–43.

Brown, B. E., & Anema, M. A. (2007). Student issues. The road to excellence for minority graduate students. *Nurse Educator, 32*(6), 234–235.

Burnette, M. (2008). Celebrating excellence: Past, present and future. *Minority Nurse, 2008*(Winter), 36–41.

Curtis, E. A. (2008). The effects of biographical variables on job satisfaction among nurses. *British Journal of Nursing, 17*(3), 174–180.

de Leon-Siantz, M. L., & Meleis, A. (2007). Integrating cultural competence into nursing education and practice: 21st century action steps. *Journal of Transcultural Nursing, 18,* 86S–90S.

Goldberg, C. B., & Allen, D. G. (2008). Black and white and read all over: Race differences in reactions to recruitment Web sites. *Human Resource Management, 47*(2), 217–236.

Halfer, D., & Saver, C. (2008). Bridging the generation gaps. *NurseWeek (S. Central), 15*(9), 36–41.

Hira, N. (2007). You raised them, now manage them. *Fortune, 155*(10), 38–46.

Loughrey, M. (2008). Just how male are male nurses? *Journal of Clinical Nursing, 17*(10), 1327–1334.

Lyons, S. M., OKeeffe, F. M., Clarke, A. T., & Staines, A. (2008). Cultural diversity in the Dublin maternity services: The experiences of maternity service providers when caring for ethnic minority women. *Ethnicity & Health, 13*(3), 261–276.

Managing across the generations: Best practices for managing four age groups (2008). *OR Manager, 24*(4), 11. [Reprinted from Martin, C. A., & Tulgan, B. *Managing the Generation Mix.* 2nd ed. Amherst, MA: HRD Press, 2006.]

Minority student leaders: 40 students chosen for 2007 leadership program (2007). *ASHA Leader, 12*(15), 25.

National League for Nursing convenes innovative think tank on expanding diversity in nurse educator workforce (2008). *Maryland Nurse, 9*(3), 19.

Pardue, K. T., & Morgan, P. (2008). Millennials considered: A new generation, new approaches, and implications for nursing education. *Nursing Education Perspectives, 29*(2), 74–79.

Ratnaike, D. (2007). Breaking through the glass ceiling. *RCM Midwives, 10*(9), 407.

Riley, W. J. (2008). Diversity in the health professions matters: The untold story of Meharry Medical College. *Journal of Health Care for the Poor and Underserved, 19*(2), 331–342.

Smith, T. C., Ingersoll, G. L., Robinson, R., Hercules, H., & Carey, J. (2008). Recruiting, retaining, and advancing careers for employees from underrepresented groups. *Journal of Nursing Administration, 38*(4), 184–193.

Sullivan, L. W. (2007). Missing Persons in the Health Professions, *A Report of the Sullivan Commission on Diversity in the Healthcare Workforce* (2004).

Theodore, R. (2008). Advancing diversity in nursing: An interview with Dr. Catherine Alicia Georges. *Policy, Politics, and Nursing Practice, 9*(1), 22–26.

Tweddel, L. (2007). Analysis. Is nursing sexist? *Nursing Times, 103*(23), 8.

Walker, D. (2008). The Institute for Nursing and the Sylvia C. Edge Endowment Sponsors LaVern Allen RN for participation in the Rutgers College of Nursing Minority Nurse Leadership Institute. *Institute for Nursing Newsletter, 4*(2), 5.

Yee, K. C., Mills, E., & Airey, C. (2008). Perfect match? Generation Y as change agents for information communication technology implementation in healthcare (pp. 496–501). In: S. K. Andersen, G. O. Klein, S. Schulz, J. Aarts, & M. C. Mazzoleni (Eds.), *Studies in Health Technology and Informatics,* Vol. 136. Amsterdam: IOS Press.

WEB RESOURCES

American Assembly for Men in Nursing	http://aamn.org/
American Medical Student Association, Diversity in Medicine	www.amsa.org/div
Asian & Pacific Islander Nurses Association	http://www.aapina.org
Diversity Rx	http://www.diversityrx.org
The Center for Cross-Cultural Health	http://www.crosshealth.com
Center for Healthy Families and Cultural Diversity, Department of Family Medicine, University of Medicine and Dentistry of New Jersey, Robert Wood Johnson Medical School	http://www2.umdnj.edu/fmedweb/chfcd/
Commission on Graduates of Foreign Nursing Schools	http://www.cgfns.org
Men in Nursing	http://www.nursingcenter.com/library/journalissue.asp?Journal_ID=606912&Issue_ID=798200#allissues
Male Nurse Magazine	http://www.malenursemagazine.com/
Men in Nursing, Historical Information	http://www.nurses.info/history_men.htm
Minority Nurse	http://www.minoritynurse.com
National Alaska Native American Indian Nurses Association	www.nanaina.com
National Association of Hispanic Nurses	http://www.thehispanicnurses.org
National Black Nurses Association	http://www.nbna.org
National Coalition of Ethnic Minority Nurse Associations	http://www.ncemna.org/officers.html
The Office of Minority Health, Department of Health and Human Services	http://www.omhrc.gov
Philippine Nurse's Association of America	http://www.philippinenursesaa.org/
Sigma Theta Tau, International Honor Society of Nursing, Position Statement on Diversity	http://www.nursingsociety.org/aboutus/GlobalInitiatives/Pages/diversity.aspx
Sullivan Commission on Diversity in the Healthcare Workforce Report	http://www.wkkf.org/default.aspx?tabid=94&CID=1&ItemID=10415&NID=85&LanguageID=0
U.S. Equal Employment Opportunities Commission (EEOC)	http://www.eeoc.gov/

CHAPTER 10

Mandatory Minimum Staffing Ratios: Are They Working?

• CAROL J. HUSTON •

Learning Objectives

The learner will be able to:

1. Explore factors driving legislative mandates for minimum registered nurse (RN) representation in the staffing mix.
2. Summarize current research findings regarding the effect of staffing ratios and staffing mix on patient outcomes.
3. Debate driving and restraining forces for legislating minimum licensed staffing ratios.
4. Assess the efficiency and effectiveness of the processes used by the state of California Department of Health Services to determine initial minimum RN–patient staffing ratios for different types of hospital units.
5. Describe challenges to staffing ratio implementation in California, including the need to define "licensed nurses," legal challenges to the "at all times clause," and strategies directed at delaying or rescinding the mandate altogether.
6. Investigate the movement and/or progress of states other than California to adopt minimum RN staffing ratios.
7. Discuss the effect of the current nursing shortage on the likelihood of successful passage of proposed staffing ratio legislation in states other than California.
8. Argue for or against the appropriateness of the "at all times clause" as part of California's staffing ratio mandate.
9. Assess whether California's 2004 implementation of mandatory minimum RN staffing ratios has met its intended goals.
10. Identify alternatives to staffing ratio mandates that seek to assure that staffing resources are adequate to provide safe patient care.
11. Reflect on the staffing ratios used in his or her work setting and assess, using clearly defined criteria, whether they are adequate to provide quality patient care.

For some time now, economics has been the primary driver in dictating changes in the RN skill mix in hospitals. As a result, the trend for at least the last decade has been to reduce RNs in the staffing mix and to replace them with less expensive alternatives. Empirical research increasingly concludes, however, that the number of RNs in the staffing mix has a direct effect on quality care and, in particular, patient outcomes. In response, legislators, health care providers, and the public are increasingly demanding adequate staffing ratios of RNs in acute care settings.

Indeed, a national movement to mandate minimum staffing ratios has begun. Many states in the United States, with the backing of some nursing organizations, have moved toward imposing mandatory licensed staffing requirements, and one state (California) has enacted legislation requiring mandatory staffing ratios that affect hospitals and long-term care facilities. In fact, as of 2008, 11 states (California, Connecticut, Florida, Illinois, Maine, New Jersey, Ohio, Oregon, Rhode Island, Texas, and Vermont) plus the District of Columbia had enacted legislation and/or adopted regulations addressing nurse staffing (American Nurses Association [ANA], 2008a), and a total of 18 states had pursued initiatives to ensure safe hospital nurse staffing (Keeler & Cramer, 2007). In addition, according to McGillis-Hall et al. (2006), Canada has expressed interest in adopting standardized ratios similar to those in place in California and Victoria, Australia, but concerns and disagreements have halted forward progress.

This chapter explores both the driving and restraining forces for legislative mandates for minimum RN representation in the staffing mix. California's experience, as the first state to implement minimum staffing ratios, is detailed, as well as its struggle to define appropriate ratios and implement staffing ratios in an era of limited fiscal and human resources. The chapter concludes by looking at the movement of other states toward the adoption of minimum staffing ratios and strategies that have been suggested as alternatives to mandatory staffing ratios.

CONSIDER

The literature continues to suggest that increasing the number of RNs in the staffing mix leads to safer workplaces for nurses and a higher quality of care for patients.

STAFFING RATIOS AND PATIENT OUTCOMES

Numerous studies in the last decade have examined the link between staffing mix and patient outcomes. Much,

but not all, of the research has suggested a link between the increased representation of RNs in the staffing mix and improved patient outcomes. For example, a recent study by Sochalski, Konetzka, Zhu, and Volpp (2008) of acute myocardial infarction (AMI) patients ($n = 348,720$) and surgical failure-to-rescue (FTR) ($n = 109,066$) patients discharged between 1993 and 2001 from 343 California acute care general hospitals found significant cross-sectional associations between higher nurse staffing and reductions in AMI mortality. These improvements, however, were smaller in hospitals with higher baseline staffing. There were no significant cross-sectional associations between higher nurse staffing and FTR. (See Research Study Fuels the Controversy.)

In addition, Kane, Shamliyan, Mueller, Duval, and Wilt (2007b), in their meta-analysis of 28 studies, found that increased RN staffing was associated with lower hospital-related mortality in intensive care units, as well as for patients in surgical and in medical units, when just one additional full-time-equivalent (FTE) RN was added per patient day. Such an increase was also associated with a decreased odds ratio of hospital-acquired pneumonia, unplanned extubation, respiratory failure,

---

Research Study Fuels the Controversy: Do Mandatory Minimum Staffing Ratios Improve Quality of Care?

Because mandatory minimum hospital nurse staffing ratios are under consideration in a number of states without strong empirical evidence of the optimal ratio, the researchers completed cross-sectional and fixed-effects regression analyses using a 1993–2001 panel of patient and hospital data from California to determine whether increases in medical-surgical licensed nurse staffing levels

were associated with improvements in patient outcomes for hospitals having different baseline staffing levels. Subjects were adult patients who had suffered an acute myocardial infarction (AMI) ($n = 348,720$) and surgical failure-to-rescue (FTR) ($n = 109,066$) patients discharged between 1993 and 2001 from 343 California acute care general hospitals.

STUDY FINDINGS

There were significant cross-sectional associations between higher nurse staffing and reductions in AMI mortality; however, they were reduced in the fixed-effects analyses. Improvements in outcomes were smaller in hospitals with higher baseline staffing; for each RN and RN + LVN increase, respectively, AMI mortality declined by 0.71 ($p < 0.05$) and 2.75 percentage points for hospitals with more than 7 patients per nurse, compared with

0.19 ($p = NS$) and 0.28 percentage points ($p < 0.05$) in hospitals with more than 4 patients per nurse. There were no significant cross-sectional associations between higher nurse staffing and FTR. The researchers concluded that strong diminishing returns to nurse staffing improvements and lack of significant evidence that staffing uniformly increases improved outcomes raise questions about the cost-effectiveness of implementing state-wide mandatory nurse staffing ratios.

Sochalski, J., Konetzka, R. T., Zhu, J., & Volpp, K. (2008). Will mandated minimum nurse staffing ratios lead to better patient outcomes? *Medical Care*, 46(6). Available at: http://www.lww-medicalcare.com/pt/re/medcare/abstract.00005650-200806000-00008.htm;jsessionid=LQmd1p41xgQkvwsyX63C5gQcvWV1D5b99q2FdJPhnGTn5C2mpSTL!982088527!181195629!8091!-1. Accessed July 30, 2008.

and cardiac arrest and with a lower risk of failure to rescue in surgical patients in intensive care units (ICUs). In addition, length of stay was 24% shorter in ICUs and 31% shorter for surgical patients when the additional FTE RN was added.

However, Kane, Shamliyan, Mueller, Duval, and Wilt (2007a), in their review of nearly 100 studies by the Agency for Healthcare Quality and Research, found an association between staffing levels, patient mortality, and patient outcomes but concluded that these relationships are not causal. Research by Burnes Bolton et al. (2007) also failed to find the anticipated significant improvements expected in the incidence of falls and the prevalence of hospital-acquired pressure ulcers following the implementation of mandated staffing ratios in California. A summary of these studies and several other studies completed since 2007 is included in Table 10.1.

> CONSIDER
> There is wide variation in the skill mix (percentage of licensed to unlicensed workers) and RN-to-patient ratios across the United States.

Few studies, however, have had as much effect on determining safe staffing ratios as two research studies published in 2002. The first study was the work of Needleman, Buerhaus, Mattke, Stewart, and Zelvinksy (2002). This study of 799 hospitals in 11 states found a higher prevalence of infections, such as pneumonia and urinary tract infections, failure to rescue, and shock or cardiac arrest when the nurses' workload was high.

The second study, which is often cited as the seminal work in support of establishing minimum staffing ratio legislation at the federal or state level, was completed by Aiken Clarke, Sloane, Lake, and Cheney (2002). This study of more than 10,000 nurses and 230,000 patients in 168 hospitals concluded that in hospitals with higher patient-to-nurse ratios, surgical patients had a greater likelihood of dying within 30 days of admission. In addition, they experienced increased odds of failure to rescue (mortality following complications). This occurred because the time nurses have for surveillance, early detection, and timely intervention—particularly with patients who are not at high risk but who are vulnerable to other unfavorable outcomes—has a direct effect on patient outcomes.

The study found that staffing at 6 patients per nurse rather than 4 would result in an additional 2.3 deaths per 1,000 patients and an additional 8.7 deaths per 1,000 patients with complications. Staffing at 8 patients per nurse rather than 6 would incur an additional 2.6 deaths per 1,000 patients and 9.5 deaths per 1,000 patients with complications. Uniformly staffing at 8 patients per nurse rather than 4 was expected to entail 5 excess deaths per 1,000 patients and 18.2 complications per 1,000 patients. In addition, patients had a 31% higher chance of dying within 30 days of admission (Aiken et al.).

Within days of the study's release, Aiken's study results were summarized, repeated, and analyzed in detail in almost all relevant public forums and by most professional health care organizations. The message was clear: There is a direct link between nurse-to-patient ratios and mortality rates from preventable complications, and having an inadequate number of RNs places the public at risk.

> **DISCUSSION POINT**
> Why did the study by Aiken et al. (2002) garner so much national attention in so many public forums? Were the findings significantly different than those of earlier studies? Was it timing? Was it how "the message" was managed?

ARE MANDATORY MINIMUM STAFFING RATIOS REALLY NEEDED?

It is little surprise, then, that one proposed solution to Aiken's research findings was the implementation of minimum mandatory RN–patient staffing ratios in acute care hospitals. Numerous articles have appeared in the media attesting to grossly inadequate staffing in hospitals and nursing homes, and professional nursing organizations, such as the ANA, have continued to express concern about the effect poor staffing has both on nurses' health and safety and on patient outcomes.

Proponents of mandated minimum staffing ratios argue that such ratios are absolutely essential to assuring that staffing is adequate to promote patient safety and to achieving desired patient outcomes. They also suggest that the use of standardized ratios provides a more consistent approach than acuity-based staffing and that it has appeal to nurses on the front lines because it offers some protection against overburdening assignments (McGillis-Hall et al., 2006). Greenberg (2006, p. 16) agreed, arguing that minimum staffing ratios clearly save

TABLE 10.1 | Selected Research on Nurse Staffing Levels and Patient Clinical Outcomes Since 2007

Citation	Description
Sochalski, J., Konetzka, R. T., Zhu, J., & Volpp, K. (2008). Will mandated minimum nurse staffing ratios lead to better patient outcomes? *Medical Care, 46*(6), 606–613.	There were correlations between increased licensed nurse staffing and reduced mortality rates associated with acute myocardial infarction. No relationship was found between increased nurse staffing and failure to rescue in adult surgical patients.
Burnes Bolton, L., Aydin, C., Donaldson, N., Brown, D., Sandhu, M., Fridman, M., & Aronow, HU. (2007). Mandated nurse staffing ratios in California: A comparison of staffing and nursing-sensitive outcomes pre- and postregulation. *Policy, Politics, & Nursing Practice, 8*(4), 238–250.	Anticipated significant improvements in two key nurse-sensitive indicators of patient care quality and safety—the incidence of falls and the prevalence of hospital-acquired pressure ulcers— were not observed.
Kane, R. L., Shamliyan, T., Mueller, C., Duval, S., & Wilt, T. (2007). The association of registered nurse staffing levels and patient outcomes. Systematic review and meta-analysis. *Medical Care, 45*(12), 1195–1204.	Adding just one full-time-equivalent registered nurse (RN) position per patient-day resulted in lower hospital-related mortality in intensive care and medical surgical units. In addition, hospital-acquired pneumonia, unplanned extubation, respiratory failure, and cardiac arrest declined, as did failure to rescue in surgical patients in intensive care units.
Thungjaroenkul, P., Cummings, G., & Embleton, A. (2007). The impact of nurse staffing on hospital costs and patient length of stay: A systematic review. *Nursing Economics, 25*(5), 255–265.	Significant reductions in cost and length of stay may be possible with higher ratios of nursing personnel in hospital settings. Sufficient numbers of RNs may prevent patient adverse events that cause patients to stay longer than necessary. Patient costs were also reduced with greater RN staffing because RNs have higher knowledge and skill levels to provide more effective nursing care, as well as to reduce patient resource consumption.
Kane, R. L., Shamliyan, T., Mueller, C., Duval, S., & Wilt, T. (2007). *Nursing staffing and quality of patient care. Evidence Report/Technology Assessment, No. 151* (AHRQ Publication No. 07-E005). Rockville, MD: AHRQ.	More RN hours spent on direct patient were associated not only with a reduction in hospital-related death but also with shorter lengths of stay. Decreased nosocomial bloodstream infections, urinary tract infections, failure to rescue, and other adverse events also were noted when more RN hours were spent on direct patient care.
Aiken, L. H., Clarke, S. P., Sloane, D. M., Lake, E. T., & Cheney, T. (2008). Effects of hospital care environment on patient mortality and nurse outcomes. *Journal of Nursing Administration, 38*(5), 223–229.	Surgical mortality rates were more than 60% higher in poorly staffed hospitals with the poorest patient care environments than in hospitals with better health care environments, the best nurse staffing levels, and the most highly educated nurses. The researchers conclude that if these three factors could be optimized, the actual number of patient deaths that could be averted annually is somewhere in the range of 40,000.

lives and keep nurses in the nursing profession, so "we can no longer ignore the evidence on staffing ratios."

Critics, however, suggest that the overall cost of care would increase exponentially if mandatory ratios were imposed nationally, and that no guarantee of quality improvement or positive outcomes exists with such ratios (Welton, 2007). Welton argued that reimbursement likely will not cover the increased cost of having more registered nurses, and this will result in unfunded mandates.

In addition, McGillis-Hall et al. (2006) suggested that predetermined staffing ratios overlook the level of experience and knowledge of the nurse and do not translate as easily for medical and/or surgical units as they do for specialty units, given the greater variability in the patient population needs. In addition, there is a risk that staffing may actually decline with ratios because they might be used as the ceiling or as ironclad criteria if institutions are unwilling to make adjustments for patient acuity or RN skill level.

Upenieks, Akhavan, Kotlerman, Esser, and Ngo (2007) agreed, suggesting that nurses' workload and how nurses spend their time vary across settings. They stated that this occurs in part as a result of the use of unlicensed assistive personnel (UAP) and other ancillary personnel to ensure safe and quality patient care. Upenieks et al. concluded that although staffing ratios guard against a maximum patient load per nurse, they do not specify the ideal staffing mix.

Unruh (2008) also expressed concern about the widespread adoption of minimum staffing ratios, arguing that no scientific evidence exists to support specific nurse–patient ratios in all settings. Unruh did acknowledge, however, that adequate staffing and balanced workloads are central to achieving good patient outcomes.

CONSIDER

The bottom line is that minimum staffing ratios would not have been proposed if staffing abuses and the resultant decline in the quality of patient care had not occurred in the past.

Cost is cited most often as the deterrent for implementing minimum staffing ratios. Welton (2007) warned that mandated ratios will divert resources away from patient care and into compliance, given that licensed staff are expensive. In fact, Welton pointed out that an increase of just 1 hour of additional care by a registered nurse per day at $40 per hour would increase costs by $4,000 per day and $1.4 million dollars annually for a medium-sized hospital that averaged 100 medical/surgical patients per day.

Keeler and Cramer (2007), however, in their review of staffing ratio costs, concluded that hiring more RNs, as would be expected under a federal mandatory staffing policy, would likely not create undue financial burdens in the long term for most urban hospitals. They cautioned, however, that this might not be the case in rural hospitals, and they thus suggested that mandatory staffing policy is better left to the states than the federal government.

Still others argue that it is health care professionals—not legislators or regulators—who understand health care and are best qualified to determine staffing needs. This might be the case, but given that hospitals are no longer exempt from "big business," profit-driven motives, one must question whether what is best for patients can be separated from what is best financially for the institution.

Finally, critics of staffing ratios claim that mandating specific staffing ratios during the current nursing shortage will lead to a reduction in hospital services, increased emergency room diversions, increased unit closures, and increased expenses as hospitals will need to pay additional labor costs for overtime and temporary agency nurses. Keeler and Cramer (2007), however, reported that the dire predictions about hospitals in California having to close doors if mandatory staffing ratio legislation passed never materialized. In fact, they suggested that most facilities in California did not have to hire more contracted RNs to comply with the ratios, nor was there a decrease in skill mix as a result.

In fact, Greenberg (2006) argued that the implementation of staffing ratios actually improves nurse satisfaction and, thus, retention. This improvement in the work environment should subsequently attract new nurses as well as part-time and nonemployed nurses back into the full-time nursing workforce, thus actually alleviating the nursing shortage, not making it worse. In fact, Greenberg reported that nurses from all over the country rushed to California for jobs when the staffing-ratios legislation passed and concluded that staffing ratios "can be implemented in a large and complex state without causing health care to grind to a halt" (p. 16). Trande Phillips, an RN at Kaiser Permanente's Walnut Creek (California) Hospital, agreed, stating that "before the ratios were enacted, we had complete turnover of our entire RN staff twice in three years. We were always working short staffed and patients suffered. Now the only time nurses leave is if they are moving or going back to school" (Cortez, 2008, para 20).

Research by Spetz (2008) supported Greenberg's assertions. Spetz found that California nurses' satisfaction improved between 2004 and 2006, particularly with regard to the adequacy of RN staff, time for patient education, benefits, and clerical support. In addition, there was a significant increase in overall job satisfaction between 2004 and 2006. It should be noted, however, that improvements in satisfaction with the adequacy of RN staff were not associated with the degree to which regional hospitals were expected to increase staffing.

CALIFORNIA AS THE PROTOTYPE FOR MANDATORY MINIMUM STAFFING RATIOS

Passing the Legislation

California has had a minimum ratio of licensed nurse to patient requirement (Title 22 of the California Code of Regulations) for intensive care and coronary care units for almost three decades; however, no minimums were initially established for other types of acute care units. Given increasing pressure from nursing unions in the state, increasing bad press about poor-quality care, the increased use of unlicensed assistive personnel as direct care providers, and skyrocketing patient loads for licensed nurses in acute care, California stepped forward as the first state in the nation to implement mandatory minimum staffing ratios.

Under Assembly Bill (A.B.) 394 ("Safe Staffing Law"), passed in 1999 and crafted by the California Nurses Association (CNA), all hospitals in California were to comply with the minimum staffing ratios shown in Table 10.2 by January 1, 2004. These ratios, developed by the California Department of Health Services (CDHS) with assistance from the University of California, Davis, represented the maximum number of patients an RN could be assigned to care for, under any circumstance. In addition, this legislation prohibited unlicensed personnel from performing certain procedures such as administering medication, performing venipuncture, providing parenteral or tube feedings, inserting nasogastric tubes, inserting catheters, performing tracheal suctioning, assessing patient conditions, providing patient education, and performing moderately complex laboratory tests.

TABLE 10.2	Minimum Registered Nurse Staffing Ratios for Hospitals in California Effective January 2004

Unit	Registered Nurse–Patient Ratio
Critical care/intensive care unit	1:2
Neonatal intensive care unit	1:2
Operating room	1:1
Labor and delivery	1:2
Antepartum	1:4
Postpartum couplets	1:4
Postpartum women only	1:6
Pediatrics	1:4
Step-down (initial)	1:4
Step-down (as of 2008)	1:3
Medical/surgical (initial)	1:6
Medical/surgical (as of 2005)	1:5
Oncology (initial)	1:5
Oncology (as of 2008)	1:4
Psychiatry	1:6
Emergency Room	1:4

Source: California Nurses Association (2008a).

The Struggle to Determine Appropriate Ratios

Developing draft regulations for minimum staffing ratios was challenging for the CDHS because data were not readily accessible regarding the distribution of nurse staffing in California hospitals, the number of hospitals likely to be affected by the minimum staffing requirements, or the expected costs of this legislation. In addition, the ratios were meant to supplement valid and reliable patient classification systems (PCS), which had been required in California hospitals since 1996. The problem was that although California hospitals had been required to submit their PCS data to the state, there was no standardization and little guidance about what characterized a valid PCS or what criteria should be used in determining the PCS. Therefore PCS data yielded little if any helpful information to the CDHS for determining appropriate ratios.

DISCUSSION POINT

The California Healthcare Association advocated the use of PCS as the gold standard for staffing decisions rather than staffing ratios. The CNA argued for the reverse. What motives may have driven these positions?

Cost was also an unknown. Initial projections by the Public Policy Institute of California (PPIC) in July 2001 suggested that many hospitals in California would experience sharp increases in cost associated with the increase in numbers of licensed staff. At least in part as a result of limited empirical data, proposals received by CDHS suggested a wide range of minimum staffing ratios and even more widely differing estimates of cost. The California Hospital Association (CHA), a hospital trade group representing the interests of nearly 500 hospital and health system members in California, called for a minimum staffing ratio of 1 nurse to 10 patients on medical-surgical units, whereas the unions representing the largest numbers of nurses in the state argued for minimum ratios in medical-surgical units of 1 to 4. The CNA recommended a 1 to 3 ratio in medical-surgical units.

Following months of waiting and almost 2 years of wrangling, the final minimum staffing ratios were announced in January 2002. Governor Gray Davis, in a press conference at St. Vincent's Medical Center in Los Angeles, announced that his administration supported a ratio of 1 nurse to every 6 patients in medical-surgical units—twice the number of patients supported by the CNA and 4 fewer than that favored by the CHA. Regulations were released later that spring with 45 days allocated for public comment. Hospitals in California were also required to continue to keep a PCS in place and to staff according to the PCS if it called for a larger number of nurses than the minimum ratios set by the CDHS.

Delays in Implementation

Implementing the ratio legislation proved to be just as difficult as determining what the ratios should be. The first challenge that arose was interpreting the meaning and intent of the legislation's language in regard to what constituted "licensed nurses." Almost immediately, questions were raised about whether the minimum mandatory ratios had to reflect RN representation in the staffing mix or whether licensed vocational/practical nurses (LVNs/LPNs) would meet the requirement.

The CNA argued that the intent of the law was to regulate minimum RN staffing, which inflamed the labor unions representing LVNs. Amid much controversy, the issues were aired at a public hearing before the Department of Health Services in San Francisco, and a determination was provided that the ratios referred to RNs only, and that LVNs/LPNs would be authorized to practice only under the direction of an RN or licensed physician.

Questions were then raised as to whether hospitals could eliminate or reduce their nonlicensed staff in an effort to save costs, given that the number of RNs would be increased. The CNA argued that the ratios were based on CDHS surveys of existing hospital staffing patterns, and that nonlicensed staff should not be cut if safe patient care was to be assured. The state, however, chose not to weigh in, arguing that its position was to regulate minimum RN–patient ratios; as a result, many hospitals immediately began reducing the number of support personnel to offset the increased cost of RN staff. Indeed, Mitchell (2007) suggested that many hospitals decreased the number of support staff, including unlicensed assistive personnel and housekeepers, and this placed additional burdens on registered nurses, who were forced to assume nonnursing care tasks.

Finally, the CHA, with the help of State Senator Sam Aanestad, introduced new legislation (A.B. 847) to the California State Senate Health and Human Services committee in April 2003 in an attempt to delay implementation of the 1 to 5 minimum nurse–patient staffing ratio on medical-surgical units until it could be ascertained that adequate RNs were available to meet the ratios. Opponents of the delay argued that this was simply an effort to preclude implementation of the mandate altogether. The bill failed.

Then the hospitals persuaded Governor Arnold Schwarzenegger to issue an emergency regulation in November 2004 to overturn emergency room ratios and the improved medical-surgical ratios, citing financial crises (Cortez, 2008). In response, the CNA and the National Nurses Organizing Committee (NNOC) launched more than 100 protests against Schwarzenegger, which resulted in a massive grassroots movement and the stinging defeat of four Schwarzenegger-ballot initiatives in a 2005 special election (Cortez). The emergency regulation was ruled illegal in March 2005 by a state Superior Court Judge and overturned. The judge argued that the financial state of hospitals did not give the state the right to delay implementing the law because the law's intent was to improve patient safety. Hospitals were told to comply immediately.

Still, resistance to staffing ratio implementation continued. Hospitals were accused of encouraging management staff to undermine and avoid compliance with the new RN staffing ratios. Nursing unions responded with threats to close down units with inadequate staffing, to delay elective surgeries, and to wage a public relations campaign to garner public support for the nurses.

The Struggle to Implement the Ratios

Despite these efforts and a pervasive, ongoing resistance to staffing ratio implementation, the staffing ratio mandate did become effective January 1, 2004. But were hospitals ready and willing to implement these changes?

By and large, bigger hospitals in the state were ready to meet the mandate by the time of its implementation. Many smaller hospitals, however, had existing budget deficits and had to seek waivers from the CDHS because of their difficulty in meeting ratios. Waivers were allowed; however, hospitals had to be rural and meet very strict conditions.

> **DISCUSSION POINT**
> Should small rural hospitals be given waivers for the mandatory staffing ratios? Is this justified by the patient population characteristics, or is it simply an economic incentive to keep these hospitals viable?

The "At All Times" Clause

In addition, almost immediately after implementation, legal clarification became necessary regarding interpretation of the law with regard to ratio coverage "*at all times.*" A ruling by the CDHS blindsided many hospitals in its strict interpretation that ratios had to be maintained at all times, including breaks and lunches. For many hospitals, this meant hiring additional rotating staff to fill in for nurses when they leave the bedside for short periods (breaks, lunch, transporting patients, etc.) or face being noncompliant.

As a result, the CHA filed a lawsuit on December 30, 2003, challenging the ruling and arguing that the "at-all-times" ruling was impossible to implement. The motion was heard in a Sacramento court on May 14, 2004. In a 10-page ruling issued May 26, 2004, the judge dismissed the hospital association lawsuit, saying that not adhering to the "at all times" clause would make the nurse-to-patient

ratios meaningless. Again, the ruling was an effort to maintain the intent of the law—to protect patients.

> **DISCUSSION POINT**
> Is an "at all times" ruling necessary to assure quality health care?

Assuring Compliance: The Role of the California Department of Health Services

The CDHS is charged with compliance oversight of mandatory minimum staffing ratios in California acute care hospitals and enforces these regulations in the same general manner in which they have enforced intensive care and critical care unit staffing regulations for the last three decades. The CDHS (2004) Web site details the following procedures for verifying compliance, responding to complaints, and addressing compliance violations:

- Compliance with the regulations may be verified during a periodic survey or in response to a complaint. Although there is no statutory time frame within which CDHS must initiate an on-site investigation in response to a complaint against an acute care hospital, by existing policy, CDHS will initiate an investigation within 48 hours if a credible allegation of serious and immediate jeopardy to patients is received. If the allegation does not constitute serious and immediate jeopardy, the complaint will be investigated during the next periodic survey or along with the next "serious" complaints.

- If a violation of the ratio requirements occurs, CDHS will issue a deficiency notice to the hospital and require an acceptable plan of correction. CDHS may verify that the plan of correction has been implemented and the deficiency corrected during any subsequent complaint investigation or periodic survey.

- There is no penalty or monetary fine for a violation of the ratio regulations itself; however, as of 2007, hospitals can be fined up to $25,000 for staffing violations that result in serious injury or death to patients (Leighty, 2008) (the law has yet to be tested). If the CDHS concludes that the violation of the ratio regulations is so severe that it poses an immediate and substantial hazard to the health or safety of patients, CDHS may also order the hospital to reduce the number of patients or to close a unit until additional staffing is obtained.

CONSIDER

If there are no monetary fines from the CDHS for noncompliance, what will motivate California hospitals to continue to comply with mandated staffing ratios?

The Bottom Line: Has Registered Nurse Staffing Improved in California Hospitals as a Result of Mandatory Minimum Staffing Ratios?

As of January 1, 2008, California's historic staffing law for registered nurse staffing ratios completed its phase-in period (Cortez, 2008). Five years of data now exist regarding compliance with the staffing ratios, as well as changes in patient outcomes.

In terms of compliance, Conway, Konetzka, Jingsan, Volpp, and Sochalski (2008) reported that nurse staffing ratios in California were relatively unchanged from 1993 to 1999 but increased significantly from 1999 to 2004 in preparation for the implementation of mandated minimum staffing ratios. The largest increase was in 2004. Hospitals most likely to be below minimum ratios had a high Medicaid/uninsured patient population and were government owned, nonteaching, urban, and in more competitive markets. Similarly, research by Burnes Bolton et al. (2007) found that changes in California nurse staffing have been consistent with the expected increases in licensed staffing as a result of the mandate.

The California Hospital Association, however, suggested that although the number of nurses in California has increased as a result of staffing mandates, many of these nurses are now traveler nurses (Thrall, 2008). Leighty (2008) agreed, suggesting that to comply with the January 1, 2008, requirements to lower nurse-to-patient ratios in step-down units, telemetry, and other specialty units, many California hospitals had to resort to traveling nurses to fill basic staffing needs.

SIMILAR INITIATIVES IN OTHER U.S. STATES

The U.S. federal government has established minimum standards for licensed nursing in certified nursing homes but not in acute care hospitals. Welton (2007) suggested that there have been several attempts in the last few years in both the House of Representatives and the Senate to address and enact hospital nurse staffing laws; however, none have come close to fruition. Section 42 of the Code of Federal Regulations [42CFR 482.23(b)] does require Medicare-certified hospitals to "have adequate numbers of licensed registered nurses, licensed practical (vocational) nurses, and other personnel to provide nursing care to all patients as needed"; however, this "nebulous language and failure of Congress to enact a quality nursing care staffing act to date, has left it to the states to ensure that staffing is appropriate to patients' needs" (ANA, 2008d, para 1).

Many states are in fact actively pursuing minimum staffing ratio legislation, and Stephanie Dodge, a labor and employment attorney in the Chicago area, predicted that within 5 years, staffing legislation will have been at least introduced in all 50 states, with a significant number having passed some type of legislation involving staffing plans (Thrall, 2008).

For example, in June 2008, Governor Ted Strickland of Ohio signed safe nurse staffing legislation into law (ANA, 2008b). This legislation establishes hospital-wide nursing care committees at each hospital that must recommend a nursing services staffing plan that is "at minimum, consistent with current standards established by private accreditation organizations or governmental entities" (ANA, 2008b, para 4). The legislation also calls for at least annual evaluation of the staffing plan in terms of patient outcomes, clinical management, and costs.

Similarly, in May 2008, Governor Mary Jodi Rell of Connecticut signed legislation requiring the establishment of hospital-wide staffing plans at hospitals in that state. In doing so, Connecticut joined six other states (Illinois, Ohio, Oregon, Rhode Island, Texas, and Washington) that require hospital-wide staffing plans by committees with membership comprised of at least 50% direct care RNs ("the Texas requirement is included in regulations") (ANA, 2008c).

Florida also passed legislation addressing minimum staffing requirements for nursing homes in 2006. The rules to be developed called for "2.7 hours of direct care/resident/day as of January, 2007; with at least one certified nursing assistant per 20 residents and a minimum of one licensed nurse for 1.0 hour of direct care/resident/day and never below one nurse for 40 residents" (ANA, 2008d, para 11). That same year, Florida also enacted a law requiring a registered nurse to be present in the operating room during the entire surgical procedure (ANA, 2008d).

It should be noted, however, that many of the states that adopted legislation requiring safe staffing committees originally sought staffing ratio legislation. In 2007 alone, Illinois, Kentucky, Michigan, Missouri, New York, New Jersey, and West Virginia introduced staffing ratio legislation (ANA, 2008d). In addition, a bill to enact minimum staffing levels for hospital nurses in Massachusetts failed in July 2008 when a coalition of hospital leaders banded together to defeat the bill (Ring, 2008). Steven F. Bradley, a vice president for Baystate Health in Springfield, Massachusetts, put the price tag for implementation of mandatory minimum staffing ratios in Massachusetts at between $250 million and $500 million (Ring). Instead, a "patient safety" bill was passed that allows hospitals to set staffing standards that would then be overseen and enforced by the state.

Thrall (2008) also noted that not all state nursing groups—even those that are unions—embrace staffing ratios. In 2007, the Oregon Nurses Association (ONA) came out against a ratio bill backed by another state union. The ONA argued that it was difficult to establish one staffing standard for hospitals in Oregon or any other state because of the great variability that exists among hospitals.

New York has been debating the implementation of staffing ratios for more than 15 years (Gerardi, 2006). As early as 1993, some New York State Nursing Association (NYSNA) bargaining units were negotiating staffing provisions in their contracts. However, as nursing shortages waxed and waned in the state, so too did the emphasis on mandating minimum staffing ratios at the state level (Gerardi).

OTHER ALTERNATIVES

Efforts are also under way, in both California and the rest of the nation, to explore alternatives to improving nurse staffing that do not require legislated minimum staffing ratios. The staffing plans outlined earlier in this chapter are examples of such efforts.

The reality is that many leading health care and professional nursing organizations do not support the need for legislated minimum staffing ratios. For example, the ANA does not support fixed nurse–patient ratios. Instead,

it advocates a workload system that takes into account the many variables that exist to ensure safe staffing (Trossman, 2008). ANA President Rebecca Patton suggested that it is possible to identify principles that guide staffing on a given day for a particular unit, and these principles include patient safety, quality control, and access to care (Trossman).

Buchan (2005) also believed that staffing ratios are too inflexible and potentially inefficient if calibrated incorrectly. He argued that their strength, however, is their transparency and their simplicity. He concluded that although mandated minimum staffing ratios are only a "blunt instrument for achieving employer compliance," nonetheless "reliance on alternative, voluntary (and often more sophisticated) methods of determining nurse staffing have not been effective" (para 4).

The Joint Commission (2008, para 4), one of the most powerful accrediting bodies for hospitals in the United States, "has long had standards that require hospitals to establish organization-specific staff-to-patient ratios based upon the organization's assessment of patient care needs." Yet it has been reluctant to endorse nationally mandated minimum staffing ratios, suggesting that this would not be flexible enough to encompass the diversity represented in hospitals across the United States. Instead, the Joint Commission has advocated a "simple concept"—*staffing effectiveness*—and a "time tested methodology"—*continuous quality improvement* (CQI)—for addressing a hospital's needs to have adequate staff to care for patients (Joint Commission, para 7). Staffing effectiveness is defined as "the number, competency, and skill mix of staff in relation to the provision of needed services," and CQI "simply involves the selection and application of sensitive measures to identify potential patient care problems, the analysis of underlying factors that are contributing to the problem, and system re-design (or resource allocation) to resolve the problem" (Joint Commission, para 7).

Welton (2007) also suggested another alternative to staffing ratios: offering hospitals market-based incentives to optimize nurse staffing levels by "unbundling nursing care from current room and board charges, billing for nursing care time (intensity) for individual patients, and adjusting hospital payments for optimum nursing care" (para 2). He suggested that "the revenue code data, used to charge for inpatient nursing care, could be used to benchmark and evaluate inpatient nursing care performance by case mix across hospitals" (para 2). Efforts to implement this model nationwide within the next few years have already been initiated (Welton).

CONCLUSIONS

The literature suggests that increasing RN representation in the staffing mix improves at least some patient outcomes. What is less clear is what the optimal staffing levels are for various patient populations and when costs associated with staffing mix become unreasonable in terms of attempting to improve patient outcomes. In addition, given the lessons that have already been learned with the "RN/LVN debate" and the "at-all times" requirement, more thought must be given to how strictly staffing ratio regulations are to be interpreted and how enforcement can be effective when there are no monetary consequences for breaking rules.

In addition, the intermingling roles of state government as a legislator of minimum staffing ratios, compliance officer, disciplinary enforcer, and potential funding source to assist with mandated ratio implementation need further examination and clarification.

Finally, it must be recognized that patient acuity is continuing to rise, and the mandatory minimum staffing ratios adopted in California in 2003 were arguably inadequate just 5 years later, especially when hospitals refused to staff above the ratios when census and acuity call for it (Cortez, 2008). In fact, the CNA and the NNOC proposed even lower ratios as part of the CNA/NNOC's Hospital Patient Protection Act (CNA, 2008b). If implemented, these ratios will likely pose even greater fiscal and human resource challenges to California hospitals in terms of their implementation (Table 10.3).

TABLE 10.3 Proposed California Nurses Association (CNA)/National Nurses Organizing Committee (NNOC) Minimum Registered Nurse Staffing Ratios for Hospitals in California: CNA/NNOC's Hospital Patient Protection Act

Unit	Registered Nurse–Patient Ratio
Critical care/intensive care unit	1:2
Neonatal intensive care unit	1:2
Operating room	1:1
Labor and delivery	1:1
Antepartum	1:3
Postpartum couplets	1:3
Postpartum women only	1:4
Pediatrics	1:3
Step-down and telemetry	1:3
Medical/surgical	1:4
Other specialty care units	1:4
Psychiatry	1:4
Rehab unit and skilled nursing	1:5
Emergency room	1:4
Intensive care unit patient in emergency room	1:2
Trauma patient in emergency room	1:1

Source: California Nurses Association (2008b).

The implementation and subsequent evaluation of mandatory staffing ratios in California should, however, provide some insight into these ongoing issues that will be helpful to other states that choose to follow in California's footsteps. Clearly the enactment of California's nurse-to-patient ratio law was far from smooth, and concerns continue about whether there are enough registered nurses to meet the ratios, the costs of hiring additional licensed staff, and the need to meet the "at all times" clause.

It is not clear yet whether California has the resources (both human and fiscal) it needs to make successful staffing ratio implementation a success. Some of the implementation struggles may be related to the normal issues that arise whenever a new law takes effect; however, the reality may be that California lacks the nursing resources needed to implement its law. The struggles California has experienced thus far in implementing the mandate have been significant. The fact that it took 5 years from passage of the legislation to mandated implementation is telling. What is even more telling are the number of hospitals in California that report difficulty in meeting staffing ratio requirements and the pervasive resistance that continues to be a part of its implementation.

Keepnews (2007) suggested that it is premature to declare that California's ratios "experiment" has been unsuccessful. He pointed out that mandated staffing ratios have raised overall staffing levels, even though research has not definitively proven that mandated ratios have improved patient outcomes. He concluded that "continued research is needed to yield a clearer picture of the impact of staffing ratios and to arrive at more definitive conclusions" (p. 236).

FOR ADDITIONAL DISCUSSION

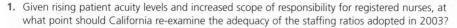

1. Given rising patient acuity levels and increased scope of responsibility for registered nurses, at what point should California re-examine the adequacy of the staffing ratios adopted in 2003?

2. In an effort to cut the costs associated with implementing minimum RN staffing ratios, many hospitals have eliminated their support staff. Have RNs gained anything when this is the case?

3. Should LVNs be counted to meet minimum mandatory staffing ratio requirements?

4. Is allowing hospitals to determine their staffing needs a little like having the "fox guard the chicken coop"?

5. Does the implementation of mandatory staffing ratios in the midst of a severe national nursing shortage make sense? Why or why not?

6. At what point does cost related to staffing mix become so prohibitive that society will be willing to accept some increase in patient morbidity and mortality?

7. What critical lessons should other states learn from California's experience thus far in implementing mandatory staffing ratios?

REFERENCES

Aiken, L. H., Clarke, S. P., Sloane, D. M., Lake, E. T., & Cheney, T. (2008). Effects of hospital care environment on patient mortality and nurse outcomes. *Journal of Nursing Administration, 38*(5), 223–229.

Aiken, L. H., Clarke, S. P., Sloane, D., Sochalski, J., & Silber, J. (2002). Effects of nurse-staffing on nurse burnout and job-dissatisfaction and patient deaths. *Journal of the American Medical Association, 288*, 1987–1993.

American Nurses Association (ANA) (2008a). *Safe staffing saves lives.* Available at: http://www.safe staffingsaveslives.org/WhatisANADoing/State Legisla tion.aspx. Accessed July 30, 2008.

American Nurses Association (ANA) (2008b). *Latest nurse staffing legislation enacted in Ohio.* Available at: http://www.safestaffingsaveslives.org/What isANADoing/StateLegislation/OhioLatestLegislation. aspx. Accessed July 30, 2008.

American Nurses Association (ANA) (2008c). *Connecticut secured nurse staffing legislation.* Available at: http://www.safestaffingsaveslives.org/Whatis ANADoing/StateLegislation/ConnecticutNurse Staffing.aspx. Accessed July 30, 2008.

American Nurses Association (ANA) (2008d). *Nurse staffing plans and ratios.* Available at: http://www. safestaffingsaveslives.org/WhatisANADoing/State Legislation/StaffingPlansandRatios.aspx. Accessed July 30, 2008.

Buchan, J. (2005). A certain ratio? The policy implications of minimum staffing ratios in nursing. *Journal of Health Services Research and Policy, 10*(4), 239–244. Available at: http://jhsrp.rsmjournals.com/cgi/ content/abstract/10/4/239. Accessed July 30, 2008.

Burnes Bolton, L., Aydin, C., Donaldson, N., Brown, D., Sandhu, M., Fridman, M., & Aronow, HU. (2007). Mandated nurse staffing ratios in California: A comparison of staffing and nursing-sensitive outcomes pre- and postregulation. *Policy, Politics, & Nursing Practice, 8*(4), 238–250.

California Department of Health Services (CDHS) (2004). *Nurse-to-patient staffing ratios for general acute care hospitals. Frequently asked questions.* Available at: http:// www.cdph.ca.gov/services/DPOPP/regs/Documents/ R-37-01_FAQ2182004.pdf. Accessed July 30, 2008.

California Nurses Association (2008a). *RN ratios alert. Ratio basics.* Available at: http://www.calnurses.org/ assets/pdf/ratios/ratios_basics_unit_0704.pdf. Accessed July 30, 2008.

California Nurses Association (2008b). *CNA/NNOC RNs across the nation take up the fight.* Available at: http://www.calnurses.org/assets/pdf/ratios/ratios_ booklet.pdf. Accessed July 30, 2008.

Conway, P. H., Konetzka, T. R., Jingsan, Z., Volpp, K. G., & Sochalski, J. (2008). Nurse staffing ratios: Trends and policy implications for hospitalists and the safety net. *Journal of Hospital Medicine, 3*(3), 193–199.

Cortez, Z. (2008). *California's nurse-patient ratio law. Saving lives, reducing the nursing shortage.* Available at: http://www.californiaprogressreport.com/2008/01/ californias_nur.html. Accessed July 29, 2008.

Gerardi, T. (2006). Staffing ratios in New York: A decade of debate. *Policy, Politics & Nursing Practice, 7*(1), 8–10.

Greenberg, P. B. (2006). Nurse-to-patient ratios: What do we know? *Policy, Politics, & Nursing Practice, 7*(1), 14–16.

Joint Commission (2008). *On Capitol Hill. Staffing effectiveness.* Available at: http://www.joint commission.org/NewsRoom/OnCapitolHill/ testimony_112002.htm. Accessed July 30, 2008.

Kane, R. L., Shamliyan, T., Mueller, C., Duval, S., & Wilt, T. (2007a). *Nursing staffing and quality of patient care. Evidence Report/Technology Assessment, No. 151* (AHRQ Publication No. 07-E005). Rockville, MD: AHRQ.

Kane, R. L., Shamliyan, T., Mueller, C., Duval, S., & Wilt, T. (2007b). The association of registered nurse staffing levels and patient outcomes. Systematic review and meta-analysis. *Medical Care, 45*(12), 1195–1204.

Keeler, H. J., & Cramer, M. E. (2007). *Journal of Nursing Administration, 37*(7/8), 350–356.

Keepnews, D. M. (2007). Evaluating nurse staffing regulation. *Policy, Politics, & Nursing Practice, 8*(4), 236–237.

Leighty, J. L. (2008). The final phase: California implements the last stages of its landmark RN-to-patient ratios law. *NurseWeek California, 21*(2), 24–25.

McGillis-Hall, L., Pink, L., Lalonde, M., Tomblin Murphy, G, O'Brien-Pallas, L., Laschinger, H., Tourangeau, A., Besner, J., White, D., Tregunno, D., Thomson, D., Peterson, J., Seto, L., & Akeroyd, J. (2006). Decision making for nurse staffing: Canadian perspectives. *Policy, Politics, and Nursing Practice, 7*(4), 261–269.

Mitchell, L. (2007). *Enloe, unions disagree on layoff impacts.* Available at: http://www.orovillemr.com/portlet/ article/html/fragments/print_article.jsp?article Id=5081630&siteId. Accessed July 30, 2008.

Needleman, J., Buerhaus, P., Mattke, S., Stewart, M., & Zelevinsky, K. (2002). Nurse-staffing levels and the quality of care in hospitals. *New England Journal of Medicine, 346,* 1715–1722.

Ring, D. (2008). *State Senate rejects patient nurse ratios.* Masslive.com. Available at: http://www.masslive.com/ news/index.ssf/2008/07/state_senate_rejects_ patientnu.html?category=Statehouse. Accessed July 29, 2008.

Sochalski, J., Konetzka, R. T., Zhu, J., & Volpp, K. (2008). Will mandated minimum nurse staffing ratios lead to better patient outcomes? *Medical Care, 46*(6). Available at: http://www.lww-medicalcare.com/pt/re/medcare/abstract.00005650-200806000-00008.htm;jsessionid=LQmd1p41xgQkvwsyX63C5gQcvWV1D5b99q2FdJPhnGTn5C2mpSTL!982088527!181195629!8091!-1. Accessed July 30, 2008.

Spetz, J. (2008). Nurse satisfaction and the implementation of minimum nurse staffing regulations. *Policy, Politics, & Nursing Practice, 9*(1), 15–21.

Thrall, T. H. (2008). Nurse staffing laws: Should you worry? *Hospitals & Health Networks, 82*(4), 36–39.

Thungjaroenkul, P., Cummings, G., & Embleton, A. (2007). The impact of nurse staffing on hospital costs and patient length of stay: A systematic review. *Nursing Economics, 25*(5), 255–265.

Trossman, S. (2008). A case for safe staffing. ANA brings together RNs, other stakeholders for summit. *American Nurse, 40*(2), 1.

Unruh, L. (2008). Nurse staffing and patient, nurse, and financial outcomes. *American Journal of Nursing, 108*(1), 62–72.

Upenieks, V. V., Akhavan, J., Kotlerman, J., Esser, J., & Ngo, M. J. (2007). Value-added care. A new way of assessing nursing staffing ratios and workload variability. *Journal of Nursing Administration, 37*(5), 243–252.

Welton, J. M. (2007) Mandatory hospital nurse to patient staffing ratios: Time to take a different approach *OJIN: The Online Journal of Issues in Nursing, 12*(3). Available at: http://cms.nursingworld.org/MainMenuCategories/ANAMarketplace/ANAPeriodicals/OJIN/TableofContents/Volume122007/No3Sept07/MandatoryNursetoPatientRatios.aspx. Accessed July 30, 2008.

BIBLIOGRAPHY

Berg, C. (2008). Upfront. Show me the data: How have the California staffing ratios affected patient care? *NurseWeek California, 21*(2), 10.

Byrd, J. (2007). *Nurses rally for bill to boost staffing.* Available at: http://dwb.thenewstribune.com/news/northwest/v-printer/story/6355696p-5672053c.html. Accessed July 30, 2008.

California's historic RN-to-patient hospital staffing ratios upgraded again with new year (2008). Available at: http://findarticles.com/p/articles/mi_m0EIN/is_2008_Jan_2/ai_n27487163. Accessed July 30, 2008.

DeGuzman, P. (2008). Legislated nurse staffing ratios: What you need to know. *Virginia Nurses Today, 16*(1), 3.

Evans, M. (2006). Nurse-ratio fight goes national. *Modern Healthcare, 36*(11), 20.

Frolich, A., Talavera, J. A., Broadhead, P., & Dudley, R. A. (2007). A behavioral model of clinician responses to incentives to improve quality. *Health Policy, 80,* 179–193.

Gerdtz, M. F., & Nelson S. (2007). 5-20: A model of minimum nurse-to-patient ratios in Victoria, Australia. *Journal of Nursing Management, 15*(1), 64–71.

Goulette, C. (2008). Data set. CalNOC study inconclusive on staffing numbers. *Advance for Nurses (Northern California and Northern Nevada), 5*(8), 21–22.

Gordon, S., Buchanan, J., & Bretherton, T. (2008). *Safety in Numbers: Nurse-to-Patient Ratios and the Future of Health Care.* Ithaca, NY: Cornell University Press.

Harrington, C., & O'Meara, J. (2006). Assessing California's nursing home staffing standards. *Policy, Politics & Nursing Practice, 7*(1), 11–13.

Hawkins, C. T., Flynn, L., & Clarke, S. P. (2008). Relationships between registered nurse staffing, processes of nursing care, and nurse-reported patient outcomes in chronic hemodialysis units. *Nephrology Nursing Journal, 35*(2), 123–131, 145.

Ho, B. (2007). Texas ratio bill introduced. *Registered Nurse: Journal of Patient Advocacy, 103*(2), 4.

Reeves, K. (April, 2007). *New evidence report on nurse staffing and quality of patient care.* Medsurg nursing. Available at: http://findarticles.com/p/articles/mi_m0FSS/is_2_16/ai_n19170739. Accessed July 29, 2008.

Rutherford, P. (2007). Campaign on staffing ratios would be better use of money. *Nursing Standard, 22*(5), 33.

Safe staffing for school nurses. (2008). *Nursing Voice, 13*(2), 1.

Safety in numbers: Nurse-to-patient ratios and the future of health care: MNA goes one-on-one with award-winning health care journalist Suzanne Gordon (2008). *Massachusetts Nurse, 79*(4), 6–7.

Spetz, J., Donaldson, N., Aydin, C., & Brown, D. S. (2008). How many nurses per patient? Measurements of nurse staffing in health services research. *Health Services Research*. Available at: http://www3.interscience.wiley.com/journal/120120488/abstract?CRETRY=1&SRETRY=0. Accessed January 17, 2009.

Upenieks, V. (2007). Value-added care: A new way of assessing nursing staffing ratios and workload variability. *Journal of Nursing Administration, 37*(5), 243–252.

Upenieks, V. V., Kotlerman, J., Akhavan, J., Esser, J., & Ngo, M. J. (2007). Assessing nursing staffing ratios: Variability in workload intensity. *Policy, Politics, & Nursing Practice, 8*(1), 7–19.

WEB RESOURCES

American Federation of Teachers (AFT) AFL-CIO, Policy Statement on Safe Staffing	http://www.aft.org/topics/healthcare-staffing/policy.htm
American Nurses Association, Safe Staffing Saves Lives	http://www.safestaffingsaveslives.org/
American Organization of Nurse Executives, Policy Statement on Mandated Staffing Ratios	http://www.hospitalconnect.com/aone/advocacy/ps_ratios.html
California Department of Health Services	http://www.dhs.ca.gov
California Hospital Association	http://www.calhealth.org
Emergency Nurses Association, Position Statement on Staffing and Productivity in the Emergency Care Setting	http://www.ena.org/about/position/PDFs/Staffing-Productivity.PDF
New York State Nurses Association, Position Statement on RN Staffing Effectiveness and Nursing Shortage	http://nysna.org/practice/positions/position13_a.htm
Society of Gastroenterology Nurses and Associates, Position Statement on Minimal RN Staffing for Patient Care in the Gastrointestinal Endoscopy Unit	http://www.sgna.org/Resources/StaffingFinalPostProofVersion4061.pdf

CHAPTER 11

Mandatory Overtime in Nursing: How Much? How Often?

• CAROL J. HUSTON •

Learning Objectives

The learner will be able to:

1. Identify limitations of the Fair Labor Standards Act (FLSA) of 1938 in terms of protecting workers against mandatory overtime.
2. Identify how 2004 changes to federal overtime rules and more recent court rulings have affected traditional "white collar" employees, including salaried nurses in the United States.
3. Investigate current federal and state legislative efforts to regulate overtime limits for nurses.
4. Explore the current extent of mandatory overtime in nursing as identified in the literature.
5. Identify consequences of mandatory overtime in nursing, including fatigue, increased error rates, increased legal liability, threats to the nurse's personal safety, and increased staff turnover rates.
6. Know and understand the provisions of the Nurse Practice Act in his or her state, as well as

the position statements or advisory opinions that have been issued by his or her state board of nursing regarding mandatory overtime and patient abandonment.
7. Discuss the limits of the nurse's professional duty and assess how much risk a professional nurse should assume in fulfilling a professional duty.
8. Identify driving and restraining forces for the use of shift bidding as an alternative to mandatory overtime.
9. Explore the efficacy of alternatives to mandatory overtime, including pay enhancement programs, use of internal and external per diem staffing agencies, use of traveler nurses, and management of patient volume.
10. Reflect on the number of hours he or she can safely work before quality of care is potentially compromised.

One short-term means of dealing with the current nursing shortage has been to require nurses to work extra shifts, often under threat of "patient abandonment" or punitive measures. *Mandatory overtime*, also called *compulsory* or *forced overtime*, occurs when employees are required to work more hours than are standard (generally 40 hours per week) or risk employer reprisals as a result of their refusal to do so. Mandatory overtime may result from a number of unexpected events such as natural or human-caused disasters, sudden job vacancies, staff absences due to illness, or rapid changes in patient care requirements.

A review of the literature suggests that the use of mandatory overtime in nursing varies greatly from institution to institution and from state to state. Some

health care employers suggest that the current nursing shortage is the cause of mandatory overtime in their facilities. Increasingly, however, nurses are reporting that mandatory overtime has become standard operating procedure instead of a last resort to short staffing. Indeed, in some hospitals, mandatory overtime is routinely used in an effort to keep fewer people on the payroll, as well as to alleviate immediate shortage needs.

The American Federation of State, County, and Municipal Employees, AFL-CIO (AFSCME), agreed, suggesting that there has been a growing reliance on the use of mandatory overtime by nurses to meet routine staffing needs: "In many workplaces, overtime is no longer an occasional requirement prompted by an emergency or unforeseen event. Rather, it is a routinized alternative to proper staffing" (AFSCME, 2008a, para 1).

Indeed, a recent American Nurses Association (ANA) survey of nearly 5,000 nurses across the United States revealed that more than 67% work unplanned overtime every month (ANA, 2008b). A similar picture emerges from a survey of nurses done by the Wisconsin Federation of Nurses and Health Professionals in Milwaukee. Forty-two percent of the nurses surveyed were forced to work overtime at least twice a month, and 12% said that overtime was forced on them at least once a week (Cunningham, 2008).

Some nursing specialty units are known to have more mandatory overtime than others, such as the operating room and postanesthesia care units. In fact, Garrett (2008) reported that many nurses in the perioperative unit consider it normal to work a 40-hour week and then take mandatory call for an additional 4 to 72 hours each week. Garrett suggested that the fatigue of nurses working in this setting and under these conditions might actually approximate that of being under the influence of alcohol. She noted research done by Rosekind and colleagues that demonstrated that after 17 hours without sleep, performance degrades to the equivalent of having a blood alcohol concentration of 0.05%, and after 24 hours without sleep, the effect on performance is equivalent to having a blood alcohol level of 0.10%. Garrett concluded that although mandatory overtime is commonplace in the perioperative setting, it leads to staff-member fatigue that might adversely affect patient safety.

In an effort to create guidelines for safe practice in the perioperative setting, the Association of Perioperative Registered Nurses (AORN) created a Position Statement on Safe Work/On-Call Practices (AORN, 2007). Excerpts from this document are shown in Box 11.1.

BOX 11.1 | EXCERPTS FROM THE 2007 AORN POSITION STATEMENT: SAFE WORK/ON-CALL PRACTICES

The AORN, recognizing the potential negative consequences of sleep deprivation and sustained work hours and further recognizing that adequate rest and recuperation periods are essential to patient and perioperative personnel safety, suggests the following strategies:

1. Perioperative registered nurses should not be required to work in direct patient care more than 12 consecutive hours in a 24-hour period and not more than 60 hours in a 7-day period.

2. Sufficient transition time is required for appropriate patient handoff and staff relief. Under extreme conditions exceptions to the 12-hour limit may be required (e.g., disasters). Organization policy should outline exceptions to the 12-hour limitation. All worked hours (i.e., regular hours and call hours worked) should be included in calculating total hours worked.

3. Off-duty periods should be inclusive of an uninterrupted 8-hour sleep cycle, a break from continuous professional responsibilities, and time to perform individual activities of daily living.

4. Arrangements should be made, in relation to the hours worked, to relieve a perioperative registered nurse who has worked on-call during his or her off shift and who is scheduled to work the following shift to accommodate an adequate off-duty recuperation period.

5. The number of on-call shifts assigned in a 7-day period depends on the type of facility and should be coordinated with the number of sustained work hours and adequate recuperation periods mentioned above.

6. An individual's ability to meet the anticipated work demand should be considered for on-call assignments. Limited research indicates older people are more likely than younger people to be adversely affected by sleep deprivation; however, there is no research specific to the effects of on-call assignment and a person's age.

| 183 |

CHAPTER 11 • MANDATORY OVERTIME IN NURSING: HOW MUCH? HOW OFTEN?

DISCUSSION POINT

Is mandatory overtime simply part of the work culture in the operating room or postanesthesia care units? Should there be different expectations or rules regarding mandatory overtime in these units?

MANDATORY OVERTIME AS A WAY OF LIFE IN THE UNITED STATES

Although nurses bemoan the increasing commonality of mandatory overtime in the profession, the reality is that mandatory overtime is not new, nor is it restricted to nursing. Gelb (2008) suggested that Americans typically work more hours and take fewer vacations than workers in other advanced economies. In fact, the International Labor Organization (ILO) suggested that about 80% of Americans work 40 hours or more each week, as compared to fewer than half of Danes, Finns, the French, or Germans (Gelb). Moreover, the ILO states that "Americans spend about 1,800 hours a year at work, compared to 1,600 hours or fewer in Belgium, Denmark, France, Germany, the Netherlands and Sweden" (Gelb, para 14). In contrast, South Koreans work about 2,400 hours per year (Gelb).

Gelb (2008) suggested that for many Americans hard work is a badge of honor. However, it may well be that Americans are working this hard because they are afraid not to. In the United States, unlike most European countries, employment is *at will*, meaning that employers can dismiss employees for any reason (aside from those of gender, race, age, or disability) or for no reason at all. Thus, employees who refuse to work overtime can lose their jobs or face other reprisals.

Nurses argue, however, that mandatory overtime in nursing is not comparable to mandatory overtime in other fields because the consequences of being overly fatigued for the nurse may literally have life-and-death consequences. Proponents of mandatory overtime argue that it is an economic reality, given how limited labor health care resources are, particularly in light of the international nursing shortage. The problem is that both positions are correct.

CONSIDER

Many nurses report a dramatic increase in the use of mandatory overtime to solve staffing problems and fear potential consequences for safety and quality of care for their patients.

This chapter will define mandatory overtime, examine the extent of its use in nursing, discuss the consequences of mandatory overtime in nursing as identified in the literature, and look at staffing alternatives that might alleviate the problem.

LEGISLATING MANDATORY OVERTIME

The Fair Labor Standards Act

The definition of what constitutes overtime in the United States or how it should be calculated has historically varied from state to state and from industry to industry. There are, however, national standards in terms of the Fair Labor Standards Act (FLSA) of 1938. This act, which regulates overtime, imposes no limits on overtime hours, nor does it prohibit dismissal or any other sanction for declining overtime work. It does, however, require that payroll employees (those who are not "exempt" from the overtime requirements of the FLSA) be paid an overtime premium of at least one and one-half times the regular rate of pay for each hour worked more than 40 in a week (U.S. Department of Labor, 2008).

CONSIDER

Labor laws such as the FLSA need to be amended to protect workers against excessive work hours and mandatory overtime and to protect the public from the dangers of an overburdened, stressed workforce.

Recent Changes to Federal Overtime Rules

There have been changes, however, to the federal overtime rules in the last decade. These changes, which became effective August 23, 2004, defined exemptions from the FLSA for what were traditionally called "white-collar" employees. The new rules increased the amount of money employees could earn before they were no longer eligible to receive overtime pay; however, employees who directed and supervised two or more other full-time employees fell under the executive exemption (Overtime Pay and White-Collar Exemptions, 2008).

Similarly, the new rules excluded employees from the FLSA who have the authority to hire, fire, and promote employees or if their primary duties involve the performance of office or nonmanual work and the exercise of discretion and independent judgment (Overtime Pay and White-Collar Exemptions, 2008). In addition, employees who have primary duties requiring either knowledge of an advanced type were excluded because the rules no longer distinguished advanced knowledge from "knowledge obtained from a general academic education, an apprenticeship or from training in the performance of routine, manual, or physical process" (Overtime Pay and White-Collar Exemptions, para 4).

Almost immediately, nursing leaders expressed concern that the language in the new rules opened the door for employer attempts to reclassify nurses as exempt from overtime protections historically given to workers under the FLSA. This occurred because under the new regulations, "learned professionals" earning fairly low salaries (anything above $455 per week) could not earn overtime pay.

Nurses meet the criteria of *learned professional*, which is defined in part as "employees who perform work that requires advanced knowledge (work which is predominantly intellectual in character and which includes work requiring the consistent exercise of discretion and judgment" (U.S. Department of Labor, 2007, para 6). In addition, the learned professional must have advanced knowledge in a field of science or learning, and the advanced knowledge must be customarily acquired by a prolonged course of specialized intellectual instruction (U.S. Department of Labor).

Concerns about the exemption of health care workers from protection under the FLSA were borne out in a June 2007 Supreme Court ruling that the U.S. Department of Labor had acted appropriately in denying FLSA protection to 10 home care workers even when employed by large, third-party home care agencies (Dawson, 2007). In the case of *Long Island Care at Home, LTD. v. Coke*, "the Court ruled that Ms. Evelyn Coke, a home care aide from Queens, New York, deserved neither overtime pay nor minimum wage, although she was frequently asked to work up to 70 hours per week" (Dawson, para 1).

The *Legal Eye Newsletter* (Home Health, 2008) suggested that this ruling occurred because of an exemption to the FLSA that applies to companions and housekeepers who work in the homes of their clients. The *Newsletter* went on to note that the U.S. District Court for the Southern District of Florida recently clarified the law, suggesting that licensed staff who go into clients'

homes to perform nursing assessments and to provide treatments are not home companions or housekeepers and thus are entitled to overtime.

In addition, it is important to note that nurses are eligible for overtime pay and protection under the FLSA if they are classified by employers as hourly—not salaried—employees, because salaried employees are not eligible for overtime. Thus, salaried employees and nurses who are considered to be exempt under the FLSA have virtually no rights under these new overtime rules. They are entitled only to their base salary, less deductions, by law and may be held to whatever schedule an employer demands because there are no restrictions on mandatory overtime in the FLSA.

Legislating Limits on Nursing Overtime

Despite multiple efforts over the last decade to introduce national legislation directed at prohibiting employers from requiring licensed health care employees to work more than 8 hours in a single workday or 80 hours in any 14-day work period—except in the case of a natural disaster or declaration of emergency by federal, state, or local government officials—no such legislation has passed.

States are, however, increasingly taking a role in both defining mandatory overtime and putting limits to its use. Every nurse should know and understand the provisions of the Nurse Practice Act in his or her state, as well as the position statements or advisory opinions that have been issued by the state board of nursing on mandatory overtime and patient abandonment.

> **DISCUSSION POINT**
> What position statement or advisory opinion has your state board of nursing issued regarding mandatory overtime and patient abandonment? Do you feel that it is adequate to protect both nurses and patients from unsafe working conditions?

In addition, the ANA has added the mandatory overtime issue to its Nationwide State Legislative Agenda, supporting the enactment of mandatory overtime legislation by state legislatures and the attention to such issues by regulatory agencies (ANA, 2008a). As of early 2009, 15 states had restrictions on the use of mandatory overtime for nurses, 11 states by enacting legislation (Connecticut, Illinois, Maryland, Minnesota, New Jersey, New Hampshire, New York, Oregon, Pennsylvania,

| 185 |

CHAPTER 11 • MANDATORY OVERTIME IN NURSING: HOW MUCH? HOW OFTEN?

Rhode Island, Washington, and West Virginia) and 3 by including such provisions in regulations (California, Missouri, and Texas) (ANA, 2008a).

For example, New York enacted legislation in 2008 that prohibits health care employers (excluding home care facilities) from forcing nurses to work overtime, except during health care disasters that increase the need for health care personnel unexpectedly or when a health care employer determines that there is an emergency and has made a good faith effort to have overtime covered on a voluntary basis (ANA, 2008a). Another exception includes an ongoing medical or surgical procedure in which the nurse is actively engaged, such as in surgery, and whose continued presence through completion is essential to the health and safety of the patient (ANA).

Although the New York legislation provides a good example of how states can reduce the risk of mandatory overtime for nurses, it should be noted that the New York Nurses Association first proposed legislation to ban mandatory overtime in 2000. Eight years were required to gain enough support from patient advocacy groups and other unions that represent nurses (such as the New York State Public Employees Federation and the New York State United Teachers) for the legislation to pass (Nurses Welcome Agreement, 2008; Nurses Win Ban, 2008).

Minnesota successfully passed legislation in 2007 that prohibits nurses from being required to work more than a "normal work period," meaning 12 or fewer consecutive hours, consistent with their predetermined work shift, but again excludes an emergency (ANA, 2008a):

The definition of emergency refers to a period when replacement staff are not able to report for duty for the next shift or increase patient need, because of unusual, unpredictable, or unforeseen circumstances such as, but not limited to, an act of terrorism, a disease outbreak, adverse weather conditions, or natural disasters which impact the continuity of patient care (ANA, para 5).

Similar legislation became effective in New Hampshire in 2008. This legislation prohibited an employer from disciplining or removing any right, benefit, or privilege of a registered nurse, licensed practical nurse, or licensed nursing assistant for refusing to work more than 12 consecutive hours, except under specific circumstances, such as those identified in the New York and Minnesota legislation (ANA, 2008a). A nurse might be disciplined for refusing to work mandatory overtime in these situations.

PATIENT ABANDONMENT

One of the most common reasons nurses cite for working mandatory overtime is the threat that refusal to do so could be construed as *patient abandonment*, a charge that can result in loss of licensure. Therefore, many nurses believe that they have no choice when confronted by a request for overtime, despite the fact that they might be working a shift in excess of 12 hours.

CONSIDER
In some facilities, nurses are being threatened with dismissal or with the charge of patient abandonment if they refuse to accept overtime.

Despite this perception, the ANA does not support the forced overtime of nurses, and their position is that a nurse should not be held accountable for patient abandonment if the nurse turned down an assignment that could be unsafe to patients or self. In fact, generally speaking, most state boards of nursing suggest that refusal to work mandatory overtime is not patient abandonment; in a situation in which a nurse has accepted a patient or assignment, the nurse must simply notify the supervisor that he or she is leaving and report off to another nurse.

Usually, however, nurses have less likelihood of losing their license if an assignment (mandatory overtime) is never accepted in the first place than if the assignment is accepted and then the nurse changes his or her mind. This is because accepting the assignment suggests that a nurse–patient relationship has been established. Cady (2008, para 15) agreed, suggesting

When the nurse accepts a patient assignment, the nurse maintains responsibility for that patient until the nurse–patient relationship is ended by the patient's discharge, the transfer of responsibility to another nurse, or the patient's refusal of the nurse's services. If no nurse is available for the transfer of responsibility, then the presently assigned nurse is legally and morally obligated to continue to care for the patient until the time that another nurse becomes available to take over that patient assignment.

Scudder and Edmunds (2007, para 11) also agreed, suggesting that patient abandonment requires three things: (1) that there be an established provider–patient relationship (duty) in which the patient *reasonably* expected that care would be provided, (2) that the provider negligently failed to carry out his or her obligation (breach of duty), and (3) that an injury (damage) was caused (actual and proximate) by the abandonment.

In addition, boards of nursing in several states have developed clear statements differentiating patient abandonment from *employee abandonment*. Typically, these statements define *employment abandonment* as nurses leaving their places of work to avoid injury to patients or to themselves.

Cady (2008) also distinguished between the refusal to accept a patient assignment and patient abandonment. Cady suggested that patient abandonment occurs when the nurse engages in a patient assignment and ceases to provide nursing care without appropriately transferring the responsibility for the patient to another professional nurse.

This definition is similar to language used by the Maryland Board of Registered Nursing (BRN) in defining patient abandonment; however, the Maryland BRN (2007) suggested that there are many variables to be examined in determining whether patient abandonment has actually occurred. The definition of patient abandonment and these variables are shown in Box 11.2.

CONSIDER

Although boards of nursing often rule that refusing mandatory overtime is not patient abandonment and thus is not cause for loss of licensure, they have no jurisdiction over employment and contract issues. Refusing to work mandatory overtime may still result in termination of a nurse's employment.

BOX 11.2

THE LINK BETWEEN NURSE–PATIENT RELATIONSHIPS AND PATIENT ABANDONMENT AS OUTLINED BY THE MARYLAND BOARD OF REGISTERED NURSING

Abandonment occurs when a licensed nurse terminates the nurse–patient relationship without reasonable notification to the nursing supervisor for the continuation of the patient's care.

The nurse–patient relationship begins when responsibility for nursing care of a patient is accepted by the nurse. Nursing management is accountable for assessing the capabilities of personnel and delegating responsibility or assigning nursing care functions to personnel qualified to assume such responsibility or to perform such functions.

The Variables that Need to be Examined in Each Alleged Incident of Abandonment Include but are not Limited to:

1. What were the licensee's assigned responsibilities for what time frame? What was the clinical setting and resources available to the licensee?

2. Was there an exchange of responsibility from one licensee to another? When did the exchange occur, i.e., shift report, etc.?

3. What was the time frame of the incident, i.e., time licensee arrived, time of exchange of responsibility, etc.?

4. What was the communication process, i.e., whom did the licensee inform of his or her intent to leave, and was it lateral, upward, downward, etc.?

5. What are the facility's policies, terms of employment, and/or job description regarding the licensee and call-in, refusal to accept an assignment, reassignment to another unit and mandatory overtime, etc.?

6. What is the pattern of practice/events for the licensee and the pattern of management for the unit/facility, i.e., is the event of a single isolated occurrence, or is it one event in a series of events?

7. What were the issues/reasons why the licensee could not accept an assignment, continue an assignment or extend an original assignment, etc.?

Source: Maryland Board of Registered Nursing (2007). *Abandonment*. Available at: http://www.mbon.org/main.php?v=norm&p=0&c=practice/abandonment.html. Accessed August 6, 2008.

| 187 |

CHAPTER 11 • MANDATORY OVERTIME IN NURSING: HOW MUCH? HOW OFTEN?

THE CONSEQUENCES OF MANDATORY OVERTIME

Research on the effects of overtime has been largely limited to studies of individuals working scheduled 12-hour shifts. According to a study by the Division of Biomedical and Behavioral Science of the National Institute for Occupational Safety and Health, when staff *plan* to work 12-hour shifts or additional shifts on a volunteer basis, they are more likely to get plenty of rest immediately before working the extended shift. Overtime mandated by an employer, however, occurs with little or no prior notice, so higher levels of fatigue may occur. In addition, many nurses report working far more than 12 hours when mandatory overtime is involved.

How long can nurses work safely? Given the variability in each situation, there is no one answer to this question. There is little doubt, however, that after a certain point of protracted worktime, fatigue becomes a factor and the likelihood of errors, near errors, mistakes, and lapses in judgment increases.

Other industries, such as airlines and trucking, have recognized this for years and have limited the hours employees in these industries can work without breaks (ANA, 2008d). The ANA (2006) argued that nursing employers should do the same by ensuring that sufficient system resources exist to (1) provide the individual registered nurse in all roles and settings with a work schedule that provides for adequate rest and recuperation between scheduled work and (2) provide sufficient compensation and appropriate staffing systems that foster a safe and healthful environment in which the registered nurse does not feel compelled to seek supplemental income through overtime, extra shifts, and other practices that contribute to worker fatigue.

> ### CONSIDER
> Federal regulations have used transportation laws to place limits on the amount of time that can safely be worked in aviation and trucking. It seems appropriate that Congress needs to go beyond the FLSA and at least examine the need to create safety parameters around mandatory overtime in nursing.

The reality, however, is that mandatory overtime is very much a part of contemporary nursing practice, and the literature increasingly suggests that fatigue resulting in errors is a consequence. A literature review by Garrett (2008) found that hospital administrators frequently rely on the use of mandatory or voluntary overtime to cover staff nurse vacancies. This leads to staff-member fatigue that may adversely affect patient safety as well as nurse burnout. (See Research Study Fuels the Controversy.)

Research Study Fuels the Controversy: The Effect of Mandatory Overtime on Medical Errors and Nurse Burnout

This literature review explored the effect of nurse staffing patterns on the frequency of medical errors, fatigue, and nurse burnout.

STUDY FINDINGS
This review of the literature suggested that nurse staffing patterns can have positive and negative effects on patient care and that low levels of nurse staffing can result in medical errors, adverse outcomes, and nurse burnout. The author concluded that nurses who suffer fatigue as a result of working mandatory overtime or call are set up for the potential to make medical mistakes, which not only have a negative effect on nurses and their coworkers, but also may result in adverse outcomes for patients.

In addition, Garrett pointed out that the financial burden associated with adverse events typically raises the cost of total treatment dramatically. Garrett concluded that when adverse outcomes occur as a result of low staffing, that blame is often placed on nurses and no solutions are explored to the problems that managed care and budget cuts have caused. Instead, she suggested that hospital administrators should invest in adequate nurse staffing to improve patient safety and increase nurse retention.

Garrett, C. (2008). The effect of nurse staffing patterns on medical errors and nurse burnout. *AORN Journal, 87*(6), 1191–1192, 1194, 1196–2000.

Similarly, a recent study by Warren and Tart (2008) at a non-for-profit magnet community hospital found that fatigue caused by long work hours, working on call, and insufficient rest periods led to perioperative documentation errors. When a reduced call schedule was implemented, a significant reduction in nursing documentation errors was observed, with the greatest reduction in errors seen among nurses working 12-hour or call shifts.

In another recent study of 2,273 registered nurses in the United States, Jeanne Geiger-Brown of the University of Maryland found that adverse work schedules negatively affect sleep quality and work performance (Study Reveals Sleep Problems, 2008). The research analyzed work schedule variables including hours per day, days per week, weekends per month, quick returns (less than 10 hours off between shifts), mandatory overtime, on-call, and circadian mismatch, and found that the worse the schedule, the worse was the sleep for most nurses. Geiger-Brown suggested that the inadequate sleep that occurs as a result of adverse work schedules has both short-term (needle-stick injuries and musculoskeletal disorders) and long-term (cardiovascular and metabolic diseases) health consequences for nurses and possibly for the patients for whom they care (Study Reveals Sleep Problems).

Similarly, a benchmark study by Rogers, Wei-Ting, Scott, Aiken, and Dinges (2004) found that the risk of making an error greatly increased when nurses had to work shifts that were longer than 12 hours, when they worked significant overtime, or when they worked more than 40 hours per week. Nurses who worked shifts of 12.5 hours or longer were three times more likely to make errors than those who worked an 8.5-hour day. Working overtime increased the odds of making at least one error, regardless of how long the shift was originally scheduled.

In addition, logbooks completed by the 393 hospital staff nurses in Rogers et al.'s study revealed that participants usually worked longer than scheduled and that approximately 40% of the 5,317 work shifts they logged exceeded 12 hours. Fourteen percent of respondents worked at least 16 consecutive hours at least once during the 4-week period studied, suggesting that double shifts or longer are not confined to rare emergencies. The longest shift worked was nearly 24 hours, and 65% of respondents suggested that they had a hard time staying awake during at least one shift of work during the

study period, and 20% said that they fell asleep at least once during their work shift (Rogers et al.).

A 2007 study by the U.S. Agency for Healthcare Research and Quality (AHRQ) also found that overtime was one of the components of working conditions that influenced elderly patients' outcomes in intensive care settings (Collins-Sharp & Clancy, 2008). Research by the AHRQ also found that there are significantly greater risks to patient safety when nurses work beyond their regularly scheduled work hours (Collins-Sharp & Clancy).

These findings reinforced those of a report of the Board on Health Care Services (HCS) and the Institute of Medicine (IOM), *Keeping Patients Safe: Transforming the Work Environment of Nurses*, which said that nurses' long working hours pose a serious threat to patient safety. In fact, the report argued that "limiting the number of hours worked per day and consecutive days of work by nursing staff, as is done in other safety-sensitive industries, is a fundamental safety precaution" (PA Nurses Also Address, 2007, para 3). Similarly, Marquis and Huston (2009) argued that certain minimum criteria should always be met for safe staffing. These criteria are shown in Box 11.3.

DISCUSSION POINT

How many hours can the typical nurse work before she or he might be considered unsafe? How much individual leeway is feasible in making this determination?

In contrast to the studies already cited, Berney and Needleman (2006), in their study of 161 acute care general hospitals in New York State from 1995 to 2000, found an association between RN overtime and lower rates of mortality in medical and surgical patients. In other words, as overtime increased, mortality decreased. The researchers suggested this might be a result of increased overtime by permanent nursing staff who would be less inclined to make errors than increased hours by temporary staff. They cautioned, however, that their findings were suggestive, not definitive. In addition, they expressed concern that their findings might have been due to random variation rather than an actual association.

The link between mandatory overtime and nurse dissatisfaction and turnover, however, has little controversy. In fact, working conditions are often cited as the primary cause for nurses leaving the profession or

| 189 |

CHAPTER 11 • MANDATORY OVERTIME IN NURSING: HOW MUCH? HOW OFTEN?

| BOX 11.3 | MINIMUM CRITERIA FOR STAFFING DECISIONS |

- Decisions made must meet state and federal labor laws and organizational policies.
- Staff must not be demoralized or excessively fatigued by frequent or extended overtime requests.
- Long-term as well as short-term solutions must be sought.
- Patient care must not be jeopardized.

Source: Marquis, B., & Huston, C. (2009). *Leadership Roles and Management Functions* (6th ed.). Philadelphia: Lippincott Williams & Wilkins.

reducing work hours. A study by the Ohio Nurses Association reported that approximately 60% of the nurses it surveyed had considered leaving nursing because of mandatory overtime (Widowfield, 2004).

Similarly, the United Steel Workers of America (n.d.) reported that recent studies showed that one in five nurses were considering leaving nursing; when polled on their reasons for leaving, mandatory overtime was always listed in the top 10 reasons. Mandatory overtime also discourages nurses from accepting employment in the first place. Perhaps that is why mandatory overtime is almost universally banned by magnet hospitals.

> **DISCUSSION POINT**
> Is increasing the use of mandatory overtime perpetuating the nursing shortage? Do you think nurses who no longer work in nursing roles would return to work if mandatory overtime was banned?

Finally, although mandatory overtime may be thought of as a cost-saving measure, it often generates very large costs, even if sometimes unaccounted for, in the form of increased turnover, lower productivity, longer patient stays, and higher rates of treatment errors that in turn necessitate more extended and costly solutions (AFSCME, 2008b). This was certainly supported in Garrett's (2008) literature review. Clearly, mandatory overtime must be eliminated or the nursing shortage will worsen and the quality of patient care will further erode. In addition, mandatory overtime erodes morale and poses threats to both patients and their caregivers. One source went so far as to suggest that mandatory overtime is linked to a host of patient problems and that it is perhaps the worst practice to emerge from the era of downsizing and managed care (AFSCME, 2008b).

> **CONSIDER**
> In an age of severe nursing shortages, creating an environment that promotes safe work environments is critical to nurse retention.

PROFESSIONAL DUTY AND CONSCIENCE

Mandatory overtime and patient abandonment must also be examined in terms of professional duty. A *professional duty* is the direct result of others having welfare rights, such as the right to safe care. Because people have a right to such care, nurses have an associated duty to ensure that they accept patient care assignments only if they are mentally and physically able to provide, at minimum, safe care.

The problem is that there is great variability in terms of how many hours a nurse can work and still provide competent safe care. For example, the practice of mandatory overtime is grounded in the commitment to prevent harm to patients by guaranteeing adequate nurse–patient ratios, yet the overfatigued nurse may pose even greater risk of harm to patients by agreeing to work. The ANA (2008a) agreed, suggesting that "regardless of the number of hours worked, each registered nurse has an ethical responsibility to carefully consider his/her level of fatigue when deciding to accept any assignment extending beyond the regularly scheduled work day or week, including mandatory or voluntary overtime assignment."

> **DISCUSSION POINT**
> Who bears the risk or the consequences of risk when an overworked nurse makes errors that contribute to patient harm?

Cady (2008) added that there are many reasons why a nurse might refuse to care for a patient. She suggested that nurse managers must be aware of the nexus between moral dilemmas in health care and the right of providers to refuse a patient care assignment.

Cady went on to say that one option nurses should consider if they do not want to work mandatory overtime is to file for *conscientious objection*. The purpose of conscientious objection is to protect the rights of employees who refuse to participate in procedures on the basis of conscience. The issue of whether a nurse can refuse mandatory overtime on the basis of conscience, however, has limited case law precedent.

The ANA's *Code of Ethics* (ANA, 2001) might also be helpful to some nurses in resolving potential ethical conflicts between their professional duty to provide care and conscience, or the realization that providing such care may actually place patients at risk for harm. The *Code of Ethics*, however, might actually potentiate the dilemma because it states that nurses should care for all people without discrimination and maintain and foster nursing competence and professional development. The problem is that it also says that the nurse is to maintain conditions of employment that are conducive to high-quality nursing care.

The ANA also recommends a Bill of Rights as a tool for dialogue to resolve concerns that nurses may have about work environments that might not support professional practice. The Bill of Rights was actually conceived to support nurses in an array of workplace situations, including mandatory overtime, and suggests that nurses must bring these workplace issues to the attention of employers to meet their responsibilities to their patients and to themselves (ANA, 2008c).

UNIONS AND MANDATORY OVERTIME

Because collective bargaining agreements can require greater protections beyond those outlined in the FSA, the position of most collective bargaining agents is that the practice of mandatory overtime should be eliminated entirely. However, there are differences among union contracts, and the strategies used by unions to reduce mandatory overtime vary greatly.

The American Federation of Teachers (AFT) (n.d.) has been working with its state affiliates to ban the practice of mandatory overtime through a twofold approach—legislation and contract language: "At the state level, AFT Healthcare affiliates in Connecticut, Maryland, New Jersey and Oregon have won legislative and regulatory bans on the use of mandatory overtime. The New Jersey legislation is the strongest in the nation, and covers all healthcare workers—not just nurses" (AFT, para 5 and 6).

The Service Employees International Union (SEIU) (2008) has also consistently spoken out against mandatory overtime. In 2007, the SEIU endorsed passage of proposed federal legislation known as the Safe Nursing and Patient Care Act of 2007 (HR 2122), which amended Title XVIII of the Social Security Act to limit the number of mandatory overtime hours a nurse could be required to work for providers paid by the Medicare Program. Unfortunately, this bill stalled in the Senate in October 2007. In addition, the SEIU, in partnership with the Nurse Alliance, created an Overtime Report Form for nurses, union or nonunion, to document mandatory or pressured overtime (SEIU).

The American Federation of State, County and Municipal Employees (AFSCME) is also working to eliminate mandatory overtime in response to inadequate staff to operate public agencies such as prisons, veterans homes, and mental health and developmental centers. For example, AFSCME union leaders stated "significant cutbacks in the number of state employees in Illinois have forced current workers to take on extra overtime hours, sometimes being forced to work double shifts with little advance notice. Those who can't pick up the required overtime shifts are disciplined" (Wiehle, 2008, para 2). To address the issue, AFSCME held a news conference to highlight the plight of affected workers. In addition, the union is backing legislation to ban forced overtime except in emergency situations. This legislation passed the House of Representatives and awaits Senate action (Wiehle).

ALTERNATIVES TO MANDATORY OVERTIME

There are many successful alternatives to mandatory overtime that share commonalities—providing incentives that induce employees to willingly work extra hours and giving employees some degree of control over when they work.

One alternative intended to reduce staffing shortages is *shift bidding*. In shift bidding, a health care organization

| 191 |

CHAPTER 11 • MANDATORY OVERTIME IN NURSING: HOW MUCH? HOW OFTEN?

posts available shifts online as well as maximum pay rate, and then nurses bid their price to work on that shift. If the organization receives more offers to work than are needed, the nurses requesting the highest rate of pay are typically notified and given an option to re-submit a lower bid (Foster, 2006).

Generally speaking, in shift bidding, managers select qualified nurses who put in the lowest hourly rate. Yet the "lowest bids" do not come cheap. Robert Blake, Assistant Vice President of the Internal Staffing Division of Memorial Hermann in Houston, Texas, suggested that the average hourly rate for nurses who shift bid there is $39.00 (Foster, 2006). This still represents a significant cost reduction for the hospital, however, because outside agency nurses average $59.00/hour. Blake reported that Memorial Hermann has saved nearly $22 million between 2001 and 2005 since launching online shift bidding (Foster).

Similarly, Kulma and Springer (2006) detailed an online shift bidding program implemented in 2004 at a southern regional medical center in Georgia. Employees can access the shift bidding system anywhere there is Internet capability, to find available shifts that match their interest, skills, and experience: "The system shows only shifts that employees are qualified to work, ensuring that the right resources with the right skills are matched as appropriate to open shifts" (p. 93).

Kulma and Springer argued that shift bidding eliminates the dissatisfaction that occurs with the high use of contract labor because employees often resent working side by side with individuals doing the same job but being paid significantly more. Sixty percent of the staff actively bid on shifts, a number that doubled between 2005 and 2006. In addition, Kulma and Springer noted that although the number of staff in the as-needed temporary pool base stayed relatively constant, the average number of hours that nurses picked up per pay period increased by 8.8 hours. This is equivalent to increasing nurse staffing by 15 full-time equivalents or 30%.

Critics of shift bidding suggest that although this alternative gives nurses more control over their work scheduling, it should not be a replacement for having full-time, qualified staff who can provide better continuity of care. It also encourages nurses to work more than they should. In addition, the idea that nurses would bid against each other in an online auction, with each subsequent bid lowering the price of their services, is repugnant to some.

DISCUSSION POINT

Do you believe that shift bidding is in the best interest of RNs? Does the need for flexibility and choice in scheduling outweigh the idea that the "cheapest" RN is the one who should work?

Lambrinos, LaPosta, and Cohen (2004) described another alternative successfully used at an academic medical center that increased nursing hours while decreasing costs. This *Pay Enhancement Program* included a monetary incentive program and a new premium pay structure. The incentive program was based on committed hours, as well as the actual number of hours worked each pay period by full-time and 0.9-status nurses. Nurses who worked 80 or more hours in a 2-week period received bonuses of $150 to $200 per pay period.

Premium pay for last-minute call-ins was redesigned so that full-time nurses were eligible for a premium rate of 2.0, whereas nurses at 0.9 status could receive premium pay at a rate of 1.75 times normal. Nurses working between 0.5 and 0.8 status were limited to premium pay of 1.5 times their normal rate of pay. Both the incentive program and premium pay options were reported to have encouraged nurses to work more, meaning that mandatory overtime would be decreased.

Another alternative to mandatory overtime was reported at Borgess Medical Center in Michigan (Borgess RNs Win, 2007). This alternative created a *nurse resource team* to supplement the full-time nursing staff. The nurse resource team provides a pool of per diem nurses who are already familiar with the hospital and appropriately trained to fill in as needed.

CONSIDER

All nurses should be involved in creating proactive, beneficent staffing policies at the unit or institutional level, as well as through state and national organizations and governmental venues.

CONCLUSIONS

The mandatory overtime dilemma, like so many in nursing, comes down to a conflict regarding how best to use limited resources (fiscal and human) to provide safe, quality health care. Most nurses and administrators can agree on two goals: (1) staffing should be at least minimally adequate to assure that all patients receive safe care, and (2) nursing staff should not be placed at personal or legal risk to provide that care.

The problem is that the onus is on management to ensure that there is appropriate staffing, and most health care institutions state that there simply are not enough resources to meet the first goal without jeopardizing the second. Clearly, more alternatives such as shift bidding and pay enhancement programs need to be explored. Neither health care administrators nor nurses should have to choose between meeting the needs of patients and meeting the needs of nurses.

The bottom line is that workers should have the right to refuse overtime without fear of repercussion, especially when staffing shortages and mandated overtime are the norm and not the exception. Unfortunately, given the severity and duration of the current nursing shortage, the use of mandatory overtime as a means of meeting minimum staffing needs is an issue that will plague the nursing profession for some time to come. The AFSCME (2008a) agreed, and suggested that unless legislation to stop mandatory overtime is passed, the practice will continue.

FOR ADDITIONAL DISCUSSION

1. How does the presence of a collective bargaining agreement affect a hospital's ability to require mandatory overtime? How much power do unions have in negotiating this aspect of working conditions?

2. Would passage of a national ban on mandatory overtime tie the hands of hospitals to assure that staffing is at least minimally adequate during periods of acute nursing shortages?

3. Does the use of mandatory overtime really save hospitals money in terms of recruitment and benefits?

4. How do the rates of mandatory overtime in nursing compare with those in other professions?

5. Why is nursing the only profession at risk for loss of licensure if an individual is found guilty of patient abandonment?

6. Are charges of patient abandonment legally and morally appropriate if a nurse works his or her required shift but refuses to stay and work longer?

7. Given the severity and scope of the nursing shortage, what is the likelihood that mandatory staffing will continue to be used for both emergency and routine staffing needs?

REFERENCES

American Federation of State, County and Municipal Employees, AFL–CIO (AFSCME) (2008). *Stop mandatory overtime.* Available at: http://www.afscme.org/workers/6569.cfm. Accessed August 1, 2008.

American Federation of State, County and Municipal Employees, AFL–CIO (AFSCME) (2008b). *Worst practices. Mandatory overtime.* Available at: http://www.afscme.org/una/sns10.htm. Accessed August 6, 2008.

American Federation of Teachers (n.d.) *Mandatory overtime.* Available at: http://www.aft.org/topics/mandatory-overtime/. Accessed August 6, 2008.

American Nurses Association (ANA) (2001). *Code of Ethics for Nurses with Interpretive Statements.* Washington, DC: American Nurses Publishing. Available at: http://www.nursingworld.org/ethics/code/protected_nwcoe303.htm. Accessed August 6, 2008.

American Nurses Association (ANA) (2006). *Position statement: Assuring patient safety: The employers' role in promoting healthy nursing work hours for registered nurses in all roles and settings.* Available at: http://www.nursingworld.org/MainMenuCategories/The PracticeofProfessionalNursing/workplace/Workforce/NurseFatigue/EmployersRole.aspx. Accessed August 6, 2008.

| 193 |

CHAPTER 11 • MANDATORY OVERTIME IN NURSING: HOW MUCH? HOW OFTEN?

American Nurses Association (ANA) (2008a). *Mandatory overtime*. Nursing World. Available at: http://www.nursingworld.org/MainMenuCategories/ANAPoliticalPower/State/StateLegislativeAgenda/MandatoryOvertime.aspx. Accessed August 1, 2008.

American Nurses Association (ANA) (2008b). *ANA government affairs on mandatory overtime*. Available at: http://www.nursingworld.org/MainMenuCategories/ANAPoliticalPower/Federal/Issues/MandatoryOvertime.aspx. Accessed August 5, 2008.

American Nurses Association (ANA) (2008c). *Bill of rights FAQs*. Available at: http://www.nursingworld.org/EspeciallyForYou/stafftesting/FAQs.aspx. Accessed August 6, 2008.

American Nurses Association (ANA) (2008d). *Nurse fatigue*. Available at: http://www.nursingworld.org/MainMenuCategories/ThePracticeofProfessionalNursing/workplace/Workforce/NurseFatigue.aspx. Accessed August 6, 2008.

Association of Perioperative Registered Nurses (AORN) (2007). AORN position statement: Safe work/on-call practices (pp. 409–412). In: *Standards, Recommended Practices, and Guidelines*. Denver, CO: AORN. Available at: http://ioivw.aorn.org/PracticeResources/AORNPositionStatements/Position_SafeWorkOnCallPractices/. Accessed August 6, 2008.

Berney, B., & Needleman, J. (2006). Impact of nursing overtime on nurse-sensitive patient outcomes in New York hospitals, 1995–2000. *Policy, Politics & Nursing Practice, 7*(2), 87–100.

Borgess RNs win with elimination of mandatory overtime (2007). *American Nurse, 39*(3), 4.

Cady, R. F. (2008). Refusal to care. *JONA's Healthcare Law, Ethics, & Regulation, 10*(2), 46–47.

Collins-Sharp, B. A., & Clancy, C. M. (2008). *Journal of Nursing Care Quality, 23*(20), 97–100.

Cunningham, D. (2008). *Wisconsin Federation of Nurses: Mandatory overtime hurts patient care*. Workers Independent News. Available at: http://www.laborradio.org/node/8652. Accessed August 5, 2008.

Dawson, S. L. (2007). Taking a cue from the Supreme Court. *Nursing Homes: Long Term Care Management, 56*(10), 8–10.

Foster, R. (2006). The bidding begins. *Hospitals & Health Networks, 80*(9), 26.

Garrett, C. (2008). The effect of nurse staffing patterns on medical errors and nurse burnout. *AORN Journal, 87*(6), 1191–1192, 1194, 1196–2000.

Gelb, M. (2008). For many Americans, hard work is badge of honor. Americans skimp on vacations; economists say work ethic can pay off. Available at: http://www.america.gov/st/econ-english/2008/July/20080703151840berehellek0.7706415.html. Accessed August 1, 2008.

Home health: Professional staff get overtime pay (2008). *Legal Eagle Eye Newsletter for the Nursing Profession, 16*(4), 4.

Kulma, M., & Springer, B. (2006). Easing the bottom-line impact of staffing shortages: A case study in shift bidding. *Healthcare Financial Management, 60*(4), 92–97.

Lambrinos, J., LaPosta, M. J., & Cohen, A. (2004). Increasing nursing hours without increasing nurses. *Journal of Nursing Administration, 34*(4), 195–199.

Marquis, B., & Huston, C. (2009). *Leadership Roles and Management Functions* (6th ed.). Philadelphia: Lippincott Williams & Wilkins.

Maryland Board of Registered Nursing (2007). *Abandonment*. Available at: http://www.mbon.org/main.php?v=norm&p=0&c=practice/abandonment.html. Accessed August 6, 2008.

Nurses welcome agreement to ban mandatory overtime, New York (2008). Available at: http://www.medicalnewstoday.com/articles/112051.php. Accessed July 31, 2008.

Nurses win ban on mandatory overtime in New York (2008). Available at: http://www.silobreaker.com/DocumentReader.aspx?Item=5_877935894. Accessed August 1, 2008.

Overtime pay and white-collar exemptions: Seeking clarification in light of recent revisions (2008). *Illinois Business Law Journal*. Available at: http://iblsjournal.typepad.com/illinois_business_law_soc/2008/02/have-the-dols-n.html. Accessed August 1, 2008.

PA nurses also address mandatory overtime (2007). *American Nurse, 39*(3), 4.

Rogers, À., Wei-Ting, H., Scott, L. D., Aiken, L. H., & Dinges, D. F. (2004). The working hours of hospital staff nurses and patient safety. *Health Affairs, 23*(4), 202–212.

Scudder, L., & Edmunds, M. W. (2007). Nurses journal scan. Termination: Ethical and legal implications. *Journal for Nurse Practitioners, 3*, 379–383. Available at: http://www.medscape.com/viewarticle/561232. Accessed August 5, 2008.

Service Employees International Union (SEIU) (2008). *Working to limit mandatory overtime.* Available at: http://www.seiu.org/health/nurses/madatory_overtime/. Accessed August 5, 2008.

Sleep study reveals sleep problems with shift work (2008). New South Wales Nurses' Association. Available at: http://www.nswnurses.asn.au/news/13865.html. Accessed August 6, 2008.

United Steelworkers of America (n.d.). *Facts on mandatory overtime.* Available at: http://www.uswa.org/uswa/program/content/515.php. Accessed June 25, 2004.

U.S. Department of Labor (2007). *Fact sheet #17D: Exemption for professional employees under the Fair Labor Standards Act (FLSA).* Available at: http://www.dol.gov/esa/whd/regs/compliance/fairpay/fs17d_professional.pdf. Accessed August 1, 2008.

U.S. Department of Labor (2008). *Overtime pay.* Available at: http://www.dol.gov/dol/topic/wages/overtimepay.htm. Accessed August 1, 2008.

Warren, A., & Tart, R. C. (2008). Fatigue and charting errors: The benefit of a reduced call schedule. *AORN Journal, 88*(1), 88–95.

Widowfield, J. (2004). Safer nurses; safer care: Ban on mandatory overtime proposed. *Ohio Nurses Review, 79*(2), 1, 10.

Wiehle, A. (2008). *Union for state workers wants mandatory overtime eliminated.* Available at: http://www.chicagotribune.com/news/local/chi-union-no-overtime-09may09,0,3271345.story?track=rss. Accessed August 6, 2008.

BIBLIOGRAPHY

Blegen, M. A., Vaughn, T., & Vojir, C. P. (2008). Nurse staffing levels: Impact of organizational characteristics and registered nurse supply. *Health Services Research, 43*(1 Part 1), 154–173.

Desrosiers, G. (2007). Mandatory overtime: This has gone on too long! *Perspective Infirmiere, 4*(5), 10–14.

Ellerbe, S. (2007). Practice matters. Staffing through web-based open-shift bidding. *American Nurse Today, 2*(4), 32–34.

FLSA: Are personal caregivers entitled to overtime? (2007). *Legal Eagle Eye Newsletter for the Nursing Profession, 15*(8), 4.

Heslin, M. J., Doster, B. E., Daily, S. L., Waldrum, M. R., Boudreaux, A. M., Smith A., Peters, G., Ragan, D. B., Buchalter, S., Bland, K. I., & Rue, L. W. (2008). Durable improvements in efficiency, safety, and satisfaction in the operating room. *Journal of the American College of Surgery, 206*(5), 1083–1089.

Nelson, R., & Kennedy, M. S. (2008). The other side of mandatory overtime. *American Journal of Nursing, 108*(4), 23–24.

Peck, R. L. (2007). Staffing fireworks! *Nursing Homes: Long Term Care Management, 56*(7), 6.

Potera, C. (2007). In the news. Patient outcomes linked to ICU nurses' working conditions. *American Journal of Nursing, 107*(8), 19.

Sharp, B. A. C., & Clancy, C. M. (2008). Limiting nurse overtime, and promoting other good working conditions, influences patient safety. *Journal of Nursing Care Quality, 23*(2), 97–100.

Stone, P. W., Mooney-Kane, C., Larson, E. L., Horan, T., Glance, L. G., Zwanziger, J., & Dick, A. W. (2007). Nurse working conditions and patient safety outcomes. *Medical Care, 45*(6), 571–578.

Stop mandatory overtime (2007). *Chart, 104*(2), 3.

Trueman, C. A. (2007). A call to arms: Having success in recruitment and retention. *Caring, 26*(2), 48–49.

Witek, M. (2007). Understaffed, overworked, and overtime.... A triple threat to nursing's health. *Nursing Spectrum (New York and New Jersey), 19A*(20), 4.

Wright, L. D. (2007). Case focus. Voluntary overtime, unsafe nursing practice, and the quest for institutional accountability. *JONA's Healthcare Law, Ethics & Regulation, 9*(2), 50–53.

| 195 |

CHAPTER 11 • MANDATORY OVERTIME IN NURSING: HOW MUCH? HOW OFTEN?

WEB RESOURCES

Academy of Medical Surgical Nurses, Official Position Statement on Mandatory Overtime	http://www.medsurgnurse.org/cgi-bin/WebObjects/AMSNMain.woa/1/wa/viewSection?wosid=SWvI5kTDdzqs2PA15Jg7Qs5qc9l&tName=positionsMandatoryOvertime&s_id=1073744079&ss_id=536873229
American Association of Critical Care Nurses, Position Statement on Mandatory Overtime	http://classic.aacn.org/AACN/pubpolcy.nsf/72fe271374e4c5338825688e00776c20/7945af78da4b2d7988256ce000660bc5?OpenDocument
American Nurses Association, Position Statement: Opposition to Mandatory Overtime	http://www.nursingworld.org/readroom/position/workplac/revmot2.htm
American Organization of Nurse Executives, Policy Statement on Mandatory Overtime	http://www.aone.org/aone/advocacy/ps_mandatory_ot.html
Arizona Nurses Association, Position Statement on Mandatory Overtime	http://www.aznurse.org/default.asp?PageID=10001160
Colorado Nurses Association, Position Statement on Mandatory Overtime	http://www.nurses-co.org/Article_feature.asp?story=272
Compliance Assistance, U.S. Department of Labor, Fair Labor Standards Act	http://www.dol.gov/esa/whd/flsa/
Emergency Nurses Association Position Statement, Mandatory Overtime	http://www.ena.org/about/position/PDFs/166A20AC32114CE0A771A448A488B1B6.pdf
Pennsylvania State Nurses Association, Position on Mandatory Overtime	http://www.panurses.org/site/resources/Position/positions.cfm?action&ID=11
Wisconsin Organization of Nurse Executives, Position Statement on Senate Bill 512, February 27, 2008	http://www.w-one.org/uploads/MandatoryOvertime2-2008.pdf

CHAPTER 12

Violence in Nursing: The Expectations and the Reality

• CHARMAINE HOCKLEY •

Learning Objectives

The learner will be able to:

1. Identify common terms used to describe workplace violence, including *horizontal violence, bullying,* and *mobbing.*
2. Explore the prevalence of workplace violence in nursing as compared to other professions.
3. Recognize workplace violence as both a national and a global problem.
4. Differentiate among nurse-to-nurse violence, patient-to-nurse violence, organization-to-nurse violence, violence perpetrated by external parties, third-party violence, the effect of mass trauma or natural disasters on nurses, and nurse-to-patient violence.
5. Compare the incidence, most frequent types, and common consequences of workplace violence for men and women.
6. Identify antisocial workplace behaviors that may lead to nurses causing each other harm.
7. Analyze common reasons that victims are reluctant to report workplace violence.
8. Describe potential long-term consequences of workplace violence, including physical, emotional, and spiritual repercussions.
9. Delineate specific strategies that can be undertaken by individuals, employers, organizations, and governments to reduce workplace violence.
10. Apply ethical and moral codes of professional practice as guides for developing best practices to guard against and respond to workplace violence.
11. Reflect on personal behaviors or attitude that might create a threatening workplace environment for others.

Violence in nursing is not a new phenomenon, but it has only been in the last two decades that the issue has been acutely recognized. This has led to a rapid growth of research on the issue, most of which reinforces the ongoing seriousness and magnitude of the problem faced by nurses in their day-to-day employment. Furthermore, these studies show that violence in nursing is not rare or isolated to a single setting but is experienced by nurses in a variety of geographical locations and service areas. In other words, the violence that nurses experience can occur wherever they might live or work.

This chapter is divided into three main sections. The first section begins by exploring what is meant by violence in nursing, the language used to describe this issue, and the types of violence that nurses might experience. The second section introduces a variety of strategies to address the issue. The third and final section showcases some of the wide-ranging projects that have been undertaken to address violence in nursing.

> **DISCUSSION POINT**
> How does violence in nursing affect patient care?

WHAT IS VIOLENCE IN NURSING?

Over the years, violence in nursing has often been a difficult concept to grasp, in part because of people's misinterpretation of what the term "violence" implies, as well as because of the language used to describe this behavior. Many people, both from within and outside the health care system, still find it difficult to accept that violence occurs to nurses in the workplace by both patients and staff. This might be in part because of the language that is used to describe the incident; it might derive from people's reluctance to expand their understanding of the meaning of violence as being more than a physical act; or it could be the result of the community's perception that such things do not happen to nurses. For example, the use of the term "bullying" to describe and define workplace incidents may conjure up a perception of schoolyard bullying and therefore minimize the effect that this behavior can have on the person involved.

Historically, different countries have used different terms to describe this violent behavior. For example, the nursing literature in the United States led the way by referring to this behavior as *horizontal violence*. In Europe, the preferred term has been *mobbing*, and in the United Kingdom, the literature refers to this behavior as *bullying*. Australian nursing literature initially used the term horizontal violence. In the last 5 to 10 years, the term *workplace violence* has become accepted as the preferred term globally, particularly since the release of papers from internationally recognized organizations such as the International Council of Nurses (ICN), the World Health Organization (WHO), the Honor Society of Nursing, Sigma Theta Tau International (STTI), the Royal College of Nursing (RCN), and the Royal College of Nursing, Australia (RCNA). Nevertheless, terms such as horizontal violence (Hurley, 2006), bullying (Lewis, 2006), and mobbing (Yildirum & Yildirum, 2008) continue to be used.

A review of the literature shows that there does not appear to be standard definitions of workplace violence, horizontal violence, bullying, or mobbing. One of the earliest references is Roberts (1983), who, in examining horizontal violence, argued compellingly that some of the salient aspects of nursing subculture and behaviors came within the framework of oppression theory. Since then, there has been an ongoing discussion and debate on what is violence in nursing and an ever-increasing number of studies from different research perspectives, including the qualitative feminist point of view (Paliadelis, Cruickshank, & Sheridan, 2007), the ethnographic viewpoint (Hodson, 2008), and grounded theory (Strandmark & Hallberg, 2007), to name a few.

In recent years research from different geographical locations, such as Hong Kong (Mak, Chung, Chan, & Cheung, 2008), Iran (Motamedi, 2008), and Turkey (Celik & Celik, 2008), and from different nursing services, such as high-security psychiatric hospitals (Jones, 2008), hemodialysis units (Jones, Callaghan, Eales, & Ashman, 2008), and accident/emergency departments (Rampersaud, 2008) have demonstrated that this violent behavior is not unique to any specific country or any specific clinical area.

Studies exploring the perspectives of students and faculty members have also been undertaken (Ferns, & Meerabeau, 2008; McLaughlin & Wellman, 2008) showing that violence toward and among nurses is not specifically unique to the health care sector but also occurs in nursing learning institutions. Each of these perspectives and nursing services brings forward language that is unique and highlights that although there is a common theme—violence in nursing—how this behavior is defined or the language used depends on the perspective of the researchers or practitioners.

> ### CONSIDER
> Violence has penetrated every sector of society, including the workplace, and yet there continues to be difficulty in defining these incidents. Who are the victims?

Although the true extent of violence in nursing is considered to be greater than the statistics indicate, studies show that violence against female nurses is greater than that against male nurses. This is not unexpected, given that nursing continues to be a predominantly female occupation.

Studies into violence against men in other contexts tend to focus on rites of initiation of apprentices, college fraternity rites of passage (hazing), and armed service "bastardization" practices. However, the question of whether workplace violence against male nurses is an outcome of the same forces identified in studies into workplace violence in female nurses is open to further research (e.g., Harding, 2008). Because the statistics show that men are often the major perpetrators of violence in society and in the workplace (except possibly for internal violence in nursing), the very fear that some male nurses might experience violence could also create more violent incidents in the workplace, generating a recurring cycle of violence.

Defining Violence in Nursing

A specific definition for violence in nursing could be as follows:

> Violence in nursing is the outcome of any act that causes harm to a nurse. Along a continuum, these acts can range from nonphysical, such as abuse of power, verbal, financial and emotional abuse, to physical, including homicide being the most extreme. Violence is not so much the act itself; it is the outcome of a harmful experience. The harm experienced can extend to third party victims such as colleagues and significant others such as family members (Modified from Hockley, 2006).

In a wider context, a succinct definition, with a strong physical focus, comes from the federal government, which defines workplace violence as "violent acts (including physical assaults and threats of assaults) directed toward persons at work or on duty" (National Institute for Occupational Health and Safety, 2002, para 3).

DISCUSSION POINT

Do you have to be harmed by these behaviors or tactics to experience violence in nursing? Is it violence in nursing if you are not harmed? What are the different types of harm a person can experience by these behaviors or the tactics used? Are some types of harm more serious than others?

In comparison to the foregoing definitions, various Australian state laws tend to avoid the term violence when describing these types of workplace behaviors, preferring the terms "inappropriate behavior" or "bullying" (Occupational Health, Safety & Welfare Act, 1986). For example, Section 55A of the Occupational Health, Safety and Welfare Act (1986) reads as follows:

Occupational Health, Safety and Welfare Act 1986 (SA)
S55A—Inappropriate behaviour towards an employee
(1) For the purposes of this section, bullying is behaviour—
  (a) that is directed towards an employee or a group of employees, that is repeated and systematic, and that a reasonable person, having regard to all the circumstances, would expect to victimize, humiliate, undermine or threaten the employee or employees to whom the behaviour is directed; and
  (b) that creates a risk to health or safety.

(2) However, bullying does not include—
  (a) reasonable action taken in a reasonable manner by an employer to transfer, demote, discipline, counsel, retrench or dismiss an employee; or
  (b) a decision by an employer, based on reasonable grounds, not to award or provide a promotion, transfer, or benefit in connection with an employee's employment; or
  (c) reasonable administrative action taken in a reasonable manner by an employer in connection with an employee's employment; or
  (d) reasonable action taken in a reasonable manner under an Act affecting an employee.

This definition clearly shows the fundamental difference between what is considered bullying and other inappropriate behaviors and what the employers' fundamental legal rights are to manage their organization effectively.

In the United States, the General Duty Clause of the Occupational Health and Safety (OHS) Act, Section 5(a)(1), states "Each employer: shall furnish to each of his employees employment and a place of employment which are free from recognized hazards that are causing or are likely to cause death or serious physical harm to his employees" (OHS Act, 1970). This act requires employers to comply with OHS standards. Therefore, when there is a high risk of violence that is recognized as a serious hazard, then under Section 5(a)(1) of the OHS Act the employer is required to take steps to minimize the risks. If the employer fails to implement reasonable steps to address the hazard, such as violence in nursing, this failure could result in the finding of an OHS violation.

DISCUSSION POINT

Is legislation the best approach to addressing violence in nursing? How frequent and severe is violence in nursing?

Violence in the workplace is a serious safety and health issue (U.S. Department of Labor, Occupational Safety and Health Administration 2007). The reporting of workplace violence is not always nursing specific. For example, homicide is the fourth-leading cause of fatal occupational injury in the United States. According to the Bureau of Labor Statistics Census of Fatal Occupational Injuries (CFOI), there were 516 workplace homicides in 2006 in the United States, out of a total of 5,703 fatal work injuries (U.S. Department of

Labor, Bureau of Labor Statistics Census, 2007). In 2006, "the number of fatal injuries in professional and business services decreased 7 percent, and the rate of fatal injury was also lower. However, the number and rate of fatal injury in both educational and health services and in leisure and hospitality services were higher" (U.S. Department of Labor, Bureau of Labor Statistics Census 2007, p. 4).

Determining how many of these homicide cases involve nurses is difficult, but homicide in nursing, although rare, does occur. North America actually has a tragic history of nurses being killed. During the 1960s, eight student nurses were murdered in Canada, and many nurses have been murdered at work or coming to and from work. At times the perpetrator is known to the nurse, and other times they are strangers. For example, the perpetrator was known to and employed at the same hospital as the murdered Canadian registered nurse Lori Dupont (Health and Safety Professional, 2008; Registered Nurses Association Ontario, 2005; Schmidt, 2007).

In a homicide case in the United Kingdom, the perpetrator was unknown to the nurse. In this instance, "A 19-year-old man described by doctors as Britain's most dangerous teenager, was found guilty of stabbing a nurse to death in a frenzied attack as she took a cigarette break last year" (Australian Broadcasting Corporation, 2007).

Data collecting agencies such as the U.S. Department of Labor and SafeWork SA of Australia do have national and state statistics of reported cases. However, because of the data processing procedures and reporting delays, many of the statistics become available only when they are already 1 to 3 years out of date.

In South Australia, SafeWork SA is a state authority charged with investigating, addressing, and reporting unsafe practices in the workplace. Following the proclamation of Section 55A of the OHS Act of 1985 in August 2005, the data collected by SafeWork SA has shown that there have been 330 matters specifically referred to SafeWork SA in the 3-year period, from a state population of 1.2 million. Eight of these matters were referred to the Industrial Relations Commission of South Australia, and six of these eight cases have been addressed, with two remaining open. There are no data available to show how many of these 330 matters involved nurses or health care agencies (SafeWork SA, 2008).

There is no doubt that nurses are experiencing various forms of violence at work. Because there are no dedicated global reporting networks, however, it is difficult to accurately assess how many nurses experience violent behaviors at work (Hahn et al., 2008). The literature shows that much of the data collected on violence in nursing, such as gender of the perpetrator and targeted person, frequency, nature, and duration of the behavior, and the different types of tactics used, are from studies undertaken by nurses in specialized clinical areas (e.g., Fudge, 2006).

An Australian nursing study (Farrell, Bobrowski, & Bobrowski, 2006) reported that a majority of respondents (63%) had experienced some form of aggression (verbal or physical abuse) in the 4 working weeks immediately prior to the survey. In comparison, an Iranian study that explored the physical aspects of violence among nurses reported that "ninety-one percent of the participants said they had been exposed to workplace violence (physical, verbal, emotional, or sexual), three times or more in the last year" (AbuAl-Rub, Khalifa, & Bakir Habbib, 2007, p. 284). In the same study,

> Forty-nine of 116 (42.2%) participants said they had been physically attacked; seven of them (14.3%) with a lethal weapon . . . . The majority of physical incidents were by relatives of patients (n = 32; 65.3%). All physical incidents occurred inside the hospital (n = 49; 100%). Twenty-four of the 49 incidents occurred between 13.00 h and 18.00 h. (AbuAl-Rub et al., 2007, p. 284)

These are the types of data that assist managers to identify the need for appropriate requirements and resources to maintain safety at work.

What Types of Violence Do Nurses Experience?

Nurses experience different types of violence, often depending on the location, the service provided, and the perpetrator. Moreover, what one person considers to be harm may not be perceived as significant by another. Therefore, every nurse's experience is unique to that person. However, it is possible to categorize the different types of violence that nurses might experience. Box 12.1 lists seven basic categories specific to nursing. All of these types of violence have the potential to lead to physical, emotional, and financial harm.

BOX 12.1 — TYPOLOGY OF VIOLENCE IN NURSING

1. Nurse-to-nurse violence.
2. Patient-to-nurse violence.
3. Organization-to-nurse violence.
4. External perpetrators.
5. Third-party violence.
6. Impact of mass trauma or natural disasters on nurses.
7. Nurse-to-patient violence.

Source: Modified from Hockley (2006).

Nurse-to-Nurse Violence

Nurse-to-nurse violence occurs when the perpetrators and those they target work together in a vertical or horizontal workplace relationship. Box 12.2 lists some of the nonphysical antisocial workplace behaviors and tactics that can lead to personal harm. Although these are not limited to nurse-to-nurse violence, these behaviors are common in this violence category. These behaviors can, over a prolonged time, cause a person to develop low self-esteem, to feel worthless, or to feel frustrated. When an individual does decide to report these incidents, they are often difficult to prove unless there are

BOX 12.2 — EXAMPLES OF NONPHYSICAL VIOLENCE

1. Being uncivil, such as exhibiting rudeness, impoliteness, and silence.
2. Condoning improper behavior by being unsupportive and uncooperative.
3. Setting someone up for failure, imposing ideas, taking someone's ideas, undermining, embarrassing someone.
4. Exhibiting threatening behavior—making someone feel intimidated, threatened, or fearful.
5. Spreading rumors, making defamatory online statements.
6. Stalking.
7. Making anonymous communications.
8. Improperly taking credit.
9. Assigning blame or fault.

Source: Gale, Swain-Campbell, and Hannah (2008); RCNA (2007), Teaster and Teaster (2008).

witnesses, and even then, there is no guarantee of support from colleagues (Bailey & Jennings, 2008; Henderson, 2008; Rampersaud, 2008; Hockley, n.d.).

The nonphysical experiences just identified depend on context. For example, a customer being treated impolitely or ignored by a salesperson is considered different than a work colleague continually being treated impolitely or ignored at work. Furthermore, it is the nonphysical behavior and tactics that are often harder to prove because there are no accompanying physical signs (Hockley, n.d.). Often the nonphysical form of violence that nurses experience is characterized by a power disparity that can also occur from those lower on the hierarchy ladder than the targeted person. This behavior is at times referred to as mobbing when employees "gang up" on their manager or students on their professor. The degree of harm a nurse experiences often depends on the frequency, intensity, and duration of the behavior and/or tactic used (Hockley).

Patient-to-Nurse Violence

Patient-initiated violence originates mainly from patients, but at times it is their families or visitors who are the perpetrators, with nurses being the target of their hostility. Along a continuum from high-risk to potential low-risk areas in which patients or their family/visitors could be perpetrators are mental health facilities, locked dementia wards, remote regional facilities, and maternity and children's wards (RCNA, 2007, p. 9). The factors contributing to workplace violence, particularly in accident and emergency areas, include alcohol-related aggression and recreational drug misuse (RCNA, p. 9).

In general, the reporting from these settings shows that often a nurse is the victim of an attack simply because of being in the wrong place at that time. In other words, these attacks are not personal; the perpetrators are acting out their aggression, possibly because of stress, substance abuse, illness, or a feeling of vulnerability. Moreover, these attacks against nurses are generally one-time incidents, except in the cases of patients who are unstable (e.g., substance abuse), have a disability (e.g., brain injury), or have a long-term mental health problem (e.g., dementia).

This distinction about mental patients is often not made, is ignored, or is not reported. Hence the RCNA (2007) noted "Patients with mental health problems are often wrongly perceived to be responsible for an increased incidence of verbal abuse and aggression towards health care workers" (p. 9). Physical violence requires proximity and therefore is more likely to occur in

BOX 12.3 — EXAMPLES OF PHYSICAL VIOLENCE

1. Hitting.
2. Spitting.
3. Punching.
4. Pinching.
5. Kicking.
6. Sexual assault.
7. Rape.
8. Murder.

Source: Gale, Swain-Campbell, and Hannah (2008), RCNA (2007), Teaster and Teaster (2008).

patient-to-nurse violence or by external perpetrators than other forms of situations that a nurse might experience (see Box 12.3).

CONSIDER

The effect of antisocial workplace behaviors on a person depends on that person. Not everyone is personally or professionally harmed by these behaviors or incidents.

When patients or their families target nurses, they generally use different behaviors or tactics compared to, for example, when nurses target each other. How these aggressive behaviors are perceived and managed often depends on the context. Training programs frequently focus on the warning signs of aggression and how to manage them effectively (e.g., Nau, Dassen, Halfens, & Needham, 2008; U.S. Department of Labor, 2008).

Moreover, how a person responds to various intimidating and threatening behaviors, and whether they are personally or professionally harmed, will vary from person to person. Some nurses, despite the fact that some of these incidents can be traumatic, even aberrant in nature, believe that this is a "part of the job" (RCNA, 2007, p. 6) and putting up with it shows their degree of personal dedication and professional commitment.

Organization-to-Nurse Violence

In the recent past, the emphasis on organizational violence mainly referred to the harm that might occur to nursing staff when an organization is experiencing economic pressures resulting in restructuring, redundancy, redeployment, or resignations. However, contemporary literature shows that organizational issues that contribute to nurses feeling stressed relate to changing work environments (RCNA, 2007), such as keeping up to date with current clinical requirements and technological knowledge, insufficient staff numbers to improve nurse-to-patient ratios, and the need to create safer workplaces (Ontario Nurses Association, 2006). Consequently, a series of incidents involving violence in nursing is both an indicator of an organization in crisis and a stressed nursing workforce.

One of the characteristics of this form of violence is that it affects the whole organization—and not only the targeted person, but also the perpetrator. When violence occurs, the organization's reputation is often tarnished, with low staff morale, increased absenteeism, reduced efficiency, and spiraling recruiting, legal, and organizational costs. There is also the possibility of retaliatory violence by staff via strikes, picket lines, deliberate damage such as arson, computer hacking, and, in the worst cases, random killings.

On occasion, health care facilities that experience this type of violence may be "named" on the Internet, sometimes through various nursing chat groups or by a "whistleblower." A health care facility that receives bad publicity will find it difficult to attract qualified staff and may, in fact, attract the "wrong" type of staff to meet nursing staffing needs. This increases the potential for aggrieved staff members to take future legal action against the employer for negligent hiring.

External Perpetrators

The violence that is perpetrated by outsiders entering the workplace with criminal intent includes armed robbery for drugs or gang reprisals in emergency departments as examples. This form of violence also includes incidents that occur while a nurse is going to or returning from work. In these incidents, the assailant may not have any personal or workplace relationship. This form of violence is often random and can include rape, robbery, attempted homicide, or homicide (Australian Broadcasting Corporation, 2007).

Third-Party Violence

Until recently, legislation and research into violence in nursing mainly recognized two parties: perpetrator and victim. However, it is now recognized that there is a third party: the witnesses to these behaviors and incidents who may be affected. A definition of third-party violence is that it "is the outcome of workplace violence and can include those who directly or indirectly witness the event(s) such as those with a professional relationship (e.g., colleagues), personal relationship (e.g., family members and significant others) and indirect relationship (e.g., case managers)" (modified from Hockley, 2006).

When a nurse targets another nurse in the workplace, others may witness this behavior. Nurses, as witnesses, can support the perpetrator's actions, ignore these actions, or become third-party victims of the behavior. However, other third parties—those with a personal or indirect relationship—are also drawn into these incidents.

There is the potential for third-party witnesses to experience similar emotions and feelings of being harmed in some way to those of the primary target. Some nurses, for example, may be reluctant to be seen speaking with a nurse who has been targeted because of the fear of becoming the next target, that is, the fear of guilt by association. Nearly all of the reports on third-party violence showed that this form of workplace violence systematically undermined the individual; therefore, the perpetrator was inflicting damage not only on the primary target, but also on secondary targets—the third person (Hockley, n.d.).

In addition, there is the potential for another manifestation of third-party violence in nursing: the family member who cares about the person who is the primary target. There is the potential for family members and significant others to experience the same symptoms, as third-party victims of domestic violence. There is a high probability that the longer the person who has been targeted is being harmed by these workplace behaviors, the more probable it is that third-party relationships with that person will also experience poor health and changes in financial status and socialization.

CONSIDER
The effects of violence in nursing extend far beyond the workplace.

Effect of Mass Trauma or Natural Disasters on Nurses

This type of violence focuses on the nurse's experience in times of extreme emergency, such as biochemical assaults, terrorist attacks, attacks on civil society, or violence related to armed conflict or other major disasters. This form of violence may occur once (e.g., a terrorist attack; schoolyard or workplace massacres) or at special events (e.g., the final games of a sports season). Natural disasters such as the tsunami the day after Christmas 2005 or Hurricane Katrina in 2006 can have a huge effect on the nurses involved that lasts for many years after the event. Many trauma-related issues are emerging, in part because of the changing trends in the different types of violence that are occurring and being experienced in society. There is a scarcity of nursing research on the effect on nurses managing large numbers of trauma cases caused by exceptionally violent acts.

Little is known about the effect of this type of violence on nurses. What can be assumed from studies of workers traumatized by events—for example, service personnel in Vietnam, Afghanistan, and Iraq; firefighters and police officers in New York, Washington, D.C., and Pennsylvania following the September 11, 2001, attacks; rescue workers after the Bali bombing on October 11, 2002, the train bombing in Madrid in 2004, and the London underground bombings in 2005, to name a few—is the potential for serious health and mental health issues to arise, such as posttraumatic stress disorder (PTSD).

For many years the International Council of Nurses has recognized "the need for information resources to assist in coping with the aftermath of these attacks and the climate of fear and uncertainty they have created" (ICN, 2002, p.1). However, until further research is undertaken, the strategies used to address this type of violence must be taken from other contexts. That is not to say that they are not appropriate, but many of the strategies are from predominantly male-oriented occupations, such as law enforcement. With nursing being a predominantly female occupation, the health and mental health issues might be different from those in male-oriented occupations.

Clearly, nursing work associated with violent situations can be very stressful. What is missing from scholarly writing are the voices of nurses working in highly volatile areas of practice and the traumatizing effects this might have on them following mass trauma or natural disasters. The lack of acknowledgment of nurses working in extremely violent and traumatizing situations in the long term is apparent in the literature.

Nurse-to-Patient Violence

This form of violence occurs when nurses are violent toward those in their professional care. Although there have been studies on the various forms of violence toward nurses, there has been little research into the causes and effects of nurse-initiated violence toward patients.

Earlier work by Hockley (2005) reported extreme cases of nurse-to-patient violence—in particular, nurses who murdered their patients. A recent study by Field (2007, p. 2) reported

> The opportunities for nurses to murder a patient or patients would be largely constrained by the proximity of other staff. However, the cases that do exist clearly demonstrate that this is not always so. Where a patient (or a number of patients) is murdered by a nurse, the nursing staff working in the ward or unit typically find themselves sharply criticized for not having identified the problem before the patient was killed.

Violence by nurses against people in their care goes against the professional code of ethics, and it is important to identify the issues that cause nurses to act in this way. Over the last decade there has been a significant increase in the reporting of nurses transgressing professional boundaries. This is, in part, a response to professional bodies such as the Honor Society of Nursing, Sigma Theta Tau International (STTI), drawing attention to unprofessional behavior.

CONSIDER
Further work needs to be done to develop an instrument that can accurately predict which nurses are at risk of causing harm to those in their care.

What Can Be Done to Stop Workplace Violence?

There are a variety of organizational, legal, and ethical strategies that can be used to address violence in nursing.

Organizational Approach
An organization may address violence in nursing through policies and procedures, education, and training, as well as by having an organizational culture that does not condone this behavior. For example, there are many educational programs that have been developed

to address different aspects of violence in nursing (e.g., Benson, Allen, Miller, Rogers, & Paterson, 2008; Kritek, Zager, & Manning, 2008; McIntosh, 2008b).

In addition, the counseling services that are offered to nursing staff often depend on who the perpetrators are and their behaviors, as well as on the tactics that are used. Although many of these services are provided with the best of intentions, staff offered these services, particularly if they relate to nurse-to-nurse violence, are wary and concerned that the information will "get back to the workplace" (Hockley, n.d.). When counseling is not successful, some complaints can be addressed through conciliation. If the perpetrator is a nurse, he or she may be referred to an appropriate statutory organization for disciplinary action, as discussed later.

Legislative Approach
OHS Legislation
Many countries have national occupational health and safety (OHS) statutory bodies, including the United States, Canada, and the United Kingdom. Australia does not have a national approach to OHS, but each Australian state and territory has its individual OHS legislation. Nevertheless, whether an international, national, or individual state/territory approach is used, the OHS legislations have as a common goal to mandate that employers provide employees with a safe working environment. There is an expectation that when a person enters the workplace, he or she will be safe and free from harm. That is, the employer has a duty of care to its employees.

In most jurisdictions, there will be similar legislation to deal with sexual harassment and racism based on equal opportunity (EO) principles. EO legislation, in the main, has been well established for many years and therefore it could be argued that an employee might have better success with a complaint under the equivalent EO act than if he or she chose to follow the organization's grievance procedure for violent behavior situations.

The legal protection of employees through these statutory bodies has been created with a range of roles, including enforcement of their various acts and education and training relating to the various provisions. If any of these provisions are breached, legal action may be taken.

Nurses Act

Each country (or state in the United States) has an equivalent document to a Nurses Act that gives legislative power to a nurse registration board—for example, the California Nurses Practice Act. A typical board's role is to endorse professional standards and ensure that the highest standards are achieved and maintained. Disciplinary action can range from requiring mediation and education to address the problem (e.g., managing aggressiveness) to requiring registration restrictions; in very severe cases, a nurse may be deregistered.

In Australia, each state's Nurses Board has a self-regulatory system that gives it the power to set standards, and if these standards are breached, it has the power to discipline its members and if necessary to report breaches of a criminal nature. These powers are delegated through legislation—for example, the South Australia Nurses Act of 1999. Under this act, all employers have an obligation to report unprofessional conduct to the Board. Failure for an employer to comply with this obligation may incur a maximum penalty (Nurses Act, 1999, Section 45). In addition, members of the public, nurses, or any other professional group can make complaints about unprofessional conduct or nurses, which the Board must investigate. In follow-up, the Nurses Board of South Australia (NBSA) must provide annual reports to the Minister of Health regarding complaints received and action taken (Nurses Act, 1999, Section 15).

The growing interest in the area of violence in nursing has given rise to various interpretations of what these behaviors involve. For example, the South Australia Nurses Act states that unprofessional conduct includes improper and unethical conduct in relation to nursing, incompetence or negligence, and contravening or failing to comply with the provision of the Act, the code of conduct or professional standard, as well as to their registration (Nurses Act, 1999, Section 45).

Generally the legislation does not specifically illustrate the range of behavior that constitutes unprofessional behaviors, and therefore many professional bodies have provided fact sheets and brochures educating their members and patients about what could constitute such behavior. For example, the NBSA Standard Therapeutic Relationships and Professional Boundaries fact sheet defines sexual misconduct as applying "to the full range of behaviors, actions and attitudes from a naive understanding of the therapeutic relationship to predatory behaviour" (NBSA, 2003, p. 6).

When, for example, the NBSA completes an investigation and there is sufficient evidence on the balance of probabilities to prove a complaint of unprofessional conduct, "the investigation file is forwarded to the Crown Solicitor's Office requesting that a legal document known as a 'Complaint' be drafted in order for the matter to be formally heard by a panel of the Board" (NBSA, 2008a, p. 7). Alternatively, the NBSA's representative, the Registrar, "may elect to obtain advice from the Crown Solicitor's Office to determine whether the evidence is sufficient to proceed" (NBSA, 2008b, p. 10). There are other options the Board might follow. For example, the Board is empowered to take notice and adopt any decisions or judgments from any other jurisdiction that might be appropriate to the relevant proceedings.

How prevalent unprofessional conduct is among the nursing profession is identified in annual reports. The 2006 to 2007 NBSA *Annual Report* showed that the Board received 173 new complaints, of which there were 124 complaints relating to unprofessional conduct under Section 22 of the Nurses Act of 1999. The types of unprofessional conduct were not specifically broken down into categories, so it is not possible to determine which complaints were of a violent nature or led to criminal or civil action being taken. However, the state can begin prosecution if it considers that the breach is criminal.

Tribunal Case Studies

In Australia, a variety of serious professional misconduct cases can be referred to an appropriate tribunal. For example, in Western Australia (WA), a nurse was refused renewal of her practicing certificate by the WA Nurses Board because she failed to disclose that she was on parole from a prison sentence. She appealed to the Administrative Appeals Tribunal for a review of the Board's decision, and the Tribunal affirmed the refusal to renew her license on the grounds that the conviction undermined her claim to be of good character and integrity, which was essential in her profession (Chan and the Nurses Board of Western Australia WASAT 115, 2005).

In this case, the tribunal played a major role in the disciplinary process. However, in Australia, tribunals do not have the same power as constituted judicial bodies, and therefore their processes and decisions are not binding on the parties concerned. In other words, one ignores it at one's peril, but the determination is not as binding as if the case had been heard before a judicial court.

Case Law

A review of cases identifies the emergence of two separate role standards against which nurses can be judged. First, there is their practice role, and second, there is their professional responsibility role. In personal and professional transgressions, a nurse's public and professional reputation may suffer. In a personal transgression, for example, an off-duty nurse might commit a serious physical assault at a party, which is a crime. The nurse's professional competence is not in question, but his or her nonpractice behavior has importance against which his or her overall practice can be judged. This may affect the nurse's future professional standing and licensing.

On the other hand, a nurse might seriously assault a patient at work. In this situation the nurse's professional competence is in question.

If the nurse's behavior is considered of such a serious nature that the state uses its power to punish or deter that behavior, then a criminal action might arise. The range of criminal behaviors in which a nurse might be involved either as a perpetrator or a victim covers areas such as sexual offences, serious assault, murder, rape, and so on.

A nurse could have a civil case against the perpetrator for assault if he or she was threatened or physically attacked and fears for his or her life. The perpetrator could be a patient, a colleague, or a person unknown to the nurse. Often a civil case may be brought against a person when a criminal charge has been unsuccessful or the nurse is suing for damages. The O. J. Simpson case demonstrated this.

A nurse who has experienced any of the various forms of violence at work could take the organization to court for negligent hiring if it can be proved that the perpetrator has a prior history of workplace violence. A civil action might also be taken when, for example, the patient seeks redress or compensation for wrongs committed by a nurse, such as in malpractice cases or a serious breach of professional boundaries.

The legal protection of those targeted in the workplace is primarily based on their rights to sue somebody for damages. Unfortunately, studies show that the chances of being successful in a court of law are minimal. With legal fees being high and compensation low and the length of time it takes for a case to come to court, nurses who have decided to take this route often change their minds and prefer to settle out of court (Gregersen, 2008; Hockley, n.d.).

CONSIDER

The use of legal services is often the best approach to addressing violence in nursing.

WHAT IS BEING DONE TO ADDRESS VIOLENCE IN NURSING?

Global Approaches

One of the earliest and most significant international studies on workplace violence was the International Labour Office (ILO), International Council of Nurses (ICN), World Health Organization (WHO), and Public Services International (PSI) (2002) paper entitled "Framework Guidelines for Addressing Workplace Violence in the Health Sector: Joint Program on Workplace Violence in the Health Sector."

Another highly successful international joint project was the sponsoring of the Inaugural International Workplace Violence in Health Care Conference held in Amsterdam in 2008. The sponsoring organizations were the Honor Society of Nursing, Sigma Theta Tau International; the Dundalk Institute of Technology; Oud Consultancy; the Connecting Partnership for Consult and Training; Public Service International; the International Labour Organization; the International Hospital Federation; and the International Council of Nurses. The focus of the conference was violence against health care workers. The aims of the conference included sensitizing stakeholders to the issue of workplace violence, to understand the manifestations and the human, professional, and economic implications of workplace violence, and to promote effective policies and strategies to create safe work environments.

In addition, different countries undertook or are undertaking various ongoing reviews to establish the extent, nature, and effect of violence in the workplace. In the United States, for example, one of the research goals to be accomplished by 2010 for the National Occupational Research Agenda (NORA) for Occupational Safety and Health Research and Practice is to identify effective strategies and develop programs that support emergency medical system personnel who witness critical incidents (e.g., traumatic accidents, on-the-job death of co-workers) (National Occupational Research Agenda [NORA] for Occupational Safety and Health Research and Practice, Goal 15.5.2, 2008).

The American Nurses Association (ANA), among its many goals, aims to reduce violence in nursing through health care reform and public policy, such as distributing a model Workplace Prevention Bill for all relevant member associations to use as a format when seeking legislative approaches to reduce violence and require employers to implement prevention programs (ANA, 2007). The assessment tool that has been developed by the ANA aids in the systematic collection of data so as to better understand and address workplace violence, such as reducing workplace abuse and harassment through legislative efforts (ANA).

In Australia, the RCNA (2007) issued a paper entitled "National Overview of Violence in the Workplace." The aim of this paper was to explore the issues affecting Australian nurses in the workforce (RCNA, p. 5). Similarly, the United Kingdom's Health and Safety Executive Commission (HSE) strategic plan entitled "A Strategy for Workplace Health and Safety in Great Britain to 2010 and Beyond" was designed to achieve a record of workplace health and safety that would lead the world (HSE, 2008).

Individual Research

In the last 5 years there has been a rapid growth in research into violence in the workplace generally and into nursing workplaces specifically. A review of the literature shows that research into workplace violence is branching out into a variety of themes, including online forums with participants discussing their experiences of workplace violence (Frankish, 2008), forensic nursing (Markowitz & Chasson, 2008), the development of staff training and education modules (Candela & Bowles, 2008), and the auditing of training programs (Benson et al., 2008). Other areas being studied include exploring the legal and ethical aspects of workplace violence (Constantino, 2008; Gregersen, 2008); gaining insight into breaching professional boundaries (McIntosh, 2008a); examining the legal and ethical implications of workplace violence and bullying in the aged-care sector (Timo, Carter, & Anderson, 2008); and studying the professional services used by primary target and third-party witnesses of workplace violence (Hockley, n.d.). Evaluative studies such as those of the experience of violence and the perception of risk of lone working community nurses in the United Kingdom following the RCN campaign to protect lone workers (Sunley, 2008) have also gained attention in the literature. (See Research Study Fuels the Controversy on page 208.)

CONCLUSIONS

There has been a growing interest in violence in nursing as researchers interested in the health care sector have become increasingly aware that this phenomenon is not only an individual or organizational problem but is also a public health and human rights issue. Although there have been many changes made to minimize this unconscionable behavior in the health care culture and environment, there is still some way to go. The outcome of the studies undertaken has highlighted the need for more research and understanding of the causes and conditions that generate violence in nursing.

An important area that appears to be missing in the literature is the perpetrator's perspective of workplace violence in the health sector. In other words, why do nurses act inappropriately in the workplace? How can nurses become self-aware of their inappropriate behavior? What causes nurses to act in this way? What can be done to prevent this behavior?

One approach is to move the focus away from the individual and to consider that most people who bully have wide organizational support or tacit approval. Without that support, these people would not be tolerated as long as they are. Therefore it is important to examine why this behavior is tolerated and what strategies should be implemented to counter organizational support.

Research Study Fuels the Controversy: How Do Nurses and Their Families Survive?

This project was a part of a series of studies to establish the extent, nature, and effect of the various forms of inappropriate behavior in the workplace on primary targets and third-party victims. An exploratory study was undertaken into the methods that victims and family members use to survive the effect of workplace violence and associated inappropriate behaviors such as bullying and mobbing. This study focused on how people select support strategies during this stressful period in their lives. The emphasis was on success stories, especially the strengths of those who are, or have been, affected by workplace violence. However, it was important for participants to tell their story, including the "ups and downs" of seeking support.

STUDY FINDINGS

The first of this series, commencing in the early 1990s, identified that nurses targeted at work mainly relied on themselves during this stressful period in their lives, in part because people with whom they discussed their experience either did not believe them or did not understand what they were experiencing. From the targeted person's perspective, family members were generally unsupportive.

Later studies in this series found that although organizations offered counseling services for critical incidents in the workplace, they rarely offered counseling services when a nurse was being bullied at work. The organizational option was instead to offer aggression management training or leadership courses to the perpetrator. Nearly a decade on, an interim report in this study continues to show the lack of organizational support in cases of nurse-to-nurse violence, although there has been some improvement in this area.

The current phase of this study is examining whether, in spite of the fact that there has been an increase in the awareness of violence in nursing, there is a change in the services that targeted nurses and their families use, and if there is, what they are and how helpful they have been.

Source: Hockley, C. (n.d.). *An exploratory study into the methods victims and family members use to survive the impact of workplace violence and associated inappropriate behaviors such as bullying and mobbing.* Unpublished.

FOR ADDITIONAL DISCUSSION

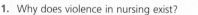

1. Why does violence in nursing exist?
2. How important is the language used to address violence in nursing?
3. What are the advantages and disadvantages of having general definitions of violence included in legislation?
4. Is it possible to experience violence in nursing without being professionally or personally harmed?
5. Are education and training programs the most cost-effective approach to addressing violence in nursing?
6. How can legislation or organizations assist third-party witnesses, such as family members, when they are harmed by the outcome of violence in nursing?
7. What role do professional nursing organizations play in addressing violence in nursing?
8. Should nurses take civil action against patients that attack them?
9. Is it paradoxical that those whose responsibility it is to provide care and promote an environment in which the human rights, values, customs, and spiritual beliefs of those in their care are respected should commit heinous crimes against those individuals?
10. Is zero tolerance of violence in nursing achievable?

REFERENCES

AbuAlRub, R. F., Khalifa, M. F., & Bakir Habbib, M. (2007). Workplace violence among Iraqi hospital nurses. *Journal of Nursing Scholarship, 39*(3), 281–288.

American Nurses Association (ANA) (2007). *ANA 2007 annual report.* Available at: http://www.nursing world.org/FunctionalMenuCategories/AboutANA. aspx. Accessed July 4, 2008.

Australian Broadcasting Corporation (2007). UK's 'most dangerous teen' murdered nurse. Available at: http://www.abc.net.au/news/stories/2007/06/29/1965238.htm. Accessed July 4, 2008.

Bailey, K. E., & Jennings, M. W. (2008). *The development of crises negotiation to forensic mental health—Staff training and policies to deal with extreme violence in the workplace.* Presented at the International Conference on Workplace Violence in the Health Sector, Together, Creating a Safe Work Environment, 22–24 October, Amsterdam, The Netherlands.

Benson, R., Allen, J., Miller, G., Rogers, P., & Paterson, B. (2008). *Motor skills learning in breakaway training using the evidence base of sports science.* Presented at the International Conference on Workplace Violence in the Health Sector, Together, Creating a Safe Work Environment, 22–24 October, Amsterdam, The Netherlands.

Candela, L., & Bowles, C. (2008). *Developing learning modules to address interpersonal violence among nurses.* Presented at the International Conference on Workplace Violence in the Health Sector, Together, Creating a Safe Work Environment, 22–24 October, Amsterdam, The Netherlands.

Celik, S. P., & Celik, Y. (2008). *Positive working environment: Violence against nurses in Turkey.* Presented at the International Conference on Workplace Violence in the Health Sector, Together, Creating a Safe Work Environment, 22–24 October, Amsterdam, The Netherlands.

Chan and the Nurses Board of Western Australia WASAT 115 (2005). Available at: http://decisions. justice.wa.gov.au/SAT/SATdcsn.nsf. Accessed January 19, 2009.

Constantino, R. (2008). *Ethical, legal and sociocultural issues (ELSI). Principles for the employer in workplace violence.* Presented at the International Conference on Workplace Violence in the Health Sector, Together, Creating a Safe Work Environment, 22–24 October, Amsterdam, The Netherlands.

Farrell, G. A., Bobrowski, C., & Bobrowski, P. (2006). Scoping workplace aggression in nursing: Findings from an Australian study. *Journal of Advanced Nursing, 55*(6), 778–787.

Ferns, T., & Meerabeau, L. (2008). *The reporting behaviors of student nurses who have experienced verbal abuse.* Presented at the International Conference on Workplace Violence in the Health Sector, Together, Creating a Safe Work Environment, 22–24 October, Amsterdam, The Netherlands.

Field, J. G. (2007). *Caring to death: A discursive analysis of nurses who murder patients.* Ph.D. Thesis. School of Population Health and Clinical Practice: Nursing, University of Adelaide, South Australia.

Frankish, J. (2008). *Nurses and workplace violence: Online information exchange for nurses to report on, reflect on, and act on aggressive behavior in the workplace.* Presented at the International Conference on Workplace Violence in the Health Sector, Together, Creating a Safe Work Environment, 22–24 October, Amsterdam, The Netherlands.

Fudge, L. (2006). Why, when we are deemed to be careers, are we so mean to our colleagues? Horizontal and vertical violence in the workplace. *Canadian Operating Room Nurse, 24*(4), 13–16.

Gale, C., Swain-Campbell, N., & Hannah, A. (2008). *A modification of the perception of patient aggression scale: Does this measure one factor, and what does it mean?* Presented at the International Conference on Workplace Violence in the Health Sector, Together, Creating a Safe Work Environment, 22–24 October, Amsterdam, The Netherlands.

Gregersen, J. (2008). *What is workplace bullying supposed to be? A case study based on court judgements.* Presented at the International Conference on Workplace Violence in the Health Sector, Together, Creating a Safe Work Environment, 22–24 October, Amsterdam, The Netherlands.

Hahn, S., Needham, I., Hantikainen, V., Muller, M., Kok, G., Dassen, T., & Halfens, R. (2008). *Violence against health care staff in general hospitals: An underestimated problem?* Presented at the International

Conference on Workplace Violence in the Health Sector, Together, Creating a Safe Work Environment, 22–24 October, Amsterdam, The Netherlands.

Harding, T. (2008). *Why don't you just leave? Horizontal violence and the experience of men who are nurses.* Presented at the International Conference on Workplace Violence in the Health Sector, Together, Creating a Safe Work Environment, 22–24 October, Amsterdam, The Netherlands.

Health and Safety Professional (2008). *Workplace violence. How will you recognize it?* Available at: http://www.hspinc.ca/images/UserUploaded/Newsletters/Issue%2016%Spring%20Summer%202009. pdf. Accessed July 4, 2008.

Health and Safety Executive Commission (HSE) (2008). *A strategy for workplace health and safety in Great Britain to 2010 and beyond.* Available at: http://www.hse.gov.uk/consult/condocs/strategycd.pdf. Accessed July 4, 2008.

Henderson, A. (2008). *Nurses and workplace violence: Towards an effective intervention.* Presented at the International Conference on Workplace Violence in the Health Sector, Together, Creating a Safe Work Environment, 22–24 October, Amsterdam, The Netherlands.

Hockley, C. (2005). Staff violence against those in their care (pp. 77–96). In: V. Bowie, B. S. Fisher, & C. L. Cooper (Eds.), *Workplace Violence. Issues, Trends and Strategies.* Cullompton, Devon, U.K.: Willan.

Hockley, C. (2006). Violence in nursing: The expectations and the reality (pp. 226–247). In: C. Huston (Ed.), *Professional Issues in Nursing: Challenges and Opportunities.* Philadelphia: Lippincott Williams & Wilkins. Philadelphia.

Hockley, C. (n.d.). *An exploratory study into the methods victims and family members use to survive the impact of workplace violence and associated inappropriate behaviors such as bullying and mobbing.* Unpublished.

Hodson, R. (2008). The ethnographic contribution to understanding co-worker relations. *British Journal of Industrial Relations, 46*(1), 169–192.

Hurley, J. E. (2006). Nurse-to-nurse horizontal violence: Recognizing and preventing it. *Imprint, 53*(4), 68–71.

International Council of Nurses (ICN) (2002). *Terrorism and bioterrorism: Nursing preparedness.* Available at: http://www.icn.ch/matters_bio.htm. Accessed January 19, 2009.

International Council of Nurses (ICN) (2008). *Workplace bullying in the health sector.* Available at: http://www.icn.ch/matters_bullying.htm. Accessed January 19, 2008.

International Labour Office (ILO), International Council of Nurses (ICN), World Health Organization (WHO), & Public Services International (PSI) (2002). *Framework guidelines for addressing workplace violence in the health sector. Joint program on workplace violence in the health sector.* Available at: http://www.who.int/violence_injury_prevention/violence/interpersonal/en/WVguidelinesEN.pdf. Accessed January 19, 2009.

Jones, D. (2008). *The incidence of violence and aggression in a high security psychiatric hospital: A one year study examining the types and frequency of aggression and violence exhibited by high security psychiatric patients.* Presented at the International Conference on Workplace Violence in the Health Sector, Together, Creating a Safe Work Environment, 22–24 October, Amsterdam, The Netherlands.

Jones, J., Callaghan, P., Eales, S., & Ashman, N. (2008). *Violence and aggression in haemodialysis units in general hospitals.* Presented at the International Conference on Workplace Violence in the Health Sector, Together, Creating a Safe Work Environment, 22–24 October, Amsterdam, The Netherlands.

Kritek, P., Zager, L., & Manning, L. (2008). *A workplace violence training program that works.* Presented at the International Conference on Workplace Violence in the Health Sector, Together, Creating a Safe Work Environment, 22–24 October, Amsterdam, The Netherlands.

Lewis, M. A. (2006). Nurse bullying: Organizational considerations in the maintenance and perpetration of health care bullying cultures. *Journal of Nursing Management, 14*(1), 52–58.

Mak, Y. L. E., Chung, K. L., Chan, W. L., & Cheung, C. Y. (2008). *Creating a safe working environment in emergency department of Tuen Mun Hospital in Hong Kong.* Presented at the International Conference on Workplace Violence in the Health Sector, Together, Creating a Safe Work Environment, 22–24 October, Amsterdam, The Netherlands.

Markowitz, J., & Chasson, S. (2008). *Responding to workplace sexual violence: Utilizing forensic nurses and other victim service professionals.* Presented at the International Conference on Workplace Violence in the Health Sector, Together, Creating a Safe Work Environment, 22–24 October, Amsterdam, The Netherlands.

Motamedi, B. (2008). *Violence in the workplace, the experience of nurses in Isfahan, Iran.* Presented at the International Conference on Workplace Violence in the Health Sector, Together, Creating a Safe Work Environment, 22–24 October, Amsterdam, The Netherlands.

McIntosh, W. (2008a). *The relationship between workplace violence and professional boundaries—Exploring the impact on client care.* Presented at the International Conference on Workplace Violence in the Health Sector, Together, Creating a Safe Work Environment, 22–24 October, Amsterdam, The Netherlands.

McIntosh, W. (2008b). *Workplace bullying is the solution, so what is the problem?* Presented at the International Conference on Workplace Violence in the Health Sector, Together, Creating a Safe Work Environment, 22–24 October, Amsterdam, The Netherlands.

McLaughlin, S., & Wellman, N. (2008). Verbal aggression—What is the impact on student nurses? Presented at the International Conference on Workplace Violence in the Health Sector, Together, Creating a Safe Work Environment, 22–24 October, Amsterdam, The Netherlands.

McNally, M. J. (2008). *An urban acute care hospital's response to workplace violence.* Presented at the International Conference on Workplace Violence in the Health Sector, Together, Creating a Safe Work Environment, 22–24 October, Amsterdam, The Netherlands.

National Institute for Occupational Health and Safety (2002). *Violence occupational hazards in hospitals* [DHHS (NIOSH) Publication No. 2002-101]. Available at: http://www.cdc.gov/niosh/2002-101.html. Accessed July 4, 2008.

National Occupational Research Agenda (NORA) (3/21/08). Draft Preliminary Public Comment Version. National Public Safety Sub-Sector Agenda for Occupational Safety and Health Research and Practice in the U.S. Research Goal 15.2.2 (2008). Available at: http://74.125.95.132/search?q=cache:93G6qGHs4fEJ:www.cdc.gov/niosh/nora/comment/public/pubsafsubdraftmar2008/pdfs/PubSafSubDraft-Mar2008.pdf_3/21/08_draft_preliminary_public+comment_version&hl_en&ct_clnk&cd_6&gl_us. Accessed January 19, 2009.

Nau, J., Dassen, T., Halfens, R., & Needham, I. (2008). *Nursing students' experiences in managing patient aggression.* Presented at the International Conference on Workplace Violence in the Health Sector, Together, Creating a Safe Work Environment, 22–24 October, Amsterdam, The Netherlands.

Nurses Act (1999). South Australian Consolidated Acts. Available at: http://www.austlii.edu.au/au/legis/sa/consol_act/na1999111/. Accessed January 19, 2009.

Nurses Board of South Australia (2003). *Therapeutic relationships and professional boundaries.* Available at: http://www.nursesboard.sa.gov.au/pdf/Standards_Ther_Rel_Prof_Boundaries.pdf. Accessed January 19, 2009.

Nurses Board of South Australia (2006–2007). *Nurses Board of South Australia Annual Report 2006–2007.* Available at: http://www.nursesboard.sa.gov.au/documents/Annual_Report_2006-07.pdf. Accessed July 27, 2008.

Nurses Board of South Australia (2008a). *Nursing and midwifery. NBSA Bulletin 25,* April 2008. Available at: http://www.nursesboard.sa.gov.au/documents/Bulletin_25.pdf. Accessed July 27, 2008.

Nurses Board of South Australia (2008b). *Nursing and midwifery. NBSA Bulletin 26,* July 2008. Available at: http://www.nursesboard.sa.gov.au/documents/Bulletin_26.pdf. Accessed January 19, 2009.

Occupational Health, Safety and Welfare Act (1986). South Australian Consolidated Acts. Available at: http://www.austlii.edu.au/au/legis/sa/consol_act/ohsawa1986336/. Accessed January 19, 2009.

Occupational Health and Safety Act (1970). Available at: http://www.osha.gov/pls/oshaweb/owadisp.show_document?p_table=OSHACT&p_id=2743. Accessed January 19, 2009.

Ontario Nurses Association (2006). ONA spotlights safety gaps in health-care facilities. Available at: http://www.ona.org/search/node/safety+gaps. Accessed July 4, 2008.

Paliadelis, P., Cruickshank, M., & Sheridan, A. (2007). Caring for each other: How do nurse managers 'manage' their role? *Journal of Nursing Management, 15*(8), 830–837.

Rampersaud, P. (2008). *New emergency nurse description of transitioning to an experienced emergency nurse: The impact of workplace factors.* Presented at the International Conference on Workplace Violence in the Health Sector, Together, Creating a Safe Work

Environment, 22–24 October, Amsterdam, The Netherlands.

Registered Nurses Association Ontario (2005). *Inquest probing death of Ontario nurse slain in hospital makes 26 recommendations.* Available at: www.longwoods.com/view.php?aid+19440. Accessed July 4, 2008.

Roberts, S. (1983). Oppressed group behavior: Implications for nursing. *Advances in Nursing Science, 5*(4), 21–30.

Royal College of Nursing, Australia (RCNA) (2007). *National overview of violence in the workplace* (Issues Paper, March). ACT, Australia: Author.

SafeWork SA (2008). Appendix 1. Review of Section 55A. Inappropriate behaviour towards an employee. Terms of Reference, Review Process and Issues Paper. In: *Final Report on the Review of Section 55A. Inappropriate behavior towards an employee. Occupational Health, Safety and Welfare Act 1986 (SA).* Available at: http://www.safework.sa.gov.au/uploaded_files/FINAL_Report_Review_Section_55A_(September%202008).pdf. Accessed January 19, 2009.

Schmidt, D. (2007). Dupont jury returns with 26 recommendations. *The Windsor Star,* Tuesday, December 11. Available at: http://www.canada.com/windsorstar/story.html?id=5d433e6e-15ca-4baa-8ce7-081757cbc8e5. Accessed July 4, 2008.

Strandmark, M. K., & Hallberg, L. M.-R. (2007). The origin of workplace bullying: Experiences from the perspective of bully victims in the public service sector. *Journal of Nursing Management, 15*(3), 332–341.

Sunley, K. (2008). *You're not alone—The Royal College of Nursing's campaign to protect lone workers.* Presented at the International Conference on Workplace Violence in the Health Sector, Together, Creating a Safe Work Environment, 22–24 October, Amsterdam, The Netherlands.

Taylor, L. (2008). *UK Nurses' perceptions of violence: A case study within an accident and emergency department.* Presented at the International Conference on

Workplace Violence in the Health Sector, Together, Creating a Safe Work Environment, 22–24 October, Amsterdam, The Netherlands.

Teaster, L.O'D., & Teaster, S. (2008). *Prevention and early intervention of violence at work.* Presented at the International Conference on Workplace Violence in the Health Sector, Together, Creating a Safe Work Environment, 22–24 October, Amsterdam, The Netherlands.

Timo, N., Carter, G., & Anderson, A. (2008). *Legal and ethical implications of workplace bullying and violence: Evidence from the Australian aged care industry.* Presented at the International Conference on Workplace Violence in the Health Sector, Together, Creating a Safe Work Environment, 22-24 October, Amsterdam, The Netherlands.

U.S. Department of Labor (2008). *Hospital eTool. Emergency department (ED) module. Workplace violence.* Available at: http://www.osha.gov/SLTC/etools/hospital/er/er.html#WorkplaceViolence. Accessed January 19, 2009.

U.S. Department of Labor, Bureau of Labor Statistics Census (2007). *National census of fatal occupational injuries in 2006.* Available at: www.bls.gov/news.release/pdf/cfoi.pdf. Accessed July 14, 2008.

U.S. Department of Labor, Occupational Safety and Health Administration (2004). *Guidelines for preventing workplace violence for health care & social service workers.* Available at: www.osha.gov/index.html. Accessed July 4, 2008.

U.S. Department of Labor, Occupational Safety and Health Administration (2007). *Safety and health topics. Workplace violence. Fact sheets.* Available at: www.osha.gov.html. Accessed July 4, 2008.

Yildirum, A., & Yildirum, D. (2008). *Mobbing behaviors encountered by academic staff in university and their responses to them.* Presented at the International Conference on Workplace Violence in the Health Sector, Together, Creating a Safe Work Environment, 22–24 October, Amsterdam, The Netherlands.

BIBLIOGRAPHY

Hoobler, J. M., & Brass, D. J. (2006). Abusive supervision and family undermining as displaced aggression. *Journal of Applied Psychology, 91*(5), 1125–1133.

Meglich-Sespico, P., Faley, R. H., & Knapp, D. E. (2007). Relief and redress for targets of workplace bullying. *Employee Responsibilities and Rights Journal, 19*(1), 31–43.

Saunders, P., Huynh, A., & Goodman-Delahunty, J. (2007). Defining workplace bullying behavior. Professional and lay definitions of workplace bullying. *International Journal of Law and Psychiatry, 30*(4–5), 340–354.

Steinman, S. (2003–2007). *My Hyena Journal. The Survival Toolkit for Victims of Workplace Violence.* Available at: www.worktrauma.org/susanstore.htm. Accessed July 20, 2008.

Tracy, S. J., & Alberts, J. K. (2007). Burned by bullying in the American workplace: Prevalence, perception, degree and impact. *Journal of Management Studies, 44*(6), 837–862.

WEB RESOURCES

International Council of Nurses	http://www.icn.ch
International Labour Organization	http://www.ilo.org
National Institute for Occupational Safety and Health, Violence in the Workplace	http://www.cdc.gov/niosh/violcont.html
Royal College of Nursing, Australia	http://www.rcna.org.au
Worktrauma Organization, South Africa	http://www.worktrauma.org/
World Health Organization	http://www.who.org

CHAPTER 13

Technology in the Health Care Workplace: Benefits, Limitations, and Challenges

• CAROL J. HUSTON •

Learning Objectives

The learner will be able to:

1. Describe emerging opportunities for robotic technology in health care, including surgery, diagnostics, and therapy, the provision of direct care, assistance with pharmaceutical applications/dispensing, and as couriers in supply chain automation.
2. Reflect on the degree to which technologically sophisticated, emotion-sensing, mental service robots will be able to replace professional nurse caregivers in the future.
3. Discuss how different types of biometric technology can be used to increase the likelihood that access to health care information is both targeted and appropriate.
4. Identify current "smart object'" applications in health care.
5. Detail how point-of-care bar coding is being implemented and potential benefits for its use.
6. Explore the effect of computerized physician/prescriber order entry on the reduction of medication errors and adverse drug events, as well as current barriers to widespread implementation of its use.
7. Provide examples of expanding electronic and wireless communication technologies that assist in personal organization, as well as data management.
8. Identify how electronic health records (EHRs), telehealth/telenursing, and point-of-care testing can be used to overcome geography-of-care issues.
9. Identify barriers to the widespread implementation of EHRs despite governmental encouragement to develop this technology.
10. Analyze how the Internet has changed the relationship between providers and their patients in terms of the power of information.
11. Recognize emerging roles for nurse informaticists (also known as clinical nurse informaticists).
12. Engage in futuristic thinking regarding how technology will further alter 21st-century health care and the roles of health care providers.
13. Examine his or her degree of "technophobia" and complete a personal assessment of technology skills deficits and strengths.

Technology is everywhere and it is continually transforming health care, particularly nursing care. Indeed, both consumer and provider expectations of health care are being shaped by experiences with more technologically advanced enterprises, such as the travel and banking industries: "Healthcare is just now beginning to develop the information systems that would improve transactions among providers, consumers, and financiers of healthcare" (Vlasses & Smeltzer, 2007, p. 376).

With advances in technology come new challenges, opportunities, and problems. Clearly, technology can cut costs, improve patient outcomes, streamline workflow, and improve information accessibility. Determining what technology should be developed in an era of limited resources and how it should be used, however, raises all kinds of issues. In addition, many questions exist as to how to educate health care providers about using new technology.

CONSIDER
Technology is like a rolling freight train—it's very difficult to stop it and even more dangerous to get in the way.

This chapter addresses many of the technology advances being used in 21st-century health care, including robotics, computers, and wireless communication, to improve the utilization of human resources. Biometrics, point-of-care testing, and computerized data access/entry are presented as technological approaches for improving documentation and knowledge acquisition. Electronic health records and telehealth are introduced as strategies for overcoming geography-of-care issues, and provider computer order entry and clinical decision support (CDS) systems are discussed both as strategies for improving existing care processes and as a means for high-quality clinical decision making. Finally, the Internet's effect on both patients and providers is explored, including the concept of "expert patient" and the resultant need for nurses trained in consumer health informatics.

NEW TECHNOLOGIES IN HEALTH CARE

Most Baby Boomers remember the TV show *Star Trek*, in which the spaceship crew and aliens dematerialized into tiny atoms for transport between locations and sensors were waved over patients in the sick bay, rendering an immediate diagnosis and treatment. Although technology has not yet reached this point, much of the futuristic thinking envisioned on *Star Trek* is likely to some day become a reality.

Noor (2007) suggested that *biomechatronics*, which merges the human with the machine, will continue to increase in prominence in the near future. He pointed out that by drawing from an interdisciplinary field encompassing biology, neurosciences, mechanics, electronics, and robotics, "biomechatronic devices have been developed that interact with human muscle, skeleton, and nervous systems with the goals of restoring human motor control impaired by trauma, disease, or birth defects" (p. 23). He went on to say that future biomechatronics applications may eventually include pancreas pacemakers for diabetics, "mentally controlled electronic muscle stimulators for stroke and accident survivors, as well as miniature cameras

and microphones that can be wired into the brain, allowing blind people to see and deaf people to hear" (p. 23).

DISCUSSION POINT
Do you believe that technology will someday eliminate "disease" as we know it today? If so, what are the implications in terms of life span and the prevalence of chronic disease?

Nelson (2003) also provided a glimpse into such a future, suggesting that some day, computer-based diagnostic tools will give unprecedented images of soft and hard tissues in the body, eliminating exploratory surgery and invasive procedures. Biologic markers of disease and genetic markers will facilitate the forecasting of disease and disability, and patients will wear "health watches" to detect new signs and symptoms before they develop into emergencies. In addition, health monitoring devices will be installed in showers to complete daily body scans and full-body examinations, and microbots and nanodevices will circulate in the body and repair systems early in the disease process.

Nelson went on to report that room sensors will be developed that will automatically charge for all health care–related supplies. In addition, such sensors will charge for human health care resources based on the number of minutes health providers interact with patients. Automated voices will announce the exact time that providers will see patients. All assessments and diagnostics will be automatically recorded in the patient's record, and automated recognition systems will reduce errors (Nelson).

Finally, Nelson (2003) suggested that health care teams will cover all specialties and will be aided by *expert systems* (defined as computer applications that perform tasks otherwise performed by human experts) that both constrain decisions and improve patient outcomes. In addition, synthetic life forms (robots) will have developed to the point that there will be few differences between what these life forms and humans can do.

Robots and Health Care
Robots in Surgery

The use of robots as described by Nelson may not be as futuristic as it sounds. Indeed, the use of robotics in health care is no longer science fiction. The first robotic-assisted surgery dates back to the mid 1980s when a robot was used to place a needle for brain biopsy using computed tomographic guidance (Noor, 2007). Robotic-assisted heart bypass surgery followed in 1998, and the first unmanned robotic surgery took place in May 2006 in Italy.

Recently, engineers at Duke University, using novel three-dimensional technology and a basic artificial intelligence program, guided the actions of a rudimentary tabletop robot to perform surgery (Robotics Trends, 2008). The engineers suggested that such technology will eventually allow robots to perform surgery on patients in dangerous situations or in remote locations, such as on the battlefield or in space, with minimal or no human guidance. On a more immediate level, the technology could make certain contemporary medical procedures safer for patients. Another 2008 study demonstrated that autonomous robots could successfully perform simulated needle biopsies (Robotic Trends).

Robots in Diagnostics and Therapy

Brumson (2008) suggested that robots are increasingly being used in diagnostics and therapy because their accuracy and steadiness often exceed those of human caregivers. For example, Brumson discussed the use of robotics with linear accelerators in treating tumors: "Linear accelerators are small devices mounted on the end of the robot to direct a thin beam of radiation into a tumor. Using the robot, doctors can precisely place high dose radiation inside a tumor" (para 9).

Similarly, although still in prototype development, robotic technology in cardiology is being developed that will allow a snake-like device to be inserted through a small incision below the sternum, which can then adhere to a patient's beating heart. A robot is able to access areas of the heart that normally require the patient's lungs to be deflated: "The hope for this type of robot is to inject medication, attach pacemakers or target specific points for cauterization as a treatment for cardiac arrhythmia into areas of the heart that are difficult to access" (Brumson, 2008, para 10).

Robots as Direct Care Providers

Robots are also being developed to provide direct patient care. These *service robots* are increasingly being used as care givers, particularly for the elderly. McNicol

(2008) noted that this is especially true in Japan, which is known as the "robot kingdom." In fact, more than one third of the exhibits at the November 2007 International Robotic Exhibition featured service robots. Japan has turned to service robots as a result of a burgeoning elderly population and a low birth rate, which has resulted in a severe shortage of caregivers.

According to Takanori Shibata, a senior research scientist at the National Institute of Advanced Industrial Science and Technology, "robot caregivers can be divided into *physical service* and *mental service* robots. The former are designed to help with tasks such as washing or carrying elderly people, although given the limitations of current technology, not to mention safety concerns, they are still quite a long way from commercialization" (McNicol, 2008, para 5).

Robots are also being developed that can be autonomous, with a sense of their environment. For example, autonomous wheelchairs and robotic-assisted walking devices could "provide home care, help the elderly move around, or guide blind people. Portable surgical robotics, coupled with advanced telecommunications and telepresence facilities, could provide health-care and telementoring services in remote areas, war zones, and possibly, future human space missions" (Noor, 2007, p. 24).

Mental service robots, on the other hand, are already here. According to McNicol (2008, para 6), "one of the best known is Paro, an interactive robot designed by Shibata himself. The sophisticated robot can remember its name and change its behavior depending on how it is treated. It has been extensively tested in homes for elderly people and in hospitals." The 2002 *Guinness Book of Records* named Paro "the world's most therapeutic robot" (McNicol, para 6). Paro retails for about $3,000, and more than 1,000 have been produced since 2004.

Many consumers and health care providers have expressed concern, however, about the lack of emotion in robots, suggesting that this is the element of human caregivers that can never be replaced. Boivin and Williams (2008, p. 38) stated that robots will never replace nurses, "since even the most optimistic roboticists recognize that no combination of metallic parts, microchips, and binary files could replace the empathetic touch or clinical intuition of a human nurse."

New technology developed by scientists at Meiji University in Tokyo, however, has resulted in a kind of robot intelligence known as "*kansei*," which means "emotion or feeling" (McNicol, 2008; Christensen, n.d.). *Kansei* robots use vision systems to monitor human expressions, gestures, and body language and voice sensors to pick up on intonation and individual words and sentences. In addition, *kansei* robots sense human emotion through wearable sensors that monitor pulse rate and perspiration.

DISCUSSION POINT

To what degree can nurses be replaced by technology? Can therapeutic "caring" be demonstrated by robots? Do you feel that you could have a therapeutic conversation with a robot?

Christensen (n.d.) noted that when the *kansei* robot hears a word it searches through its database of more than 500,000 words to find common associations. The robot then matches the results to emotional categories and, using its 19 movable parts, generates 1 of 36 expressions on its polyurethane face. The *kansei* robot can make 36 different facial expressions (using the 19 different movable parts underneath its silicon face mask). For example, the word "sushi" elicits expressions of enjoyment, whereas the word "war" brings about fear or disgust (Christensen).

Service robots are also being used as robot couriers for supply chain automation. Aethon Inc. has produced mobile robots called *TUGs* that can locate assets as well as transport them, including medications, supplies, equipment, and other goods that rely on scarce, valuable human resources for pushing carts (Service Robotics, 2008):

> All of Aethon's robots can be equipped with RFID [radio frequency identification antennas], giving them the ability to track assets over very large areas with very few antennas. Additionally, TUGs can provide automated transportation, ensuring that clinicians not only know where the equipment is, but can have it brought directly to the point of care so they don't have to leave the patient care area (Service Robotics, para 4).

FirstHealth Moore Regional Hospital in Pinehurst, North Carolina, recently introduced such technology. Their robotics technology include

> one HOMER, a specialized TUG dedicated to only asset tracking, three pharmacy TUGs and two materials handling TUGs for par stock replenishment to the floors from the warehouse. Both the HOMER and

> TUGs sport mobile antennas that track key hospital assets tagged with RFID tags. Once the robots identify where equipment is located, the data is passed to an asset utilization software program that provides overall visibility into the location of hospital assets. This translates into more efficient organization and location of the assets without adding costly hospital infrastructure (Service Robotics, 2008, para 5).

Robots in the Pharmaceutical Industry

Another application of robotics was developed for use in the pharmaceutical industry. Jeff Burnstein, executive vice president of the Robotic Industries Association, suggested that life sciences/pharmaceutical/biomedical/medical devices are among the best-performing nonautomotive markets, and that the majority of robotic equipment sales growth in this sector stems from pharmaceutical packaging applications (Healthcare Packaging, 2008).

For example, AstraZeneca's Global Technical Services employs nine robotic cells and 16 robots on several of its packaging lines at its plant in Södertälje, Sweden. A company spokesperson says the he "expects the company's use of robotics to continue, as they provide 'flexibility and 'digital' changeover. They're also more ergonomic, requiring no [manual] lifting or handling of boxes" (Healthcare Packaging, 2008, para 7).

In addition, robots (in the form of automated drug-dispensing devices and related technology) are being used in central fill pharmacies around the world:

> The trend is moving increasingly towards automating pill dispensing in hospitals and at the retail level. This interest at the retail level is fueled by a shortage of pharmacists in the United States and by a desire to get pharmacists out from behind the counter to allow them to interact with patients (Brumson, 2008, para 14).

Biometrics

The health care environment is also being rapidly transformed by new technology as a result of the need to comply with the Health Insurance Portability and Accountability Act of 1996 (HIPAA). HIPAA calls for a tiered approach to data access in which staff members have access to only the information that they need to know to perform their jobs, and so new technology to assure that access is both targeted and appropriate is being developed.

One such new technology is *biometrics*, the science of identifying people through physical characteristics such as fingerprints, handprints, retinal scans, voice recognition, facial structure, and dynamic signatures. Biometrics can be used to "either identify or authenticate computer users before they can gain access to sensitive data. Proponents maintain that it is far superior to typing in passwords—not only does it positively authenticate the user, it eliminates the burden of having to carry around lists of passwords" (Andrews, 2006, para 12).

Fingerprint biometrics is still the most common type of biometrics in health care, primarily because of its ease of use, small size, and affordable price. Andrews (2006) suggested that 45,000 to 50,000 caregivers currently use fingerprint technology on a regular basis, making the health care industry the largest user of fingerprint scanning technology for identification and authentication purposes.

Detection of facial geometry is also beginning to make inroads into health care. Facial geometry "builds biometric recognition of each user by capturing facial landmarks and storing them for future encounters" and then fine tunes recognition accuracy by adding new data, such as approach angles and facial variations such as hairstyles and eyeglasses (Andrews, 2006, para 18).

Smart Cards and Smart Objects

Health care organizations are also increasingly integrating biometrics with "*smart cards*" to ensure that an individual presenting a secure ID credential really has the right to use that credential. Smart cards are credit card–sized devices with a chip, stored memory, and an operating system that record a patient's entire clinical history. Although still in the early development stage, the integration of biometrics with smart cards eliminates the need for multiple identification requirements, so no time is lost in retrieving passwords or keys (Analysis: Integrated Smart Card, 2008). The market for such integrated cards was $249.1 million in 2007 and is expected to reach $822.2 million by 2013 (Smart Cards Integrated, 2008).

An example of successful smart card integration was unveiled by Community Health Network, an Indianapolis-based hospital system, in August 2008 (Lee, 2008). The hospital offered free tech tools to patients who signed up to receive a credit-card–sized "my-

Community" card. Patients swipe their "myCommunity" cards at kiosks and use touch screens to complete the inpatient and outpatient check-in process. The technology, which took about 3 years and cost $1.2 million to develop, also allows patients to keep track of their conditions and medications and includes a blog for new parents or long-term patients (Lee).

Smart objects are everyday objects injected with easy-to-use software that give devices a degree of intelligence (Nelson, 2003). For example, the University of Pittsburgh Medical Center recently introduced a "smart hospital room" (Fahy, 2008), which includes computer screens that display vital signs, medications, and other personal information and even identify the health professionals entering the room. In addition, the computer system reminds patients to ask for help in getting out of bed if they are at risk for falls and focuses a spotlight on the hand sanitizer dispenser when people enter or leave, reminding them to wash their hands.

Hatler (2008, p. 21) described the use of "smart beds" at St. Joseph's Hospital and Medical Center in Phoenix. The smart bed offers "continuous, noncontact, noninvasive, real time monitoring of heart and respiratory rate and potential early detection of bed exit." The smart bed actually consists of two components: a passive sensor array embedded in a coverlet that zips over the existing matter and a bedside unit: "The bedside unit accommodates digital signal processing algorithms used to calculate heart and respiratory rates and displays the data" (Hatler, p. 21).

Preliminary outcomes from the smart bed use at St. Joseph's Hospital and Medical Center suggest that smart bed use did not result in lower fall rates on the unit; however, when fall rates were compared to those of other patients receiving care in the unit, the fall rate did show a significant downward trend. Hospital length of stay and costs were also not significantly affected by use of the vigilance system. Hatler (2008) reported, however, that there were a significantly smaller number of emergent returns to the intensive care unit, declining from 11% to 1% during the study period. This was attributed to the enhanced ability of the smart bed to detect early changes in patients' conditions.

Point-of-Care Testing

Point-of-care testing (POCT), which has evolved into a multibillion dollar industry, is another technological advance that is improving bedside care and promoting more positive outcomes, as a result of more timely decision making and treatment. The College of American Pathologists defines POCT as testing designed to be used at or near the site where the patient is located, that do not require permanent dedicated space, and that is performed outside of the physical facilities of the clinical laboratories (Express Healthcare, 2008). Two primary types of POCT instruments exist: small bench-top analyzers (e.g., blood gas and electrolyte systems) and handheld, single-use devices (such as urine albumin, blood glucose, and coagulation tests) (Express Healthcare).

In POCT, caregivers gather and test specimens near the patient or at the bedside using handheld analyzers, pulse oximeters, and blood glucose monitoring systems. Then, by networking via the Internet and downloading results to a central clinical lab, manual documentation of test results can be eliminated. Many clinicians feel that "point-of-care testing (POCT) is a prerequisite for early recognition of life-threatening conditions as they require that laboratory results are made available in real-time and, if possible, at the critically ill patient's point of care" (Express Healthcare, 2008, para 2).

POCT testing also works for consumer use in the home. Patients can precisely monitor their laboratory values, submit them electronically to the lab, and then have results in minutes. POCT testing represents only a small portion of clinical laboratories' total testing volume, however, and evaluation challenges exist for all POCT programs in terms of accuracy, ease of use, quality control, and accurate data management. Indeed, delivering diagnostic tests at the bedside may be prone to errors as a result of failure to follow procedures, inappropriate documentation, improper patient identification, and failure to perform required quality control tests. More pilot programs are needed to evaluate the use of POCT testing.

Automated Medication Administration: Point-of-Care Bar Coding and Intravenous Smart Pumps

Automated medication administration is another technology that shows great promise for reducing medication errors and improving quality of care. *Point-of-care bar coding*, the least expensive method of electronic patient labeling, has been developed to help caregivers ensure the right medication, in the right dose, is given to the right patient at the right time and by the right route (the "*five rights*"). Bar coding works by requiring the nurse to match, with a handheld scanner, his or her name tag, the bar code on the patient's identification band, and the medication to be given. When one of the five "rights" does not match, an alert is issued or the medication will not be dispensed from its storage system. In using point-of-care bar coding, then, nurses become "the last line of defense" in preventing medication errors made by pharmacists and physicians (Hurley et al., 2007).

Goldstein (2008) reported that about one third of the nation's hospitals currently have a bar-code medication-dispensing system, but most if not all hospitals are expected to install such a system within a few years. The cost to implement such a system is hundreds of thousands of dollars, so the cost may be prohibitive for smaller rural hospitals.

> **DISCUSSION POINT**
> Given that rural hospitals often cannot afford the expensive technological innovations that larger hospitals can, will this limitation result in a two-tiered system of health care quality?

In addition, implementation of point-of-care bar coding is not without problems. A recent study by the *Journal of the American Medical Informatics Association* found that nurses often develop workarounds that undermine bar coding's safeguards. For example, if a nurse needed to go to another unit or floor to pick up a drug for several patients, he or she might choose to just scan all the patients' barcodes to pick up the doses, even though these scans would be done far from the patients' bedsides (Goldstein, 2008). In fact, research by Ross Koppell from the University of Pennsylvania found that "nurses overrode patient ID scans 4.2 percent of the time, often because bar codes were unreadable for reasons ranging from the child who chewed on hers to the patient with dementia who tore his off to the ones smudged and soggy from blood, urine or feces" (Goldstein, para 20). In addition, caregivers encountered numerous other obstacles, including wireless dead spots, dead batteries in handheld scanners or on the computer, and an inability to take the handheld scanner into rooms where contagious diseases are an issue.

Hurley et al.'s (2007) research also found that although bar coding clearly decreases medication errors and promotes nursing satisfaction, procedural features were sometimes problematic. For example, bar coding was viewed as being more time consuming; however, nurses recognized that the extra time was needed for verification, which translates to safety.

In addition, hospitals are increasingly turning to so called "*smart" pumps* for intravenous (IV) therapy infusions. These smart pumps have safety software inside an advanced infusion therapy system that prevents IV medication errors by setting minimum and maximum dose limits, as well as preset limits that cannot be overridden at a clinician's discretion. A study by Nuckols et al. (2008), however, found that the smart pumps used in their study facility eliminated only 4% of IV adverse drug events (ADEs). The researchers concluded that smart pump capabilities must be expanded before more IV ADEs can be prevented.

CONSIDER

The Institute for Safe Medication Practices suggested that smart pumps are not smart on their own: "They need careful programming for dose limits and staff need a commitment to use the technology as intended" (Hahn & Whitbeck, 2007, p. 27).

Computerized Physician/Providers Order Entry

Computerized physician/provider order entry (CPOE) is also a rapidly growing technology. Part of this growth has occurred as a result of its designation as one of three key patient safety initiatives by the Leapfrog Group, a conglomeration of non–health care Fortune 500 company leaders committed to modernizing the current health care system. In addition, the 1999 Institute of Medicine study *To Err Is Human* recommended the use of CPOE to address medical errors.

CPOE is a clinical software application designed specifically for providers to write patient orders electronically rather than on paper. With CPOE, providers produce clearly typed orders, reducing medication errors based on inaccurate transcription.

CPOE also gives providers vital *clinical decision support* (CDS) via access to information tools that support a health care provider in decisions related to diagnosis, therapy, and care planning of individual patients. For example, physicians might access evidence-based medicine databases electronically for CDS when writing medication orders. If the provider has ordered a test or treatment that is contraindicated for a particular patient or condition, the CDS will inform that provider of the potential danger at the time the order is entered.

DISCUSSION POINT

Should health care organizations require prescribing providers to write their orders electronically, or should this be left to the discretion of the provider?

Translating CPOE into action has not been without challenges. The literature suggests that there are unintended consequences of CPOE, which can be positive, negative, or both, depending on one's perspective (Ash et al., 2007). These consequences are reported as relating to work/more work, workflow, system demands, communication, emotions, and dependence on the technology, as well as shifts in the power structure and the introduction of a new possible source of error (Ash et al.). Aggressive detection and management of these adverse unintended consequences is vital for CPOE success. (See Research Study Fuels the Controversy on page 222.)

In addition, although many health care organizations see the value in CPOE technology, they do not consider it an immediate necessity. A majority of the 145 participants in Modern Healthcare's latest information technology (IT) survey confirmed that CPOE is an important element in their IT plans, but when asked if their organization had either a CPOE system in operation or currently being implemented, only 58.3% of respondents indicated that they did (CPOE Still A Priority, But. . ., 2008). Of those who said they did not, 45.6% said that they planned to contract for a CPOE system in the next 12 months.

These adoption rates are higher than penetration rates reported in other surveys based on random samples. For example, a survey by the Leapfrog Group in August 2007, found that just 10% of its respondents had met that organization's standards for having a functioning CPOE system (CPOE Still a Priority, But. . . ., 2008):

> *Karen Linscott, chief operating officer for the Leapfrog Group, concedes even a 10% CPOE adoption rate is much higher than what would be realized if all 5,000 or so of U.S. hospitals were polled. Linscott says the prospects of picking up the current, glacial pace of CPOE adoption aren't good if things don't change (CPOE Still a Priority, But. . ., p. S5).*

Research Study Fuels the Controversy: Challenges to CPOE Implementation

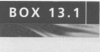

The literature clearly suggests that there are unintended consequences of using CPOE, which extends beyond errors. This study examined the extent and importance of eight types of CPOE-related unintended adverse consequences at 176 U.S. hospitals using CPOE.

STUDY FINDINGS

Hospitals experienced all eight types of unintended adverse consequences, although some were considered more important than others. Those related to new work/more work, workflow, system demands, communication, emotions, and dependence on the technology were ranked as most severe, with at least 72% of respondents ranking them as moderately to very important. Hospital representatives were less sure about shifts in the power structure and the possibility of CPOE as a new source of errors. There was no relationship between kinds of unintended consequences and number of years CPOE has been used. Despite the relatively short length of time most hospitals have had CPOE (median 5 years), it is highly infused, or embedded, within work practice at most of these sites.

The researchers concluded that the unintended consequences of CPOE are widespread and important. In addition, they can be positive, negative, or both, depending on one's perspective, and they continue to exist over the duration of use. Aggressive detection and management of adverse unintended consequences is vital for CPOE success.

Source: Ash, J. S., Sittig, D. F., Poon, E. G., Guappone, K., Campbell, E., & Dykstra, R. H. (2007). The extent and importance of unintended consequences related to computerized provider order entry. *Journal of the American Medical Informatics Association, 14*(4), 415–423.

There also may be cultural obstacles to CPOE; for example, a physician might prefer to write orders by hand instead of using a computer. In addition, the requirements to fully meet Leapfrog's CPOE standards are stringent (Box 13.1). Still, institutional and clinician adoption of CPOE is crucial to helping caregivers to reduce medical errors and enhance patient safety, and health care institutions must commit the necessary human and financial resources to make this technological innovation a reality.

Clinical Decision Support

Clinical decision support is defined broadly as "a clinical system, application or process that helps health professionals make clinical decisions to enhance patient care" (Healthcare Information and Management Systems Society, 2008, para 1). Like CPOE, CDS will likely be commonplace by 2020, giving providers the promise for access at the point of care to cutting-edge research, best practices, and decision-making support to improve patient care. For example, Isabel Health, an online diagnosis decision support application, "combats diagnosis error by reminding clinicians of potential diagnoses. After users input free-text symptoms, Isabel searches published literature for possible diagnoses, with relevance attached. Isabel also provides access to annotated images for visual confirmation as well as suggestions for next steps, and can integrate with a hospital EMR" (The Advisory Board Company, 2006).

BOX 13.1 | **REQUIREMENTS FOR FULL COMPLIANCE WITH LEAPFROG'S CPOE STANDARD**

1. Hospitals must ensure that physicians enter at least 75% of medication orders via a computer system with prescribing-error prevention software.

2. Hospitals must demonstrate that their inpatient CPOE system can alert physicians to at least 50% of common, serious prescribing errors, using Leapfrog's CPOE Evaluation Tool. (Note: For the 2008 survey, the scored results from the CPOE Evaluation Tool will not be used in the publicly reported survey results, only the fact that the hospital tested its system. However, in 2009, scores from the tool will be used.)

Source: Leapfrog fact sheet. Computerized physician order entry (2008). Available at: http://www.leapfroggroup. org/media/file/Leapfrog-Computer_Physician_Order_ Entry_Fact_ Sheet.pdf. Accessed August 14, 2008.

Electronic and Wireless Communication

Electronic communication technologies are also expanding at an exponential pace (Meneses & McNees, 2007). Computers are increasingly a part of interdisciplinary team communication and care documentation in acute care hospitals, although futurists predict that computers in the not too distant future will essentially be invisible, replaced with *smart objects.*

Computerized charting is commonplace, with more institutions moving toward the use of *tablet personal computers*—flat-panel laptops that use a stylus pen or touch screen technology. For example, these wireless tablets are being used at Lowell General Hospital in Massachusetts (Most Wired, 2008). Nurses carry the wireless tablets into patient rooms when making rounds. This gives them more direct time with their patients because notes can be recorded at the time of the assessment. In addition, the nurses have access to all the chart data, including test results and radiology images. As part of its multimillion dollar commitment to technology, the hospital reports having 200 tablets housed in locked wall units throughout the hospital. In addition, wall units in the room fold down to become work tables, holding a full-size keyboard and mouse as well. There are also 100 computers on wheels (COWs), providing health care providers access to patient records and information at the click of a mouse (Most Wired).

In addition, *personal digital assistants* (PDAs)—mobile, handheld devices such as the Palm series and Handspring Visors—that give users access to text-based information are becoming common. Advances include institution-wide documentation systems in which everyone uses the same documentation software, and the information is transferred to and retrieved from a central server via "hot synching" (putting the PDA into a cradle or connecting it via cable to the central server). In addition, the PDA can serve as a reference library, especially for drug information, and as a calculator for computing drug doses.

PDAs, however, are not cheap, typically costing between $100 for a barebones glorified calculator and up to $800 for a device that uses Microsoft or Palm operating systems. In addition, PDAs can be lost or stolen, posing concerns about patient confidentiality. Finally, some nurses feel uncomfortable using such technology in front of patients and some just feel uncomfortable with the technology itself. However, the quality and number of PDA applications continue to grow, as does their use.

The use of *wireless local area networking* (WLAN) is also growing rapidly. WLAN uses a spread-spectrum radio frequency to link two or more computers or devices without using wires. This allows caregivers to access, update, and transmit critical patient and treatment information despite moving between or being located at multiple sites of care. The area of outreach in the network is called the *basic service set.* For example, wireless technology at the Baylor College of Medicine in Houston, Texas, allows

> the transmission of 12-lead electrocardiogram (ECG) waveforms from remote locations to handheld computers of cardiologists. There is no significant difference in the interpretation of the results using the handheld liquid crystals display (LCDs) screens and the traditional paper but the immediate accessibility of the results leads to a reduction in treatment time (Igbokwe, 2007, para 5).

Similarly, *Bluetooth* technology creates a small wireless network (called a *piconet*) between two pieces of hardware through short-range radio signals. This allows devices such as keyboards to link with personal computers and headsets to link with cell phones. Igbokwe (2007) suggested that Bluetooth technology can allow health care providers in hospitals to stay in touch with each other at all times, arrange their schedules instantaneously, and receive results of procedures and investigations not just at any time, but also almost anywhere within the hospital's vicinity.

Electronic Health Records

Even health records have changed as a result of technology. The *electronic health record* (EHR) is a digitalized record of a patient's health history that may be made up of records from many locations and/or sources, such as hospitals, providers, clinics, and public health agencies. For example, an EHR might include immunization status, allergies, patient demographics, lab test and radiology results, advanced directives, current medications taken, and current health care appointments. The EHR is available 24 hours a day, 7 days a week and has built in safeguards to assure patient health information confidentiality and security.

BOX 13.2 | EIGHT CORE FUNCTIONS OF AN ELECTRONIC HEALTH RECORD

1. Health information and data.
2. Results management.
3. Order entry/management.
4. Decision support.
5. Electronic communication and connectivity.
6. Patient support.
7. Administrative processes.
8. Reporting and population health management.

Source: Bordowitz, R. (2008). Electronic health records: A primer. *Laboratory Medicine, 39*(5), 301–307.

In May 2003, the U.S. Department of Health and Human Services asked the Institute of Medicine (IOM) to provide guidance on the key care delivery–related capabilities of an EHR system. According to Bordowitz (2008), the IOM report stated that an EHR system has eight core functions (Box 13.2) and should include the following:

■ Longitudinal collection of electronic health information for and about people, in which health information is defined as information pertaining to the health of an individual or health care provided to an individual.

■ Immediate electronic access to person- and population-level information by only authorized users.

■ Provision of knowledge and decision support that enhance the quality, safety, and efficiency of patient care.

■ Support of efficient processes for health care delivery. Critical building blocks of an EHR system are the EHRs maintained by providers (e.g., hospitals, nursing homes, ambulatory settings) and by individuals (also called personal health records).

In addition, in January 2004, President George Bush set a goal that most Americans would have an EHR by 2014 (Office of the Assistant Secretary of Defense (Health Affairs) and the TRICARE Management Activity, 2008). Similarly, Canada Health Infoway predicted that 50% of Canadians will be able to access their EHRs by 2009 (Pooley, 2006). Indeed, most developed countries are actively moving toward the establishment and implementation of EHRs. Australia has proposed a

strategy known as Health Connect to facilitate the adoption of common standards by all e-health systems in the Australian national, state, and territory governments (Health Connect, 2006). The National Health Service in the United Kingdom began an EHR system in 2005 and has developed a national system to transfer records directly and securely from one general practitioner (GP) to another. More than 100,000 patients in 4,000 GP practices in the United Kingdom are using this system (NHS Connecting for Health, 2008).

It is not easy, however, to make such system-wide changes. Nor is it cheap. A lack of funding, debates about who "owns" the data in the system, and the challenges of getting computers to "talk to each other" will exist for some time (Pooley, 2006). Indeed, a review of the literature suggests limited success regarding the use of EHR. Perhaps this simply reflects normal resistance to change, given the number of behavioral and procedural changes required to rework such a fundamental aspect of normal operations; however, further research is needed to examine the benefits and the drawbacks of using EHRs.

Physicians have been especially slow to adopt EHRs. A recent study by DesRoches et al. (2008) of 2,758 physicians revealed that only 4% had an extensive, fully functional electronic records system as part of their practice and only 13% reported having a basic system. Primary care physicians and those practicing in large groups, in hospitals or medical centers, and in the Western region of the United States were more likely to use electronic health records. Financial barriers were viewed as the most significant variable affecting the adoption of electronic health records.

In addition, Bordowitz (2008) noted that some studies have suggested that the use of an EHR may interfere with the patient–provider encounter, preventing quality information from being attained. Patients felt less satisfied when providers were using a computer in the exam room because the visits typically took longer and seemed less personal to them.

CONSIDER

"While the implementation of the electronic record has resulted in significant improvements in patient safety, it is not a single panacea for all medical errors, rather it is a supporting tool that requires an organizational culture of safety and an awareness of the new generation of errors that are emerging" (Malloch, 2007, p. 160).

Other Electronic Data Repositories and Intranets

Many electronic data repositories have been created within organizations as a way of cataloging internal reference materials, such as policy and procedure manuals. This increases the likelihood that staff will be able to find such resources when they need them and that they are as up to date as possible. In such a system, references are typically converted to the portable document format and launched electronically via an Intranet.

Intranets are internal networks (not normally accessible from the Internet) that allow workers and departments to share files, use Web sites, and collaborate. Scharfe-Pretino and Von Bacho (2008) described the creation of such an intranet at Strong Memorial Hospital in Rochester, New York. The purpose of creating the intranet was to enhance communication and feedback, a goal identified by the institution's gap analysis early in the American Nurses Credentialing Center Magnet Application process. The hospital created a "one-stop-shopping" intranet for nursing resources," including "real-time information and updates, feedback to management, meeting minutes and agenda items for the shared governance council, quality improvement information, cultural diversity, and career options" (p. 104). In addition, the site included links to the Joint Commission on Accreditation of Healthcare Organizations, the National Patient Safety Goals site, patient satisfaction initiatives, an online work force engagement survey (supported by a grant through the Hospital Association of New York State), and information about performance improvement and best practices.

TELEHEALTH AND TELENURSING

Given declining reimbursement, the current nursing shortage, and an increasing shift in care to outpatient settings, home care agencies are increasingly exploring technology-aided options that allow them to avoid the traditional 1:1 nurse–patient ratio with face-to-face contact. *Telehealth*, also called remote monitoring technology, telemedicine, telenursing, telecare, telehomecare, telemanagement, e-health, and telephone care, allows nurses to care for patients over a distance, using a combination of telecommunication and multimedia technologies. Harrison and Lee (2006, p. 291) suggested it is through even greater investments in telecommunica-

tions equipment and supporting information technology, that the "full potential of e-health will be realized." For example, if technology such as the electronic health record is not available to capture telehealth data, the full potential of not only immediate data transfer, but also permanent storage, may be lost. Many rural communities may lack the bandwidth to support telehealth and must adopt new software systems before such programs can become viable (Prinz, Cramer, & Englund, 2008).

> ### CONSIDER
> If the benefits of telemedicine are to be fully realized, providers need to be able to merge telehealth data with information from other clinical systems. Electronic health records may be one means of accomplishing this goal.

Nelson (2003) also looked to the future in his prediction that most health care in the future will essentially be removed from traditional office environments and be provided either virtually through videophones and monitoring equipment or at ambulatory centers in places such as shopping centers and kiosks. The focus of primary care then will become "forecast, prevent, and manage" (Nelson, p. S28).

For nurses, telehealth has meant greater ubiquity—nurses can now practice across geographic boundaries and be directly involved in patient care, even when they are not directly on site with patients. For patients, telehealth has meant increased flexibility and, often, more personalized care. For health care providers, telehealth has typically resulted in improved quality of care and lower costs. It has also provided new strategies for dealing with the health disparities created by geographic location, age, and homebound status. Indeed, Prinz et al. (2008, p. 152) suggested that "with increasing demands on the healthcare system to provide care to an ever-growing number of chronically ill and aging populations, especially in rural sectors of the United states, serious consideration must be given to how—or if—telehealth presents a viable solution for extending care."

> ### CONSIDER
> Telehealth provides greater opportunities for nurse–patient encounters, particularly for homebound, geographically isolated individuals.

How Telehealth Works

In more advanced telehealth, providers interact with patients through computer stations hooked up in the patient's home that typically include a video monitor, a moveable color video camera, a speakerphone and microphone, and one or more medical peripherals for patient self-monitoring, such as blood pressure and pulse meter, stethoscope, pulse oximeter, scale, and glucometer. Patients record their heart rates, blood pressures, blood glucose levels, and other readings periodically and then transmit these data to a provider with a computer station similar to theirs. This gives the provider a real-time picture of the patient's health status. In less sophisticated telehealth programs, assessment, intervention, and evaluation occur by fax, e-mail message, or simply by telephone.

DISCUSSION POINT
What, if anything, is "lost" when there is no face-to-face meeting between the nurse and the patient? Can technology overcome this loss? What does technology offer that face-to-face visits do not?

Telehealth and Telenursing Outcomes

Because telehealth and telenursing are relatively new, performance indicators and appropriate measures of quality are still being determined. More research also is needed to determine what telehealth system—or mix of telehealth and in-home visits—adds the most value both clinically and financially. In addition, Harrison and Lee (2006, p. 291) suggested that further study is needed to "determine whether barriers to e-health in rural communities, such as lack of resources, lower education levels, or large Medicare populations impact the implementation of e-health programs."

Desired patient outcomes for telehealth nursing are a little better defined. They include patient satisfaction, increased involvement in health care decision making, reduced travel time and expense, increased time with health care providers, improved health care, improved quality of life, and increased medical record data for clinical decision making.

CONSIDER
The practice of telephone nursing has not yet been standardized, and there are limited standardized tools to assess outcomes.

Despite a need to continue to further clarify what constitutes quality in telenursing, researchers are examining outcomes. A meta-analysis of 130 studies about home telehealth by Bensink, Hailey, and Wotton (2007) suggested there are a number of high-quality studies supporting the use of home telehealth in the areas of diabetes, the general area of mental health, high-risk pregnancy monitoring, heart failure, other cardiac conditions, and smoking cessation.

One such study, done by Bonnie Wakefield of the University of Missouri Sinclair School of Nursing, found that patients who received a telehealth intervention had significantly delayed hospital readmission rates than those who received traditional care (Telehealth Cuts Readmissions, 2008). Patients in the study were randomly selected to receive follow-up by telephone or videophone after hospitalization for heart failure. Wakefield noted that "people who suffer from chronic illnesses usually wait three to six months between office appointments with their care providers. With video and telephone technology, nurses have the ability to interact regularly with patients and provide a sense of security" (p. 63).

Similarly, Fonda et al. (2007) found that participation in a telehealth eye care program was significantly correlated with whether diabetic patients later obtained standard eye care, improvement in hemoglobin A1c, and improvement in low-density lipoprotein. Fonda et al. concluded that telehealth eye care programs that incorporate evaluation, education, and care planning improve certain diabetes-related health outcomes.

In contrast, research by Whitten and Mickus (2007) found that the addition of telehealth to chronic obstructive pulmonary disease/congestive heart failure patient care was not a significant predictor of health and well-being, either positively or negatively. Although those receiving telehealth had worse ratings on the general health subscale after the intervention, this measure was only significant when controlling for a number of key variables in the model. In regard to patient perceptions of home telecare, patients were satisfied with the technology and the way that care was delivered via this modality.

In addition, Prinz et al. (2008) suggested that reimbursement is not always guaranteed for telehealth and that sometimes telehealth is more expensive than other health care delivery systems that result in the same patient outcomes. Nonetheless Prinz et al. concluded that "telehealth will undoubtedly play an even more significant role in the near future, as the health system grapples with the nursing shortage and a concomitant need to extend care and overcome access barriers created by geography and age" (p. 156).

IS TECHNOLOGY WORTH THE COSTS?

Most health care economists would agree that the rapid introduction of new technologies is a significant factor in high health care costs. Domrose (2004) agreed that state-of-the-art technology is expensive and requires more education but suggested that it also generally saves time, creates less room for error, reduces the amount of pushing and lifting that nurses must do, and gives nurses more time to do nursing. Vlasses and Smeltzer (2007) agreed, suggesting that "although new technology may actually increase the cost of care up front, that this same technology has the potential to improve health and eventually decrease care costs" (p. 375).

In addition, it appears that hospitals that adopt more technology applications are more likely to have desirable quality outcomes. In a study of 98 Florida hospitals, Menachemi, Chukmaitox, Saunders, and Brooks (2008) found that hospitals that had adopted a greater number of IT applications were significantly more likely to have desirable quality outcomes on seven inpatient quality indicators. (See Research Study Fuels the Controversy)

Not all critics agree, however. Some argue that technology is not only expensive (both initially and in terms of maintenance and technical support), but also needs constant upgrades, and the education needed to truly be competent in the use of all this technology is never ending.

In addition, not all nurses embrace technology. This may simply represent a resistance to change, or it might be that nursing input has not historically been used in technology acquisition decisions. In addition, it is possible that many health care providers, including nurses, have received inadequate orientation to the technology in place. One must also remember that not all technology is worth the cost. Cost must always be weighed against possible benefits of the technology, effect on health care provider satisfaction, and projected utilization patterns.

THE INTERNET AND HEALTH CARE

The Exponential Growth of the Internet

The growth of the Internet as an information source for all types of information, including health, has grown exponentially and will continue to do so. Cisco Systems predicted that traffic on the world's networks will increase 46% annually from 2007 to 2012, nearly doubling every 2 years. As a result, there will be an annual bandwidth demand of approximately 522 exabytes (1 exabyte

---

Research Study Fuels the Controversy: The Link between Information Technology and Quality of Care

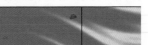

This study explored the relationship between information technology (IT) adoption and quality of care in acute care hospitals. Data from 98 hospitals in Florida were available for analyses. Sources of data included an IT survey of hospitals between May and October 2003 and hospital administrative discharge data obtained from the Florida agency responsible for hospital licensure.

STUDY FINDINGS
In multivariate regression analyses, hospitals that had adopted a greater number of IT applications were significantly more likely to have desirable quality outcomes on seven inpatient quality indicators, including risk-adjusted mortality from percutaneous transluminal coronary angio-plasty, gastrointestinal hemorrhage, and acute myocardial infarction. An increase in clinical IT applications was also inversely correlated with utilization of incidental appendectomy, and an increase in the adoption of strategic IP was inversely correlated with risk-adjusted mortality from craniotomy and laparoscopic cholecystectomy.

Source: Menachemi, N., Chukmaitov, A., Saunders, C., & Brooks, R. G. (2008). Hospital quality of care: Does information technology matter? The relationship between information technology adoption and quality of care. *Health Care Management Review, 33*(1), 51–59.

equals 10^{18} bytes) (Malik, 2008). In addition, Cisco predicts that "monthly global internet provider (IP) traffic in December 2012 will be 11 exabytes higher than in December 2011, a single-year increase that will exceed the amount by which traffic has increased in the eight years since 2000" (para 1) and that "mobile data traffic will roughly double each year from 2008 through 2012" (para 4).

The Effect of the Internet on Provider–Patient Relationships

Historically, providers were recognized as the keepers of medical information. This allowed them to be the primary health care decision maker, often relegating patients to a somewhat passive and dependent role. The Internet has, however, changed these dynamics because it has expanded the power and control of health information from providers alone to patients themselves. Indeed, the Internet, which is growing faster than any other medium in the world, has great potential to improve Americans' health by enhancing communications and improving access to information for care providers, patients, health plan administrators, public health officials, biomedical researchers, and other health professionals.

Indeed, Tanaka (2008) suggested that there are 2,265 health information Web sites for consumers to explore in attempting to answer their health-related questions. This number doubled since 2005, and, all told, such health sites had 69 million U.S. visitors in the month of July 2008 alone (Tanaka).

Lorence and Park (2008) warned, however, that little research has been done to differentiate levels of health information access on the Web by different subgroups, linking online socioeconomic characteristics and health-seeking behaviors. Their analysis of a landmark Pew Foundation survey suggested that a persistent "digitally underserved group" does exist that must be addressed. Until then, they argued, the chances for implementation of a consumer-focused, shared decision-making model are limited.

The "Expert Patient"

The Internet has also changed health care access, education, and information sharing. Most individuals with Internet access use the Internet to search for health care information. In fact, a study by Harrison and Lee (2006) found that "86% of adults with Internet access have used it for health-related information, and health queries represent 37% of their total internet usage" (p. 283). In addition, 50% of the respondents in Harrison and Lee's study "demonstrated significant interest in accessing their own medical information via the Internet" (p. 283).

The end result is that patients have electronic access to medical information on virtually any topic, any time. This suggests that many consumers have at least the opportunity to be better informed about their health care problems and needs than in the past. In fact, this increased opportunity for consumers to access information has resulted in the creation of what is known as the "*expert patient*"—a patient who has the confidence, skills, information, and knowledge to participate in his or her health care.

Theoretically, expert patients are better informed and thus better able to be active participants in decision making. Although most providers appreciate well-informed patients who have demonstrated the initiative to learn more about their health care needs and problems, there are concerns regarding the accuracy and currency of information patients find on the Internet. In addition, many patients do not fully understand the information that is available to them, even when it is accurate. Some providers are concerned that patients will inappropriately self-diagnose, leading them to seek inappropriate treatment or no treatment at all. A smaller number of providers simply do not want to share decision-making power with patients.

> ### DISCUSSION POINT
> Empowering patients and involving them in their health care decision making is a socially encouraged value in health care today. Do you believe that most providers value and appreciate having increased numbers of "expert patients"?

Students in health care programs must be taught to not only recognize patient expertise, but also to actively encourage and support it. Finally, patients will need to become experts at retrieving health care information and deciphering it to better empower themselves in health care decision making.

Nursing Informatics

Handling access to virtually unlimited information via the Internet has been a challenging transition for both patients and providers. As a result, new nursing specialties have emerged, including *nursing informatics* (NI). In fact, the use of nursing informatics (NI) was identified by the Institute of Medicine as one of the skills and competencies required by health care professionals in the 21st century (McDaniel and White Delaney, 2007).

NI is a specialty that integrates nursing science, computer science, and information science to manage and communicate data, information, and knowledge in nursing practice. The International Medical Informatics Association Interest Group on Nursing Informatics (2007, para 1) defined NI as "the integration of nursing, its information, and information management with information processing and communication technology, to support the health of people worldwide."

Kreimer (2007) suggested that *nurse informaticists,* also known as *clinical nurse informaticists,* are typically involved in the implementation of EHRs and that at least 75% of nurse informaticists are developing or implementing clinical information or documentation systems. Kreimer (para 11) also pointed out that such "carefully crafted electronic systems help improve interdisciplinary communication, whereas poorly designed systems can contribute to prescription errors and other medical mistakes." The competency of the informatics nurse is critical.

Such competency, has not, however, historically been guaranteed by advanced education. Before the American Nurses Associations' designation of NI as a specialty in 1992, most nurses involved in informatics were self-educated. Many NI specialists simply adopted the title when they were appointed to serve as a nurse member of a hospital information system team (The HIMSS Nursing Informatics Awareness Task Force, 2008). In 1988, however, the first graduate program in nursing informatics was established at the University of Maryland School of Nursing in Baltimore, and numerous other graduate programs have proliferated since then.

Most nurse informaticists, however, do not hold graduate degrees. Many do hold an informatics nurse specialist certification, which became available from the American Nurses Credentialing Center in 1995. Requirements to take the certification exam include a baccalaureate or higher degree; an active Registered Nurse license with at least 2 years of professional practice; and experience of at least 2,000 hours of NI within the last 3 years, or 12 hours of graduate work and 1,000 hours of NI practice, or completion of a graduate program in NI that includes at least 200 clinical hours or practicum (The HIMSS Nursing Informatics Awareness Task Force, 2008).

> ### CONSIDER
> Informatic theories and competencies are now being incorporated into many basic nursing associate degree and baccalaureate curriculums (The HIMSS Nursing Informatics Awareness Task Force, 2008).

Brokel (2007) stated that three approaches are being used to promote NI competency: the first is an academic education at the master's or doctorate level with focused courses in health and NI; the second is professional membership education, including attendance at workshops, institutes, and certification programs; and the third is self-education that includes networking opportunities available through vendor-user conferences, list serves, or Web sites where members of professional informatics organizations share experiences (p. 12).

McDaniel and White Delaney (2007) suggested, however, that this multipronged approach and not requiring NI scholars to earn graduate degrees has been costly and suboptimal and has resulted in a low output of research-productive scholars:

> *For over 15 years, nurses who sought research training in nursing informatics had only two options; an apprenticeship model of training with one of the few informatics scholars at a PhD granting institution, or training within a Medical Informatics PhD program. At best, the apprenticeship model produces 2–3 graduates a year nationally (McDaniel and White Delaney, p. 115).*

The majority of Medical Informatics programs are in locations without doctoral programs in nursing, although Columbia University was noted as an exception (McDaniel and White Delaney).

The TIGER Initiative
In an effort to enable all nurses and student nurses to fully engage in health care's emerging digital era, the first Technology Informatics Guiding Education Reform (TIGER) Summit was held in fall 2006. Seven critical components for enabling nurses to use informatics in practice and education to provide safer, higher-quality care were defined and ranked (Sensmeier, 2007).

The seven recommendations and action steps were as follows:

1. Fully engaging in health information technology (HIT) standards and interoperability development

2. Fully engaging in the national HIT agenda, working specifically with the Office of the National Coordinator

3. Creating comprehensive informatics competencies for all areas of nursing

4. Reforming educational curriculum, faculty, and program development

5. Creating innovative and effective staff development/continuing education programs

6. Improving clinical applications used by nurses

7. Creating a demonstration gallery/center to showcase best practices

Sensmeier (2007, p. 8) suggested that "the TIGER Initiative has the potential to transform nursing education and practice into an automated, information-rich, consumer-driven healthcare environment" but warned that all nurses must get involved for this to happen.

CONCLUSIONS

Noor (2007) suggested that 21st-century cyber-infrastructure will likely evolve into an electronic care continuum with pervasive access to global, accurate,

and timely medical knowledge for individuals about their health needs in an era of rapid change and expanding knowledge. Clearly, evolving technologies offer great opportunities to improve the quality of patient care, but technology alone is not the answer. Regardless of the system that is deployed, health care organizations must consider what technology can best be used in each individual setting and how it should be used. In addition, successfully adopting and integrating new technology will require that care providers understand that technology's limitations as well as its benefits.

Debates about how best to merge the human element of care (caring) and technology will continue. Historically, machines have been unable to demonstrate caring, although the development of new robotic devices is challenging this long-held belief.

Nurses also need to overcome their "technophobia" because, clearly, care can be improved with the appropriate use of technology and, ironically, it is technology that will likely give nurses more time to do "nursing." Nurses must therefore keep the improvement of patient care first and foremost in their technology development agenda. In addition, nurses must embrace the use of technology as part of the skill set that will be expected of nurses in the 21st century.

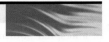

FOR ADDITIONAL DISCUSSION

1. Is there a place for technology development in health care, even when it does not contribute to the improvement of patient outcomes? In other words, should the technology itself ever be the desired goal?

2. Are nursing schools adequately preparing students with the skill sets and competencies they will need to function successfully in a progressively more technological workplace?

3. How should organizations deal with "technophobic" nurses? Should health care employers let nurses decide what level of expertise they wish to acquire?

4. What safeguards are in place to assure confidentiality of the electronic health record? Do you believe confidentiality is greater with electronic or paper records?

5. What technology do you believe has the greatest potential to reduce the current nursing shortage? Why?

6. What technologies currently in use would you predict to be obsolete in 10 years?

7. What barriers exist in health care environments that will impede the development of technology in years to come?

8. What safeguards do consumers have that the health information they find on the Internet is accurate and appropriate?

REFERENCES

Andrews, J. (2006). *Biometrics leaves imprint on healthcare.* Available at: http://www.healthcareitnews.com/story.cms?id=4916. Accessed August 12, 2008.

Analysis: Integrated smart card, biometric technology market expected to soar. (2008). Available at: http://www.secprodonline.com/articles/59570/. Accessed August 13, 2008.

Ash, J. S., Sittig, D. F., Poon, E. G., Guappone, K., Campbell, E., & Dykstra, R. H. (2007). The extent and importance of unintended consequences related to computerized provider order entry. *Journal of the American Medical Informatics Association, 14*(4), 415–423.

Bensink, M., Hailey, D., & Wotton, R. (2007). A systematic review of successes and failures in home telehealth. Part 2: Final quality rating results. *Journal of Telemedicine & Telecare, 2007,* S3:10–S3:14.

Boivin, J., & Williams, S. (2008). From toyland to the real world. *NurseWeek (California), 21*(5), 38–39.

Bordowitz, R. (2008). Electronic health records: A primer. *Laboratory Medicine, 39*(5), 301–307.

Brokel, J. Creating sustainability of clinical information systems (2007). *Journal of Nursing Administration, 37*(1), 10–13.

Brumson, B. (2008). Robots for life. *Laboratory, medical and life science applications.* Available at: http://www.robotics.org/content-detail.cfm/Industrial-Robotics-Feature-Articles/Robots-for-Life:-Laboratory-Medical-and-Life-Science-Applications/ content_id/605. Accessed August 12, 2008.

Christensen, B. (n.d.) Kansei robot reacts to words like 'president,' 'pushi'. Available at: http://www.technovelgy.com/ct/Science-Fiction-News.asp?NewsNum=1072. Accessed August 7, 2008.

CPOE still a priority, but... .... adoption rates vary according to who's asking (2008). *Modern Healthcare, 38*(8), S5.

DesRoches, C. M., Campbell, E. G., Rao, S. R., Donelan, K., Ferris, T. G., Jha, A., Kaushal, R., Levy, D. E., Rosenbaum, S., Shields, A. E., & Blumenthal, D. (2008). Electronic health records in ambulatory care—A national survey of physicians. *New England Journal of Medicine, 359*(1):50–60.

Domrose, C. (2004). Working smart. *NurseWeek, 17*(6), 13–15.

Express Healthcare (2008). *Point of care testing.* Available at: http://www.expresshealthcaremgmt.com/200805/market26.shtml. Accessed August 11, 2008.

Fahy, J. (2008). UPMC testing 'smart' rooms; Six rooms at UPMC Shadyside are equipped with computer screens that keep doctors and patients informed. *Pittsburgh Post-Gazette,* January 16, 2008, p. A.1.

Fonda, S. J., Bursell, S. E., Lewis, D. G., Garren, J., Hock, K., & Cavallerano, J. (2007). The relationship of a diabetes telehealth eye care program to standard eye care and change in diabetes health outcomes. *Telemedicine Journal and e-Health, 13*(6), 635–644.

Goldstein, J. (2008). Hospital bar codes not a perfect Rx. *The Philadelphia Inquirer.* Available at: http://www.philly.com/inquirer/front_page/20080701_Hospital_bar_codes_not_a_perfect_Rx.html. Accessed August 13, 2008.

Hahn, T., & Whitbeck, E. (2007). Smart pumps and synergy. *IT Solutions. Supplement, 2007*(September), 27–28.

Harrison, J. P., & Lee, A. (2006). The role of e-health in the changing health care environment. *Nursing Economics, 24*(6), 283–289.

Hatler, C. (2008). How intelligent are smart beds? *Nursing Management, 39*(2), 20–26.

Health Connect (2006). *Introduction.* Available at: http://www.health.gov.au/internet/hconnect/publishing.nsf/Content/intro. Accessed April 20, 2008.

Healthcare Information and Management Systems Society (2008). *Clinical decision support.* Available at: http://www.himss.org/ASP/topics_clinicalDecision.asp. Accessed April 21, 2008.

Healthcare Packaging (2008). *Robotic Rx for pharmaceutical packaging.* Available at: http://www.healthcare-packaging.com/archives/2008/03/robotic_rx_for_pharmaceutical_1.php. Accessed August 11, 2008.

Hurley, A. C., Bane, A., Fotakis, S., Duffy, M. E., Sevigny, A., Poon, E. G., & Gandhi, T. K. (2007). Nurses' satisfaction with medication administration point-of-care technology. *Journal of Nursing Administration, 37*(7/8), 343–349.

Igbokwe, O. (2007). *Wireless technology and healthcare.* Available at: http://www.biohealthmatics.com/Articles/0000000016.aspx. Accessed August 14, 2008.

Kreimer, S. (2007) *Nurses bridge gap between IT, care.* Available at: http://www.dallasnews.com/sharedcon tent/dws/classifieds/news/jobcenter/news/stories/ DN-informatics_29emp.ART.State.Edition1.4320696. html. Accessed August 13, 2008.

Leapfrog fact sheet. Computerized physician order entry (2008). Available at: http://www.leapfroggroup.org/ media/file/Leapfrog-Computer_Physician_Order_ Entry_Fact_Sheet.pdf. Accessed August 14, 2008.

Lee, D. (2008). *Improving healthcare with a card. Community health program offers patients tech tools, convenience.* Available at: http://www.indystar.com/ apps/pbcs.dll/article?AID=/20080807/BUSI NESS/808070393. Accessed August 17, 2008.

Lorence, D., & Park, H. (2008). Group disparities and health information: A study of online access for the underserved. *Health Informatics Journal, 14*(1), 29–38.

Malik, O. (2008). *Big growth for the internet ahead, Cisco says.* Available at: http://gigaom.com/2008/06/16/ big-growth-for-internet-to-continue-cisco-pre dicts/. Accessed August 13, 2008.

Malloch, K. (2007). The electronic health record: An essential tool for advancing patient safety. *Nursing Outlook, 55*(3), 159–161.

McDaniel, A. M., & White Delaney, C. (2007). Training scientists in the nursing informatics research agenda. *Nursing Outlook, 55*(2), 115–116.

McNicol, T. (2008). *Robots lend a hand in Japan.* Available at: http://www.roboticstrends.com/personal_ robotics/article/robots_lend_a_hand_in_japan/. Accessed August 7, 2008.

Menachemi, N., Chukmaitov, A., Saunders, C., & Brooks, R. G. (2008). Hospital quality of care: Does information technology matter? The relationship between information technology adoption and quality of care. *Health Care Management Review, 33*(1), 51–59.

Meneses, K. D., & McNees, P. (2007). Transdisciplinary integration of electronic communication technology and nursing research. *Nursing Outlook, 55*(5), 242–249.

Most wired (2008). TMCNet.com. Available at: http://www.tmcnet.com/usubmit/2008/08/14/ 3600707.htm. Accessed August 14, 2008.

NHS Connecting for Health (2008). *GP2GP reaches 100,000 transfers.* Available at: http://www.connect ingforhealth.nhs.uk/newsroom/news-stories/ gp2gp100k?searchterm=electronic+health+record. Accessed April 20, 2008.

Noor, A. (2007). Re-engineering healthcare. *Mechanical Engineering, 129*(11), 22–27.

Nelson, A. (2003). Using simulation to design and integrate technology for safer and more efficient practice environments. *Nursing Outlook, 51*(3), S27–S29.

Nuckols, T., Bower, A., Paddock, S., Hilborne, L., Wallace, P., Rothschild, J. M., Griffin, A., Fairbanks, R. J., Carlson, B., Panzer, R. J., & Brook, R. H. (2008). Programmable infusion pumps in ICUs: An analysis of corresponding adverse drug events. *Journal of General Internal Medicine, 23*(S1), 41–45.

Office of the Assistant Secretary of the Defense (Health Affairs) and the TRICARE Management Activity (2008). *AHLTA—Electronic health records.* Available at: http://www.ha.osd.mil/AHLTA/. Accessed April 13, 2008.

Pooley, E. (2006). Health's digital divide: Electronic health records. *Canadian Business Magazine.* Available at: http://www.canadianbusiness.com/technology/ companies/article.jsp?content=20060213_ 74576_74576. Accessed April 21, 2008.

Prinz, L., Cramer, M., & Englund, A. (2008). Telehealth: A policy analysis for quality, impact on patient outcomes, and political feasibility. *Nursing Outlook, 56*(4), 152–258.

Robotics Trends (2008). *First steps toward autonomous robot surgeries.* Available at: http://www.robotic strends.com/home/features/first_steps_toward_ autonomous_robot_surgeries/. Accessed August 7, 2008.

Scharfe-Pretino, T., & Von Bacho, S. (2008). Nursing intranet web site: A critical communication tool. *Journal of Nursing Care Quality, 21*(2), 104–109.

Sensmeier, J. (2007). The future of IT? Aggressive educational reform. *IT Solutions. Supplement, 2007,* 2–8.

Service Robotics (2008). *Aethon's autonomous mobile robotic system provides complete asset utilization solution.* Available at: http://www.roboticstrends.com/ service_robotics/article/aethons_mobile_robotic_ system/. Accessed August 6, 2008.

Smart cards integrated with biometrics to provide cost-effective and secure solutions... (2008). Reuters, February 21, 2008. Available at: http://www.reuters.com/ article/pressRelease/idUS31045+22-Feb-2008+ BW20080222. Accessed August 13, 2008.

Tanaka, W. (2008). *Health tips on your iPhone.* Available at: http://www.forbes.com/technology/ 2008/08/25/healthy-web-sites-tech-personal- cx_wt_0825health.html. Accessed August 26, 2008.

Telehealth cuts readmissions of patients with chronic illness. (2008). *Hospitals & Health Networks, 82*(6), 63.

The Advisory Board Company. (2006). *Wired hospital 2020. Diagnosis decision support.* Clinical Advisory Board Interviews and Analysis. Available at: http://us.isabelhealthcare.com/info/images/14461_CAB_44-47.pdf. Accessed April 21, 2008.

The HIMSS Nursing Informatics Awareness Task Force (2008). An emerging giant: Nursing informatics. *Nursing Management, 38*(3), 38–42.

The International Medical Informatics Association Interest Group on Nursing Informatics (2007). *Definition–Informatics.* Available at: http://www.imiani.org/. Accessed August 28, 2008.

Vlasses, F. R., & Smeltzer, C. H. (2007). Toward a new future for healthcare and nursing practice. *Journal of Nursing Administration, 37*(9), 375–380.

Whitten, P., & Mickus, M. (2007). Home telecare for COPD/CHF patients: Outcomes and perceptions. *Journal of Telemedicine and Telecare, 13*(2), 69–73.

BIBLIOGRAPHY

Alegent Health Home Care and Hospice, Omaha, NE (2008). Home health outcomes in a CHF population: A study of patients on telehealth vs. patients not on telehealth. *Remington Report, 16*(3), 22–24.

Banks, M. R., Willoughby, L. M., & Banks, W. A. (2008). Animal-assisted therapy and loneliness in nursing homes: Use of robotic versus living dogs. *Journal of the American Medical Directors Association, 9*(3), 173–177.

Barker, K., Amaral, E., & Idleman, D. (2007). Long-range planning and physician involvement lead to a successful CPOE implementation at a Maryland Health System. *Health Management Technology, 28*(11), 30–31.

Boissy, P., Corriveau, H., Michaud, F., Labonte, D., & Royer, M. (2007). A qualitative study of in-home robotic telepresence for home care of community-living elderly subjects. *Journal of Telemedicine & Telecare, 13*(2), 79–84.

Buckles Prince, S., & Herrin, D. M. (2007). The role of information technology in healthcare communications, efficiency, and patient safety. *Journal of Nursing Administration, 37*(4), 184–187.

Denmark, D. (2008). The evidence-based advantage: The proper use of EBM in CPOE can enhance physician decision-making and improve patient outcomes. *Health Management Technology, 29*(3), 22, 24–25, 29. Available at: http://findarticles.com/p/articles/mi_m0DUD/is_3_29/ai_n24923700?tag=artBody;col1. Accessed January 20, 2009.

Doc spearheads adoption of CPOE, early-warning system (2008). *Modern Healthcare, 38*(28), 34.

Fuji, L. (2008). Robotic telepresence for collaborative clinical outreach. *Studies in Health Technology and Informatics, 132,* 233–235.

Goedert, J. (2008). *The role document management will play in EHRs.* Health Data Management. Available at: http://www.healthdatamanagement.com/issues/2008_55/26712-1.html?CMP=OTC-RSS. Accessed August 17, 2008.

Koch, N., Racela, J., & Ruiz, S. (2008). Jumping to solutions: Implementing a structured "look before you leap" discovery process can lead to successful IT adoption. *Health Management Technology, 29*(3), 28, 30–31.

Koeniger-Donohue, R., & Bisbee, S. L. (2007). Optimizing clinical use of handheld technology: PDAs for NPs. *American Journal for Nurse Practitioners, 11*(5), 22–23.

Mace, S. (2008). Getting the message. *NurseWeek, 21*(14), 20.

Meyers, S. (2007). Robots become RN's little helpers. *NurseWeek, 8*(3), 12–13.

McGowan, J. J., Cusack, C. M., & Poon, E. G. (2008). Formative evaluation: A critical component in EHR implementation. *Journal of the American Medical Informatics Association, 15*(3), 297–301.

McGraw, A. (2008). A nurse's informatics wish list. *Computers, Informatics, Nursing, 26*(3), 129–131.

Mitchell, G. J. (2007). Picturing the nurse-person/family/community process in the year 2050. *Nursing Science Quarterly, 20*(1), 43–44.

Moses, G. R., & Doarn, C. R. (2008). Barriers to wider adoption of mobile telerobotic surgery: Engineering, clinical and business challenges.

Studies in Health Technology and Informatics, 132, 308–312.

Ross, C., & Banchy, P. (2007). They key to CPOE: Thoughtful planning, flexible training and strong staff involvement leads to a successful CPOE implementation. *Health Management Technology, 28*(11), 22, 24, 28.

Scollin, P., Healey-Walsh, J., Kafel, K., Mehta, A., & Callahan, J. (2007). Evaluating students' attitudes to using PDAs in nursing clinicals at two schools. *Computers, Informatics, Nursing, 25*(4), 228–235.

Shamir, L. (2008). Evaluation of face datasets as tools for assessing the performance of face recognition methods. *International Journal of Computer Vision, 79*(3), 225–230.

Sroga, J., Patel, S. D., & Falcone, T. (2008). Robotics in reproductive medicine. *Frontiers in Bioscience, 13,* 1308–1317.

Sunil, K., Kashyap, K., Fei, H., Mark, L., & Yang, X. (2008). Ubiquitous computing for remote cardiac patient monitoring: A survey. *International Journal of Telemedicine and Applications.* Article ID 459185. Available at: http://www.hindawi.com/GetArticle. aspx?doi=10.1155/2008/459185. Accessed January 20, 2009.

Vasquez, M. (2008). Down to the fundamentals of telehealth and home healthcare nursing. *Home Healthcare Nurse, 26*(5), 280–289.

Vincent, A., Caitlin, M., Pan, E., Hook, J. M., Kaelber, D., & Middleton, B. (2007). A new taxonomy for telehealth technologies. *AMIA 2007 Annual Symposium Proceedings, 2007*(October 11), 1145.

Websites on pain a minefield of misinformation (2008). *Bone & Joint, 14*(7), 82.

WEB RESOURCES

American Nursing Informatics Association	http://www.ania.org
American Telemedicine Association	http://www.atmeda.org
Association of Telehealth Service Providers	http://www.atsp.org
Canadian Society of Telehealth	http://www.cst-sct.org
Health Care and Intellectual Property	http://www.cptech.org/ip/health/
Healthcare Information and Management Systems Society	http://www.himss.org/ASP/index.asp
Health Technology Advisory Committee	http://www.health.state.mn.us/htac/
HIPAAdvisory	http://www.hipaadvisory.com
HIPAAlert	http://www.hipaadvisory.com/alert/
Medical Privacy	http://www.epic.org/privacy/medical/
Medical Records Institute	http://medrecinst.com
HRSA Office for the Advancement of Telehealth	http://telehealth.hrsa.gov
TelehealthNet	http://telehealth.net
Telemedicine Information Exchange	http://tie.telemed.org

CHAPTER 14

Medical Errors: An Ongoing Threat to Quality Health Care

• CAROL J. HUSTON •

Learning Objectives

The learner will be able to:

1. Differentiate among the terms *medical error*, *medication error*, and *adverse event*.
2. Described highly publicized patient cases from the mid to the late 1990s, as well as seminal research studies that brought national attention to the problem of medical errors in the United States.
3. Explore current research studies examining the scope, common causes, and financial/human costs of medical errors in the United States.
4. Summarize key findings of the 1999 Institute of Medicine (IOM) report *To Err is Human*, as well as the multipronged approach identified by the IOM to address the problem of medical errors in the United States.
5. Identify the national committees and groups formed as a result of governmental or legislative intervention after the 1999 IOM report to address the problem of medical errors.
6. Describe the intent and impact of Medicare's Pay for Performance (P4P) initiatives, as well as Medicare's 2008 decision to no longer reimburse health care providers for care needed as the result of "never events" or other preventable errors.
7. Differentiate between workplaces that emphasize a "culture of blame" and those that seek to provide a "culture of safety management."

8. Identify the meaning of a six-sigma error failure rate and determine how commonly acceptable error rates in health care compare with other industries such as banking and the airlines.
9. Analyze the effect of the medical liability system on systematic efforts to uncover and learn from mistakes that are made in health care.
10. Differentiate among the three evidence-based standards identified by Leapfrog as having the greatest potential to reduce medical errors: computerized physician order entry (CPOE), evidence-based hospital referral (EHR), and intensive care unit physician staffing (IPS).
11. Track current federal and state legislative efforts that encourage the voluntary reporting of health care errors by affording confidentiality protections for such reports.
12. Review current research to determine whether organizational, governmental, and national efforts to reduce the incidence of medical errors in the United States have resulted in desired outcomes.
13. Reflect on the likelihood that he or she would self-report his or her medical errors to his or her employer, as well as to the involved patients and families.

Quality health care has emerged as a critically important yet underachieved goal in the United States. Among the most significant threats to achieving quality health care are the scope and prevalence of medical errors.

Although medical errors have surely occurred since medicine began, the problem in the United States did not receive nationwide attention until several highly publicized cases in the mid 1990s. One such case involved Betsy Lehman, a *Boston Globe* reporter who died following multiple chemotherapy administration errors. The news media jumped on the story because it demonstrated repeated widespread communication and dispensing errors, despite multiple safeguards in place to keep them from happening.

Libby Zion's case occurred about this same time. Zion, 18 years old, died 8 hours after entering a New York emergency department with seemingly minor complaints of fever and earache. Her death from drug interactions brought attention both to the all-too-narrow range between effective and toxic doses of some drugs and the danger of drug–drug interactions, even when all drugs are administered in doses that are considered safe when administered individually. The case also brought attention to the lack of supervision of residents and interns in the United States, as well as the excessive work hours forced on them and the errors that occur as a result.

Finally, there was the story of Willie King, a diabetic man from Tampa, Florida, who had the wrong leg amputated. This case, which became known as the "wrong leg" case, captured the collective dread of wrong-site surgery, but it is a medical error that occurs too frequently as a result of the symmetry of the human body.

DISCUSSION POINT

Do you believe that the general public considers itself to be at risk for harm when receiving health care? Do you personally know someone who has been harmed by a medical error?

Perhaps it was the clustering of these high-profile cases that made Americans stop and look at the problem of medical errors, or maybe it was just time to do so. The end result was that an unprecedented number of seminal research studies delving into medical errors were undertaken in the late 1990s that attempted to discover how many errors were occurring, what was causing them, and what their financial and human costs were.

The results were disconcerting, to say the least. Most studies highlighted multiple concerns about quality of care, including high rates of provider-induced injury, unnecessary care, and inappropriate care. Many studies found the number of errors in health care to be unacceptably high. The seminal study of this time, *To Err Is Human*, published in 1999 by the Institute of Medicine (IOM), a congressionally chartered independent organization, provided evidence that the public was highly vulnerable to human error

in U.S. health care institutions, an arena in which many thought they were safe.

In addition, unlike most health care research, which generally receives little if any national press, medical error research findings in the late 1990s were published and analyzed in almost every media forum in the country. Consumers were barraged with study findings suggesting that the quality of health care was inadequate and that medical errors were a significant problem leading to increased morbidity and mortality.

DISCUSSION POINT

Do you believe that the quality of health care has declined in the last few decades, or is it simply better monitored and more openly reported today?

As a result, consumers, providers, and legislators stepped forward to voice their concerns and to demand, at minimum, a safer health care system. The government listened and directed providers to re-examine how quality health care was provided, measured, and monitored so that cultures of safety could be developed in all health care organizations.

This chapter examines seminal and current research on medical errors, medication errors, and adverse events, as well as the directives that emerged as a result of their findings. Mechanisms for achieving four goals put forth by the IOM as part of *To Err Is Human* are identified. Finally, strategies for creating a culture of safety management in health care are identified, as are the challenges of changing a system that all too often focuses on individual errors rather than on the need to make system-wide changes.

DEFINING TERMS: MEDICAL ERRORS, MEDICATION ERRORS, AND ADVERSE EVENTS

In reviewing the literature on medical errors, medication errors, and adverse events in health care, it is helpful to first define common terms. *Medical errors* are defined as "incorrect actions or plans that may or may not cause harm to a patient" (Ghimire, 2008, para 4). A Henry J. Kaiser Family Foundation (2008, para 3) study showed that "after being read a common definition of medical errors, about one-third of Americans (34%) reported that they had been personally involved in a situation where a preventable medical error was made in their own care or that of a family member."

Medication errors are defined by the National Coordinating Council for Medication Error Reporting and Prevention (NCC MERP) as:

Any preventable event that may cause or lead to inappropriate medication use or patient harm while the medication is in the control of the health care professional, patient, or consumer. Such events may be related to professional practice, health care products, procedures, and systems, including prescribing; order communication; product labeling, packaging, and nomenclature; compounding; dispensing; distribution; administration; education; monitoring; and use" (NCC MERP, 1998-2008, para 1).

The Joint Commission (2008a) reported that errors associated with medications are believed to be the most common type of medical error and are a significant cause of preventable adverse events. A recent IOM study confirmed this report, suggesting that 7,000 patients die each year from medication errors, and another 450,000 adverse drug events are linked to preventable medication errors (Aspden, Wolcott, Bootman, & Cronenwett, 2007).

Finally, *adverse events* are defined as "injuries to patients occurring during medical management, not necessarily because of an error" (Ghimire, 2008, para 4). A recent study by Weissman et al. (2008) suggested that postdischarge, patients in interviews report many adverse events that are not documented in the medical record; some are serious and preventable.

SEMINAL RESEARCH ON MEDICAL ERRORS: 1990 TO 2000

The last decade of the 20th century was marked by a rapid increase in research on medical errors. One of the earliest large-scale studies suggesting that medical errors were a significant problem in health care was published by Brennan et al. (1991) in the *New England Journal of Medicine*. This benchmark study involved more than 30,000 hospital patients in New York State. Nearly 5 of every 100 patients suffered an adverse event caused by a medical error of omission or commission. Of these adverse events, approximately one in four involved negligence. The overwhelming majority of iatrogenic

occurrences, however, resulted from organization, system, or process failures.

This study, extrapolated to the national population, suggested that 1.3 million people were injured each year in hospitals; of that number, 180,000 would die from those injuries. Providing additional cause for alarm, the report also suggested that most of those injuries were actually preventable.

Leape et al. (1991) also reported that drug complications represented 19% of these adverse events, and that 45% of these adverse events were caused by medical errors. In this study, 30% of the individuals with drug-related injuries died.

In another study, Leape (1994) reported that the average intensive care unit (ICU) patient experienced almost two errors per day. One of five of these errors was potentially serious or fatal. In fact, this translates into a level of proficiency of approximately 99%, which seems reasonable. However, if performance levels of 99.9%—substantially better than those found in the ICU by Leape—were applied to the airline and banking industries, it would equate to two dangerous landings per day at Chicago's O'Hare International Airport, or 32,000 checks deducted hourly from the wrong account (Leape).

CONSIDER
The safety record in health care is a far cry from the enviable record of the similarly complex aviation industry.

DISCUSSION POINT
Should the health care industry be willing to accept higher error rates than the banking or airline industries? Why or why not? Is the public willing to do so?

Another seminal study in the late 1990s involving medical errors was completed by Thomas et al. (1999). Their research, based on a chart review of 14,732 medical records from 28 hospitals in Colorado and Utah, found that 265 of 459 (57%) adverse events were preventable. The total cost of adverse events was $661,889,000, with preventable adverse events costing an additional $308,382,000. In addition, the study estimated the national costs of all preventable adverse events to be just under $17 billion (in 1996 dollars).

A recent study by Pappas (2008) of 3,200 inpatients also underscored the cost of medical errors. This study found that the actual direct cost of an adverse event was $1,029 per case in congestive heart failure cases and $903 in surgical cases. There was also a significant increase in the cost per case in medical patients with urinary tract infections and pressure ulcers.

> ### CONSIDER
> Patient safety incidents cost the federal Medicare program alone $8.8 billion between 2004 and 2006 and resulted in 238,337 potentially preventable deaths (HealthGrades, 2008).

To Err Is Human

Many of the studies done in the 1990s laid the foundation for what is perhaps the best-known and largest study ever done on the quality of health care: *To Err Is Human* (Kohn, Corrigan, & Donaldson, 2000). This report, which represented a compilation of more than 30 studies completed by the IOM, found that:

- At least 44,000 Americans die each year as a result of medical errors, and the number may be as high as 98,000.

- Even when using the lower estimate, deaths due to medical errors could be considered the eighth-leading cause of death in 1999.

- More people die in a given year as a result of medical errors than from motor vehicle accidents, breast cancer, or AIDS.

The IOM study also examined the types of errors that were occurring. Many of the adverse events were associated with the use of pharmaceutical agents and were potentially preventable. Medication errors alone, both in and out of the hospital, were estimated to account for more than 7,000 deaths in 1993, and 1 of every 854 inpatient hospital deaths was the result of a medication error. Children experienced harmful medication errors three times more often than adults (5.7% of medication orders for pediatric patients), and the rate was higher yet for neonates in the neonatal intensive care unit. In addition, ICU patients suffered more life-threatening medication errors than any other patient population.

> ### CONSIDER
> "Experts agree that medication errors have the potential to cause harm within the pediatric population at a higher rate than in the adult population. For example, medication dosing errors are more common in pediatrics than adults because of weight-based dosing calculations, fractional dosing (e.g., mg vs. Gm), and the need for decimal points" (Joint Commission, 2008a, para 1).

Within a short time of the IOM report's release, some people began to question the numbers, asking whether the problem of medical errors could be as serious as it seemed. The first study to reliably confirm the IOM figures was a 2004 study by the health care ratings company HealthGrades (2004). This study looked at 3 years of Medicare data in all 50 states and Washington, D.C., and reported that approximately 1.14 million patient safety incidents (PSIs) occurred among the 37 million hospitalizations in the Medicare population for the study period. The most commonly occurring PSIs were failure to rescue, decubitus ulcer, and postoperative sepsis.

Of the total 323,993 deaths among Medicare patients in those years who developed one or more patient-safety incidents, 263,864, or 81%, of these deaths were directly attributable to the incidents (HealthGrades, 2004). In addition, one in every four Medicare patients who were hospitalized from 2000 to 2002 and experienced a patient-safety incident died. Perhaps most startling, however, was the conclusion that the United States loses more lives to patient safety incidents every 6 months than it did in the entire Vietnam War. This also equates to three fully loaded jumbo jets crashing every other day for the last 5 years. Finally, the study noted that if the Centers for Disease Control and Prevention's annual list of leading causes of death included medical errors, it would show up as number six, ahead of diabetes, pneumonia, Alzheimer's disease, and renal disease (HealthGrades).

A follow up report by the IOM in 2006 also confirmed the scope of medical errors identified in *To Err is Human*. This report, *Preventing Medication Errors*, suggested that medication errors were surprisingly common and costly to the nation. The report concluded that at least 1.5 million preventable adverse drug events occur in the United States each year and that "changes from doctors, nurses, pharmacists, and others in the health care industry, from the Food and Drug Administration (FDA) and other government agencies, from hospitals and other health-care organizations, and from patients" would be necessary to decrease the prevalence of these errors (National Conference of State Legislatures, 2008, para 1).

DISCUSSION POINT

Is the U.S. public aware of the prevalence of medical errors? If not, what should be done to galvanize them to take action?

The Response to the Institute of Medicine Report

Within weeks of the release of *To Err is Human*, the Senate held its first hearings on the issue, and additional hearings were conducted by committees of both the House of Representatives and the Senate. Local, state, and national leaders, as well as private and public sector leaders, took immediate action. The significance of the IOM report as a catalyst for change cannot be overstated.

That said, however, it is important to note that the problems of medical errors and patient safety were not completely unrecognized before *To Err Is Human* was published. Perhaps the most significant aspect of the IOM study was that it summarized the high human cost of medical errors in language that was understandable by the general public. In addition, previously, an assumption was made that most patient injuries were the

result of negligence, incompetence, or corporate greed. The IOM report indicated, however, that errors are simply a part of the human condition and that the health care system needed to be redesigned so that fewer errors would occur.

As a result of these findings, the IOM recommended a national goal of reducing the number of medical errors by 50% over 5 years (Kohn et al., 2000). To that end, it outlined a four-pronged approach to reducing medical mistakes nationwide (Box 14.1). The strategies needed to achieve this national goal and attend to each of the four approaches are numerous, however, and only a few are detailed in this chapter.

WORKING TO ACHIEVE THE INSTITUTE OF MEDICINE GOALS

The first of the IOM's four-pronged approach to reducing medical errors was to "establish a national focus to create leadership, research, tools, and protocols to enhance the knowledge base about safety" (Kohn et al., 2000, p. 6). The second was to "raise standards and expectations for improvements in safety through the actions of oversight organizations, group purchasers, and professional groups" (p. 6). Work to achieve both of these goals began almost immediately after the IOM report was published. Indeed, a number of national committees and groups were formed as a result of governmental or legislative intervention. Some of the committees, groups, and legislative efforts spearheading the task to reduce medical errors are outlined here.

BOX 14.1 | **THE IOM'S FOUR-PRONGED APPROACH TO REDUCING MEDICAL MISTAKES NATIONWIDE**

- Establish a national focus to create leadership, research, tools, and protocols to enhance the knowledge base about safety.
- Identify and learn from medical errors through both mandatory and voluntary reporting systems.
- Raise standards and expectations for improvements in safety through the actions of oversight organizations, group purchasers, and professional groups.
- Implement safe practices at the delivery level.

Source: Kohn, L. T., Corrigan, J. M., & Donaldson, M. S. (Eds.) (2000). Executive summary (pp. 1–6). In: *To Err Is Human: Building a Safer Health System.* Available at: **http://books.nap.edu/openbook.php?record_id=9728&page=R1.** Accessed August 15, 2008.

Quality Interagency Coordination Task Force

The Quality Interagency Coordination (QuIC) Task Force was established by President Bill Clinton in 1998 to coordinate federal agencies that provided health care services. In December 1999, the task force began to evaluate the IOM recommendations and develop strategies for identifying threats to patient safety and reducing medical errors.

The final report, *Doing What Counts for Patient Safety: Federal Actions to Reduce Medical Errors and Their Impact*, was delivered to the president in February 2000. The report proposed taking strong action on all of the IOM recommendations to reduce errors, implementing a system of public accountability, developing a robust knowledge base about medical errors, and changing the culture in health care organizations to promote the recognition of errors and improvement in patient safety.

The National Forum for Health Care Quality Measurement and Reporting

Consistent with the QuIC's recommendations, the National Forum for Health Care Quality Measurement and Reporting was launched by Vice President Al Gore in 2000. Known as the National Quality Forum (NQF), it is a broad-based, private, not-for-profit body that establishes standard quality measurement tools to help people better ensure the delivery of quality services (NQF, 2008a). The mission of the NQF is "to improve the quality of American healthcare by setting national priorities and goals for performance improvement, endorsing national consensus standards for measuring and publicly reporting on performance, and promoting the attainment of national goals through education and outreach programs" (NQF, 2008b, para 2).

Since its inception, the NQF has endorsed about 400 performance measures and practices, and many more are either in the early stages of development or moving through the NQF endorsement process. NQF also was the first to create a list of 27 *serious reportable events*, a list that was expanded to 28 events in 2006. In addition, the NQF Board of Directors approved expansion of their mission in 2008 to include working in partnership with other leadership organizations to establish national priorities and goals for performance measurement and public reporting (NQF, 2008c). The resultant National Priorities Partnership (NPP) includes representatives from 27 major national organizations. The first draft of their core set of national priorities is shown in Box 14.2.

Floyd D. Spence National Defense Authorization Act of 2001

In October 2000, President Clinton signed into effect the Floyd D. Spence National Defense Authorization Act (NDAA) of fiscal year 2001, specifically requiring the Department of Defense to establish a centralized process for reporting, compiling, and analyzing errors in health care within the defense health program. It also mandated the creation of a Patient Safety Center at the Armed Forces Institute of Pathology to analyze patient

---

BOX 14.2 | THE NATIONAL QUALITY FORUM'S NATIONAL PRIORITIES PARTNERSHIP GOALS

1. Engage patients and their families in managing their health and making decisions about their care.
2. Improve the health of the U.S. population.
3. Improve the safety of the U.S. health care system.
4. Guarantee appropriate and compassionate care for patients with life-limiting illnesses.
5. Ensure patients received well-coordinated care across all providers, settings, and levels of care.
6. Guarantee high-value care across acute and chronic episodes.
7. Eliminate waste while assuring the delivery of appropriate care.

Source: National Quality Forum (2008d). *National priorities partnership. Priority areas and corresponding goals*. Available at: http://www.qualityforum.org/about/NPP/assets/NPP_Goals_07_03_08.pdf. Accessed August 15, 2008.

care errors and to develop and execute plans to reduce and control those errors.

The National Patient Safety Foundation

The National Patient Safety Foundation (NPSF) was also formed in response to the IOM report. The mission of the NPSF, as amended in 2003, is to measurably improve patient safety in the delivery of health care by its efforts "to identify and create a core body of knowledge; identify pathways to apply the knowledge; develop and enhance the culture of receptivity to patient safety; raise public awareness and foster communications about patient safety; and improve the status of the Foundation and its ability to meet its goals" (NPSF, 2008, para 2). Basic tenets of the NPSF are shown in Box 14.3.

The Joint Commission

New organizations were not the only ones that responded to the recommendations of the IOM. The Joint Commission (formerly known as the Joint Commission for Accreditation of Healthcare Organizations [JCAHO]), in existence since 1951, accredits hospitals, long-term care facilities, psychiatric facilities, ambulatory care programs, and home health operations.

The Joint Commission's National Patient Safety Goals, implemented in January 2003, set forth clear, evidence-based recommendations to focus health care organizations on significant documented safety problems. These goals are updated annually for ambulatory care settings, behavioral health settings, hospitals, home care disease-specific care, laboratories, home-based care, and office-based surgery (Joint Commission, 2008b). The goals for hospitals in 2009 are shown in Box 14.4.

The Joint Commission also maintains one of the nation's most comprehensive databases of sentinel (serious adverse) events by health care professionals and their underlying causes. A *sentinel event* is defined by the Joint Commission (2008c, para 1) as "an unexpected occurrence involving death or serious physical or psychological injury, or the risk thereof. Serious injury specifically includes loss of limb or function. The phrase, 'or the risk thereof' includes any process variation for which a recurrence would carry a significant chance of a serious adverse outcome." Such events are called "sentinel" because they signal the need for immediate investigation and response. Information from the JCAHO sentinel database is regularly shared with accredited organizations to help them take appropriate steps to prevent medical errors.

Another JCAHO priority is the development of a *root cause analysis* with a plan of correction for the

---

BOX 14.3 | BASIC BELIEFS: NATIONAL PATIENT SAFETY FOUNDATION

- Patient safety is central to quality health care as reflected in the Hippocratic Oath: "Above all, do no harm."
- Prevention of injury, through early and appropriate response to evident and potential problems, is the key to patient safety.
- Continued improvement in patient safety is attainable only through establishing a culture of trust, honesty, integrity, and open communication.
- An integrated body of scientific knowledge and the infrastructure to support its development are essential to advance patient safety significantly.
- Patient involvement in continuous learning and constant communication of information among caregivers, organizations, and the general public will improve patient safety.
- The system of health care is fallible and requires fundamental change to sustainably improve patient safety.

Source: National Patient Safety Foundation (2008). *About us.* Available at: http://www.npsf.org/au/. Accessed August 16, 2008.

BOX 14.4   JOINT COMMISSION 2009 NATIONAL PATIENT SAFETY
GOALS FOR HOSPITALS

1. Improve the accuracy of patient identification.
2. Improve the effectiveness of communication among caregivers.
3. Improve the safety of using medications.
4. Reduce the risk of health care–associated infections.
5. Accurately and completely reconcile medications across the continuum of care.
6. Reduce the risk of patient harm resulting from falls.
7. Reduce the risk of influenza and pneumococcal disease in institutionalized older adults.
8. Reduce the risk of surgical fires.
9. Encourage patients' active involvement in their care as a patient safety measure.
10. Prevent health care–associated pressure ulcers (decubitus ulcers).
11. Have the organization identify safety risks inherent in its patient population.
12. Improve recognition and response to changes in a patient's condition.

Source: Joint Commission (2008b). *2009 national patient safety goals hospital program.* Available at:
http://www.jointcommission.org/PatientSafety/NationalPatientSafetyGoals/09_hap_npsgs.htm.
Accessed August 15, 2008.

---

errors that do occur. The Joint Commission's (2008d) Sentinel Event Policy provides that organizations that are either voluntarily reporting a sentinel event or responding to the Joint Commission's inquiry about a sentinel event submit their related root cause analysis and action plan electronically to the Joint Commission whenever such events occur. The sentinel event data are then reviewed, and recommendations are made. The Joint Commission (2008c) defends the confidentiality of the information, if necessary, in court.

Similarly, some organizations use a *failure mode and effects analysis* (FMEA) to "examine processes in detail—including sequencing of events, assessing the actual and potential risk, failure, or points of vulnerability; and logical prioritizing areas for improvement based on actual or potential patient care impact" (Riehle, Bergeron, & Hyrkas, 2008, p. 29). In hospitals, FMEA is typically used by interdisciplinary teams and multiple professions to identify steps in the care process that might fail (Riehle et al.).

CONSIDER

National legislation designed to keep such error analyses confidential is a critical but still-unrealized step. This discourages error reporting.

Centers for Medicare and Medicaid Services

The Centers for Medicare and Medicaid Services (CMS), formerly the Health Care Financing Administration (HCFA), also plays an active role in setting standards and measuring quality of health care. With the introduction of the Medicare Quality Initiatives (MQIs) in November 2001, a new era of public reporting on quality began. These diverse initiatives encourage the public reporting of quality measures for nursing homes, home health agencies, hospitals, and kidney dialysis facilities. These data are then made available to consumers on the Medicare Web site to assist them in making health care choices or decisions.

Medicare also established *pay for performance (P4P)*, also known as *quality-based purchasing*, in the middle of the first decade of the 21st century. P4P initiatives were created to "align payment and quality incentives and to reduce costs through improved quality and efficiency" (University Health System Consortium, 2007, p. 2).

For example, the 2007 Physician Quality Reporting Initiative (PQRI) allowed for payments to health professionals who satisfactorily reported quality information to Medicare. The PQRI is a voluntary program that allowed eligible health care professionals to "receive bonus payments of 1.5 percent of their total allowed Medicare charges, subject to a cap, by satisfactorily submitting quality information for services they furnished between July and December of 2007" (Medicare Quality Reporting, 2008, para 5). The CMS announced bonus payments of more than $36 million to the more than 56,700 health professionals who responded (Medicare Quality Reporting).

Research by the University Health System Consortium (2007) suggested that P4P activity in the Medicaid sector has focused on health plans, with a few states providing physician incentives through P4P programs. Hospital Medicaid P4P programs have yet to be implemented. The University Health System Consortium went on to say that the administrative burden involved in data collection and reporting appears to be the most significant obstacle for participants in any P4P program, but especially in the Medicaid P4P initiatives. They also suggested that there is a lack of provider buy-in and feedback on the design and implementation of the P4P program in general.

Unruh, Hassmiller, and Reinhard (2008, p. 71) agreed, suggesting that

> although little is known about how P4P will affect clinical and financial performance of health care organizations, even less is known about its impacts on nursing. Nursing leaders then are called on to lead the way in finding answers to these questions and in promoting policies that will lead to positive change (Unruh et al., p. 69).

DISCUSSION POINT
Should it be necessary to pay health care professionals bonuses to submit quality information?

In addition, in an effort to reduce the number of preventable medical errors, including "*never events*" (errors that should never happen, such as removing the wrong limb in surgery, leaving a foreign object inside a patient during surgery, or sending a baby home with the wrong parents), Medicare announced that effective October 1, 2008, it will no longer pay for care that is required as a result of eight specific preventable errors or "never events" (see Box 14.5). The CMS is already proposing to add an additional nine hospital-acquired conditions to the initial list of eight (Kurtzman & Buerhaus, 2008), including hospital-acquired ventilator-associated pneumonia (VAP), beginning in October 2009 (Kirchheimer, 2008). Beneficiaries of care cannot be charged either. In addition, Medicare is also requiring all hospitals to report never events or receive a reduced annual payment update (CMS, 2007).

In addition, the number of states that said their hospitals would not bill patients for the worst kinds of medical mistakes, including operating on the wrong body part or the wrong person or giving someone the wrong blood type, grew from 11 in February 2008 to almost half of all states in August 2008 (Aleccia, 2008, para 1): "Hospitals in another eight states have agreed to general guidelines that advise eliminating bills on a case-by-case basis for errors proven to be both serious and preventable" (para 4).

BOX 14.5 | EIGHT HOSPITAL ACQUIRED CONDITIONS THAT ARE NO LONGER COVERED BY MEDICARE AS OF OCTOBER 1, 2008

1. Pressure ulcers
2. Preventable injuries such as fractures, dislocations, and burns
3. Catheter-associated urinary tract infections
4. Vascular catheter–associated infections
5. Certain surgical-site infections
6. Objects mistakenly left inside surgical patients
7. Air emboli
8. Blood incompatibility reactions

Source: Kurtzman, E. T., & Buerhaus, P. I. (2008). New Medicare payment rules: Danger or opportunity for nursing? *American Journal of Nursing (AJN), 108*(6), 30–35.

In addition, in April 2008, legislation was introduced in California that would eliminate Medi-Cal (California's version of Medicaid) reimbursement to hospitals for care associated with medical errors (Goulette, 2008). This state movement to no longer bill for "never errors" began in September 2008, when Minnesota became the first state to announce that its hospitals would no longer charge patients or insurers for avoidable errors. Within weeks, others states began following suit (Aleccia, 2008).

Private insurance companies are expected to follow suit. According to Goulette (2008, p. 8), "Wellpoint, parent company of Anthem Blue Cross in California, has announced it will no longer pay for care to repair mistakes or additional care needed as a result of preventable mistakes." Aetna insurance has begun requiring hospitals to report errors and to waive costs associated with those errors but has not yet announced intent for nonreimbursement (Goulette).

DISCUSSION POINT
Should private insurance plans also refuse to pay for care that is extended as the result of medical errors, even if the state has no such legislation?

These new policies will require hospitals to maintain meticulous documentation about what conditions are present on admission to differentiate between pre-existing conditions and those that are acquired during the hospital stay (Keefe, 2007). It will also require comprehensive head-to-toe assessments, particularly in regard to skin assessments (Keefe).

The CMS has also announced plans to require hospitals to publicly report data on 43 new quality measures in fiscal year 2009, including failure to rescue, pressure ulcer prevalence, patient falls, and patient falls with injury, in order to get their full payment update in fiscal year 2010 (Kirchheimer, 2008). This payment will continue to be based on diagnosis-related groups (DRGs).

Patient Safety Task Force

Another government-appointed group to address the IOM goals was the Patient Safety Task Force (PSTF). This task force, established in April 2001, is composed of representatives from the Agency for Healthcare Research and Quality (AHRQ), the Centers for Disease Control and Prevention (CDC), the Food and Drug Administration (FDA), and the CMS. This group was responsible for coordinating both the integration of data collection on medical errors and adverse events and the research and analysis efforts. In addition, the PSTF was charged with promoting collaboration within the Department of Health and Human Services in an effort to improve health care quality by preventing the adverse events associated with health care delivery.

The PSTF completed several projects. First, a series of "demonstration projects" was funded to study medical errors. Then, the demonstration projects were used to develop national benchmarks and other comparative data to create accurate assessments of certain classes of adverse events.

CONSIDER
Although few organizations would argue against the benefits of well-developed and well-implemented quality control programs, quality control in health care organizations has evolved primarily from external effects and not as a voluntary monitoring effort.

Mandatory Report Cards

In response to the demand for objective measures of quality, including the number and type of medical errors, many health plans, health care providers, employer purchasing groups, consumer information organizations, and state governments have begun to formulate health care quality report cards. Most states have laws requiring providers to report some type of data. According to Gearon (2006), more than half of all states in the United States have developed health maintenance organization (HMO) report cards or list complaint-related information to help consumers compare the performance of competing health plans in their area. The AHRQ also is exploring the development of a report card for the nation's health care delivery system, and the National Committee for Quality Assurance's Health Plan Report Card lets an individual create a health plan report card online.

It is important to remember, however, that many report cards do not contain information about the quality of care rendered by specific clinics, group practices, or physicians in a health plan's network. In addition, most report cards focus on service utilization data and patient satisfaction ratings and have minimal data regarding medical errors.

Critics of health care report cards also point out that health plans may receive conflicting ratings on different report cards. This results from using different performance measures, as well as how each report card pools and evaluates individual factors. Report cards might also not be readily accessible or might be difficult for the average consumer to understand.

This clearly was the case in research done by Der-Gurahian (2008), which suggested that publicly released performance data lacked rigorous evaluation of reporting systems and the influence that such data had on patient behavior was unclear. The study concluded that poorly constructed report cards may actually impair consumers' comprehension of the measures and may cause consumers to make decisions that are inconsistent with their goals.

Still, in August 2008, *USA Today* posted "the government's best estimates of heart attack, heart failure and pneumonia death rates for every U.S. hospital for the past two years on its website" (Sternberg & Debarros 2008, para 7). Immediate reactions to the article by readers were mixed, with many readers expressing frustration that data were not available for locations they searched, and others suggesting that death rates are a poor measure of hospital performance, given that the acuity of patients varies dramatically. Others shared personal stories of poor care that they or a family member received in a hospital, and still others encouraged the development of additional Web sites similar to the one given. What was perhaps most apparent about this Web site launch was that consumers wanted more access to meaningful quality-of-care information and that such data, which have long been kept secret, are now becoming public.

CONTEMPORARY RESEARCH ON MEDICAL ERRORS

Despite all the interventions that came out of the IOM study, current literature suggests that only minimal progress has been made in addressing the problem and that medical errors continue to occur at an alarming rate. Only several current studies are discussed here due to space constraints.

A large study by HealthGrades (2008) that reviewed 41 million Medicare patient records between 2004 and 2006 in virtually all of the nation's nearly 5,000 nonfederal hospitals reported 238,337 potentially preventable deaths. The overall incident rate was approximately 3% of all Medicare admissions, accounting for 1.1 million patient safety incidents during the 3 years studied. Medicare patients who experienced a patient safety incident had a one-in-five chance of dying as a result of the incident. The study concluded that if all of the hospitals had performed at the level of Distinguished Hospitals for Patient Safety, approximately 220,106 patient safety incidents and 37,214 Medicare deaths could have been prevented, saving the U.S. $2.0 billion during the study period.

Similarly, a study by Robert Holloway of 1,440 stroke patients admitted to Strong Memorial Hospital at the University of Rochester Medical Center in Rochester, New York, between July 2001 and December 2004 found that 12%, or 173 patients, experienced an adverse event (Ghimire, 2008). A total of 201 events were reported for the 173 patients. Holloway concluded that "if these figures were applied to the nearly one million patients admitted to U.S. hospitals each year for stroke, 50,000 to 100,000 patients may experience an adverse event related to an error" (Ghimire, para 3).

Troubling statistics were also reported in a 2007 *Los Angeles Times* article, which reported that instances in which a patient was injured after receiving the wrong medication or dose from a hospital doubled between 1997 and 2007, and that at least 1.5 million U.S. residents are involved in such incidents each year (Bar Code Technology, 2007). In addition, the *Times* reported that serious injuries reported to the FDA due to hospital drug errors increased from about 35,000 in 1998 to about 90,000 in 2005 (Bar Code Technology).

A study by Takata, Mason, Taketomo, Logsdon, and Sharek (2008) also reaffirmed the continuing problem of medical errors in children, finding that pediatric patients experience an 11.1% rate of adverse drug events, a figure far higher than that reported in earlier studies. The study also showed that 22% of those adverse drug events were preventable, 17.8% could have been identified earlier, and 16.8% could have been mitigated more effectively. In addition, only 3.7% of the errors were identified by using traditional voluntary reporting methods. The medication class most frequently associated with an adverse drug event was analgesics/opioids, and the diagnostic category (based on principal discharge diagnosis) most commonly associated with an adverse drug event was congenital anomalies.

Piscone et al.'s (2008) findings were equally disturbing. In this retrospective study of 10,187 hospitalizations of elderly patients admitted to a Midwest teaching hospital between July 1, 1998, and December 31, 2001, 861 medication errors occurred. Ninety-six percent of those errors might have been preventable. The most common errors were omissions errors (48.8%), and the primary sources were administration (54%) and transcription errors (38%).

The "human element" as a factor in pharmaceutical dispensing medication errors was reinforced in a recent study reported by Parshuram et al. (2008). In this study, 118 health care professionals who were involved in the preparation of intravenous medication infusions as part of their regular clinical activities prepared 464 morphine infusions under simulated conditions with direct observation. The morphine concentration in each prepared infusion was then measured using chromatography. Almost 35% of the infusions deviated from the intended concentration by more than 10%. In addition, 3% of drug-volume calculations had 2-fold errors and 1.2% had 10-fold errors. This study supported previous findings of high error rates in the preparation of intravenous medications. The researchers concluded that reducing provider fatigue and producing pediatric-strength solutions or industry-prepared infusions might reduce future medication errors.

Another recent study examined problems that family practice clinics experience in receiving critical lab work, imaging, and heart monitoring results (Minority Patients Get Slow Test Results, 2008). About one fourth of the mistakes made at the clinic represented a failure to get results to doctors: "One-quarter of the errors resulted in delays in care for patients, and 13 percent caused pain or suffering. Eighteen percent resulted in actual harm" (Minority Patients Get Slow Test Results, para 5). What was even more alarming was that the rate of test implementation errors was nearly double for minority groups, at 32% versus 18% for whites. In addition, minority patients were twice as likely to experience physical harm and almost three times more likely to experience adverse consequences as a result of the errors (Minority Patients Get Slow Test Results).

Finally, Encinosa and Hellinger (2008), in their nationwide study of more than 161,000 patients between the age 18 to 64 years in employer-based health plans who underwent surgery between 2001 and 2002, found high mortality associated with medical errors. The study found that 1 of every 10 patients who died within 90 days of surgery did so because of a preventable error, and that one third of the deaths occurred after the initial hospital discharge. In addition, the researchers concluded that the financial effect of patient safety events might be underestimated by up to 30%. (See Research Study Fuels the Controversy.)

Research Study Fuels the Controversy: The Cost of Surgical Errors

The study was based on a nationwide sample of more than 161,000 patients, ages 18 to 64 years, in employer-based health plans who underwent surgery between 2001 and 2002. The authors used AHRQ's patient safety indicators to identify medical errors.

STUDY FINDINGS

The study found that 1 of every 10 patients who died within 90 days of surgery did so because of a preventable error, and that one third of the deaths occurred after the initial hospital discharge. In addition, potentially preventable medical errors that occur during or after surgery likely cost employers nearly $1.5 billion a year. Insurers paid an additional $28,218 (52% more) for surgery patients who experienced acute respiratory failure and an additional $19,480 (48% more) for postoperative infections, compared with patients who did not experience either error. Nursing care associated with medical errors, including pressure ulcers and hip fractures, cost an additional $12,196 (33% more).

Because the consequences of medical errors extend beyond the acute care hospitalization, the researchers concluded that the financial effect of patient safety events might be underestimated by up to 30%. The researchers concluded that the cost savings from reducing medical errors are much larger than previously thought.

Source: Encinosa, W. E., & Hellinger, F. J. (2008). Impact of medical errors on 90-day costs and outcomes: An examination of surgical patients. *Health Services Research*. Available at: http://www3.interscience.wiley.com/journal/120855828/abstract/. Accessed August 16, 2008.

CREATING A CULTURE OF SAFETY MANAGEMENT

In response to public forces and professional concerns, patient safety has become one of the nation's most pressing challenges and a mandate for every health care organization. Indeed, the final recommendation of the IOM report was to implement safe practices at the delivery level. The strategies that have been recommended to achieve this goal are overwhelming both in scope and quantity.

Strategies discussed in this chapter include the "six-sigma" approach (a customer-based, management philosophy) to error management; the mandatory/voluntary reporting of errors; attempts to increase confidentiality of reporting to reduce the fear of legal liability for reporting errors that do occur; the Leapfrog recommendations; the use of bar coding; a change in organizational cultures from that of "individual blame" to error identification and system modification; the development of patient safety solutions by the World Health Organization's World Alliance for Patient Safety; and the 100,000 Lives and 5 Million Lives campaigns.

A Six-Sigma Approach

One approach that has been taken to create a culture of safety management at the institutional level has been the implementation of the "*six-sigma*" *approach. Sigma* is a statistical measurement that reflects how well a product or process is performing. Higher sigma values indicate better performance. Historically, the health care industry has been comfortable striving for three-sigma processes (all data points fall within three

standard deviations) in terms of health care quality instead of six. This is one reason why health care has more errors than the banking and airline industries, in which achieving six sigmas is the expectation. Organizations aim for this lofty target by carefully applying six-sigma methodology to every aspect of a particular product or process.

Mandatory Reporting of Errors

The third prong of the IOM's four-pronged approach to creating a safer health care system is "to identify and learn from medical errors through both mandatory and voluntary reporting systems" (Kohn et al., 2000, p. 6). To accomplish this, the IOM report recommended developing a mandatory reporting system for medical errors and adverse events at both the state and national levels.

State mandates for reporting medical errors and adverse events have been slow to materialize, although at least 15 states have passed laws aimed at reducing prescription drug errors, including Arizona, Colorado, Delaware, Florida, Idaho, Illinois, Louisiana, Maryland, Massachusetts, Michigan, Montana, South Dakota, Tennessee, Texas, and Washington (National Conference of State Legislatures, 2008).

Some states have reporting mandates that apply only to specific types of errors. For example, from 2002 through 2006, 16 states enacted legislation requiring the reporting of data on hospital acquired infections (HAIs) (Arias, 2008). As of September 2007, an additional 17 states had proposed or enacted HAI-reporting legislation. Of the 21 states that have requirements for infection-related reporting, 19 of them make rates public and 2 report data only to their state agencies (Arias).

It is important to note that the IOM report did suggest, in addition to mandatory reporting, that more options be created for limited voluntary reporting systems in all 50 states. The IOM also recommended that more research be conducted on how best to develop voluntary reporting systems that complement proposed mandatory reporting systems.

Increased mandatory and voluntary reporting must also occur at the institutional level, as well as by individual providers. As a result, the IOM report suggested that mandatory adverse event reporting should initially be required of hospitals and eventually of other institutional and ambulatory care delivery facilities. This was the impetus for the subsequent JCAHO action for sentinel event reporting as part of the accreditation process.

It is difficult, however, to enforce greater disclosure and reporting at the individual provider level. Ethical and professional guidelines suggest that providers have a responsibility to disclose medical errors. Yet the literature continues to suggest that this does not happen, because of fear of legal suits or disciplinary measures by employers. A 2007 survey found that many nurses worry that they would be fired if they reported an error (Gaskill, 2008). In another multimethod study of 29 small rural hospitals in nine western states over 3 years, Cook, Hoas, Guttmannova, and Joyner (2004) found that even when there was overwhelming agreement (97%) among participants that an error had occurred, only 64% stated that they would disclose the error to the patient affected.

The ironic part is that a study by Mazor et al. (2004), suggested that full disclosure after a medical error actually reduced the likelihood that patients would change physicians, improved patient satisfaction, increased trust in the physician, and resulted in a more positive emotional response. Full disclosure was also apt to reduce the likelihood that patients would seek legal advice under some, but not all, circumstances; the specifics of the case and the severity of the clinical outcome also affected patients' responses (Mazor et al.).

DISCUSSION POINT

Do you believe that error disclosure rates differ between nurses and physicians? If so, which professional group is more likely to disclose errors and why?

Perhaps this failure to disclose medical errors is a major contributor to the disconnect that exists between consumers' perceptions of the quality of their health care and the actual quality provided. Even consumers who are aware of medical error statistics often report that they believe medical errors to be a problem but believe that such errors will not happen to them because they trust and believe in their health care provider.

DISCUSSION POINT

Do you consider the care you receive from your primary care provider to be high quality? Are your perceptions subjective, or do you have objective data to back up your impression? Have you actively searched for such data on your primary care provider?

Legal Liability and Medical Error Reporting

If quality health care is to be achieved, the medical liability system and our litigious society must be recognized as potential barriers to systematic efforts to uncover and learn from mistakes that are made in health care. One recommendation of the IOM panel was to encourage learning about safety from cross-institutional reporting systems for errors. This reporting is inhibited by fears that such data will be discovered in liability lawsuits.

DISCUSSION POINT

Have you ever encouraged a family member, friend, or colleague to seek compensation for medical errors? If so, do you think this was the most appropriate means of redress?

The provision of stronger confidentiality protections likely would improve the voluntary sharing of data. In 2002, the Patient Safety Improvement Act was introduced to the House of Representatives. This bill provided legal protections for medical error reporting, stating that error information voluntarily submitted to patient safety organizations could not be subpoenaed or used in legal discovery. It also generally required that the information be treated as confidential. After multiple revisions, the final legislation, called the Patient Safety and Quality Improvement Act of 2005, was signed into law by President George W. Bush in July 2005.

Federal legislation has also been proposed to protect the voluntary reporting of ordinary injuries and "*near misses*"—errors that did not cause harm this time but easily could the next time. This would be like what is done in aviation, in which near misses are confidentially reported and can be analyzed by anyone.

Leapfrog Group

The Leapfrog Group is a conglomeration of non–health care Fortune 500 leaders dedicated to reducing preventable medical mistakes and improving the quality and affordability of health care (Leapfrog Group, 2007a). The group has advised the health care industry that big leaps in patient safety and customer value can occur if specific evidence-based standards are implemented, including (1) computerized physician (or prescriber) order entry (CPOE), (2) evidence-based hospital referral (EHR), and (3) intensive care unit physician staffing (IPS).

CPOE, which was discussed in Chapter 13, is a promising technology that allows physicians to enter orders into a computer instead of handwriting them:

> *Recent research shows that if this Leapfrog practice was implemented in all urban hospitals in the U.S., we could prevent as many as 907,600 serious medication errors each year. Studies have also shown that CPOE reduces length of stay; reduces repeat tests; reduces turnaround times for laboratory, pharmacy and radiology requests; as well as delivering cost savings (Leapfrog, 2007c, para 1).*

EHR involves making sure that patients with high-risk conditions are treated at hospitals whose characteristics are associated with better outcomes. Indeed, HealthGrades' (2008) analysis of 41 million Medicare patient records found that patients treated at top-performing hospitals had, on average, a 43% lower chance of experiencing one or more medical errors compared to the poorest-performing hospitals.

IPS considers the level of training of ICU medical personnel. Evidence suggests that quality of care in hospital ICUs is strongly influenced by whether "*intensivists*" (those familiar with ICU complications) are providing care and how the staff is organized (Leapfrog Group, 2007b): "Mortality rates are significantly lower in hospitals with ICUs managed exclusively by board-certified intensivists. Research has shown that in ICUs where intensivists manage or co-manage all patients versus low intensity there is a 30% reduction in hospital mortality and a 40% reduction in ICU mortality" (Leapfrog, 2007b, para 1).

Bar Coding Medications

In addition, Leapfrog has endorsed the use of bar coding to reduce point-of-care medication errors (see Chapter 13 for a further discussion of bar coding medications). Per a U.S. Food and Drug Administration (FDA) rule adopted in April 2004, all prescription and over-the-counter medications used in hospitals must contain a national drug code number. The FDA suggested that a bar code system coupled with a CPOE system would greatly enhance the ability of all health care workers to follow the "five rights" of medication administration—that the *right* person receives the *right* drug, in the *right* dose, via the *right* route, at the *right* administration time. Perschke (2008), warned, however that the five rights alone, even when used with CPOE, do not guarantee safety. Critical thinking is required by nurses, as is an ongoing need to identify and address system weaknesses and human factors that adversely affect medication safety (Perschke).

In addition, JCAHO originally proposed in its 2005 National Patient Safety Goals and Requirements that accredited organizations would have to implement bar code technology to identify patients and match them to their medications or other treatments by January 2007. Because of implementation concerns, especially in terms of costs, this proposal was abandoned by JCAHO in July 2004. Fewer than 20% of U.S. hospitals had installed the bar code systems to read the labels as of 2007 (Bar Code Technology, 2007). See Chapter 13 for additional discussion on bar coding medications at the point of care.

Changing Organizational Cultures

Perhaps the most significant change that must occur before a nationwide culture of safety management can exist is that organizational cultures must be created that remove blame from the individual and instead focus on how the organization can be modified to reduce the likelihood of such errors occurring in the future. Stumpf (2007, p. 61) agreed, arguing that safety aspects of care should be discussed at every opportunity, "on rounds, at department meetings, in discussions with administrators, and in teaching residents and medical students." In addition, Stumpf suggested that creating or supporting protocols and guidelines and improving communication among all members of the health care team would reduce the chance of errors occurring.

Gaskill (2008) also agreed, suggesting that the implementation of a "*just culture*" in work settings will be needed to encourage voluntary reporting and reduce the prevalence of errors. Just cultures exhibit "giving constructive feedback and critical analysis in skillful ways, during assessments based on facts, and having respect for the complexity of the situation" (p. 14). This type of intervention encourages people to reveal the errors they have made so that the organization can learn from them. In addition, the just culture philosophy suggests rewarding staff that report errors or near-errors to help them to overcome the fear of reporting (Gaskill).

Similarly, Jessee (2006) suggested that an organizational climate must be created in which safety is an integral part of day-to-day operations, that adequate resources must be devoted to patient safety, and that organizational policies must be in place to support patient safety. White (2006) suggested that the significant leaders in the 21st century would be those that lead in identifying and adopting innovative safety and quality improvement approaches.

Clearly, a punitive approach to medical errors is not productive, and errors will not be reported if workers fear the consequences. Employees and patients need to feel comfortable and without fear of personal risk in reporting hazards that can affect patient safety.

CONSIDER

Ignoring the problem of medical errors, denying their existence, or blaming the individuals involved in the processes does nothing to eliminate the underlying problems.

Patient Safety Solutions

Recognizing that health care errors affect 1 in every 10 patients around the world, the World Health Organization's (WHO) World Alliance for Patient Safety and the Collaborating Centre packaged nine effective solutions, called *patient safety solutions,* to reduce such errors (WHO, 2007, para 1). A patient safety solution is defined as "any system design or intervention that has demonstrated the ability to prevent or mitigate patient harm stemming from the processes of health care" and is based on interventions and actions that have reduced problems related to patient safety in some countries (WHO Collaborating Centre for Patient Safety Solutions, 2008, para 2).

In 2006 and 2007, more than 50 recognized leaders and experts in patient safety from around the world came together to identify and adapt the nine solutions to different needs. An international field review of the solutions was then conducted to gather feedback from leading patient safety entities, accrediting bodies, ministries of health, international health professional organizations, and other experts. In April 2008, the International Steering Committee approved the inaugural solutions and initiated the process for developing the second round of patient safety solutions (WHO Collaborating Centre for Patient Safety Solutions, 2008). The patient safety solutions adopted in 2008 are shown in Box 14.6.

The 100,000 Lives and 5 Million Lives Campaigns

In addition, the Institute for Health Improvement (IHI) in the United States launched a campaign to close the quality gap and save patient lives with its *100,000 Lives* campaign. Dr. Donald Berwick, a Harvard professor and president of the Massachusetts-based nonprofit IHI, issued a challenge to hospital officials nationwide in December 2004 to implement six types of changes, including using rapid response teams, ensuring that heart attack patients receive correct care, preventing medication errors, preventing hospital-acquired infections, and preventing pneumonia in patients on ventilators by 2007 (American Society for Quality, 2005).

More than 3,100 facilities enrolled before the campaign ended in December 2006 (Pastorius, 2008). Preliminary reports suggest that 122,342 lives were saved in the first 18 months of implementation alone (Tanne, 2006), despite the fact that only about one third of the hospitals reported diligence in all six interventions (Healthblog, 2006). This leads one to wonder what improvement would be possible if 100% participation and compliance were assured.

The *5 Million Lives* campaign was a separate IHI initiative to protect patients from five million incidents of

BOX 14.6 | WHO'S COLLABORATING CENTRE'S PATIENT SAFETY SOLUTIONS (2008)

Patient safety solutions that demonstrate the ability to prevent or mitigate patient harm stemming from the processes of health care include the following:

1. Look-alike, sound-alike medication names: Look-alike and sound-alike drug names are among the most common causes of medication errors and is a worldwide concern.

2. Patient identification: Failure to correctly identify patients often leads to medication, transfusion, and testing errors; wrong-person procedures; and the discharge of infants to the wrong families.

3. Communication during patient hand-overs: Gaps in hand-over (or hand-off) communication can cause serious breakdowns in the continuity of care and result in inappropriate treatment and patient harm.

4. Performance of correct procedure at correct body site: Cases of wrong procedure or wrong-site surgery are largely the result of miscommunication and unavailable or incorrect information.

5. Control of concentrated electrolyte solutions: Biologics, vaccines, and contrast media have a defined risk profile, and concentrated electrolyte solutions that are used for injection are especially dangerous.

6. Ensuring medication accuracy at transitions in care: Medication reconciliation is a process designed to prevent medication errors at patient transition points.

7. Avoiding catheter and tubing misconnections: The design of tubing, catheters, and syringes currently in use is such that it is possible to inadvertently cause patient harm through connecting the wrong syringes and tubing and then delivering medication or fluids through an unintended wrong route.

8. Single use of injection devices: One of the biggest global concerns is the spread of human immunodeficiency virus (HIV), the hepatitis B virus (HBV), and the hepatitis C virus (HCV) because of the reuse of injection needles.

9. Improved hand hygiene to prevent health care–associated infection: Effective hand hygiene would prevent many of the infections acquired by more than 1.4 million people worldwide at any given time.

Source: Excerpted and adapted from WHO Collaborating Center for Patient Safety Solutions (2008). *Patient safety solutions.* Available at: **http://www.ccforpatientsafety.org/30723/**. Accessed August 16, 2008.

medical harm between December 2006 and December 2008 (IHI, 2007). This initiative challenged hospitals to "even more rapidly improve the care they provide to protect 5 million patients from harm over a 2-year period." To accomplish this, the campaign expanded its focus from reducing mortality to preventing medical harm (Pastorius, 2008, p. 14). A spokesperson for the IHI suggested that the campaign is successfully generating energy, national activity, and further awareness in meeting this lofty goal (Pastorius).

CONCLUSIONS

Medical errors are not the only indicator of quality of care. They are, however, a pervasive problem in the current health care system and one of the greatest threats to quality health care. In fact, Bob King, founder and chief executive officer of GOAL/QPC, a not-for-profit company directed at continuous improvement, quality, and organizational transformation, suggests that health care is running 10 to 20 years behind in applying the quality technology that other industries have embraced successfully (iSixSigma Europe, 2008).

Efforts to reduce medical errors over the last decade have not resulted in the achievement of desired outcomes. There is a plethora of current studies that suggest that the health care system continues to be riddled with errors and that patient and worker safety are compromised. Yet movement toward the IOM goals is occurring. It is likely that there has never been another time when the public, providers, and government have worked together so closely to achieve a shared health care goal.

Much remains to be done. Sustained public interest will be needed to create the momentum necessary to systematically change the health care system in a way that reduces patients' vulnerability to medical errors. In addition, although there has been a great deal of talk about taking a systems approach to the problem of medical errors, there has not been much discussion regarding exactly how this integration is to be accomplished. The bottom line is that "dramatic change must take place before all consumers will be able to consistently receive health care of the quality and safety they deserve" (Mastal, Joshi, & Schulke, 2007, p. 323).

FOR ADDITIONAL DISCUSSION

1. If cost containment and quality goals conflict, which do you think will take precedence in health care organizations today?

2. Why do so many providers, despite stated dissatisfaction levels, state that they feel helpless about reducing medical errors and improving the quality of health care?

3. Why have quality control efforts in health care organizations evolved primarily from external requirements and not as voluntary monitoring efforts?

4. Where does individual provider responsibility and accountability begin and end in a culture in which medical errors are recognized as being a failure of the system?

5. How common is it that medical error documentation is used against employees as part of the performance appraisal process? If so, does this discourage reporting?

6. Does the average consumer have access to and an accurate understanding of health care report cards?

7. Given that most individuals can quickly identify medical errors that have happened to them, a friend, or a family member, why does the U.S. public seem so reluctant to accept that medical errors constitute a threat to the quality of their health care?

8. Has your fear of legal liability ever influenced your decision to report a medical error?

REFERENCES

Aleccia, J. N. (2008). *More states shred bills for awful medical errors. Patients in 23 states will no longer pay for certain mistakes, hospitals say.* MSNBC. Available at: http://www.msnbc.msn.com/id/26081421. Accessed August 17, 2008.

American Society for Quality (2005). *Rapid response teams big part of 100,000 lives campaign.* Available at: http://www.asq.org/qualitynews/qnt/execute/displaySetup?newsID=221. Accessed February 27, 2007.

Arias, K. M. (2008). Mandatory reporting and pay for performance: Health care infections in the limelight. *AORN Journal.* BNet. Available at: http://findarticles.com/p/articles/mi_m0FSL/is_4_87/ai_n25333583. Accessed August 16, 2008.

Aspden, P., Wolcott, J. A., Bootman, J. L., & Cronenwett, L. R. (2007). *Preventing Medication Errors.* Washington, DC: National Academies Press.

Bar code technology could help curb drug errors at hospitals (2007). iHealthBeat. Available at: http://www.ihealthbeat.org/articles/2007/11/26/Bar-Code-Technology-Could-Help-Curb-Drug-Errors-at-Hospitals.aspx?topicID=59. Accessed August 17, 2008.

Brennan, T. A., Leape, L. L, Laird, N. M, Hebert, L., Localio, A. R., Lawthers, A. G., Newhouse J. P., Weiler, P. C., & Hiatt, H. H. (1991). Incidence of adverse events and negligence in hospitalized patients. Results of the Harvard Medical Practice Study 1. *New England Journal of Medicine, 324*(6), 370–376.

Centers for Medicare and Medicaid Services (CMS) (2007). *Medicare and Medicaid move aggressively to encourage greater patient safety in hospitals and reduce never events.* Available at: http://www.cms.hhs. gov/apps/media/press/release.asp?Counter=3219 &intNumPerPage=10&checkDate=&checkKey=&srch Type=1&numDays=3500&srchOpt=0&srch Data=&keywordType=All&chkNewsType=1%2C+ 2%2C+3%2C+4%2C+5&intPage=&showAll=& pYear=&year=&desc=&cboOrder=date. Accessed August 16, 2008.

Cook, A. F., Hoas, H., Guttmannova, K., & Joyner, J. C. (2004). An error by any other name. *American Journal of Nursing, 104*(6), 38–39.

DerGurahian, J. (2008). More doubts over reporting: New study shows medical-error reporting systems can lead to confusion, frustration among patients and some providers. *Modern Healthcare, 38*(6), 32–33.

Encinosa, W. E., & Hellinger, F. J. (2008). Impact of medical errors on 90-day costs and outcomes: An examination of surgical patients. *Health Services Research.* Available at: http://www3.interscience. wiley.com/journal/120855828/abstract/. Accessed August 16, 2008.

Gaskill, M. (2008). Learning from mistakes. "Just culture" is replacing blame in some California hospitals. *NurseWeek (California), 21*(8), 14–15.

Gearon, C. J. (2006). *State-by-state guide to health care provider performance.* AARP. Available at: http:// www.aarp.org/health/doctors/articles/statebystate_ guide_healthcare_provider_performance.html. Accessed August 29, 2008.

Ghimire, L. V. (2008). Preventing medical errors in managing stroke patients. *The Journal of Young Investigators, 19*(2). Available at: http://www.jyi.org/ news/nb.php?id=924. Accessed August 15, 2008.

Goulette, C. (2008). From the hill. Never say never. State looks to follow CMS lead in 'never event' legislation. *Advance for Nurses (Northern California and Northern Nevada), 5*(17), 8–9.

Healthblog (2006). *Evidence based medicine saves more than 100,000 lives.* Available at: http://blogs.msdn. com/healthblog/archive/2006/06/14/631127.aspx. Accessed February 27, 2007.

HealthGrades (2004). *HealthGrades quality study. Patient safety in American hospitals.* Available at: http:// www.healthgrades.com/media/english/pdf/ hg_patient_safety_study_final.pdf. Accessed August 15, 2008.

HealthGrades (2008). *Medical errors cost U.S. $8.8 billion, result in 238,337 potentially preventable deaths according to HealthGrades Study.* Available at: http:// www.healthgrades.com/media/DMS/pdf/ HealthGradesPatientSafetyRelease2008.pdf. Accessed August 15, 2008.

Henry J. Kaiser Family Foundation (2008). *Spotlight. Public opinion on medical errors.* Available at: http://www.kff.org/spotlight/mederrors/index.cfm. Accessed August 15, 2008.

Institute for Health Improvement (IHI) (2007). *Protecting 5 million lives.* Available at: http://www.ihi.org/ IHI/Programs/Campaign/. Accessed February 27, 2007.

iSix Sigma Europe (2008). *GOAL/QPC leader will help healthcare professionals use quality, creativity and innovation tools to boost productivity.* Valeocon Management Consulting. Available at: http://europe. isixsigma.com/library/content/n080328a.asp. Accessed April 23, 2008

Jessee, W. (2006). What patient safety looks like. Six steps that mark an organization that really cares about medical errors. *Modern Healthcare, 36*(42), 18.

Joint Commission (2008a). *Preventing pediatric medication errors.* Available at: http://www.jointcommission. org/SentinelEvents/Sentinel EventAlert/sea_39.htm. Accessed August 15, 2008.

Joint Commission (2008b). *2009 national patient safety goals hospital program.* Available at: http://www. jointcommission.org/PatientSafety/National PatientSafetyGoals/09_hap_npsgs.htm. Accessed August 15, 2008.

Joint Commission (2008c). *Sentinel event.* Available at: http://www.jointcommission.org/SentinelEvents/. Accessed August 16, 2008.

Joint Commission (2008d). *Alternatives for sharing sentinel event-related information with the Joint Commission.* Available at: http://www.jointcommission. org/SentinelEvents/ReportingAlternatives/. Accessed August 16, 2008.

Keefe, S. (2007). Ahead of the game. *Advance for Nurses (Northern California and Northern Nevada), 4*(26), 23–24.

Kirchheimer, B. (2008). Wrestling with a new reality. *NurseWeek, 21*(14), 34–35.

Kohn, L. T., Corrigan, J. M., & Donaldson, M. S. (Eds.) (2000). Executive summary (pp. 1–6). In: *To Err Is Human: Building a Safer Health System.* Available at: http://books.nap.edu/openbook.php?record_id=9728&page=R1. Accessed August 15, 2008.

Kurtzman, E. T., & Buerhaus, P. I. (2008). New Medicare payment rules: Danger or opportunity for nursing? *American Journal of Nursing (AJN), 108*(6), 30–35.

Leape, L. L. (1994). Error in medicine. *Journal of the American Medical Association, 272,* 1851–1857.

Leape, L. L., Brennan, T. A., Laird, N., Lawthers, A. G., Localio, A. R., Barnes, B. A., Hebert, L., Newhouse, J. P., Weiler, P. C., & Hiatt, H. (1991). The nature of adverse events in hospitalized patients: Results of the Harvard Medical Practice Study II. *New England Journal of Medicine, 324*(6), 377–384.

Leapfrog Group (2007a). *Homepage.* Available at: http://www.leapfroggroup.org/. Accessed August 16, 2008.

Leapfrog Group (2007b). *ICU physician staffing.* Available at: http://www.leapfroggroup.org/for_hospitals/leapfrog_hospital_survey_copy/leapfrog_safety_practices/icu_physician_staffing. Accessed August 16, 2008.

Leapfrog Group (2007c). *Computerized physician order entry.* Available at: http://www.leapfroggroup.org/for_hospitals/leapfrog_hospital_survey_copy/leapfrog_safety_practices/cpoe. Accessed August 16, 2008.

Mastal, M. F., Joshi, M., & Schulke, K. (2007). Nursing leadership: Championing quality and patient safety in the boardroom. *Nursing Economics, 25*(6), 323–331.

Mazor, K. M., Simon, S. R., Yood, R. A., Martinson, B. C., Gunter, M. J., Reed, G. W., & Gurwitz, J. H. (2004). Health plan member's views about disclosure of medical errors. *Annals of Internal Medicine, 140,* 409–418.

Medical quality reporting initiative pays over $36 million to participating physicians from the 2007 PQRI reporting period (2008). Available at: http://www.medicalnewstoday.com/articles/115276.php. Accessed August 16, 2008.

Minority patients get slow test results. Testing problems can slow treatment, cost money (2008). Available at: http://www.wnbc.com/health/17188334/detail.html. Accessed August 17, 2008.

National Conference of State Legislatures (2008). *State initiatives to avoid prescription drug errors.* Available at: http://www.ncsl.org/programs/health/RxErrors.htm. Accessed August 17, 2008.

National Coordinating Council for Medication Error Reporting and Prevention (NCC MERP) (1998–2008). *About medication errors.* Available at: http:// www.nccmerp.org/aboutMedErrors.html. Accessed August 15, 2008.

National Patient Safety Foundation (NPSF). (2008). *About us.* Available at: http://www.npsf.org/au/. Accessed August 16, 2008.

National Quality Forum (NQF) (2008a). *About us.* Available at: http://www.qualityforum.org/about/. Accessed August 15, 2008.

National Quality Forum (NQF) (2008b). *Mission.* Available at: http://www.qualityforum.org/about/mission.asp. Accessed August 15, 2008.

National Quality Forum (NQF) (2008c). *NQF national priorities partnership.* Available at: http://www.qualityforum.org/about/NPP/. Accessed August 15, 2008.

National Quality Forum (NQF) (2008d). *National priorities partnership. Priority areas and corresponding goals.* Available at: http://www.qualityforum.org/about/NPP/assets/NPP_Goals_07_03_08.pdf. Accessed August 15, 2008.

Pappas, S. H. (2008). The cost of nurse-sensitive adverse events. *Journal of Nursing Administration, 38*(5), 230–236.

Parshuram, C. S., To, T., Seto, W., Trope, A., Koren, G., & Laupacis, A. (2008). Systematic evaluation of errors occurring during the preparation of intravenous medication. *Canadian Medical Association Journal, 178*(1). Available at: http://www.cmaj.ca/cgi/content/abstract/178/1/42?ijkey=03478e5f53d2cf31c56127a06f6e46dbd8bc2a2d&keytype2=tf_ipsecsha. Accessed August 17, 2008.

Pastorius, D. (2008). Update: 5 million lives campaign. *Nursing Management, 39*(5), 13–18.

Perschke, A. L. (2008). *Building on the five rights. How the foundation for safe medication delivery gets stronger.* Nurse.com. Available at: http://include.nurse.com/apps/pbcs.dll/article?AID=/20080825/DC02/108250078. Accessed August 26, 2008.

Picone, D. M., Titler, M. G., Dochterman, J., Shever, L., Kim, T., Abramowitz, P., Kanak, M., & Qin, R. (2008). Predictors of medication errors among elderly hospitalized patients. *American Journal of Medical Quality, 23*(2),115–127.

Riehle, M. A., Bergeron, D., & Hyrkas, K. (2008). MFEA and medication administration. *Nursing Management, 39*(2), 28–33.

Sternberg, S., & Debarros, A. (2008). Hospital death rates unveiled for first-time comparison. *USA Today.* Available at: http://www.usatoday.com/news/health/2008-08-20-hospital-death-rates_N.htm?loc=interstitialskip. Accessed August 21, 2008.

Stumpf, P. G. (2007). Taking aim at the top 3 patient safety errors in ob/gyn. *Contemporary OB/GYN, 52*(1), 58–62.

Takata, G. S., Mason, W., Taketomo, C., Logsdon, T., & Sharek, P. J. (2008). Development, testing, and findings of a pediatric-focused trigger tool to identify medication-related harm in U.S. children's hospitals. *Pediatrics, 121*(4), e927–e935. Available at: http://pediatrics.aappublications.org/cgi/content/full/121/4/e927. Accessed August 15, 2008.

Tanne, J. H. (2006). U.S. campaign to save 100,000 lives exceeds its target. *BMJ,* 2006(332), 1468. Available at: http://www.bmj.com/cgi/content/extract/332/7556/1468-b. Accessed February 27, 2007.

Thomas, E. J., Studdert, D. M, Newhouse, J. P., Zbar, B. I. W., Howard, K. M., Williams, E. J., & Brennan, T. A. (1999). Costs of medical injuries in Colorado and Utah in 1992. *Inquiry, 36,* 255–264.

University Health System Consortium (2007). *Medicaid pay for performance programs slow to gain traction.* Available at: http://www.naph.org/naph/publications/MedicaidPayForPerformanceProgramsSlowToGainTraction. pdf. Accessed August 17, 2008.

Unruh, L. Y., Hassmiller, S. B., & Reinhard, S. C. (2008). The importance and challenge of paying for quality nursing care. *Policy, Politics & Nursing Practice, 9*(2), 68–72.

Weissman, J. S., Schneider, E. C., Weingart, S. N., Epstein, A. M., David-Kasdan, J., Feibelmann, S., Annas, C. L., Ridley, N., Kirle, L., & Gatsonis, C. (2008). Comparing patient-reported hospital adverse events with medical record review: Do patients know something that hospitals do not? *Annals of Internal Medicine, 149*(2), 100–108.

White, K. M. (2006). Be a best-in-class organization. *Nursing Management, 37*(9), 53–57.

WHO Collaborating Center for Patient Safety Solutions (2008). *Patient safety solutions.* Available at: http://www.ccforpatientsafety.org/30723/. Accessed August 16, 2008.

World Health Organization (2007). *WHO launches 'nine patient safety solutions.'* Available at: http://www.who.int/mediacentre/news/releases/2007/pr22/en/index.html. Accessed August 16, 2008.

BIBLIOGRAPHY

Adams, M., Bates, D., Coffman, G., & Everett, W. (2008). *Saving lives, saving money: The imperative for computerized physician order entry in Massachusetts hospitals.* Available at: http://www.nehi.net/publications/8/saving_lives_saving_money_the_imperative_for_computerized_physician_order_entry_in_massachusetts_hospitals. Accessed January 21, 2009.

Fung, C. H. (2008). *The public reporting of performance data: An intervention in need of more evaluation.* National Quality Measures Clearinghouse. Available at: http://www.qualitymeasures.ahrq.gov/resources/commentary.aspx?file=PublicReporting.inc. Accessed August 16, 2008.

Gross, P. A., & Bates, D. W. (2007). A pragmatic approach to implementing best practices for clinical decision support systems in computerized provider order entry systems. *Journal of the American Medical Informatics Association, 14*(1), 25–28.

Hoffmann, B., Beyer, M., Rohe, J., Gensichen, J., & Gerlach, F. M. (2008). "Every error counts": A web-based incident reporting and learning system for general practice. *Quality and Safety in Health Care, 17*(4), 307–312.

Kuo, G. M., Phillips, R. L., Graham, D., & Hickner, J. M. (2008). Medication errors reported by U.S. family physicians and their office staff. *Quality and Safety in Health Care, 17*(4), 286–290.

Lawrence, D. (2008). Closing the loop: CIOs are finding that CPOE is only one (imperfect) tool in the fight against medical errors. *Healthcare Informatics, 25*(6), 90–91.

Levine, S. L., & Cohen, M. R. (2007). Preventing medication errors in pediatric and neonatal patients (pp. 469–492). In: M. R. Cohen (Ed.), *Medication Errors*. Washington, DC: American Pharmacists Association.

Madegowda, B., Hill, P. D., & Anderson, M. A. (2007). Medication errors in a rural hospital. *Medsurg Nursing, 16*(3), 175–180.

Moore, M. L., & Putman, P. A. (2008). Cultural transformation towards patient safety. One conversation at a time. *Nursing Administration Quarterly, 32*(2), 102–108.

Obsy, L. (2008). *Medicare won't pay for errors.* Greenvilleonline.com. Available at: http://www.greenvilleonline.com/apps/pbcs.dll/article?AID=/20080727/YOURUPSTATEHEALTH/807270314/-1/OPINION. Accessed August 16, 2008.

Pukk-Härenstam, K., Ask, J., Brommels, M., Thor, J., Penaloza, R. V., & Gaffney F. A. (2008). Analysis of 23,364 patient-generated, physician-reviewed malpractice claims from a non-tort, blame-free, National Patient Insurance System: Lessons learned from Sweden. *Quality and Safety in Health Care, 17*(4), 259–263.

Reducing med errors in the PACU (2008). *Advance for Nurses (Northern California and Northern Nevada), 5*(16), 19–20.

Rinke, M. L., Shore, A. D., Morlock, L., Hicks, R. W., & Miller, M. R. (2007). Characteristics of pediatric chemotherapy medication errors in a national error reporting database. *Cancer, 110*(1),186–195.

Shamliyan, T. A., Duval, S., Du, J., & Kane, R L. (2008). Just what the doctor ordered. Review of the evidence of the impact of a computerized physician order system on medication errors. *Health Services Research, 43*(1), 32–53.

Shapiro, E. (2008). Disclosing medical errors: Best practices from the "leading edge": Part II. *Care Management, 14*(3), 11–15.

Shur, R., & Simons, N. (2008). Quality issues in health care research and practice. *Nursing Economics, 26*(4), 258–262.

Small patients, big risk. Alert reveals children at higher risk for med errors (2008). *Advance for Nurses (Northern California and Northern Nevada), 5*(14), 34.

The second victim: Supporting staff members after a medical error: Emotional needs often remain unmet (2008). *Briefings on Patient Safety, 9*(6), 1–4.

Use of tool kits may reduce medical errors (2008). *AORN Journal, 87*(6), 1076.

WEB RESOURCES

Agency for Healthcare Research and Quality	http://www.ahcpr.gov
American Nurses Association, National Center for Nursing Quality, National Database of Quality Nursing Indicators	http://www.nursingworld.org/quality
Council for Affordable Quality Healthcare	http://www.caqh.org
Department of Veterans Affairs	http://www.va.gov
Institute for Healthcare Improvement	http://www.ihi.org/IHI
Institute for Healthcare Improvement, 5 Million Lives Campaign	http://www.ihi.org/IHI/Programs/Campaign/
Institute for Safe Medication Practices	http://www.ismp.org
Joint Commission on Accreditation of Healthcare Organizations	http://www.jcaho.org
Joint Commission on Accreditation of Healthcare Organizations, 2009 Patient Safety Goals	http://www.jointcommission.org/PatientSafety/NationalPatientSafetyGoals/

Leapfrog Group	http://www.leapfroggroup.org
National Association for Healthcare Quality	http://www.nahq.org/
National Committee for Quality Assurance	http://www.ncqa.org
National Guideline Clearinghouse	http://www.guideline.gov
National Patient Safety Foundation	http://www.npsf.org/
National Quality Forum	http://www.qualityforum.org
National Quality Measures Clearinghouse	http://www.qualitymeasures.ahrq.gov
Quality Healthcare Network—Canada	http://www.qualityhealthcarenetwork.ca
U.S. Food and Drug Administration	http://www.fda.gov

CHAPTER 15

Whistle-Blowing in Nursing

• CAROL J. HUSTON •

Learning Objectives

The learner will be able to:

1. Define whistle-blowing and differentiate between internal and external whistle-blowing.
2. Identify conditions that should be met before whistle-blowing occurs, as well as situations in which whistle-blowing is clearly indicated.
3. Examine how cultural background may affect a nurse's willingness to blow the whistle on unsafe practices.
4. Identify risks and retaliatory consequences frequently experienced by whistle-blowers as a result of their actions.
5. Explore why reactions to whistle-blowers are often mixed and why the courage to speak out is something we honor more often in theory than in fact.
6. Differentiate among the consequentialist, deontological, and utilitarian viewpoints regarding the purposes of whistle-blowing.
7. Analyze how whistle-blowing could be considered a failure of organizational ethics.
8. Delineate strategies to create an organizational climate that both discourages the need for whistle-blowing and supports the whistle-blower when it is necessary for him or her to come forward.
9. Identify strategies that whistle-blowers should use to reduce the likelihood of retaliation and to reduce their legal liability.
10. Analyze existing and proposed federal and state legal protections for whistle-blowers.
11. Identify the process used by a whistle-blower to file a *qui tam* or whistle-blower lawsuit under the False Claims Act and the potential benefits of dong so.
12. Reflect on his or her willingness to assume the personal risks associated with whistle-blowing, should the need arise.

Watergate break-in . . . Enron and the artificial manipulation of energy prices . . . Martha Stewart and insider trading . . . WorldCom and accounting fraud . . . Bridgestone and Firestone tires . . . Dow Corning and silicone breast implants . . . Morgan Stanley and overcharging customers. All of these high-profile cases, involving some degree of ethical malfeasance, have led the U.S. public to an increased sense of moral awareness about what is right and what is wrong. In addition, these cases have all come to the attention of the public as the result of "whistle-blowing."

Lachman (2008, p. 126) defines whistle-blowing in the nursing context as the "action taken by a nurse who goes outside the organization for the public's best interest when it is unresponsive to reporting the danger through the organization's proper channels." Similarly, Bainbridge (2008, para 1) defines a whistle-blower "as a person who reveals any wrongdoings or malpractices that are taking place within an organization. These revelations could be made either to the general public or to those who are in a position of authority." Likewise, the Free Online Dictionary (2008, para 2) defines a whistle-blower as "an informant who exposes wrongdoing within an organization in the hope of stopping it."

It is generally accepted that there are two types of whistle-blowing: internal and external. *Internal whistle-blowing* typically involves reporting concerns up the chain of command within an organization in the hope that whatever the problem is, it will be resolved. *External whistle-blowing* involves reporting concerns outside the organization and, in particular, to the media. In many cases, whistle-blowing becomes external only if inadequate action is taken at the organizational level to address the concerns of the whistle-blower. In some cases, however, whistle-blowing becomes external in an effort to embarrass an organization publicly or to seek financial redress.

DISCUSSION POINT
Is it ever appropriate to whistle-blow externally before attempting to resolve the problem internally?

In an era of managed care, declining reimbursements, and the ongoing pressure to remain fiscally solvent, the risk of fraud, misrepresentation, and ethical malfeasance in health care organizations has never been higher. As a result, the need for whistle-blowing has also likely never been greater.

This chapter explores the effect of "groupthink" on the likelihood that whistle-blowers will come forward. In addition, it presents select cases of whistle-blowing. Personal risks associated with whistle-blowing are described, as are the mixed feelings many individuals hold about whistle-blowing. Whistle-blowing is also explored as a failure of organizational ethics, and strategies are identified to create an organizational climate that both discourages the need for whistle-blowing in the first place and supports the whistle-blower when it is necessary for him or her to come forward. Finally, legal protections for whistle-blowing are discussed.

GROUPTHINK AND WHISTLE-BLOWING

Being a whistle-blower takes great courage and self-conviction because it requires the whistle-blower to avoid *groupthink*—an inappropriate conformity to group norms. Going outside of groupthink often carries significant personal and professional risks.

Colvin (2002) recounted how Sherron Watkins, an accountant, first blew the whistle on Enron's complex "special-purpose entities." She detailed them in a memo to Chief Executive Officer Ken Lay, her boss's boss's boss. She understood that something wrong was going on—something everyone else seemed to think was perfectly okay—and that public revelation would be disastrous.

What Colvin argued was most important in this scandal was that Watkins had access to the same facts as many other people inside Enron, yet somehow she was able to escape the groupthink that ensnared her colleagues. Soon after writing the memo, she identified herself as its author and met with Mr. Lay. When her memo eventually became public, the wrongness of what happened was apparent even internally (Colvin, 2002).

Colvin recounts a similar story at WorldCom, where Cynthia Cooper, another internal auditor, saw something that did not look right and took matters into her own hands. In this case, Cooper began investigating some of the company's capital expenditures and discovered bookkeeping entries that would eventually uncover what is likely the largest accounting fraud in U.S. history.

Faced with disturbing facts, Cooper discussed her findings with the company's controller and with Scott Sullivan, the chief financial officer. Sullivan tried to explain to her why costs that had previously been expensed were suddenly being capitalized. Then he asked her to stop the audit, which was being conducted early, and to put it off until the third quarter. She did not. Instead, she continued—and immediately went over her boss's head and called the chairman of the board's audit committee. He arranged to meet with her and the company's new auditor, KPMG. Two weeks later, WorldCom announced that it would restate earnings by $3.9 billion—the largest restatement ever.

Again, Colvin (2002) suggested that the importance of Cooper's refusal to postpone her audit, as Sullivan had asked, is even greater than it may appear. Facts uncovered about the company, combined with the memo Sullivan wrote to the board in a last-ditch attempt to defend himself, show that if Cooper had "been a good soldier," the whole problem might have been concealed forever.

A similarly unsettling case was reported by Smith (2008), who profiled corporate whistle-blower Dana de Windt, a stockbroker at the financial services firm of Morgan Stanley. De Windt complained to government regulators that the company was cheating brokerage clients, having overcharged brokerage customers on 2,800 purchases of $59 million of bonds. De Windt repeatedly confronted his bosses with "questions tucked inside a thick, three-ring binder" for more than 4 years, and management's response was simply for "him to get over it" (para 5). Finally, de Windt reported the situation to regulators, and in August 2007, Morgan Stanley settled the resulting complaint brought by the U.S. Securities and Exchange Commission (SEC) by paying a $6.1 million fine.

In a high-profile whistle-blower case in New Mexico, six nurses at Memorial Medical Center in Las Cruces independently voiced concerns to their nurse managers over a 6-year period regarding inadequate and inappropriate care being given by an osteopathic physician on staff (Bitoun Blecher, 2001–2008.). In addition, the nurses brought the alleged shortcomings of this particular doctor to the attention of other physicians. The doctor in this case was later accused of negligence and incompetence after one of her patients died from sepsis and another suffered a serious injury.

For reasons that are still unclear, however, the hospital failed to act on the nurses' complaints. Instead, the hospital challenged the nurses' actions and disciplined them, citing state regulations that forbid sharing patient information for any reason. The hospital also retaliated after the case was filed and the nurses agreed to testify against the doctor. One of the nurses retired and later heard that she had been blackballed by the institution, whereas a second nurse allegedly was offered a management position in the hospital after being identified as a potential witness for the hospital (Hook, 2001). The American Nurses Association (ANA) responded by filing an *amicus curiae* ("friend of the court") brief on behalf of the nurses. This brief cited conflict and ambiguity in New Mexico law and urged the court to protect the nurses, who were exercising their ethical responsibility. The ANA argued that the application of the state regulation in question limited the ability of the nurse to report incompetent practice, which is a statutory mandate (Hook).

According to Judith Dunaway, member of the New Mexico Nurses Association and a clinical instructor at New Mexico State University in Las Cruces, "Sometimes the atmosphere in a hospital is set up so that you cannot work through the system, and that's what happened here—the system failed" (Bitoun Blecher, 2001–2008, para 28). "If that system refuses to address the complaints, then the process starts breaking down. We're not exactly sure where the breakdown occurred in this case. Supposedly, the complaints never got to the very top. Whether that's true or not, we don't know" (para 28).

CONSIDER

"Advocacy is the foundation and essence of nursing, and nurses have a responsibility to promote human advocacy" (Marquis & Huston, 2009, p. 122).

Perhaps the most frightening aspect of these four cases is that the responses by management at Enron, WorldCom, the Memorial Medical Center, and Morgan Stanley are not unique. Many organizations are aware of problem situations but choose to ignore them until a crisis occurs or the problem becomes public.

Some nurses take comfort in thinking that any moral professional would report substandard care. The reality, however, is often very different, and many professionals are torn between what they believe they should do and what they actually do. This is particularly disconcerting, and those who bear witness are required to overcome groupthink despite their moral distress. This is a primary reason why so many whistle-blowers delay in reporting their concerns outside the organization.

For example, Ohnishi, Hayama, Asai, Kosugi, and Hayama (2008) conducted a grounded theory study of two nursing staff members who worked in a psychiatric hospital in Japan that was convicted of large-scale wrongdoing. They found that these nurses did not immediately decide to blow the whistle when they first became suspicious and had a clear sense of wrongdoing.

Instead, they continued to work, driven by appreciation, affection, and a sense of duty. When the situation became unconscionable, they reported what was going on. However, immediately after whistle-blowing, their emotions wavered among a guilty conscience, fear of retribution, and pride, which subsequently transformed into a stable sense of relief combined with regret for delayed action.

DISCUSSION POINT

Why is speaking out often honored more in theory than in fact?

EXAMPLES OF WHISTLE-BLOWING IN NURSING

With the current nursing shortage, complaints about unsafe staffing and the use of unlicensed assistive personnel to perform nursing tasks outside their scope of practice are common. Worse yet, some nurses claim that they have been told to participate in illegal or unethical activities—things such as fraudulently altering medical records, falsifying insurance claims, and covering up the failure to meet mandated staffing ratios.

A review of the literature reveals multiple case studies of whistle-blowing by nurses. For example, in 2007, two nurses in Missouri blew the whistle on what they felt to be nursing home abuse and neglect of nursing home residents, which involved gross malpractice (McCranie, 2007). In addition, the nurses alleged that the nursing home operator was defrauding Medicare and Medicaid by providing essentially worthless care to the nursing home residents. According to the nurses, many of the patients suffered from "dehydration, weight loss, and preventable bed sores that eventually led to amputations," that "nursing home staffing was cut to unacceptable levels to save money" and that "other nurses misused patients' medicines, which were not locked securely" (McCranie, para 2).

Tariman (2007) presented the story of Barry Adams, a Registered Nurse (RN) who blew the whistle on unsafe nurse staffing and its effect on patient care. Despite reporting his concerns to his supervisors and filing an official hazards report with the director of nursing at his institution, he received no response. He was then fired for an alleged insubordination. Fortunately, Adams had documented his actions, as well as the poor patient out-

comes, including patient falls and medication errors. Adams was vindicated by the National Labor Relations Board when they ruled that he had been fired illegally for whistle-blowing (Tariman).

Whistle-blowing cases involving nurses are not limited to the United States. Myers (2008a) recounted the story of significant failings in infection control (an outbreak of *Clostridium difficile*) that caused, or probably caused, at least 90 deaths at Maidstone and Tunbridge Wells NHS Trust, Kent, England. The 2007 investigation found that although clinical staff reportedly raised concerns about the spreading infection, no effective action was taken. In short, the nurses' concerns went unheeded.

Indeed, a recent survey of 752 nurses by *Nursing Standard* and the whistle-blowing charity Public Concern at Work revealed that the number one reason that nurses cited for not raising a patient safety concern was that nothing would be done (Blowing the Whistle, 2008). The frustrating part of this is that 68% of these nurses had serious concerns about patient safety in the last 3 years. Of these, 87% said that they had reported their concerns, usually to their line managers. Only 29% of respondents thought that their manager had handled their concerns well and that patient risks had been addressed or resolved properly; 47% thought that the issues were handled "badly" and that safety concerns were overlooked; and 23% of those who had reported safety issues thought that the risks they identified went on to harm patients (Blowing the Whistle). (See Research Study Fuels the Controversy on page 263).

Another recent report from England highlights not only the difficulty that whistle-blowers face in changing bad situations, but also the personal consequences they often suffer as a result of their whistle-blowing. Scott (2008) told the story of Moi Ali, a nurse who exposed how pedophile nurses escaped punishment in the United Kingdom. As a result of her whistle-blowing, she was "pressured to quit" two top jobs, one as a board member of NHS Lothian and the second as vice president of the nurses' regulatory body—the Nursing and Midwifery Council (Scott, para 3). Ali asserted that she was asked to leave both positions because her superiors felt that "her whistle-blowing had impacted her position." Her superiors responded that the decisions to resign were entirely her own.

The same type of story comes from yet another country. In November 2002, four nurses in New South

Research Study Fuels the Controversy: When No One Listens

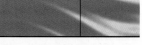

This descriptive study of 752 nurses by *Nursing Standard* and the whistle-blowing charity Public Concern at Work used a survey research design to examine the beliefs of nurses in the United Kingdom about whistleblowing.

STUDY FINDINGS

Results indicated that 68% of nurses had serious concerns about patient safety in the last 3 years. Of these, 87% said that they had reported their concerns, usually to their line managers. Forty-seven percent thought that the matter was handled "badly" and that their safety concerns had been overlooked.

Of those nurses reporting safety fears, 38% said that they had suffered serious or lasting negative professional consequences as a result of whistle-blowing. Sixty-four percent thought that their organizations would fail to support them if they faced reprisals after reporting concerns, and nurses who experienced negative professional consequences of whistle-blowing were twice as likely to say that the risks that they had identified had harmed patients as those who had not. In addition, 37% of respondents who experienced negative consequences of whistle-blowing said that their organizations had used whistle-blowing procedures to discourage staff from raising concerns. Despite all this, when asked whether they would report a risk if they noticed one the following week, 85% of survey respondents said that they would.

Blowing the whistle (2008). *Nursing Management—UK, 15*(3), 7.

Wales, Australia, went public with their concerns about how clinical incidents were managed and patient safety at two hospitals (Johnstone, 2005). Eight months later, the same thing happened in Queensland, when "Toni Hoffman, the charge nurse of the intensive care unit at Bundaberg Base Hospital, raised serious concerns about the practices of a newly appointed surgeon, Dr Jayant Patel" (Johnstone, p. 8). She believed that the surgeon's practices were placing patients at unacceptable risk of preventable adverse events, including death. After 2 years of trying to address the problem within the hospital, she went public with her concerns: "What has since been described as a 'medical scandal' of unprecedented dimensions in Australia, suddenly emerged as front-page news here and around the world, again highlighting the role and responsibility of nurses as advocates for patient safety and quality care" (Johnstone, p. 8).

In both Australian cases, the nurses took their concerns about patient safety and quality of care repeatedly to management and were ignored. In addition, nurses in both cases reported high levels of intimidation after reporting their concerns to the appropriate authorities and were dissuaded from speaking freely at inquiries established to investigate the issues. Finally, in both cases, there was an apparent failure of whistle-blower laws to protect the nurses (Johnstone).

> ### CONSIDER
> That nurses have had to resort to whistle-blowing "to try and remedy a serious wrong detected in the course of their work is a travesty, not only of the principles and practice of good clinical governance and clinical risk management, but also of justice" (Johnstone, 2005, p. 8).

Patient advocacy has a central role in nursing. So too does professional advocacy, through which nurses are committed to improving the practice of nursing and maintaining the integrity of the health care profession. Both advocacy roles suggest that the nurse is accountable for assuring that at least minimum standards are met. All of these cases depict nurses who believed that they were acting honorably in the role of patient advocate. Yet all suffered negative consequences, including job loss. Unfortunately, this is more common than not.

Clearly, whistle-blowing should never be considered the first solution to ethically troubling behavior. Indeed, it should be considered only after prescribed avenues of solving problems have been attempted. This is true, however, only if patients' lives are not at stake. In those cases, immediate action must be taken.

In addition, the employee should typically go up the chain of command in reporting his or her concerns. This process, however, must be modified when the immediate

| BOX 15.1 | GUIDELINES FOR BLOWING THE WHISTLE |

- Stay calm and think about the risks and outcomes before you act.
- Know your legal rights, because laws protecting whistle-blowers vary by state.
- First, make sure that there really is a problem. Check resources such as the medical library, the Internet, and institutional policy manuals to be sure.
- Seek validation from colleagues that there is a problem, but do not get swayed by groupthink into not doing anything.
- Follow the chain of command in reporting your concerns, whenever possible.
- Confront those accused of the wrongdoing as a group whenever possible.
- Present just the evidence; leave the interpretation of facts to others. Remember that there may be an innocent or good explanation for what is occurring.
- Use internal mechanisms within your organization.
- If internal mechanisms do not work, use external mechanisms.
- Document carefully the problem that you have seen and the steps that you have taken to see that it is addressed.
- Do not expect thanks for your efforts.

Source: Bitoun Blecher, M. (2001-2008) *What color is your whistle*? Minoritynurse.com. Available at: **http://www.minoritynurse.com/features/nurse_emp/05-03-02c.html**. Accessed August 16, 2008; Myers, A. (2008b). How to blow the whistle safely. *Nursing Standard, 22*(25), 24.

supervisor is the source of the problem (Lachman, 2008). In such a case, the employee might need to skip that level to see that the problem is addressed.

There are other general guidelines for blowing the whistle that should also be followed, including carefully documenting all attempts to address the problem and being sure to report facts and not personal interpretations. These guidelines, as well as others, are presented in Box 15.1.

DISCUSSION POINT

In the United States, there is some evidence that the events of September 11, 2001, have made people more public spirited and more inclined to blow the whistle. Do you think this inclination is driven more by fear or by a desire to promote public good?

In addition, for some minority nurses, cultural issues further complicate whether a decision is made to blow the whistle and, if so, how it should be done. For example, "nurses with certain cultural backgrounds— for example, some Asians, Filipinos, and Africans—may be more reluctant to blow the whistle because they've been raised to respect a clear chain of command and

hierarchy" (Bitoun Blecher, 2001–2008, para 12). The same goes for nurses whose first language is not English. According to Winifred Carson, nurse practice counsel for the ANA, "They fear problems related to communication —whether they accurately communicate the magnitude of the problem and whether not speaking English as a first language would be used against them if they continue to challenge authority" (Bitoun Blecher, para 14).

Bitoun Blecher (2001–2008, para 1) suggested that "reporting incidents of wrongdoing in the workplace is always a risky business—but for minority nurses who blow the whistle, the stakes are even higher." Carson stated that minority nurses are more apt to be retaliated against, especially if they are working in nonminority settings (Bitoun Blecher, para 7).

THE PERSONAL RISKS OF WHISTLE-BLOWING

Being a whistle-blower is not without risks. Indeed, it is filled with risks. Unfortunately, most whistle-blowers set out believing that their actions will be welcomed, only to discover that the problems raised go much deeper than they imagined and the personal consequences can be overwhelming.

The personal risks of whistle-blowing can take many forms, including negative reactions from coworkers, losing one's job, and, in the extreme, legal retaliation. Bainbridge (2008) suggested that whistle-blowers are often faced with employer retaliation. He went on to say that in a typical case the employer will fire the whistle-blower, who is quite often an employee who is termed an *at-will* employee. The legislatures and courts, however, have created exceptions for those whistle-blowers who are at-will employees. Therefore, whistle-blowers can combat discrimination directed at them in the face of the accusations (Bainbridge).

Bitoun Blecher (2001–2008) also pointed out that whistle-blowers often face negative sanctions and noted an Australian survey of 95 nurses that suggested that there were severe repercussions for the 70 nurses who reported incidents of misconduct but few professional consequences for the 25 nurses who remained silent: "Fourteen percent of the whistle-blowers reported being treated as traitors, 16% received professional reprisals in the form of threats, 14% were rejected by peers, 11% were reprimanded, 9% were referred to a psychiatrist and 7% were pressured to resign" (para 6).

Schulman (2007) presented the story of Leroy Smith, a safety manager at a federal prison in California, who exposed "hazardous conditions in a prison computer recycling program where inmates were smashing monitors with hammers, unleashing clouds of toxic metals" (para 1), despite being threatened with termination and other types of retaliation. Although Smith eventually went on to be named "Public Servant of the Year" by the U.S. Office of Special Counsel (the federal agency charged with protecting government employees who expose waste, fraud, and abuse), his recognition ceremony was canceled at the last minute due to what Schulman called "ludicrous" reasons. In addition, things did not change at the prison as a result of the whistle-blowing. Smith concluded that his experience "was a beacon of false hope for public servants who are trying to correct wrongdoing," and Schulman agreed, noting that "given the current climate for whistle-blowers, false hope might be all the hope there is" (para 3).

> CONSIDER
>
> Although the U.S. public wants corruption and unethical behavior to be unveiled, the individual reporting such behavior is often looked on with distrust and considered to be disloyal.

Indeed, Schulman (2007) alleged that "a series of court rulings, legal changes, and new security and secrecy policies have made it easier than at any time since the Nixon era to punish whistle-blowers" (para 3). William Weaver, a professor of political science at the University of Texas-El Paso and a senior adviser to the National Security Whistle-blowers Coalition, agreed and stated that he now counsels federal employees against coming forward in any situation (Schulman). He said that he warns them that it will destroy their lives, cost them their families and friends, and squander their life savings on attorneys.

Clearly, whistle-blowers should never assume that doing the right thing will protect them from retaliation. Instead, potential whistle-blowers should determine their legal duty for reporting and carefully research the specifics of their protection under the law. In addition, they should try to report anonymously when possible. Moreover, they must be prepared to defend their claims.

In addition, prospective whistle-blowers should always at least try to solve problems internally before going public. When that is impossible and there is a clear indication of serious harm, they must document their actions and go public. They should also seek support and counsel before taking any steps.

Bainbridge (2008) stated that "the public recognition and value for whistle-blowing has been on a marked rise. This is giving more and more people the strength and courage to come forward and blow the whistle exposing illegal activities that could otherwise have gone unnoticed" (para 2). Lachman (2008) agreed, suggesting that whistle-blowers are increasingly being seen as brave individuals who take a stand against the inappropriate practices of an organization.

It is clear, then, that whistle-blowers often face both social and work-related retaliation, and that at times this retaliation can be severe and life altering. Yet it must be noted that at least some self-satisfaction and pride must come with the recognition that unethical behavior has been exposed and that at least the potential for

| BOX 15.2 | PROS AND CONS OF WHISTLE-BLOWING |

Pros

- Protects patients
- Improves quality of care
- Meets professional expectations and standards
- Satisfies ethical duty
- Brings problems out into the open
- Provides validation of concerns and moral "rightness"

Cons

- Poses personal and professional risks
- Casts doubt on motives
- Leads to possible job loss or employer retaliation
- Is typically a tiring, anxiety-producing, and often frustrating experience

correction is possible because of the whistle-blower's actions. Box 15.2 summarizes some of the pros and cons of whistle-blowing.

CONSIDER

"Nurses raise patient safety concerns every day, but few think of themselves as whistle-blowers—they assume they are just doing their job. Whistle-blowing has a negative image: the messenger gets crucified, the message is not heard and it all ends in tears. So speaking out is often only seen as whistle-blowing if it goes wrong" (Myers, 2008b, p. 24).

ETHICAL DIMENSIONS OF WHISTLE-BLOWING

Hook (2001, para 4) suggested that "although the average patient's immediate response to whistle-blowing would probably be a resounding 'hurrah!', whistle-blowing can create considerable moral distress for nurses as they weigh the consequences of their actions against the duties of their profession." Clearly, nurses have professional commitments not only to the well being of clients, but also to their employer and to other health care professionals. All too often, these commitments to principle and duty conflict.

This tension between loyalty to employer and the need to protect patients is a major reason so many nurses delay in blowing the whistle. Ray (2006) suggested, however, that this loyalty to the employer (organization) is misplaced when it causes harm rather than good.

Davis and Konishi (2007) discussed this moral conflict in their study of 24 Japanese nurses and viewed whistle-blowing as an act of the international nursing ethical ideal of advocacy, as well as in the larger context of professional responsibility. In this study, 10 of the nurses had previously reported another nurse and 12 had reported a physician for a wrongful act. Being direct and openly discussing sensitive topics is not valued in Japan because "such behavior disrupts the most fundamental value, harmony" (p. 194). In addition, whistle-blowing challenges long-held cultural values of group loyalty and "saving face." This requires Japanese nurses to make a professional judgment based on the perceived extent of potential harm to a patient and how the individual defines professional responsibility in the light of her or his advocacy function: "It could be considered irresponsible to report every witnessed act that could be viewed as wrong, just as it would be irresponsible not to report what is judged to be a serious wrongdoing" (p. 200).

Lachman (2008) suggested that the ethics of this divided loyalty can be viewed in relation to its moral purpose, whether that is to maximize the benefit and minimize the harm (a consequentialist view) or to fulfill a duty (a deontological Kantian view). If whistle-blowing is aimed at changing a situation for the better, the consequentialist moral framework becomes paramount. If whistle-blowing is viewed as the fulfillment of a duty to keep promises or protect patients, then the deontological framework becomes paramount.

CONSIDER

"A whistle-blower must blow the whistle for the right moral reason and reasoning" (Ray, 2006, p. 439).

A strong argument can be made for the precedence of the nurse's duty to the patient over his or her duty to the employer. Indeed, Ohnishi et al. (2008) suggested that nurses must always remember that their primary professional responsibility is to their patients, not to their employers. It can even be argued that duty to the employer may in fact justify whistle-blowing by nurses in some circumstances.

The ANA *Code of Ethics for Nurses with Interpretive Statements* may also provide guidance for nurses who are considering becoming a whistle-blower. Provision 3 of the *Code of Ethics* states that the nurse "promotes, advocates for, and strives to protect the health, safety, and rights of the patient" (ANA, 2001a, para 25). In addition, Section 3.5 states

> As an advocate for the patient, the nurse must be alert to and take appropriate action regarding any instances of incompetent, unethical, illegal, or impaired practice by a member of the health care team or the health care system, or any action on the part of others that places the rights or best interest of the patient in jeopardy (ANA, para 32).

Ethical codes of conduct from Canada, the United Kingdom, Australia, and Japan mandate similar action: "The Code of Ethics for nurses developed by the Japanese Nursing Association for both registered and licensed practical nurses notes: 'The nurse protects and safeguards individuals when their care is endangered or inhibited.' This can include whistle-blowing, although this word is not in the code" (Davis & Konishi, 2007, p. 195).

Such ethical codes bind nurses to the role of patient advocacy and compel them to take action when the rights or safety of patients are jeopardized. The bottom line is that although whistle-blowing can result in negative consequences for both the employing institution and the whistle-blower, nurses must uphold a professional standard and protect their patients.

Langone (2007) suggested that encouraging ethical behavior and professional standards in nurses begins with instilling a sense of ethics in nursing students. She advocated the use of honor codes to facilitate communication about behavioral expectations between faculty and students and to emphasize the importance of ethical behavior. An example of a modified honor code implemented in 2004 within the nursing program at Pasco-Hernando Community College (PHCC) is shown in Box 15.3.

BOX 15.3 | A MODIFIED HONOR CODE: THE HIRRE PROGRAM AT PASCO-HERNANDO COMMUNITY COLLEGE

H: Honesty

I: Integrity

R: Respect

R: Responsibility

E: Ethics

Source: Langone, M. (2007). Educational innovation. Promoting integrity among nursing students. *Journal of Nursing Education, 46*(1), 45–47.

CONSIDER

"Studies have found correlations between unethical practices as a student with future professional behavior; therefore, it is important to instill a sense of ethics in all nursing students" (Langone, 2007, p. 45).

WHISTLE-BLOWING AS A FAILURE OF ORGANIZATIONAL ETHICS

Ray (2006, p. 442) stated that "the ethical climate of an organization is the prevailing perception of that organization as reflected in its practices and procedures" and argued that "organizations must create infrastructures for the formulation of a code of ethics and practice in a way that will provide the support that is critical for raising the organization's awareness of problems that may bring potential or actual harm to patients and the public." Lachman (2008) agreed, arguing that whistle-blowing is indicative of ethical failure at the organizational level because the organization is failing to address accountability for the safety and welfare of the patients. The nurse or other employees feel compelled to take action against the wrongdoing in an effort to fulfill their professional obligations.

CONSIDER

The motive of most whistle-blowers is advocacy, not troublemaking.

Myers (2008a) also agreed, pointing out

Every organization faces the risk that something can go seriously wrong, and whether this is caused by the rare case of deliberate malpractice or, as is more likely, because of substandard practice or a serious mistake, the people who are most likely to suspect it are those working in or for the relevant organization (Myers, p. 3).

It is imperative then that nurses working on the front line be encouraged to speak up and that they be supported in their actions to do so.

For example, nursing departments within hospitals should provide their nurses with an ethics committee chaired by a nurse with experience in bioethical issues (not one who has a vested interest in promoting administrative or hierarchical constraints). Nurse managers should promote the values inherent in patient advocacy, and the organization should openly support individuals who are willing to take the risk of being a whistle-blower. The reality is that if an employee is willing to go to the trouble and risk the repercussions of blowing the whistle, those concerns should be taken seriously and investigated.

General Secretary Peter Carter of the Royal College of Nursing agreed, suggesting that workplaces must strive to be more transparent so that nurses feel safe addressing problems. In addition, nurses should feel confident that all safety issues will be addressed immediately in a positive manner (Blowing the Whistle, 2008).

CONSIDER

"One person can root out corruption and abuse of power. Once he understands this, he is redeemed and can break out of the trap of fear, and break free into the light of integrity and justice. That is the effect of seeing a brave whistle-blower stand up and win; it inspires the rest of us" (Scott Bloch, director of the Office of Special Counsel, as cited by Schulman 2007, para 1).

LEGAL PROTECTION FOR WHISTLE-BLOWERS

There is no universal legal protection for whistle-blowers; however, Faunce and Jefferys (2007) noted that under the 1st and 14th Amendments to the U.S. Constitution, state

and local government officials are prohibited from retaliating against whistle-blowers. In addition,

Although they do not fall under the category of "whistle-blower" protections, the laws protecting individual employees from mistreatment in the workplace, such as Title VII of the Civil Rights Act or the Fair Labor Standards Act, also protect employees from retaliation for asserting their rights under those laws. For example, it is illegal to terminate an employee for reporting sexual harassment, or for challenging an employer's failure to pay overtime (Joseph and Herzfeld LLP, 2008, para 12).

In addition, there is some whistle-blower protection at the state level. As of July 2008, however, only 20 states (Box 15.4) had passed some type of whistle-blower legislation, although a number of other states have since at least introduced such legislation (ANA, 2008). The problem is that although some of these state laws prohibit retaliation, the standards for proving retaliation vary.

For example, in Massachusetts,

If an employee reports legitimate violations of policy or patient care standards, state law requires the employer to correct the violations and prohibits them from taking retaliatory action against the whistle-blower, including discharge, suspension, demotion, or

---

BOX 15.4	**STATES WITH WHISTLE-BLOWER PROTECTION AS OF JULY 2008**
Arizona (2003)	Nevada (2002)
California (2003/2007)	New Jersey
Colorado (2007)	(2006/2008)
Florida (2002)	New York (2002)
Georgia (2007)	Oregon (2001)
Hawaii (amended 2002)	Texas (2007)
Illinois, (2003)	Utah (2003)
Indiana (2005)	Vermont (2004/2008)
Maine (2003/2007)	Virginia (2003)
Maryland (2002)	West Virginia (2001)
Michigan (2002)	

Source: ANA (2008). *Whistle-blower protection*. Available at: http://www.nursingworld.org/MainMenuCategories/ANAPoliticalPower/State/StateLegislativeAgenda/Whistle-blower_1.aspx. Accessed August 18, 2008.

denial of promotion. If these actions occur, the employee can report the employer to the attorney general's office, which may act on the public's behalf to protect the employee (Bitoun Blecher, 2001–2008, para 53).

Joseph and Herzfeld LLP (2008) suggested, however, that employees in most states increase their likelihood of whistle-blower protection under general statutes or common law if they meet criteria similar to those established at the federal level: (1) They must be acting in good faith that the employer or its employees are breaking the law in some way, (2) they must complain about that violation either to the employer or to an outside agency, (3) they must refuse to be a party to the violation, and (4) they should be willing to assist in any official investigations of the violation.

DISCUSSION POINT

What whistle-blowing protections, if any, exist in the state where you live? Is any legislation pending?

The False Claims Act

Some whistle-blower legislation has been enacted at the federal level, however, to encourage people to report wrongdoings. One such piece of legislation is the False Claims Act (FCA), originally a Civil War statute, which encourages whistle-blowers to come forward regarding fraud committed against the federal government and to file a lawsuit seeking lost monies in the government's name. The individual would file a *qui tam* or whistle-blower lawsuit and provide knowledge that a person defrauded the government (False Claims Act, 2007).

For example, a whistle-blower may have knowledge of a colleague inappropriately billing Medicare or Medicaid. The FCA provides protection for government whistle-blowers, thereby prohibiting employers from punishing employees who report the fraud or assist in the investigation of the fraud. If the whistle-blower is dismissed or discriminated against in any way as a result of the lawsuit, the whistle-blower can file a claim against that employer for unlawful retaliation.

To have a case brought to trial under federal law, the whistle-blower must first exhaust his or her internal chain of command and then file a complaint with the Department of Health and Human Services (DHHS). If the DHHS decides that the complaint is valid, the government proceeds with litigation against the employer,

and the whistle-blower receives a percentage of the damages awarded.

The case discussed earlier in this chapter involving the two nurses in Missouri who alleged nursing home abuse and fraud was a False Claims Act *qui tam* lawsuit. McCranie (2007, p. 6) suggested that these Missouri nurses should receive a substantial share of the money recovered by the government in this whistle-blower case because it is well deserved.

One of the best-known cases involving the FCA involved four health care professionals who opened a home infusion company known as Ven-A-Care in the Florida Keys (Taylor, 2001). The company provided care to terminally ill patients who had acquired immunodeficiency syndrome (AIDS). A large national chain, National Medical Care (NMC) approached Ven-A-Care about becoming a partner. Ven-A-Care refused because they believed NMC was using fraudulent schemes as part of their business practices. As a result, NMC countered by offering allegedly illegal incentives to local physicians to refer their patients to its Key West clinic, and Ven-A-Care was forced out of business as a result (Taylor).

One of Ven-A-Care's owners contacted government regulators in 1991 about NMC's business practices, but no action was taken. In June 1994, Ven-A-Care filed a civil whistle-blower suit against NMC in Miami. The case was later transferred to the U.S. Attorney's office in Boston. The end result was that NMC was partly dismantled, sold, and absorbed by German dialysis giant Fresenius. Fresenius paid the U.S. Justice Department $486 million in civil and criminal fines to settle Ven-A-Care's civil whistle-blower lawsuit. At least three top NMC executives pleaded guilty to criminal kickback and conspiracy charges and received prison sentences and fines, and three NMC divisions pleaded guilty to criminal fraud and kickback charges and were excluded from Medicare and Medicaid programs. None of the Key West doctors ever faced charges for their role in the NMC scheme there. Under the federal FCA, Ven-A-Care and its partners were entitled to a $40 million recovery (Taylor, 2001).

A different whistle-blower suit was brought by the four Ven-A-Care partners in 1995 in Miami federal court against more than 20 pharmaceutical companies (Taylor, 2001). This suit alleged that drug manufacturers manipulated the benchmark price Medicare uses to reimburse doctors for administering a relatively small number of drugs. That standard, known as the *average wholesale price,* is set and reported by the drug manufacturers and bears little resemblance to the average selling price of a drug.

The suit alleged that drug companies set an artificially high average wholesale price to encourage doctors who administer medications to patients with cancer, hemophilia, or AIDS to prescribe their drugs. Then physicians were encouraged to bill government health programs at 95% of average wholesale price, guaranteeing a huge built-in profit. Through that practice, called "marketing the spread," physicians stood to gain hundreds of dollars in profits per dose just for administering a drug, whereas the drug companies gained a captive market share and fat profits (Taylor, 2001).

The end result was a $14 million settlement in January with New Haven, Connecticut–based drug giant Bayer Corporation. The suit rocked the pharmaceutical industry and further stirred outrage in Congress and among consumer groups about high prescription-drug prices and illegal marketing practices. It is the first of an expected 20 settlements, and it took more than 5 years from the time the suit was filed until the first drug company settled (Taylor, 2001).

An even more recent case in which a *qui tam* lawsuit was filed was the case of Thomas Kirby, a physician and former co-chair of the Cardiothoracic Surgery Department at University Hospitals and Health System (UHHS) in Cleveland (Tariman, 2007). Kirby alleged

UHHS paid kickbacks to physicians for patient referrals from 1989–2001 in the form of phony medical directorships, payments to third-party physician practices, overpayment for physician practices, no interest loans that did not require repayment, and hospital payment of staff salaries at private-physician practices (Tariman, pp. 22–23).

Kirby blew the whistle and was paid $1.5 million, plus his attorney fees, for reporting the fraud. UHHS paid a $14 million settlement (Taylor, 2006).

Because the FCA has been fairly effective in detecting fraud at the federal level, state versions of the FCA have also passed. Under these state laws, whistle-blowers can file lawsuits seeking lost monies in the state or local government's name and share in the proceeds.

Weaknesses in the federal law have come to light. Zeller (2008) stated that the FCA does not apply to subcontractors, only to companies dealing directly with the government. This prompted two senior members of the House Judiciary Committee to introduce a companion bill in 2008 to add subcontractors to the legislation in an effort to modernize the law. Immediately, trade groups spoke up against making the change, arguing that this change would raise costs and discourage contractors from working with the government due to fears of unfounded claims by whistle-blowers. Sponsors of the bill argued that contractors only need to play by the rules to avoid penalties and that "some contractors have gotten a free ride when courts threw out cases involving subcontractors or barred testimony from whistle-blowers because they weren't privy to specific details of billing documentation" (Zeller, para 7).

In contrast, a Supreme Court ruling in 2008 narrowed the application of the False Claims Act, limiting the liability of those who do not bill the government directly but go through another entity that contracts with the U.S. (Sorrel, 2008): "Justices clarified that the plaintiffs must show that the defendants intended to defraud the U.S. and not another entity, and that alleged false statements were relevant to the government's decision to pay the claim" (para 5). In other words, it is not enough to show that government money was involved in fraud; plaintiffs must show there was fraud against the government to obtain government funds. Some legal experts say the decision could make it more difficult for whistle-blowers to prove certain cases using the false claims statute as opposed to other state or federal antifraud remedies (Sorrel).

Other Federal Legislation Related to Whistle-Blowing

Another piece of legislation, the Whistleblower Protection Act of 1989, protects federal employees who disclose government fraud, abuse, and waste. The National Labor Relations Act might also protect employees in the private sector from retaliation when employees act as a group to modify working conditions or ask for better wages.

The best protection for nongovernmental employees in the United States at this time, however, is likely the Sarbanes-Oxley Act of 2002. This act dramatically redesigned federal regulation of public company corporate governance and reporting obligations and provided some protection for whistle-blowers who report fraud in publicly traded companies to the proper authorities (OSHA Fact Sheet, 2006).

Employees in these companies who experience retaliation for whistle-blowing have 90 days to file a written complaint with OSHA: "If the evidence supports an employee's claim of retaliation and a settlement cannot be reached, OSHA will issue an order requiring the employer to reinstate the employee, pay back wages" (OSHA Fact Sheet, 2006, para 11). After OSHA issues its final ruling, either party may request a full hearing before an administrative law judge of the Department of Labor. That decision can then be appealed to the Department's Administrative Review Board for final review.

WHISTLE-BLOWING AS AN INTERNATIONAL ISSUE

Perhaps the most far-reaching whistle-blower law in the world is the United Kingdom's Public Interest Disclosure Act, which passed in July 1998 and was fully implemented by 2001. Under this act, whistle-blower disclosures to employers, regulatory bodies, and the media are protected from retaliation (Goldman & Lewis, 2007). Employers who retaliate may be subject to unlimited compensation in fines. This is because whistle-blowers are viewed as witnesses acting in the public interest. The burden of proof, however, is on the employee to show that the disclosure was protected and that the disclosure was the reason for dismissal (Goldman & Lewis).

CONCLUSIONS

Nurses as health care professionals have a responsibility to uncover, openly discuss, and condemn short-cuts that threaten the clients they serve. Clearly, however, there has been a collective silence in many such cases. The reality is that whistle-blowing offers no guarantee that the situation will change or the problem will improve, and the literature is replete with horror stories regarding negative consequences endured by whistle-blowers. The whistle-blower cannot even trust that other health care professionals with similar belief systems about advocacy will value their efforts, because the public's feelings about whistle-blowers are so mixed. In addition, state laws vary and protections for the nongovernment employee whistle-blower are often limited.

For all these reasons, it takes tremendous courage to come forward as a whistle-blower. It also takes a tremendous sense of what is right and what is wrong, as well as a commitment to follow a problem through until an acceptable level of resolution is reached. Whistle-blowers are heroes and should be treated as such; their courage is nothing short of exceptional. How unfortunate that we frequently don't treat them that way.

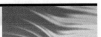

FOR ADDITIONAL DISCUSSION

1. Why do Americans have a "love–hate" relationship with whistle-blowers? Is this dichotomy prevalent in other countries as well?

2. Which is greater for you personally—your duty to your patients, your duty to your employer, or your duty to yourself? How do you sort out what you should do when these duties are in conflict?

3. Do you believe that most whistle-blowing must be external before appropriate action is taken?

4. Should whistle-blowers receive compensation under the False Claims Act?

5. Would you be willing to bear the risks of becoming a whistle-blower?

6. Do you believe that there is more, less, or the same amount of whistle-blowing in health care as in other types of industries?

7. Can you identify a whistle-blowing situation in which it might be appropriate to go outside the chain of command in reporting concerns about organizational practice?

REFERENCES

American Nurses Association (ANA) (2001a). *Code of Ethics for Nurses with Interpretive Statements*. Washington, DC: ANA Publications. Available at: http://www.nursingworld.org/ethics/code/protected_nwcoe303.htm. Accessed April 30, 2005.

American Nurses Association (ANA) (2001b). *ANA files amicus brief in support of six nurse whistleblowers*. Available at: http://www.nursingworld.org/pressrel/2001/pr0619.htm. Accessed April 30, 2005.

American Nurses Association (ANA) (2008). *Whistleblower protection*. Available at: http://www.nursingworld.org/MainMenuCategories/ANAPoliticalPower/State/StateLegislativeAgenda/Whistleblower_1.aspx. Accessed August 18, 2008.

Bainbridge, R. (2008). *Whistleblower definition*. Ezine articles. Available at: http://ezinearticles.com/?Whistleblower-Definition&id=410263. Accessed August 18, 2008.

Bitoun Blecher, M. (2001–2008) *What color is your whistle?* Minoritynurse.com. Available at: http://www.minoritynurse.com/features/nurse_emp/05-03-02c.html. Accessed August 16, 2008.

Blowing the whistle (June 2008). *Nursing Management—UK, 15*(3), 7.

Colvin, G. (2002). Wonder women of whistleblowing. *Fortune, 146*(3). Available at: http://money.cnn.com/magazines/fortune/fortune_archive/2002/08/12/327047/index.htm. Accessed August 21, 2008.

Davis, A. E., & Konishi, E. (2007). Whistleblowing in Japan. *Nursing Ethics, 14*(2), 194–202.

False Claims Act (2007). *OSHA whistleblower fact sheet*. National Whistleblower Legal Defense & Education Fund. Available at: http://www.whistleblowersblog.org/articles/faq/. Accessed August 21, 2008.

Faunce, T. A., & Jefferys, S. (2007). Whistleblowing and scientific misconduct: Renewing legal and virtue ethics foundations. *Medicine and Law, 26*(3), 567–584.

Goldman, L., & Lewis, J. (2007). Blowing the whistle. *Occupational Health, 59*(11), 16–17.

Hook, K. (Fall 2001). Toward an ethical defense of whistleblowing. *The American Nurses Association. Ethics and Human Rights Issues Update, 1*(2). Available at: http://www.ana.org/ethics/update/vol1no2a.htm. Accessed April 30, 2005.

Johnstone, M. J. (2005). Issues. Whistleblowing and accountability. *Australian Nursing Journal, 13*(5), 8.

Joseph & Herzfeld LLP (2008). *Whistleblower and Sarbanes Oxley claims*. Available at: http://www.jhllp.com/lawyer-attorney-1324989.html. Accessed August 21, 2008.

Lachman, V. D. (2008). Whistleblowers: Troublemakers or virtuous nurses? *Medsurg Nursing, 17*(2), 126–128, 134.

Langone, M. (2007). Educational innovation. Promoting integrity among nursing students. *Journal of Nursing Education, 46*(1), 45–47.

Marquis, B., & Huston, C. (2009). *Leadership Roles and Management Functions in Nursing* (6th ed.). Philadelphia: Lippincott Williams & Wilkins.

McCranie, F. (2007). *Nursing home abuse and fraud exposed by nurses in Qui Tam whistleblower case*. Whistleblower Lawyer Blog. Available at: http://www.whistleblowerlawyerblog.com/2007/06/nursing_home_abuse_and_fraud_e.html. Accessed August 17, 2008.

Myers, A. (2008a). Whistleblowing saves lives. *Nursing Management—UK, 15*(3), 3.

Myers, A. (2008b). How to blow the whistle safely. *Nursing Standard, 22*(25), 24.

Ohnishi, K., Hayama, Y., Asai, A., Kosugi, S., Hayama, Y. (2008). The process of whistleblowing in a Japanese psychiatric hospital. *Nursing Ethics, 15*(5), 631–642.

OSHA fact sheet. Filing whistleblower complaints under the Sarbanes-Oxley Act (2006). Available at: http://www.osha.gov/Publications/osha-factsheet-sox-act.pdf. Accessed August 20, 2008.

Ray, S. L. (2006). Whistleblowing and organizational ethics. *Nursing Ethics, 13*(4), 438–445.

Schulman, D. (2007). Office of Special Counsel's war on whistleblowers. *Mother Jones*. Available at: http://www.motherjones.com/news/feature/2007/05/dont_whistle_while_you_work.html. Accessed August 17, 2008.

Scott, M. (2008). *NHS whistleblower Moi Ali forced to quit over nurse row*. Sundaymall.co.uk. Available at: http://www.sundaymail.co.uk/news/newsfeed/2008/06/29/nhs-whistleblower-moi-ali-forced-to-quit-over-nurse-row-78057-20624687/. Accessed August 17, 2008.

Smith, R. (2008). A Morgan Stanley crusader; Bond-pricing issues prompt one broker's inside investigation. *The Wall Street Journal* (Eastern edition), May 24, 2008, p. B1. Available at: http://proquest.umi.com. mantis.csuchico.edu/pqdweb?index=0&did=148396 8031&SrchMode=1&sid=1&Fmt=3&VInst=PROD &VType=PQD&RQT=309&VName=PQD&TS=12 19253390&clientId=17840. Accessed August 21, 2008.

Sorrel, A. L. (2008). *Supreme Court tightens scope of False Claims Act.* amednews.com. Available at: http://www. ama-assn.org/amednews/2008/07/28/gvsa0728.htm. Accessed August 21, 2008.

Tariman, J. D. (2007). Straight talk. When should you blow the whistle for ethical reasons? *ONS Connect, 22*(2), 22–23.

Taylor, M. (2001). Four found whistleblowing the best revenge. *Modern Healthcare, 31*(24), 32–34.

Taylor, M. (2006). Settling all scores . . . UHHS to pay $14 million in kickback lawsuit. *Modern Healthcare, 36*(34), 16.

The Free Online Dictionary. (2008). *Whistleblower* (Definition). Available at: http://www. thefreedictionary.com/whistleblower. Accessed August 17, 2008.

Zeller, S. (2008). Whistleblowing pay hike? Updating a Civil War law to help whistleblowers. *CQWeekly-Vantage Point, 2008*(June 30), 1746. Available at: http:// library.cqpress.com.mantis.csuchico.edu/cqweekly/ document.php?id=weeklyreport110-000002908705& type=toc&num=161&. Accessed August 21, 2008.

BIBLIOGRAPHY

Brainard, A. H., & Brislen, H. C. (2007). Viewpoint: Learning professionalism: A view from the trenches. *Academic Medicine, 82*(11), 1010–1014.

DoBias, M. (2007). Whistle-blower law tightened: Ruling demands first hand knowledge of wrongdoing. *Modern Healthcare, 37*(14), 8.

Duffin, C. (2007). Turning a blind eye. *Nursing Older People, 19*(7), 6–7.

Dyer, C. (2008). Whistleblower who was excluded from work for five years wins apology. *British Medical Journal, 336*(7635), 63.

Finkel, E. (2007). Australian science. New misconduct rules aim to minister to an ailing system. *Science, 317*(5842), 1159.

Gray, J. (2008). Whistleblower or manipulator? *Canadian Business, 81*(12/13), 11–12.

Jackson, D. (2008). What becomes of the whistleblowers? *Journal of Clinical Nursing, 17*(10), 1261–1262.

Jones, R. (2007). Whistleblow with care. *Community Care, 2007*, 6.

Lubell, J. (2007). Few docs report peers' errors. Fears abound of litigation, ruining careers: Survey. *Modern Healthcare, 37*(49), 14.

Monin, B., Sawyer, P., Marquez, M., Sawyer, P., & Marquez, M. (2008). The rejection of moral rebels: Resenting those who do the right thing. *Journal of Personality and Social Psychology, 95*(1), 76–93.

Murray, J. S. (2008). The Paul Revere Freedom to Warn Act. *American Journal of Nursing, 108*(3), 38–39.

Tammelleo, A. D. (2006). 'Whistleblower' fired by nursing home awarded damages. *Nursing Law's Regan Report, 2006*(April 1). Available at: http://www. thefreelibrary.com/'Whistleblower'+fired+by+nursing +home+awarded+damages.-a0145474630. Accessed January 22, 2009.

Ting, M. (2008). Whistleblowing. *American Political Science Review, 102*(2), 249–267.

Whistleblower: Nursing director's suit dismissed. (2008). *Legal Eagle Eye Newsletter for the Nursing Profession, 16*(3), 7.

WEB RESOURCES

Blecher, M. B. (2001-2008). What color is your whistle? Minoritynurse.com	http://www.minoritynurse.com/features/nurse_emp/05-03-02c.html
National Whistleblower Center	http://www.whistleblowers.org
OSHA Whistleblower Fact Sheets (2008)	http://www.whistleblowersblog.org/articles/faq/
Protection for Private Sector Employee Whistleblowers	http://www.whistleblowers.org/private.htm
Whistleblowers Australia	www.whistleblowers.org.au
Whistleblower Publications	http://www.whistleblowers.org/html/publications.html

CHAPTER 16

Impaired Nursing Practice—What Are the Issues?

• JENNIFER LILLIBRIDGE •

Learning Objectives

The learner will be able to:

1. Examine the prevalence of substance misuse in the nursing profession and compare this prevalence with that in the other health care professions.
2. Reflect on possible reasons for the inadequacy of current empirical research studies examining chemical impairment in nursing.
3. Describe early risk factors that result in an increased risk for chemical addiction in the nursing profession.
4. Explore why the early identification of risk factors and substance misuse increases the likelihood of successful intervention and treatment of the impaired nurse.
5. Identify common behaviors and actions that might signify chemical impairment in an employee or colleague.
6. Analyze how personal feelings, values, and biases regarding chemical impairment might alter a colleague's or manager's ability to confront and/or help the chemically impaired employee.

7. Explore reasons why nurses with substance abuse problems often fail to receive the same caring attitude or approach from their peers that is extended to other individuals who misuse drugs and alcohol.
8. Identify state board of nursing reporting requirements for nurses suspected of chemical dependency or of diverting drugs for personal use.
9. Describe typical components of a state diversion program, as well as a "return to work" contract, for a chemically impaired nurse.
10. Identify the driving forces that compelled most state boards of nursing in the United States to move from mandatory disciplinary action for impaired nurses to diversion program treatment.
11. Reflect on personal feelings regarding the extent to which a state board of nursing has the right and/or responsibility to invade the impaired nurse's privacy to ensure recovery is ongoing.

"Helping the impaired nurse is difficult but not impossible. The choices for action are varied. The only choice that is clearly wrong is to do nothing" (National Council of State Boards of Nursing [NCSBN], 2001, p. iv). The problem of impaired nursing practice has plagued nursing for decades; however, it remains both poorly researched and poorly understood. Several explanations for the lack of recent research and the continuation of the problem can be found: (1) nurses find it difficult to talk openly about and report a situation in which "one of their own" may be engaging in behavior

that puts them and their patients at risk, (2) nurses are reluctant to self-disclose a substance abuse problem due to the stigma, and (3) there is a lack of federal funding for dealing with impaired nursing practice. The American Nurses Association's (ANA) classic definition of an impaired nurse is "one who has impaired functioning which results from alcohol or drug misuse and which interferes with professional judgment and the delivery of safe, high quality care" (ANA, 1984, p. 18).

A discussion about impaired nursing practice often raises more questions than it answers. Two key issues surround impaired nursing practice. The first is concern for patient safety. The second is concern for the health of the impaired nurse. With denial common, the problem can go without detection or treatment for years. When nurses divert drugs for personal use and make poor, often critical judgments while providing care to the vulnerable, the risk for harm to patients is high (Breier-Mackie, 2007; Fogger & McGuinness, 2006/ 2007).

Although the ANA has defined what an impaired nurse is, it is less clear what constitutes impaired practice and how to proceed when impaired practice is suspected. Can confidentiality be maintained to avoid loss of the nurse's license? What are the barriers for a nurse to report an impaired colleague; are there ethical issues? What happens to the nurse who is able to complete rehabilitation and seeks re-entry into practice? Probably the most significant and persistent question is: How can the problem be prevented in the first place? All of these questions highlight the complexity of the problem and the lack of consistent solutions.

PREVALENCE OF THE PROBLEM

Estimates on the prevalence of substance misuse in the nursing profession are varied; efforts to quantify the prevalence are fraught with problems. It has been suggested that the difficulty in part may be due to the sensitive nature of the information, and that self-disclosure is reduced due to the stigma associated with substance abuse (Saver, 2008). Prevalence was documented in a review of the literature that ended with studies from 1998 (Lillibridge, 2006). The older estimate of the ANA that 6% to 8% of nurses had a problem with drugs or alcohol was based on estimates of the problem in the broader population. There are no more recent published large-scale prevalence studies.

Shaw, McGovern, Angres, and Rawal (2004) proposed that the issue of prevalence is not as important as patterns of abuse among health professionals, such as physicians and nurses. They argued that understanding patterns of abuse might lead to more substantial outcomes than merely determining the actual numbers of health professionals with a substance abuse problem. Due to the many difficulties that surround prevalence studies, especially that of self-disclosure, perhaps it is more relevant to accept that prevalence estimations are just that—estimations—and to redirect the focus

to achieving long-term positive outcomes, especially because health care professionals, nursing organizations, and nursing education facilities do not dispute that the problem continues to exist. This may encourage researchers to explore the nature of substance use problems so that solutions can be found to bring recovered, formerly impaired individuals back into the profession.

CONSIDER

If 6% to 8% of nurses have a substance use problem, every nurse will likely work with chemically impaired colleagues at some time during his or her nursing career.

OVERVIEW OF THE LITERATURE

One of the problems in reviewing recent literature is that research about impaired nursing practice is almost nonexistent. Recent research-based literature on the topic is disappointing, and gaps about all issues related to impaired nursing practice exist. An extensive review yielded limited new material on this persistent problem. Most new articles are discussion pieces and many are anecdotal accounts about individual nurses, but very few are research based. Two literature reviews were found that were not reported in the previous edition of this book. West (2003) noted that the discussions related to impaired practice were focused mainly on prevalence, attitudes, and late symptom identification. She concluded that the problem is multifactorial, with risk increasing with a combination of factors, and left readers to ponder "what early characteristics nurses encounter that influence whether they become impaired" (2003, p. 143). The issue of early risk factor identification remains a worthy but thus far limited topic for research.

More recently Baldisseri (2007) reviewed literature on impaired practice by discussing prevalence, risk factors, treatment options, and re-entry into clinical practice. Only 2 of the 72 citations had been published within the previous 5 years. The majority represented data from the 1980s to 1990s, which supports the assertion that there is a lack of recent research; thus the review offered little in terms of new additions to solving the problem, given that the conclusions were based on dated research. The review focused on physician impairment, with statistics that are similar to those for nursing impairment. One difference between the professions is that all states in the United

States offer treatment programs for physicians, and re-entry into practice has fewer stigmas for physicians than for nurses. With limited recent empirically based research, there is little to help the profession move closer toward management and resolution of the problem, if indeed resolution is even possible.

> **DISCUSSION POINT**
> Why hasn't more nursing research been conducted that explores the experiences and perspectives of nurses who misuse substances?

Identifying Early Risk Factors for Substance Abuse

The very nature of the work of nurses seems to be challenged when risk factors are considered. Nurses have constant access to narcotics, and fatigue seems to come with the job, no matter what shift is worked. It is difficult to avoid job strain in the current health care environment, which is in the middle of the worst nursing shortage ever reported. Despite the difficulties inherent in the practice setting today, many nurses do work hard to get experience and increase knowledge so they can become specialists, only to find this, too, can put them at higher risk of turning to drugs or alcohol when coping is difficult. These issues highlight the complexity of the problem for the profession, requiring that all nurses become more aware of how to prevent it from occurring.

> **DISCUSSION POINT**
> Due to long work hours, overtime (often mandatory), and job strain, is the nursing shortage contributing to the prevalence of nurses who misuse substances?

Two recent studies addressed the issue of identification of early risk factors for the development of substance abuse problems in health care professionals. One study broadly looked at a variety of health care professionals and one specifically at nurses. Kenna and Lewis (2008) used a sample of 697 dentists, nurses, pharmacists, and physicians that was limited to one state. The aim was to look at risk factors for alcohol and other drug use in health care professionals. All data were self-reported. Several findings are noteworthy when discussing risk factors for nurses. Younger practitioners were at higher risk than their older colleagues. This is consistent with the literature about drug use in the general population. General

moderate use of alcohol was a predictor for any drug use, significant or not. Social contact was not considered a risk factor, which supports the belief that there is not a professional drug culture in the health care setting.

Several conclusions can be drawn from this study. The first is that it is imperative that new graduate and younger nurses be educated about impaired practice and their increased risk, in the hopes of facilitating positive coping strategies and increasing the focus on prevention. This means that education about impaired practice risks must start in the nursing education community. Second, alcohol should not be dismissed as a legal drug that carries less significance in the broader picture of impaired practice. Finally, impaired practitioners tend to isolate themselves from others and not seek help readily. This speaks to the issue of reporting an impaired colleague, which is discussed later in the chapter.

West (2005) explored three variables as early risk factors for substance abuse among nurses: sensation seeking, risk factors for alcohol, and family history. A study including 100 previously impaired nurses and 100 nonimpaired nurses found that these three variables could be used as predictors for impaired nursing practice. West concluded that early identification can lead to early treatment or possibly prevention. This can inform our understanding of the appropriate timeline for intervention so that early counseling and education can happen. West also stressed that education about impaired practice is critical to nursing education curricula so that nurses entering the profession can be armed with information about potential risk factors.

> **CONSIDER**
> Nurses are praised and looked up to by clients, society, and other nurses. Yet a nurse with a substance abuse problem does not seem to receive that same caring attitude from his or her peers.

National Nursing Organizations

For policies to be in place at the local level, it is imperative that the positions of leading national nursing organizations about impaired practice be clear. The ANA's policy about impaired practice can be found on its Web site, http://nursingworld.org/MainMenuCategories/ThePracticeofProfessionalNursing/workplace/ImpairedNurse.aspx. The basis for the policy is the ethical duty of the nurse to the patient, specifically Provision 3 of the ANA (2001) *Code of Ethics for Nurses.* The advocacy role all nurses have is clear; nurses must report an impaired colleague. The ANA supports treatment as opposed to discipline and a process that facilitates re-entry of the recovered nurse back into practice (ANA, 2008).

The focus of the position about impaired nursing practice of the American Association of Colleges of Nursing (AACN) is on policy development in nursing education (AACN, 1998). Their policy was written in 1994 and updated in 1998. The AACN's policy can be found on its Web site, http://www.aacn.nche.edu/publications/positions/subabuse.htm. The policy has guidelines for prevention and management of substance abuse in the nursing education community. There are specific features that address the issue for students, faculty, and staff. Critical to successful policy development is attention to confidentiality and legal perspectives. From the perspective of process and content, the necessary areas are identification, intervention, evaluation, treatment, and re-entry into practice. The AACN is in agreement with the ANA regarding the importance of treatment over a reasonable timeframe and a process for successful re-entry into practice.

The NCSBN has a *Chemical Dependency Handbook for Nurse Managers* that was published in 2001 and can be found on their Web site, https://www.ncsbn.org/524.htm. The purpose of the *Chemical Dependence Handbook* is to support nurse managers to manage chemical dependency problems with employees. As with the AACN and the ANA, the NCSBN also supports early detection and treatment of the impaired nurse with the goal of returning a recovered nurse to work. The NCSBN has a Chemical Dependency Committee with the task of rewriting the handbook and setting a research agenda for chemical dependency in nursing (K. Kenward, personal communication, July 22, 2008). A literature review has been completed, and data are being gathered about which model (peer assistance, in-house program, contractual services, etc.) and services are provided by each state board in the area of alcohol impairment.

Nurses Reporting an Impaired Colleague—Issues and Ethics

It is the responsibility of every nurse to be aware of reporting requirements when a nurse is suspected of chemical dependency or of diverting drugs for personal use. No uniform agreement exists among the states as to what those reporting requirements are. Information regarding reporting requirements can be found from each state board of nursing, which often can be easily accessed via its Web site. Before a nurse can be reported or referred to a treatment program, there must be recognition that the nurse needs help. Recognizing that a nurse is impaired might not be easy. Some common signs or behavior changes of a chemically impaired nurse are shown in Box 16.1.

In theory, reporting an impaired nurse seems like a decision that would be easy to make. The position of the ANA and other nursing organizations is clear: It is the ethical and legal duty of a nurse to advocate for public safety, their colleagues, and the profession (Saver, 2008). This means simply that it is a nurse's job to protect the patient from harm; if that means reporting an impaired colleague, that is what one must do. In practice, however, the situation is anything but clear. Some say that there is a "code of silence" (Dunn, 2005, p. 582) about impaired practice and that nurses, as professionals, need to overcome this attitude so that impaired nurses can get the help and rehabilitation they need and patients can be protected. Despite the ethical dilemma of reporting an impaired peer, early identification can mean early treatment and perhaps the maintenance of a functioning nurse in the process (Fogger & McGuinness, 2006/2007).

What are some of the barriers to fulfilling the advocacy obligation and reporting an impaired colleague? Several reasons have been suggested in the literature, including "established friendship, work history, loyalty, fear of confrontation, and fear of jeopardizing a colleague's license to practice" (Breier-Mackie, 2007, p. 227). Other reasons for not reporting a colleague could be fear of being labeled a whistle-blower or fear of retribution, such as challenges to one's work practices (Dunn, 2005). Nurse friends and peers may enable an impaired colleague due to their inability to accept that an educated and skilled practitioner is diverting drugs for personal use (Palmer & Hoffman, 2007).

CONSIDER

Whistle-blowing usually carries a negative connotation. Consider how you would feel if someone labeled you a whistle-blower for reporting an impaired peer.

BOX 16.1   SIGNS AND BEHAVIORAL CHANGES SUGGESTING CHEMICAL IMPAIRMENT

Common Signs of Impairment

- The nurse appears to be a "workaholic," arriving early, staying late, offering to work extra shifts, and offering to cover for breaks.
- The nurse often works in areas that have a high volume of commonly abused drugs; examples include the oncology department, the emergency department, and the operating room.
- The nurse volunteers to care for patients who have diminished awareness.
- There are many reports from patients that their pain medication is ineffective; narcotic count errors are common.
- Peers complain about the quality and quantity of the nurse's work.

Behavioral Changes

- Increased irritability with patients and colleagues, often followed by extreme calm.
- Social isolation; the person eats alone and avoids unit social functions.
- Extreme and rapid mood swings.
- Unusually strong interest in narcotics or the narcotic cabinet.
- Sudden dramatic change in personal grooming or any other personal habits.
- Extreme defensiveness regarding medication errors.

Source: Marquis, B. L., & Huston, C. J. (2009). *Leadership Roles and Management Functions in Nursing: Theory & Application* (6th ed.). Philadelphia: Lippincott Williams & Wilkins; Dunn, D. (2005). Substance abuse among nurses—Defining the issue. *AORN Journal, 82*(4), 573–596.

Beckstead's (2005a) work was carried out in the laboratory setting, using scenarios to study impaired nursing practice. One study explored the moderating effects of attitudes on nurses' intentions to report impaired practice. Findings include that nurses' attitudes about substance use influenced the intention to report due to a moderating effect of specific characteristics. Two characteristics studied were "use while at work" versus "use only while off duty" (p. 916). It was concluded that some nurses who used substances moderately were more critical of nurses who used substances irresponsibly. It also was found that nurses with more "permissive" attitudes placed less value on the substances involved, whereas nurses with "less permissive" attitudes placed more value on the characteristics of the offense (p. 916). Beckstead believed that these findings suggested that nurses who use substances moderately may be an asset to early identification and reporting of impaired peers.

Beckstead (2005b) also reported on the "thinking process nurses use when making decisions to report peer wrongdoing" (p. 325). The roles of incompetence and substance abuse information were the basis of analysis. The findings suggested that nurses are just as likely to report an impaired peer as they are to report technical incompetence. However, nurses used different combinations of information to make decisions and weighed the importance of cues given in the context of the case. This meant that additional information about substance abuse could alter the decision to report an incompetent colleague. Studying the thinking process of nurses as they make decisions to report impaired practice may be a critical factor in breaking down the barriers to reporting.

DISCUSSION POINT

You suspect that a coworker/friend is diverting drugs for personal use. You find yourself covering up for her because you know that she is depressed, exhausted, and having family problems. Your supervisor makes a casual comment with similar suspicions. Your first instinct is to make excuses for your friend; what would you do?

Impaired Practice Policies in the Workplace

It is a difficult and often traumatic experience for a nurse to report an impaired peer. The important consideration is that patients are not harmed, the nurse is helped, and the provider is protected. It is imperative that every health care facility and educational institution have an *Impaired Practice Policy* in place that clearly sets out the process that is to be followed if impaired practice is suspected (Palmer & Hoffman, 2007). An important component of any policy is the commitment to a drug- and alcohol-free workplace, whether that is a health care setting (Saver, 2008) or an educational environment. Another important component of any policy should include "procedures for returning to work, which normally included a signed contract, restrictions on handling of narcotics, and random urine testing for drugs" (Saver, p. 12).

A nurse who is suspected of impaired practice should not be confronted unless there is a plan in place, whether it is a referral to a person or program within the facility or a referral to the treatment program for that particular state board of nursing. Many professional associations and treatment programs have peer assistance hotlines in place that can also provide a variety of resources (Palmer & Hoffman, 2007). The key is that the nurse suspecting impaired practice and the nurse whose practice is being challenged should not feel alone in the process. Help is available and should be used.

Nondiscipline Treatment/ Diversion Programs

The disciplinary approach was the norm in most states through the 1980s. Following the ANA resolution in 1982 to support treatment of chemically dependent nurses, many states began to look at treatment and rehabilitation options instead of discipline (ANA, 1984). As of 2007, 42 states offered nondisciplinary programs for nurses with chemical dependency (K. Kenward, personal communication, July 24, 2008).

> ### CONSIDER
> Most addiction specialists and the American Medical Association view addiction as a chronic medical illness and argue that it should be approached in an analogous way to, say, diabetes or asthma.

Although most states now offer treatment options, the types of programs vary. Some programs are completely voluntary, which means that there is no threat of the nurse being reported to disciplinary authorities. Many programs, however, represent a more coercive process; that is, discipline is not implemented as long as the impaired nurse participates in the treatment program. This often requires a 2- to 5-year commitment and rigorous standards (Clark & Farnsworth, 2006). The first treatment program offered was the Intervention Project for Nurses (IPN) in Florida in 1983 (see Research Study Fuels the Controversy on page 281). The IPN has a comprehensive Web site offering information about the history of the program, including frequently asked questions and available services (http://www.ipnfl.org/faq.html).

California also offers a diversion program; information is available from the California Board of Registered Nursing (CBRN) Web site, http://www.rn.ca.gov/diversion/whatisdiv.shtml. Established in 1985, its goal is to "protect the public by early identification of impaired registered nurses and by providing these nurses access to appropriate intervention programs and treatment services" (CBRN, 2007, para 2). Impaired nurses can be self-referred or can be referred by family, coworkers, or the board. All licensed registered nurses residing in California are eligible to enter the program, but they must agree to enter the program voluntarily. Since 1985, more than 1,200 nurses have successfully completed the diversion program in California. Requirements for completion include "a change in lifestyle that supports continuing recovery and [having] a minimum of 24 consecutive months of clean, random, body-fluid tests" (para 14). Confidentiality of participants is protected by law, and nurses who successfully complete the program have their records regarding chemical impairment destroyed.

A different approach is followed in the Texas Peer Assistance Program for Nurses. This program offers services to nurses suffering from chemical dependency, as well as from anxiety and other mental health disorders. It requires abstinence, maintains confidentiality, is strictly voluntary, and is independent of the state licensing board (Texas Nurses Association [TNA], 2004). Information from the TNA Web site includes how and when to make referrals, how the program works, and important links to services and organizations (http://www.tpapn.org).

Research Study Fuels the Controversy: Nurses in Recovery

This research study explored the experiences of nine male nurses who completed Florida's Intervention Project for Nurses for nurses with a chemical dependency problem.

This study is unique in that it offers a male perspective, in a female-dominated profession, on the work pressures that might influence decisions to use substances irresponsibly in the workplace. The two overarching themes in this study were "person" and "profession." A conceptual model was developed entitled the "Caring for Nurses with Professional Impairment Model." The theme of "person" was based on how the male nurse views himself during the process of addiction. There were three aspects: predetermined risk, altered values, and sensation-seeking behavior. The theme of "profession" related to how the addicted nurse related to the profession of nursing and how individual decisions interacted with the profession during the addiction journey. The components were masterminding, professional heteronomy, getting caught, rehabilitation, spirituality, and nurse becomes the nursed. Some of the conclusions reached were that there was a decreased awareness of impaired practice in the nursing community, there was poor compliance to procedures for controlled substances, denial was common (especially among peers), and that male nurses tended to cover up stress. Some of these findings support the earlier work of Lillibridge, Cox, and Cross (2002), especially denial among colleagues that there was a problem and lack of awareness. The author of the study had many recommendations for further research, highlighting the need for research funding and interest in this professional area of nursing.

Source: Dittman, P. W. (2008). *Professional impairment: The lived experience of chemically impaired nurses.* Presented to the Joint Meeting of the Boards of Nursing, Osteopathic Medicine and Pharmacy, Tallahassee, Florida, February 29, 2008. Available at: http://www.doh.state.fl.us/MQA/osteopath/info_Prof_Impairment_Chem_Diver.pdf. Accessed August 4, 2008.

Although it initially offered a voluntary peer assistance program, Michigan has moved away from this approach and now encourages health professionals with chemical dependency problems to be admitted into a *health professional recovery program* (HPRP). To use this service, nurses must be willing to "acknowledge their impairment, agree to participate in a recovery plan that meets the criteria developed by the HPRP, and voluntarily withdraw from or limit the scope of their practice as determined necessary under the criteria established by the committee" (Fletcher, 2004, p. 92). The benefit of this program, as with the Texas approach, is that treatment reports are confidential and independent of the state licensing board.

> ### CONSIDER
> Although most states lean toward treatment rather than discipline for chemical dependency, many nurses still attach a stigma and think that impaired nurses should be punished and not allowed to return to work.

The Recovered Nurse: Re-entry into Practice

When a nurse has completed a treatment or rehabilitation program and is ready to return to work, he or she encounters a number of issues. These issues include whether the nurse's practice is limited or restricted in some way, how long the nursing board has a right to invade the nurse's privacy to ensure that recovery is ongoing, where organizational responsibility ends, who bears the cost if the nurse does not return to work at full capacity, and ensuring that confidentiality is maintained (Box 16.2).

Although many anecdotal or discussion articles were found on the topic of what constitutes a disciplinary or treatment approach to impaired practice, few recent articles could be found that addressed the concerns of re-entry of the impaired nurse to the practice setting. There are, however, some general considerations that should be taken into account when a recovered nurse returns to work.

To protect patient safety, practice restrictions may be in place for a varying time, depending on the length of

BOX 16.2 | ISSUES TO CONSIDER WHEN THE RECOVERED NURSE RETURNS TO WORK

- Should the nurse returning to work following rehabilitation have his or her practice limited or restricted in some way, such as no exposure to the drug of choice or no access to controlled substances for a period of time?
- How long does the board of nursing have a right to invade the privacy of a recovered nurse?
- Where does the organizational responsibility end?
- Who bears the cost if the recovered nurse is not able to return to work at full capacity?
- Can confidentiality be maintained?
- Should the nurse be allowed to work in stressful practice areas?
- Should the nurse initially be allowed to work full time?

the program and whether it was treatment based or disciplinary action occurred. Recovering nurses need to be reassured that their records are confidential and that they are kept separate from general personnel records. It is also important that staff nurses realize the commitment of the recovering nurse to re-establish his or her career and continue in the profession.

Most board of registered nursing Web sites offer little information about the re-entry process. Instead, they focus primarily on what should be done if someone suspects an impaired colleague, how to report it, the treatment or disciplinary action once impairment is identified, and the specific aspects of each program. A question that is left unanswered is how long the board follows a recovered nurse in terms of random drug testing. Some hospitals or health care agencies already do random drug testing, so the question of invasion of privacy has in some instances already been dealt with.

Saver (2008) suggested that a written contract is useful because it puts in writing the expectations of the nurse. This would be a voluntary agreement between the returning nurse and the employing institution. Another suggestion is for the nurse to attend a support group for chemically dependent nurses.

DISCUSSION POINT

You just came from a staff meeting at which the nurse-manager informed everyone that a recovered nurse would begin working on the unit in a few weeks. Some nurses had the attitude that the nurse not be allowed back to work because he or she could not be trusted. How would you respond to your colleagues?

Research Dissemination—Is It Happening?

Although there are limited new research findings to disseminate, the question still needs to be asked: Are the profession and education community applying/using what findings are available? Issues have been raised about student substance abuse. If you work in an educational setting or interact with students in your workplace, do you know what policies are in place if a student is suspected of impaired practice? More important, what is being done in the educational community to address the issue of alcohol and substance use by students that might be affecting their performance in the clinical setting? As suggested by the AACN, it is critical that policies regarding impaired practice be clear and in place in the educational community and that all faculty and students be aware of the content of the policy.

The literature clearly states that impaired practice policies should be in place in every health care setting. However, anecdotal evidence suggests that many nurses in clinical practice have no knowledge of such policies and would not know what to do if they suspected a colleague was impaired. Impaired practice policies should be introduced during hospital orientation for new employees and during annual renewal of hospital safety procedures. This would highlight the issue for everyone and put the problem clearly in the spotlight, especially if issues such as barriers to reporting an impaired colleague and prevalence of the problem were discussed. Nurses should be allowed to ask questions so that they are clear about the process of reporting and so that a nurse who is using substances irresponsibly knows where to go for help.

HOW CAN WE STOP LOSING NURSES TO SUBSTANCE ABUSE?

Preventative health care is finally receiving much needed attention in the media and in practice. Insurance companies are increasingly paying for prevention and screening procedures, yet many areas of health care still lag behind what would be ideal for preventative practices. The issue of preventing substance abuse is no exception to this situation. How can nurses individually and as a profession help to prevent the cycle of nurse addiction from starting?

Some of the risk factors for substance abuse that have been identified are difficult to modify. Nurses will always have easy access to narcotics, do shift work, and suffer from fatigue. The ongoing stress that has worked its way into clinical settings due to the nursing shortage seems a long way from dissipating. What, then, can be done to diminish the effects of these factors so that nurses do not turn to substances as an inappropriate coping mechanism?

Perhaps one avenue is to more fully explore the experiences of nurses who do not turn to substances. Although much has been written about self-care to prevent burnout (Marquis & Huston, 2009), no evidence could be found that linked burnout to harmful coping strategies, such as substance abuse. Do nurses who use self-care strategies to prevent burnout also use those same strategies to avoid harmful substance use? Perhaps this information about how nurses cope with difficulties of the workplace when they do not turn to drugs or alcohol will contribute to prevention. Most research focuses on the nurse who abuses drugs, when a great deal could be learned about positive coping behaviors from nurses who manage stress without abusing drugs.

Where does the education about substance abuse begin? Student nurses need not only to be made aware of the risks of substance abuse, but also to be self-aware about their attitudes and beliefs regarding those who do abuse substances, whether those people are patients or colleagues. Nursing school is an incredibly stressful time for students. Watson, Whyte, Schartau, and Jamieson (2006) reported a study of 186 nursing and midwifery students regarding alcohol consumption in the week previous to the survey. It found that 74% of students reported alcohol consumption in excess of low risk levels during the previous week. A more staggering figure was that 54.7% reported binge drinking in the previous week. Not only could appropriate education in nursing school help to prevent substance abuse from beginning, it might also allow students to explore their feelings and beliefs about impaired practice. This increased self-awareness might help students to have empathy toward impaired nurses and encourage them to take the appropriate steps to assist a nurse or fellow student in getting help.

Nursing is going through a very tumultuous time. The nursing shortage is never far from the minds of most nurses as they struggle on a daily basis with low staffing levels and a stressed work setting. How this stress is channeled can lead a nurse to have positive or negative coping strategies. What are hospitals doing to acknowledge and diffuse this stress? Are nurses too stressed to seek counsel from each other when they have a particularly bad day? Are nurses debriefing with each other or at home so they can let go of the often traumatic nature of work and move forward? Nurses and nurse-managers need to answer these questions for their particular work settings to know whether they are doing enough for themselves, their colleagues, and their staff.

CONCLUSIONS

Losing one nurse to substance misuse is losing one nurse too many. We are a profession known for its caring nature toward others, yet often we fail to care for ourselves. The harmful coping strategies that lead to substance abuse can begin even before nursing school. Educating our students may help us to increase awareness about this ever-present problem. If new graduates can bring current information to their nursing practice and be self-aware about their attitudes, beliefs, and coping strategies, then perhaps they can come armed with more positive strategies to help them when times get tough. Do we teach our students, new graduates, and seasoned nurses to ask for help when they need it, or do we expect them to "do it all"?

Nurses who suspect an impaired colleague need to take action and not engage in enabling behaviors, which have been shown to both be ineffective and further contribute to denial about the problem (Palmer & Hoffman, 2007). If all nurses are aware of the problem of chemical dependency and take the initiative to confront or intervene when they suspect a colleague of impaired practice, we are one step closer to decreasing the incidence of substance abuse in the nursing profession.

Finally, responsibility rests not just with individual nurses, but also with employers to create a positive work environment, to know employees so that confrontation can occur early, to increase awareness about substance abuse so that nurses are not afraid to ask for help, to ensure that an Impaired Practice Policy is in place, and finally to provide a process that facilitates re-entry into practice following recovery.

FOR ADDITIONAL DISCUSSION

1. Explore your attitudes and beliefs about impaired nursing practice. How would you treat a colleague suspected of diverting drugs for personal use? How would you treat a recovered nurse returning to work?

2. What kind of peer support exists in your work setting? How do staff debrief from stressful situations?

3. What do you think is the best approach to deal with impaired practice—treatment or discipline? Did moral values play a part in your decision?

4. Should recovered nurses who return to work have a limited practice? If so, for how long, and with what types of limitations? How does this affect the workload of other nurses?

5. What practices are in place in your work setting that could deter a nurse from diverting drugs for personal use?

6. Have you known a colleague who was caught stealing drugs from work? If so, how was it handled? Did the nurse seek treatment and return to work? Could it have been managed better?

7. You are a nurse-manager for an intensive care unit and have been asked to talk to student nurses about impaired practice. What key points would you make?

8. Does your workplace have an Impaired Practice Policy in place? If so, have you read it, and was it discussed during your initial hospital orientation? Is it discussed annually?

REFERENCES

American Nurses Association (ANA) (1984). *Addiction and Psychological Dysfunctions in Nursing.* Kansas City, MO: American Nurses Association.

American Nurses Association (ANA) (2001). *Code of Ethics for Nurses with Interpretive Statements.* Washington, DC: American Nurses Association. Available at: http://nursingworld.org/MainMenuCategories/ThePracticeofProfessionalNursing/EthicsStandards/CodeofEthics.aspx. Accessed August 7, 2008.

American Nurses Association (ANA) (2008). *Impaired nurse resource center.* Available at: http://nursingworld.org/MainMenuCategories/ThePracticeofProfessionalNursing/workplace/ImpairedNurse.aspx. Accessed August 7, 2008.

American Association of Colleges of Nursing (1998). *Policy and guidelines for prevention and management of substance abuse in the nursing education community.* Available at: http://www.aacn.nche.edu/publications/positions/subabuse.htm. Accessed July 28, 2008.

Baldisseri, M. R. (2007). Impaired healthcare professional. *Critical Care Medicine 35*(2, Supplement), S106–S116.

Beckstead, J. W. (2005a). The moderating effects of attitudes on nurses' intentions to report impaired colleagues. *Journal of Applied Social Psychology, 35*(5), 905–921.

Beckstead, J. W. (2005b). Reporting peer wrongdoing in the healthcare profession: The role of incompetence and substance abuse information. *International Journal of Nursing Studies, 42,* 325–331.

Breier-Mackie, S. (2007). Impaired nurses in the workplace. *Gastroenterology Nursing, 207,* 227–228.

California Board of Registered Nursing (CBRN) (2007). *What is the BRN's diversion program?* Available at: http://www.rn.ca.gov/diversion/whatisdiv.shtml. Accessed August 7, 2008.

Clark, C., & Farnsworth, J. (2006). Program for recovering nurses: An evaluation. *MEDSURG Nursing, 15*(4), 223–230.

Dittman, P. W. (2008). *Professional impairment: The lived experience of chemically dependent nurses.* Presented to the Joint Meeting of the Boards of Nursing, Osteopathic Medicine and Pharmacy, Tallahassee, Florida, February 29, 2008. Available at: http://www.doh. state.fl.us/MQA/osteopath/info_Prof_Impairment_ Chem_Diver.pdf. Accessed August 4, 2008.

Dunn, D. (2005). Substance abuse among nurses—Intercession and intervention. *AORN Journal, 82*(5), 777–799.

Fletcher, C. E. (2004). Experience with peer assistance for impaired nurses in Michigan. *Journal of Nursing Scholarship, 36*(1), 92–93.

Fogger, S., & McGuinness, T. (2006/2007). Barriers to helping impaired nurses. *Alabama Nurse, 33*(4), 5–7.

Kenna, G. A., & Lewis, D. C. (2008). Risk factors for alcohol and other drug use by healthcare professionals. *Substance Abuse Treatment, Prevention, and Policy, 3*(3). Available at: http://www.substanceabusepolicy. com/content/3/1/3. Accessed July 24, 2008.

Lillibridge, J. (2006). The chemically impaired nurse: Discipline or treatment? (pp. 314–327). In: C. J. Huston (Ed.), *Professional Issues in Nursing: Challenges and Opportunities* Philadelphia: Lippincott Williams & Wilkins.

Lillibridge, J., Cox, M., & Cross, W. (2002). Uncovering the secret: Giving voice to the experiences of nurses who misuse substances. *Journal of Advanced Nursing, 39*(3), 219–229.

Marquis, B. L., & Huston, C. J. (2009). *Leadership Roles and Management Functions in Nursing: Theory and application* (6th ed.). Philadelphia: Lippincott Williams & Wilkins.

National Council of State Boards of Nursing (2001). *Chemical dependency handbook for nurse managers.* Available at: https://www.ncsbn.org/chem_dep_hand book_intro_ch1.pdf. Accessed August 5, 2008.

Palmer, L., & Hoffman, L. A. (2007). Detecting and preventing substance abuse in health care professionals. *Critical Care Alert, 2007*(April), 5–8.

Saver, C. (2008). Substance abuse in the OR: Why managers should not ignore it. *OR Manager, 24*(5), 1, 11–12.

Shaw, M. F., McGovern, M. P., Angres, D. H., & Rawal, P. (2004). Physicians and nurses with substance use disorders. *Journal of Advanced Nursing, 47*(5), 561–571.

Texas Nurses Association (2004). *Texas peer assistance program for nurses.* Available at: http://www.tpapn.org. Accessed July 22, 2008.

Watson, H., Whyte, R., Schartau, E., & Jamieson, E. (2006). Survey of student nurses and midwives: Smoking and alcohol use. *British Journal of Nursing, 15*(22), 1212–1216.

West, M. M. (2003). A kaleidoscopic review of the literature about substance abuse impairment in nursing: Progress toward identification of early risk indicators? *Journal of Addictions Nursing, 14,* 139–144.

West, M. M. (2005). Early risk patterns in substance abuse impaired nurses. *Pennsylvania Nurse, 2005* (September), 20–21.

BIBLIOGRAPHY

Dunn, D. (2005). Substance abuse among nurses—Intercession and intervention. *AORN Journal, 82*(5), 573–596.

Grauvogl, C. (2005). Calif. program balances treatment, monitoring. *Addiction Professional, 2005*(November), 35–38.

Maher-Brisen, P. (2007). Addiction: An occupational hazard in nursing. *American Journal of Nursing, 107*(8), 78–79.

Mikos, C. A. (2008). Increased authority to discipline licenses of impaired practitioners. *Florida Nurse, 2008*(June), 10.

Pauly, B., Goldstone, I., McCall, J., Gold, F., & Payne, S. (2007). The ethical, legal and social context of harm reduction. *Canadian Nurse, 2007*(October), 19–23.

Raistrick, D., Russell, D., Tober, G., & Tindale, A. (2008). A survey of substance use by health care profession-als and their attitudes to substance misuse patients (NHS staff survey). *Journal of Substance Use, 13*(1), 57–69.

Weis, B. (2005). Winning the battle with addiction. *RN, 68*(7), 63–66.

WEB RESOURCES

Addiction Recovery Resources for the Professional	http://www.lapage.com/arr/
American Association of Colleges of Nursing	http://www.aacn.nche.edu/index.htm
American Association of Nurse Anesthetists, Peer Assistance	http://www.aana.com/Resources.aspx?ucNavMenu_TSMenuTargetID=154&ucavMenu_TSMenuTargetType=4&ucNavMenu_TSMenuID=6&id=191
American Nurses Association	http://nursingworld.org
California Board of Registered Nurses Diversion Program	http://www.rn.ca.gov/diversion/whatisdiv.shtml
Intervention Project for Nurses: Florida	http://www.ipnfl.org/faq.html
Institute for a Drug-Free Workplace	http://www.drugfreeworkplace.org
Kentucky Peer Assistance Program for Nurses	http://www.kpapn.org/information.html
Narc-Anon	http://www.nar-anon.org
National Association of State Alcohol and Drug Abuse Directors	http://www.nasadad.org
National Clearinghouse for Alcohol and Drug Information	http://www.health.org
National Council of State Boards of Nursing	http://www.ncsbn.org
National Institute on Alcohol Abuse and Alcoholism	http://www.niaaa.nih.gov/
National Institute on Drug Abuse	http://www.nida.nih.gov
Nurses in Recovery	http://brucienne.com/nir/
Nursing and Health Care Directories on: The Nursefriendly, Chemical Dependence, Substance Abuse, Impaired Nurses	http://www.nursefriendly.com/impaired/
Substance Abuse and Mental Health Services Administration	http://www.findtreatment.samhsa.gov

CHAPTER 17

Collective Bargaining and the Professional Nurse

• CAROL J. HUSTON •

Learning Objectives

The learner will be able to:

1. Define the terms *collective bargaining, union, supervisor, closed shop,* and *open shop.*
2. Explore possible motivations behind nurses' decisions to join or not join unions.
3. Describe the relationships between national economic prosperity, the existence of nursing shortages and surpluses, and unionization rates of nurses.
4. Identify major U.S. legislation that has affected the ability of nurses to unionize over time.
5. Describe the shifting balance of power between unions and management in the United States over the last century and analyze the power balance that currently exists between the two entities.
6. Identify the largest unions representing health care employees, and nurses in particular.
7. Investigate the current status of rulings by the National Labor Relations Board (NLRB) and the courts regarding the definition of "supervisor" in nursing and the effect those rulings have on

the eligibility of nurses for protection under the National Labor Relations Act (NLRA).
8. Delineate primary union organizing strategies to promote union membership, as well as specific steps for starting a union.
9. Debate the potential conflicts inherent in having the American Nurses Association serve as both a professional association for all nurses and as a collective bargaining agent.
10. Explore the impact of management has in creating a work environment that eliminates or reduces the need for unionization.
11. Reflect on whether going on strike can be viewed as an ethically appropriate action for professional nurses.
12. Explore his or her beliefs about whether belonging to unions, a practice historically reserved for blue collar workers, undermines nursings' quest for increased recognition as a profession.

There is likely no greater dichotomy than stereotypical images of nurses dressed in white uniforms and caps acting as handmaidens to physicians, and angry nurses in picket lines waving strike placards at passersby. Although both of these images are stereotypical, they are at the heart of the debate about whether nursing, long recognized as a caring and altruistic profession, should be a part of collective bargaining efforts to improve working conditions.

Collective bargaining may be defined as activities occurring between organized labor and management that concern employee relations. Such activities include

negotiation of formal labor agreements and day-to-day interactions between unions and management. A *labor union* (hereafter referred to as *union*) can be defined as "an organized association of workers, often in a trade or profession, formed to protect and further their rights and interests" (*Oxford Pocket Dictionary of Current English,* 2008, para 1).

Many nurses have strong feelings about unions and collective bargaining activities. Often these feelings have to do with their exposure to unions while they were growing up. Many nurses from working-class families were raised in a cultural milieu that promoted unionization. Other nurses know little about unions and know only what they have seen portrayed in the media. Some nurses, however, have been actively involved in collective bargaining in their place of employment and have emerged from the experience with either positive or negative impressions or a combination thereof.

Despite this tension, collective bargaining and unions are very much a part of many nurses' experiences. Although union membership in the private sector is declining, slow but steady increases have occurred in the number of nurses represented by collective bargaining agents. Still, depending on the source used, only 16% to 22% of all nurses belong to collective bargaining units (discrepancies have to do with how the numbers are calculated). The issues driving nurses to pursue unionization, however, continue to exist. Increased nursing workloads and a feeling that management does not care are significant factors encouraging increased union activity at the close of the first decade of the 21st century.

This chapter explores the historical development of unions in the United States, particularly in nursing. The motivations behind nurses' decisions to join or not join unions are explored, and the unions that represent the majority of nurses are described. Union organizing strategies are presented, as are specific steps for starting a union. Emphasis is given to the importance of management creating a work environment that eliminates or reduces the need for unionization in the first place. The chapter concludes with a discussion of the definition of "supervisor" in nursing, types of labor union–management relationships, and whether striking can be viewed as an ethically appropriate action for professional nurses.

HISTORICAL PERSPECTIVE OF UNIONIZATION IN THE UNITED STATES

Unions have been present in the United States since the 1790s. Skilled craftsmen formed early unions to protect themselves from wage cuts during the highly competitive era of industrialization:

The first American strikes in the late 1700s and early 1800s were by shoemakers, printers, and carpenters led by their trade societies and were generally effective because of the limited labor pool skilled in those

trades. The strikers simply refused to work until their pay demands were met. The strikes were generally short, peaceful, and successful (Labor Unions and Nursing, 2003, para 1).

This changed in the early 1800s, with strike activity increasing during economic prosperity and declining during less prosperous economic times. In addition, women began to participate in strikes as early as the 1820s (Labor Unions and Nursing, 2003). By the mid to late 1800s, the labor movement began to more closely resemble what we see today. Unions started negotiating with employers, addressing not only wages, but also work rules, hours, and grievances, thus arbitrating contracts between employees and employers.

Of interest, the most important labor organization of the 1800s, the Knights of Labor, discouraged strikes. Craft unions affiliated with the American Federation of Labor (AFL) in the early 1900s also questioned the usefulness of strikes, turning to private mediation groups to help settle disputes (Labor Unions and Nursing, 2003).

By the 1930s, and after 4 years of the Great Depression, repressive management was the norm, and tensions were high between workers and their employers. There were no legal protections for workers, no overtime compensation, no child labor laws, and no health or safety regulations. Workers attempted to form unions to improve working conditions, but business owners responded by blacklisting organizers and using force to prevent strikes (Franklin D. Roosevelt Presidential Library, n.d.).

President Franklin Roosevelt attempted to intervene by promoting the National Industrial Recovery Act, but he was forced to make an even bolder stand alongside labor when the Supreme Court ruled that act unconstitutional. Roosevelt promoted the National Labor Relations Act (NLRA), also known as the Wagner Act after New York Senator Robert Wagner, which was enacted in 1935. This act gave workers the right to form unions and bargain collectively with their employers (Box 17.1). It also provided for the creation of the National Labor Relations Board (NLRB) "to oversee union certification, arrange meetings with unions and employers, and investigate violations of the law" (Franklin D. Roosevelt Presidential Library, n.d, para 1).

With this rapid shift in power from management to labor, labor–management relations were turbulent throughout the 1930s and 1940s. History books are

BOX 17.1 | UNFAIR MANAGEMENT PRACTICES IDENTIFIED IN THE WAGNER ACT (1935)

1. To interfere with, restrain, or coerce employees in a manner that interferes with their rights as outlined under the act. Examples of these activities are spying on union gatherings, threatening employees with job loss, or threatening to close down a company if the union organizes.
2. To interfere with the formation of any labor organization or to give financial assistance to a labor organization.
3. To discriminate with regard to hiring, tenure, and so on, to discourage union membership.
4. To discharge or discriminate against an employee who filed charges or testified before the NLRB.
5. To refuse to bargain in good faith.

filled with battles, strikes, mass-picketing scenes, and brutal treatment by both management and employees. The balance of power, however, fell to labor unions.

Because of this, it was necessary to pass additional federal legislation to restore what was perceived to be balance of power with management. Passed in 1947, the Taft–Hartley Labor Act, also known as the Labor–Management Relations Act, retained the provisions under the Wagner Act that guaranteed employees the right to collective bargaining but added the provision that employees had the right to refrain from taking part in unions ("closed shops" were illegal) (see Box 17.2). In addition, the act permitted the union shop only after a vote of a majority of the employees. It also forbade *jurisdictional strikes* ("an illegal strike about which trade union should have the right to represent a particular group of employees in an organization" (Business Dictionary, 2008), secondary boycotts, and unions from contributing to political campaigns.

> ### DISCUSSION POINT
> The Taft–Hartley Labor Act also required union leaders to affirm they were not supporters of the Communist Party. Why was this requirement a part of the act, and how did it mesh with the culture of the time?

Eventually, federal legislation such as the Fair Labor Standards Act (1938), the Occupational Safety and Health Act (1970), and the Equal Employment Opportunity Act (1972) were passed, providing federal protection for workers. These acts were important in the history of unions because unions no longer had to be the primary source of security for workers. As a result, there has been little growth of unions in the private and blue collar sectors since membership peaked in the 1950s.

To counteract these dwindling numbers, several major unions merged, and new affiliations were formed.

BOX 17.2 | UNFAIR LABOR UNION PRACTICES IDENTIFIED IN THE TAFT–HARTLEY AMENDMENT (1947)

1. Requiring a self-employed person or an employer to join a union.
2. Forcing an employer to cease doing business with another person. This placed a ban on secondary boycotts, which were then prevalent.
3. Forcing an employer to bargain with one union when another union has already been certified as the bargaining agent.
4. Forcing the employer to assign certain work to members of one union rather than another.
5. Charging excessive or discriminatory initiation fees.
6. Causing or attempting to cause an employer to pay for unnecessary services.

In addition, new organizing tactics were developed. Nowhere is this turnaround more apparent than in the health care industry.

HISTORICAL PERSPECTIVE OF UNIONIZATION IN NURSING

Collective bargaining was slow in coming to the health care industry for many reasons. Until labor laws were amended, unionization of health care workers was illegal. In addition, nursing's long history as a service commodity further delayed labor organization in health care settings.

> **DISCUSSION POINT**
> Is it appropriate for nurses to organize into collective bargaining units, something historically reserved for blue collar workers?

Initial collective bargaining in nursing took place in government or public organizations as a result of Executive Order 10988 of President John Kennedy. This 1962 order lifted restrictions that prevented public employees from organizing. As a result, city, county, and district hospitals and health care agencies joined collective bargaining in the 1960s.

In 1974, Congress amended the Wagner Act, extending national labor laws to private nonprofit hospitals, nursing homes, health clinics, health maintenance organizations, and other health care institutions. These amendments opened the door to much union activity

for professions and the public employee sector. Indeed, a review of union membership figures shows that since 1960, most collective bargaining activity in the United States has occurred in the public and professional sectors of industry, most notably among faculty at institutions of higher education, teachers at primary and secondary levels, and physicians.

> **DISCUSSION POINT**
> Why is white collar union membership growing when the private and blue collar sectors are not? Have societal norms altered perceptions regarding the appropriateness of unionization in white collar industries?

From 1962 through 1989, there were slow but steady increases in the numbers of nurses represented by collective bargaining agents. In 1989, the NLRB ruled that nurses could form separate bargaining units, and union activity increased. However, the American Hospital Association immediately sued the American Nurses Association (ANA), and the ruling was put on hold until 1991, when the Supreme Court upheld the 1989 decision by the NLRB. A summary of the legislation affecting the development of unionization in nursing is shown in Table 17.1.

UNIONS REPRESENTING NURSES

Various unions represent nurses and other health care workers. The Service Employees International Union

TABLE 17.1	Labor Legislation	
Year	**Legislation**	**Effect**
1935	National Labor Relations Act/Wagner Act	Gave unions many rights in organizing; resulted in rapid union growth
1947	Taft–Hartley Amendment	Returned some power to management; resulted in a more equal balance of power between unions and management
1962	Executive Order 10988 (President John Kennedy)	Amended the 1935 Wagner Act to allow public employees to join unions
1974	Amendments to the Wagner Act	Allowed workers in nonprofit organizations to join unions
1989	National Labor Relations Board ruling	Allowed nurses to form separate bargaining units

(SEIU) is the largest union in the health care industry, with 900,000 members in the field, including nurses, licensed practical nurses (LPNs)/licensed vocational nurses (LVNs), doctors, lab technicians, nursing home workers, and home care workers (SEIU, 2008).

Some of the other unions that represent nurses include the ANA; the National Union of Hospital and Health Care Employees of Retail, Wholesale and Department Store Union; the American Federation of Labor–Congress of Industrial Organizations (AFL-CIO); the United Steelworkers of America (USWA); the American Federation of Government Employees, AFL-CIO; the American Federation of State, County, and Municipal Employees, AFL-CIO; the International Brotherhood of Teamsters; the American Federation of State, County, and Municipal Employees, which operates mostly in the public sector; and the United Auto Workers.

Union representation also varies by state. The states with the most union organizing for all industries, including health care, are New York, California, Pennsylvania, Michigan, and Illinois.

DISCUSSION POINT
Is it appropriate for RNs to be represented by nonnursing unions? Why would nurses seek out nonnursing unions for representation?

MOTIVATION TO JOIN UNIONS

Knowing that human behavior is goal directed, it is important to examine what personal goals union membership fulfills. Nurse-managers often tell each other that health care institutions differ from other types of industrial organizations. This is really a myth because most nurses work in large and impersonal organizations, just like workers in other industries.

CONSIDER
People are motivated to join or reject unions as a result of many needs and values.

Deciding whether or not to join a union is a personal and often complex decision because there are typically many influencing factors. Both choices can be justified, however, so both driving and restraining forces for union membership are presented here.

There are six primary motivations for joining a union (see Box 17.3). The first is to increase the power of the individual. Employees know that singly they are much more dispensable. Because a large group of employees is generally less dispensable, nurses greatly increase their bargaining power and reduce their vulnerability by joining a union. This is a particularly strong motivating force for nurses when jobs are scarce and nurses feel vulnerable. Indeed, during the massive downsizing and restructuring of the 1990s, collective bargaining priorities shifted from wages and benefits to job security.

Union activity also tends to change in response to workforce excesses and shortages. For decades, employment demand for nurses has increased and decreased periodically. High demand for nurses is tied directly to a healthy national economy, and, historically, this has been correlated with increased union activity. Similarly, when nursing vacancy rates are low, union membership and activity tend to decline.

BOX 17.3 | REASONS NURSES JOIN UNIONS

1. To increase the power of the individual.
2. To achieve wage advantages.
3. To increase their input into organizational decision making.
4. To eliminate discrimination and favoritism.
5. Because they are required to do so as part of employment (closed shop).
6. To satisfy the social need to be accepted.
7. Because they believe it will improve patient outcomes and quality of care.

A second reason for joining unions is economics. In some organizations, pay is neither fair nor competitive, and most economists agree that joining a union typically is an effective means of raising one's pay. Indeed, the American Federation of Teachers (n.d.) suggested that "in survey after survey, members say their priority issue at the bargaining table is pay" (para 17).

Bauer (2005) agreed, stating whereas there is debate about whether unionization leads to better working conditions, there is no debate about union wages being higher. He stated that unionized registered nurses (RNs) on an average earn $6,100 dollars more a year than non-union nurses. Indeed, research by Pittman (2007) found that members of collective bargaining units had higher satisfaction with their wages than nonmembers. Nonmembers, however, had higher satisfaction with nursing supervision, patient care, work setting, professional relationships, and overall job satisfaction. (See Research Study Fuels the Controversy).

Another reason nurses join unions is to communicate their aims, feelings, complaints, and ideas to others. The desire to have input into organizational decision making is a strong motivator for people to join unions. A feeling of powerlessness or the perception that administration does not care about employees is one of the most common reasons for seeking unionization.

> ### CONSIDER
> The rapid downsizing and restructuring of the 1990s left many nurses feeling that management did not listen to them or care about their needs. This discontentment provides a fertile ground for union organizers because unions thrive in a climate that perceives the organizational philosophy to be insensitive to the worker.

In addition, nurses join unions because they want to eliminate discrimination and favoritism. Unions emphasize equality and fairness. This might be an especially strong motivator for members of groups that have experienced discrimination, such as women and minorities.

The fourth primary motivation for joining a union stems from the social need to be accepted. Sometimes this social need results from family or peer pressure. Because many working-class families have a long history of strong union ties, children are frequently raised in a cultural milieu that promotes unionization.

Another reason nurses sometimes join unions is because the union contract dictates that all nurses belong to the union. This has been a big driving force among blue collar workers. However, the *closed shop*, or requirement that all employees belong to a union, has never prevailed in the health care industry. Most health care unions have *open shops*, allowing nurses to choose whether they want to join the union.

Research Study Fuels the Controversy: Union Membership and Job Satisfaction

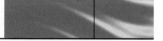

This descriptive secondary analysis used a survey database from the Minnesota Department of Health to examine differences in job satisfaction levels between registered nurses who were or were not members of a nursing collective bargaining unit. The survey, which included a job satisfaction section largely based on the Index of Work Satisfaction, was sent in 2002 to 3,645 registered nurses in Minnesota, using a random stratified sample of RNs who had renewed their RN license.

STUDY FINDINGS
Overall, all nurses reported high levels of job satisfaction; however, members of collective bargaining units had higher satisfaction with wages. Nonmembers had higher satisfaction with nursing supervision, patient care, work setting, professional relationships, and overall job satisfaction. Pittman concluded that there is a need for interventions in institutions with collective bargaining units to improve job satisfaction, nurse retention, and job recruitment.

Source: Pittman, J. (2007). Registered nurse job satisfaction and collective bargaining unit membership status. *Journal of Nursing Administration, 37*(10), 471–476.

Finally, some nurses join unions because they believe that patient outcomes are better in unionized organizations due to better staffing and supervised management practices Bruno (2005) agreed, suggesting that there is a positive relationship between unionization and safe standards of care and effective patient advocacy. Twarog (2005) echoed Bruno's claims in her assertion that mandating safe needles, limiting mandatory overtime and setting nurse-to-patient ratios have all been pushed first by unions, and that accomplishing these results was not due to employer's benevolence or goodwill. These were union-driven accomplishments.

REASONS NOT TO JOIN UNIONS

Just as there are many reasons to join unions, there also are many reasons nurses reject unions, including societal and cultural factors (see Box 17.4). Many people distrust unions because they believe that they promote the welfare state and oppose the U.S. system of free enterprise. Other individuals reject unions because they feel a need to demonstrate that they can get ahead on their own merits.

In addition, some professional employees reject unions for reasons that deal with class and education. They argue that unions were appropriate for the blue collar worker but not for the university professor, physician, or engineer. Nurses rejecting unions on this basis usually are driven by a need to demonstrate their individualism and social status.

Other employees identify with management and thus frequently adopt its viewpoint toward unions.

These nurses, therefore, reject unions because their values more closely align with management than with workers.

In addition, although employees are protected under the NLRA, some nurses reject unions because of fears of employer reprisal. Nurses who reject unions on this basis could be said to be motivated most of all by a need to keep their job.

Finally, some employees reject unions because they fear losing income associated with a strike or walkout. Strikes and walkouts are a reality of unionization; however, they are regulated by law (striking is discussed later in this chapter).

Once managers understand the needs and driving forces behind nurses' decisions to join or reject unions, they can begin to address them. Organizations with unfair management policies are more likely to become unionized. It is certainly then within managerial power to eliminate some of the needs staff feel for joining unions.

Managers can encourage feelings of power by allowing subordinates to have input into decisions that will affect their work. Managers also can listen to ideas, complaints, and feelings and take steps to ensure that favoritism and discrimination are not part of their management style. In addition, managers can strengthen the drives and needs that make nurses reject unions. By building a team effort, sharing ideas and future plans from upper management with the staff, and encouraging individualism in employees, managers can facilitate identification of the worker with management.

When nurses begin showing signs of job dissatisfaction (frustration, stress, perceived powerlessness), they

BOX 17.4 | **REASONS NURSES DO NOT WANT TO JOIN UNIONS**

1. The belief that unions promote the welfare state and oppose the U.S. system of free enterprise.
2. The need to demonstrate individualism.
3. The belief that unionization allows for mediocrity and substandard practice.
4. The belief that professionals should not unionize.
5. Identification with management's viewpoint.
6. Fear of employer reprisal.
7. Fear of lost income associated with a strike or walkout.

are sending a wake-up call to nursing management. Leaders must be alert to employment practices that are unfair or insensitive to employee needs and intervene appropriately before such issues lead to unionization. However, organizations offering liberal benefit packages and fair management practices may still experience union activity if certain social and cultural factors are present. If union activity does occur, managers must be aware of specific employee and management rights so that the NLRA is not violated by either managers or employees.

ELIGIBILITY FOR UNION MEMBERSHIP

Until recently, only *supervisors* were considered managers. As such, they were prohibited from joining unions. However, a 2006 NLRB ruling deemed that *charge nurses* might also be considered supervisors. Even part-time charge nurses are so labeled. This finding is being fought by unions, and it remains to be seen if the NLRB will change its ruling (Burger, 2006).

In addition, the definition of supervisor in nursing came into question with several administrative and court rulings in the early 1990s. These rulings came about as a result of a case involving four licensed practical nurses (LPNs/LVNs) employed at Heartland Nursing Home in Urbana, Ohio. During late 1988 and early 1989 these LPNs complained to management about what they thought were disparate enforcement of the absentee policy; short staffing; low wages for nurses' aides; an unreasonable switching of prescription business from one pharmacy to another, which increased the nurses' paperwork; and management's failure to communicate with employees (Health Care Corporation, 1992). Despite assurances from the vice president for operations that they would not be harassed for bringing their concerns to headquarters' attention, three of the LPNs were terminated as a result of their actions.

In response to what they perceived to be illegal termination, the LPNs filed for protection under the NLRA. The NLRB ruled that because the LPNs had responsibility to ensure adequate staffing, to make daily work assignments, to monitor the aides' work to ensure proper performance, to counsel and discipline aides, to resolve aides' problems and grievances, to evaluate aides' performances, and to report to management, they should be classified as "supervisors," thereby making them ineligible for protection under the NLRA.

On appeal, the administrative law judge (ALJ) disagreed, concluding that the nurses were not supervisors and that the nurses' supervisory work did not equate to responsibly directing the aides *in the interest of the employer*, noting that the nurses' focus is on the well-being of the residents rather than on the employer.

In another turnabout, the U.S. Court of Appeals for the Sixth Circuit then reversed the decision of the ALJ, arguing that the NLRB's test for determining the supervisory status of nurses was inconsistent with the statute and that the interest of the patient and the interest of the employer were not mutually exclusive. The court said that, in fact, the interests of the patient are the employer's business, and argued that the welfare of the patient was no less the object and concern of the employer than it was of the nurses. The court also argued that the statutory dichotomy the NLRB first created was no more justified in the health care field than it would be in any other business in which supervisory duties are necessary to the production of goods or the provision of services (*NLRB v. Health Care & Retirement Corp.*, 1994).

The court further stated that it was up to Congress to carve out an exception for the health care field, including nurses, should Congress not wish for such nurses to be considered supervisors. The court reminded the NLRB that the courts, and not the board, bear the final responsibility for interpreting the law. After concluding that the board's test was inconsistent with the statute, the court found that the four licensed practical nurses involved in this case were indeed supervisors and ineligible for protection under the NLRA (*NLRB v. Health Care & Retirement Corp.*, 1994).

This same interpretation, at least for full-time charge nurses, was used in another landmark court case in September 2006 to determine whether charge nurses, both permanent and rotating, at Oakwood Healthcare Inc. were "supervisors" within the meaning of the NLRA, such that they should be excluded from a unit of nurses represented by a union (Rothgerber, Johnson, & Lyons LLP, 2006):

Notably, to be a supervisor, the NLRB found that an individual must spend "a regular and substantial portion of his/her work time performing supervisory functions. Thus, individuals who sporadically fill in and perform supervisory functions on a substitute basis, such as rotating charge nurses, would not fit the definition of supervisor (Rothgerber, Johnson, & Lyons LLP, para 7).

This was not the case, however, for the full time charge nurses.

Legislation introduced in September 2007 has also obscured the issue. Sandler (2007) reported that bill HR 1644, which was approved by the House, Education, and Labor Committee, would amend the 1935 National Labor Relations Act by modifying the definition of "supervisor." The authority to "assign . . . other employees" or the "responsibility to direct them" would be removed. If this legislation moves forward, more charge nurses would be eligible for union membership, as well as protection, under the NLRA.

DISCUSSION POINT

Would the NLRB's definition of *supervisor* affect charge nurses' eligibility for union membership at the facility in which you work?

UNION ORGANIZING STRATEGIES

Haugh (2006) noted that unions use a variety of different tactics when organizing health care workers. Among the strategies he discussed are meetings, both group and one-on-one contacts are made by union representative (see Box 17.5). Other strategies used are providing literature about union benefits, writing letters, and faxing potential union members. In addition, according to Haugh, unions recently have added new methods of organizing, namely *community and corporate pressure*. This pressure is usually directed at acute care hospitals.

In corporate campaigns the union uses public events, political connections, and the local media to bring into question a hospital's quality of care, level of charity work, tax-exempt status (if nonprofit), and nurse staffing. Haugh maintained that unions are very effective in involving influential power brokers, both financiers and lawmakers. Unions are refining corporate campaigns with allegations of discrimination, boycotts, rallies, and visits to board members' homes.

Another strategy contributing to labor union wins is *activism*. Central labor councils, local labor unions, and state labor federations are reaching out to community groups, faith-based organizations, and elected officials in an effort to create unrest and change the community environment in which workers organize.

Unions often file lawsuits against employers. Labor unions maintain the goal of breaking employer resolve and demonstrate their ability to protect employees by initiating legal action on behalf of employees against targeted employers. Other corporate strategies include

---

BOX 17.5 | TEN UNION ORGANIZING STRATEGIES

1. Meetings (both group and one-on-one).
2. Leaflets and brochures.
3. Pressure on the hospital corporation through media and community contacts.
4. Political pressure on regional legislators and local lawmakers.
5. Corporate campaign strategies (raising questions in the community about the hospital's activities and commitments).
6. Activism of local employees.
7. Filing lawsuits.
8. Bringing pressure from the institution's financial supporters.
9. Lawsuits.
10. Home visits for selective one-on-one contact.

Source: Adapted from Haugh, R. (2006). The new union strategy: Turning the community against you. *Hospitals & Health Networks, 80*(5), 32–37.

union organizers establishing Web sites to enable them to keep tabs on the hospital system (Haugh, 2006). The Internet has also made accessing information about how to organize a union very accessible to interested workers. E-mail has also proven to be an inexpensive and efficient means of mass communication regarding issues critical to unions.

CONSIDER

Although, historically, unions focused heavily on wage negotiations, current issues deemed just as or more important by nurses are nonmonetary, such as guidelines for staffing, float provisions, shared decision making, and scheduling.

SEEKING UNION REPRESENTATION

The first step in seeking union representation is determining that adequate levels of desire for unionization exist. The NLRB requires that at least 30% of employees sign an interest card before an election for unionization can be held. Most collective bargaining agents, however, require 60% to 70% of the employees to sign interest cards before they begin an organizing campaign. Union representatives are generally careful to keep a campaign secret until they are ready to file a petition for election. They do this so that they can build momentum without interference from the employer.

However, legislation was introduced in the 2007 Congress called the Employee Free Choice Act (HR 800). Had it passed, unions would have been allowed to request representation from the NLRB by the use of signed cards only. This would have eliminated the need for a secret ballot election to determine union representation. This bill passed the House of Representatives but failed a cloture motion, preventing consideration of the bill in the Senate, by roll call vote (H.R. 800, n.d.).

After enough interest cards have been signed, the organization must hold an election. At that time, all employees of the same classification, such as RNs, vote on whether they desire unionization. A choice in every such election is *no representation*, which means that the voters do not want a union. During the election, 50% plus 1 of the petitioned units must vote before the union can be recognized.

Unions can also be decertified by a process similar to that of certification. *Decertification* can occur when at least 30% of the eligible employees in the bargaining unit initiate a petition asking to no longer be represented by the union. At the decertification election,

> *If no other union is involved, the choices would be between the existing exclusive representative and no representation. If another union has received a 30 percent showing of support, the choices on the ballot would be between the existing exclusive representative, the other union, and no representation. In either case, a simple majority of votes cast would determine the outcome of the decertification election (University of Minnesota, Office of Human Resources, 2008, para 2).*

There are important differences, however, between organizing in a health care facility and in other types of organizations. Generally, the solicitation and distribution of union literature are banned entirely in immediate patient care areas. Managers should never, however, independently attempt to deal with union-organizing activity. They should always seek assistance and guidance from higher-level management and the personnel department.

The entire list of rights for management and labor during the organizing and establishment phases of unionization is beyond the scope of this book. Throughout the years, Congress has amended various labor acts and laws in the attempt to balance power between management and labor. At times, the balance of power has shifted to management or labor, but Congress eventually enacts laws that attempt to restore what it judges to be the balance. The manager must ensure that the rights of management and employees are protected.

LABOR–MANAGEMENT RELATIONS

In the last 30 years, employers and unions have substantially improved their relationships. Although evidence is growing that contemporary management has come to accept the reality that unions are here to stay, businesses in the United States are still less comfortable with unions than their counterparts in many other countries. Likewise, unions have come to accept the fact that there are times when organizations are not healthy enough to survive aggressive union demands.

CONSIDER

It is possible to create a climate in which labor and management can work together to accomplish mutual goals.

Once management is faced with dealing with a collective bargaining unit, it has a choice of either accepting or opposing the union. It may actively oppose the union by using various union-busting techniques, or it may more subtly oppose the union by attempting to discredit it and win employee trust. *Acceptance* also may run along a continuum. The company may accept the union with reluctance and suspicion. Although they know that the union has legitimate rights, managers often believe they must continually guard against the union encroaching further into traditional management territory.

There also is the type of union acceptance known as *accommodation*. Increasingly common, accommodation is characterized by management's full acceptance of the union, with both union and management showing mutual respect. When these conditions exist, labor and management can establish mutual goals, especially in the areas of safety, cost reduction, efficiency, eliminating waste, and improving working conditions. Such cooperation represents the most mature and advanced type of labor–management relations.

The bottom line is that the attitudes and the philosophies of the leaders in management and the union determine what type of relationship develops between the two parties in any given organization. When dealing with unions, managers must be flexible. It is critical that they do not ignore issues or try to overwhelm others with power. The rational approach to problem solving must be used.

It is also important to remember that employees have a right to participate in union organizing under the NLRA, and managers must not interfere with this right. Prohibited managerial activities include threatening employees, interrogating employees, promising employees rewards for cessation of union activity, and spying on employees. However, if management picks up early clues of union activity, the organization may be able to take legitimate steps that will discourage unionization of its employees.

DISCUSSION POINT

When unions are present in the workplace, what should be the relationship between them and management? What is accomplished by having a competitive or hostile relationship?

AMERICAN NURSES ASSOCIATION AND COLLECTIVE BARGAINING

One difficult union issue faced by nurse-managers is the dual role of their professional organization, the ANA. The NLRB recognizes the ANA, at most state levels, as a collective bargaining agent. The use of state associations as bargaining agents is divisive among U.S. nurses. Some nurse-managers believe that they have been disenfranchised by their professional organization. Other managers recognize the conflicts inherent in attempting to sit on both sides of the bargaining table. Even for members who feel that the issue presents no real dilemma, there appears to be some conflict in loyalty.

This conflict has manifested itself in recent splitting away of state nurses associations from the parent ANA organization. Bruno (2005) suggested that the ANA has not shown leadership in a time of professional nursing crisis and that it has supported management interests over those of nurses. Since California RNs broke from the ANA, two other states, Massachusetts and Maine, have disaffiliated. In addition, two other states, New York and Pennsylvania, have declared their independence. There are no easy solutions to the dilemma created by the dual role held by the ANA.

DISCUSSION POINT

If you are a student, do you belong to the state student nurses association? If you are an RN, have you joined your state nurses association? Why or why not?

Perhaps the nursing profession should look at the experience of the American Association of University Professors (AAUP), which serves as both a professional association that promotes academic freedom and other professorial concerns and as a collective bargaining unit. In addition, there is a fundraising foundation arm. Wilson (2008) noted that their duality of mission has resulted in declining membership, budget deficits, and membership conflicts. As a result, in June 2008, AAUP leaders met to discuss restructuring the organization.

The resultant plan divides the AAUP into three separate entities: a professional association that promotes academic freedom and other academic concerns, a collective bargaining unit, and a fund-raising arm called the AAUP Foundation (Wilson). This will allow a AUP members to determine which part of the organization they wish to support with their membership dues.

CONSIDER

The ANA acts as both a *professional association* for RNs and a *collective bargaining agent*. To some nurses this dual purpose poses a conflict in loyalty.

DISCUSSION POINT

Should the ANA—the recognized professional association for nurses in the United States—also be a collective bargaining agent?

NURSES AND STRIKES

The NLRA states in part that employees shall have the right to engage in "other concerted activities" for the purpose of collective bargaining or other mutual aid or protection (Griggs, 2008). The phrase "other concerted activities" refers to "the right to effectively communicate with one another regarding self-organization at the jobsite" (Griggs, para 9).

The law then gives union members time to work together to determine whether strikes are necessary to achieve desired goals. Such strikes, however, are not allowed without giving the employer and the Federal Mediation and Conciliation Service (FMCS) 10 days notice of the intent to strike. In doing so, the facility should have a reasonable amount of time to stop admitting patients, transfer existing patients to other facilities, and reduce medical procedures that require nurse-intensive labor. Problems occur when management continues to admit new patients or maintains normal operations.

DISCUSSION POINT

Can strikes, walkouts, "blue flu epidemics," and picket lines be considered ethical actions if nurses believe that they are the only way in which they can improve working conditions or ensure safe patient care?

The controversy over whether nurses should strike is long-standing and is likely at the heart of why so many individuals fear union activity. Critics of nurses having the ability to strike suggest that it is unethical because it leaves patients without care providers. Unions argue that strikes must be supported because they are used only as a last resort and after careful consideration of every factor. The issue of striking then continues to divide the nursing profession. Ironically, both proponents and opponents of strikes in nursing argue that they aim for the same goal: safe patient care.

Indeed, the ANA has held consistently for 50 years that nurses not only have a right to strike, but also a professional responsibility and ethical duty to do so if it means maintaining work conditions conducive to providing high-quality care.

For example, the article "Court Upholds UC RNs Right to Strike" (2008) outlined a situation that occurred at the University of California (UC) hospitals in July 2005. The UC nurses called for a 1-day strike in response to what they perceived to be unwillingness by UC administrators to bargain in good faith over vital patient safety issues such as nurse-to-patient ratios. The University obtained a last-minute injunction to block the strike.

Then the University took the case to the Public Employment Relations Board (PERB) judge to see whether the RN request to strike was even legal. Administrative Law Judge Donn Ginoza ruled that

> UC had violated state law by failing to negotiate with the unions on the safe staffing proposal and by denying access to information on patient classification systems, which would have helped refine and improve staffing proposals. The ruling confirmed that under California's Higher Education Employer–Employee Relations Act, *public employees are allowed to strike against unfair labor practices (Court Upholds UC RNs Right to Strike, 2008, pp. 7–8).*

The ruling affected 10,000 UC RNs represented by the California Nurses Association (CNA) and the National Nurses Organizing Committee (NNOC), two large collective bargaining agents in the state of California.

In addition to the moral dilemmas related to the decision to strike, nurses must also determine how they feel about crossing the picket line, should a strike occur. Nurses do have a choice not to participate in strikes or to cross picket lines when strikes occur. They risk derision by their peers in doing so, however, because strikebreakers, commonly known as "*scabs*," are viewed as taking management's side on the issue and may never be fully accepted by their peers after the strike action has ended.

CONCLUSIONS

The question of whether nurses should participate in collective bargaining has been around since legislation made such organization possible. Advocates on both sides of the issues present earnest, well-reasoned arguments to support their positions. Clearly, nurses working in unionized organizations appear to have some economic advantage, and their individual vulnerability to arbitrary action on the part of their employer is reduced.

Yet, nurse's longstanding struggle to be recognized as a profession underscores concerns that the profession's involvement in collective bargaining associations, historically reserved for blue collar industries, undermines this goal. In addition, some nurses think

that union activities draw attention away from patients and patient-related activities. Union advocates argue the opposite—that improving pay, benefits, and working conditions ultimately leads to improved patient care.

There are also issues related to who can belong to a union, what the definition of "supervisor" is in nursing, and whether strikes and walkouts are ethically justified for nursing professionals. In addition, the dual role of the ANA as both the national organization for nurses and a collective bargaining agent poses ethical dilemmas for many nurses. Even unionized nurses cannot agree on the intensity and direction their unions should take, resulting in state unions breaking off from the ANA.

Finally, the relationships health care organizations have developed with their collective bargaining agents vary from direct opposition to collaboration. The effect of that relationship on working conditions and quality of patient care cannot be overstated. Unionization, then, is likely to continue to be fraught with challenges and will be one of the most passionate issues nurses will debate for some time to come.

FOR ADDITIONAL DISCUSSION

1. Does the presence of unions increase the likelihood that management will be fairer and more consistent with employers?

2. How do you feel about the AAUP dividing the organization into three distinct parts with separate activities—collective bargaining, academic support, and fund raising? Would a similar model work for the ANA?

3. Can the need for unionization be eliminated simply by management being more attentive to worker needs and being willing to provide employees reasonable working conditions and a voice in decision making?

4. Would you be willing to cross a picket line to work during an authorized strike?

5. Are there other ways nurses can increase their group power other than by unions? If so, are they as effective?

6. Some state unions are choosing to break off from the ANA. Does this further fragment nursing's collective power in the political arena by diminishing group size, or does it increase the broad-based support of nursing issues?

7. Do you believe that the current nursing shortage will accelerate the rate of unionization in nursing?

8. How does a nursing shortage affect a union's power in negotiating wages, benefits, and working conditions?

ACKNOWLEDGMENT

This chapter is reproduced, in part, with permission from Marquis, B., & Huston, C. (2009). Understanding collective bargaining, unionization, and employment laws (Chapter 22). In: *Leadership Roles and Management Functions in Nursing* (6th ed). Philadelphia: Lippincott Williams & Wilkins.

REFERENCES

American Federation of Teachers (n.d.). *Collective bargaining.* Available at: http://www.aft.org/pubs-reports/pe_advocate/junejuly08/feature.htm. Accessed August 21, 2008.

Bauer, J. (2005) Earnings survey. *RN, 68*(10), 46–53.

Bruno, E. (2005). Building a new national RN movement. *Revolution, 6*(1), 15–16, 18–21.

Burger, D. (2006). Letter from the president. *Registered Nurse, 10*(2), 2.

Business Dictionary (2008). *Jurisdictional strike. Definition.* Available at: http://www.businessdictionary.com/definition/jurisdictional-strike.html. Accessed August 21, 2008.

Court upholds UC RNs right to strike (2008). *Registered Nurse: Journal of Patient Advocacy, 104*(4), 7–8.

Franklin D. Roosevelt Presidential Library and Museum (n.d.). *Our documents: National Labor Relations Act.* Available at: http://www.fdrlibrary.marist.edu/odnlra.html. Accessed May 3, 2005.

Griggs, S. (2008). *Application of the National Labor Relations Act to non-union employers.* Find Law for Legal Professionals. Available at: http://library.findlaw.com/2000/Sep/1/128621.html. Accessed August 22, 2008.

Haugh, R. (2006). The new union strategy: Turning the community against you. *Hospitals & Health Networks, 80*(5), 32–37.

Health Care Corporation (1992). *Decisions of the National Labor Relations Board* (306 NLRB No. 11), January 21, 1992. Available at: http://www.nlrb.gov/nlrb/shared_files/decisions/306/306-11.txt. Accessed May 3, 2005

H.R. 800. Employee Free Choice Act of 2007 (n.d.) Available at: http://www.govtrack.us/congress/bill.xpd?bill=h110-800. Accessed August 21, 2008.

Labor unions and nursing (2003). Available at: http://www.freeessays.cc/db/11/bmu374.shtml. Accessed August 21, 2008.

Marquis, B., & Huston, C. (2009). *Leadership Roles and Management Functions in Nursing* (6th ed.) Philadelphia: Lippincott Williams & Wilkins.

NLRB v. Health Care & Retirement Corp. (1994). *NLRB v. Health Care & Retirement Corp.,* 114 S. Ct. 1778, May 23, 1994. Available at: http://www.law.cornell.edu/supct/html/92-1964.ZS.html. Accessed August 22, 2008.

Oxford Pocket Dictionary of Current English (2008). *Labor union. Definition.* Available at: http://www.encyclopedia.com/doc/1O999-laborunion.html. Accessed August 21, 2008.

Pittman, J. (2007). Registered nurse job satisfaction and collective bargaining unit membership status. *Journal of Nursing Administration, 37*(10), 471–476.

Rothgerber, Johnson, & Lyons LLP (2006). *Critical NLRB decision clarifies who may be a "supervisor" under the NLRA.* Available at: http://www.rothgerber.com/showarticle.aspx?Show=780. Accessed August 21, 2008.

Sandler, M. (2007). House panel approves changes to union supervisor definition. *CQ Weekly, 65*(36), 2783.

Service Employees International Union (SEIU) (2008). *About SEIU.* Available at: http://www.seiu.org/about/index.cfm. Accessed August 21, 2008.

Twarog, J. (2005). The benefits of union membership: Numerous and measurable. *Massachusetts Nurse, 76*(4), 6.

University of Minnesota, Office of Human Resources (2008). *Decertification process.* Available at: http://www1.umn.edu/ohr/er/negotiations/process/decertification/index.html. Accessed August 22, 2008.

Wilson, R. (2008). Can reorganization save the AAUP? *The Chronicle of Higher Education, 54*(42), A4.

BIBLIOGRAPHY

Adams, C. (2008). The power in the union. *Community Practitioner, 81*(4), 3.

American Federation of Teachers (n.d). *Organizing a healthcare union.* Available at: http://www.aft.org/healthcare/organizing.htm. Accessed August 21, 2008.

Are nurses safe? The spectre of workplace hazards for remote area nurses (2008). *The Queensland Nurse, 27*(2), 6–7.

Bargaining unit updates (May 2008). *Massachusetts Nurse, 79*(5), 12.

Benchmarking has put unions into very 'difficult position' (2008). *World of Irish Nursing & Midwifery, 16*(6), 21.

California nurses union makes presence known in Tennessee (2008). *Tennessee Nurse, 71*(2), 3.

Cockshaw, P. (2007). Labor needs to act to stay relevant. *Engineering News-Record, 258*(10), 70.

Greenhouse, S. (2008). Judge's ruling for union may end 6-month strike. *The New York Times,* August 15, 2008, p. 4-3.

Greenhouse, S. (2008). With contracts expired, nurses at four hospitals cite frustration. *The New York Times,* March 15, 2008, p. 2-1.

Griffing, M. (2007). Why bargaining, organizing, and politics matters. *Registered Nurse: Journal of Patient Advocacy, 103*(8), 10–11.

Kaplan, E. (2008). Labor's Growing Pains. *Nation, 286*(23), 17–23.

Labor law: Is a charge nurse a rank and file employee or a supervisor? (2007). *Legal Eagle Eye Newsletter for the Nursing Profession, 15*(7), 7.

Labor Practices: "RNs demand safe staffing" buttons may be worn on campus, court says. (2008). *Legal Eagle Eye Newsletter for the Nursing Profession, 16*(6), 6.

Non-union agreement undermines nurses (2008). *Australian Nursing Journal, 15*(11), 18.

Povich, E. (2007). Committee acts to reverse NLRB definition of supervisor. *Congress Daily,* September 19, 2007, p. 11.

Schoeff, Jr., M. (2007). 'Supervisor' bill likely to face battle in Senate. *Workforce Management, 86*(17), 18.

Twarog, J. (2008). Organizing around grievances. *Massachusetts Nurse, 79*(4), 8.

Twarog, J. (2008). Pointers on ground rules at the bargaining table. *Massachusetts Nurse, 79*(1), 13.

Unions try to hang on as open-shop laws gain ground (2007). *USA Today,* July 26, 2007, pp. 1B–2B.

Were 'striking nurses' eligible for unemployment benefits? (2008). *Nursing Law's Regan Report, 48*(10), 1.

WEB RESOURCES

American Federation of State, County, and Municipal Employees, AFL–CIO	http://www.afscme.org
American Federation of Teachers	http://www.aft.org/healthcare/index.htm
American Nurses Association	http://nursingworld.org
Australian Nursing Federation	http://www.anf.org.au
California Nurses Association	http://www.calnurse.org/
Health and Community Services Union—Australia	http://www.hacsu.asn.au/about
National Education Association	http://www.nea.org/esphome/
New York Professional Nurses Union	http://www.nypnu.org/
Nova Scotia Nurses Union	http://www.nsnu.ns.ca/
Ontario Nurses Association	http://www.ona.org/

Service Employees International Union	http://www.seiu.org/health/nurses/
International Brotherhood of Teamsters	http://www.teamster.org
United Auto Workers	http://www.uaw.org
United Food and Commercial Workers (UFCW), AFL/CIO	http://www.ufcw.org
United Nurses and Allied Professionals	http://www.unap.org
United Nurses of Alberta	http://www.una.ab.ca

CHAPTER 18

Assuring Provider Competence through Licensure, Continuing Education, and Certification

• CAROL J. HUSTON •

Learning Objectives

The learner will be able to:

1. Differentiate between *competence* and *continuing competence* in a profession.
2. Identify stakeholders that would be affected by a movement to mandate continuing competence in nursing.
3. Identify driving and restraining forces to implementing mandatory re-examination as a prerequisite for license renewal in nursing.
4. Compare support for mandatory re-examination for license renewal in nursing with that of other health professions such as medicine and pharmacy.
5. Identify arguments for and against mandated continuing education for license renewal.
6. Compare continuing education requirements for nurses with those of physicians, physician assistants, pharmacists, respiratory therapists, and other health care professionals.
7. Describe personal and professional benefits of professional certification as identified in the literature.
8. Delineate the roles/responsibilities assumed by the American Board of Nursing Specialties as the accrediting body for nursing certification.
9. Identify the strengths and weaknesses of using professional certification as an indicator of entry-level competence in advanced practice nursing.
10. Describe how portfolios and self-assessment, as tools for reflective practice, can further the goal of professional competence.
11. Explore the roles and responsibilities of the individual, employers, the state board of nursing, and professional associations in assuring both the initial and continued competence of health care practitioners.
12. Reflect on his or her beliefs regarding the need for and efficacy of mandating re-examination for licensure, continuing education, and certification for nurses to assure continuing competence.

How can one determine whether a nurse is competent? Does licensure assure competence? Does clinical performance? Does competence require clinical practice recency? Is it assured by professional certification?

Unfortunately, in many states, a practitioner is determined to be competent when initially licensed and thereafter unless proven otherwise. Yet, clearly, passing a licensing exam and continuing to work as a clinician does not assure competence throughout a career. Competence requires continual updates to knowledge and practice, and this is difficult in a health care environment characterized by rapidly emerging new tech-

nologies, chaotic change, and perpetual clinical advancements.

In 1995, the Task Force on Healthcare Workforce Regulations of the Pew Health Professions Commission recommended changing how health care professions, including nursing, were regulated and suggested that continued competence should be assured as a regulatory board function (North Carolina Board of Nursing [NCBN], 2008). The Citizens Advocacy Center, a public policy organization located in Washington, D.C., concurred, as did the 1999 Institute of Medicine (IOM) in its report *To Err Is Human*, which included a recommendation for professional licensing bodies to assume the responsibility for determining licensees' competence and knowledge.

There is little disagreement that the knowledge health care professionals need must be current and appropriate to their area of practice and that their care should be competent at the minimum. The challenge lies, however, in determining how best to assure that competence and in determining who should be responsible for its oversight.

This chapter explores definitions of *competence* with particular attention given to that of *continuing competence*. Licensure, periodic relicensure, continuing education, and professional certification are examined as potential strategies for assuring provider competence. The chapter also discusses the limitations of each of these strategies for assessing both initial and continuing competence, as well as the difficulties inherent in standardizing continuing competence requirements in a health care system composed of varied stakeholders. Finally, the chapter ends with an exploration of portfolio development and reflective practice, contemporary strategies that allow health care professionals to carry out a self-assessment of their practice and to develop a personal plan for maintaining competence.

DEFINING COMPETENCE

Competence in nursing can be defined in many ways. In a 1996 position paper entitled *Assuring Competence: A Regulatory Responsibility*, the National Council of State Boards of Nursing (NCSBN) defined continued competence as "the application of knowledge and the interpersonal, decision-making, and psychomotor skills expected for the nurse's practice role, within the context of public health, welfare and safety" (NCSBN, 2005, para 3).

In 1999, the American Nurses Association (ANA) convened an expert panel that defined three types of competence in nursing: *continuing competence, professional nursing competence,* and *continuing professional nursing competence*. Special attention was given, however, to continuing competence because so many assumptions exist regarding the rights and responsibilities of consumers, individual nurses, and employers to see that such competence is present and promulgated. Indeed, it is continuing competence that is a primary focus of this chapter, given that initial licensure suggests that at least minimum competence levels were met at that time.

In 2007, the ANA released a draft position statement on competence and competency for public review and comment. The purpose of this position paper was to define *competence* ("performing successfully at an expected level") and *competency* ("an expected level of performance that results from an integration of knowledge, skills, abilities, and judgment within the context of current and projected professional directions"). Key excerpts from this position statement are shown in Box 18.1.

Continued competence also was a focus of the NCBN (2008, para 4), which defined it as "the ongoing applica-

---

BOX 18.1 | EXCERPTS FROM THE AMERICAN NURSES ASSOCIATION (ANA) DRAFT STATEMENT ON COMPETENCE AND COMPETENCY (2007)

The ANA supports the following principles in regard to competence in the nursing profession:

- The public has a right to expect nurses to demonstrate competence throughout their careers.
- The nursing profession must shape and guide any process assuring nurse competence.
- Regulatory bodies define minimal standards for regulation of practice to protect the public.
- Employers are responsible and accountable to provide an environment conducive to competent practice.
- Nurses are individually responsible and accountable for maintaining competence.
- Assurance of competence is the shared responsibility of the profession, individual nurses, regulatory bodies, employers, and other key stakeholders.
- Competence is definable, measurable, and can be evaluated.
- Context determines what competencies are necessary.
- The measurement criteria are the competence statements for each standard of nursing practice and of professional performance.

Source: American Nurses Association (2007). *Position statement on competence and competency [Draft]*. Available at: http://www.cc-institute.org/docs_upload/anaCompetency.pdf. Accessed January 23, 2009.

tion of knowledge and the decision-making, psychomotor, and interpersonal skills expected of the licensed nurse within a specific practice setting resulting in nursing care that contributes to the health and welfare of clients served." Similarly, the Canadian Nurses Association and Canadian Association of Schools of Nursing (2004, para 1) defined continuing competence as "the ongoing ability of a nurse to integrate and apply the knowledge, skills, judgment and personal attributes required to practice safely and ethically in a designated role and setting."

Carliner et al. (2006, para 4) defined competencies as the "knowledge, skills, or attitudes that enable one to effectively perform the activities of a given occupation or function to the standards expected in employment." They also pointed out that "competencies can be considered along a spectrum, from the basic competencies needed to survive in the workforce to a range of advanced competencies needed to sustain employability and advance in one's career" (p. 29).

Finally, Tilley (2008) suggested that the defining attributes of competence are "the application of skills in all domains for the practice role, instruction that focuses on specific outcomes or competencies, allowance for increasing levels of competence, accountability of the learner, practice-based learning, self-assessment, and individualized learning experiences."

Clearly, although there is some overlap among these definitions, there is also a lack of consensus around what competence is and how it should be measured. There also appears to be difficulty in relating the continuing competence of providers with the roles they are asked to assume in the clinical setting. For example, some nurses develop high levels of competence in specific areas of nursing practice as a result of work experience and specialization at the expense of staying current in other areas of practice. Yet employers, who espouse the support of continuing competence, often ask registered nurses (RNs) to provide care in areas of practice outside their area of expertise because the current nursing shortage encourages them to do so. In addition, many current competence assessments focus more on skills than they do on knowledge.

> ## CONSIDER
> "Current competence assessment methods measure only a quarter of nurse's competence levels when they focus on skills and not knowledge" (McCready, 2007, p. 143).

In addition, professional nursing organizations decline to implement continuing competence mandates because they fear membership repercussions. For example, the American Nurses Credentialing Center (ANCC) continues to offer certification examinations for registered nurses without baccalaureate degrees, despite the recognition that such certification suggests advanced rather than basic practice.

> ## DISCUSSION POINT
> Should certification be limited to nurses with baccalaureate degrees or higher education?

The ANA advocates that states defer competence monitoring to the professional association, without governmental involvement in the process, partly because of concern about misconduct charges if state regulators are involved and partly because memberships and revenues are likely to increase if the association monitors competence. Clearly, then, stakeholders and politics continue to influence how continuing competence is defined, used, and promulgated.

The issue is also complicated by the fact that there are no national standards for defining, measuring, or requiring continuing competence in nursing. In addition, specialty nursing organizations, state nurses associations, state boards of nursing, and professional nursing organizations have not reached consensus about what continuing competence is and how to measure it, although there is little debate that it is needed. The reality is that given the multiplicity and variations of the definition of continuing competence and the number of stakeholders affected by its promulgation, identifying and mandating strategies that assure the continuing competence of health care providers will be very difficult.

> ## CONSIDER
> "A major challenge in the professional practice assessment process is objective measurement and this is difficult in the assessment of clinical competency" (McCready, 2007, p. 149).

Carliner et al. (2006) suggested that future research is needed to address the following questions regarding continuing competence:

- Do core competencies improve performance in the workplace?
- What are the benefits of developing workers' core competencies?

- How can we assess core competencies?
- What are the core competencies required to function in the changing workplace?
- Do core competencies contribute to building a learning organization?
- What core competencies are required to function in a knowledge society?
- Do core competencies improve quality of work experience?
- Do jobs match the competencies identified for them?
- Do core competencies improve workers self-efficacy and self-esteem in the workplace?
- Do core competencies acquired for one occupation transfer to other occupations?

PROFESSIONAL LICENSURE

Licensure can be defined as

The granting of permission by a competent authority (usually a government agency) to an organization or individual to engage in a practice or activity that would otherwise be illegal. Licensure is usually granted on the basis of education and examination rather than performance. It is usually permanent, but a periodic fee, demonstration of competence, or continuing education may be required (The Free Dictionary by Farlex, 2008, para 1).

Most health care professionals must be licensed, and this license is assumed to provide at least some assurance that the practitioner is competent in his or her field at the time of initial licensure.

Licensure Processes in Nursing

One of the most important purposes of the NCSBN and its 60 state boards of nursing (one in each of 46 states, 2 in 4 states, 1 in the District of Columbia, and 1 in each of 5 U.S. territories) is to protect the health, safety, and welfare of the public (Boards of Nursing, 2008; NCBSN, 2008a). This is done by having a regulatory role in the accreditation of nursing education programs, through licensure, and by implementing and enforcing the Nurse Practice Act. In addition, the NCSBN has created

and disseminated numerous nursing practice and regulation resources on nursing practice and education and maintains a database on nursing disciplinary actions taken across the nation.

It is for the licensing examinations for RNs and licensed practical nurses/vocational nurses (LPNs/LVNs), however, that the NCSBN and its state boards of nursing are probably best known. The NCSBN has developed two licensure examinations to test the entry-level nursing competence of candidates for licensure as registered nurses and as LPNs/LVNs. These examinations, the National Council Licensure Examinations (NCLEX-RN and NCLEXPN), are administered with the contractual assistance of a national test service (NCSBN, 2008b, para 1) and test integrated nursing content. Passage of the NCLEX suggests that the individual has been deemed by the state to have met minimal competence standards for entry into practice; however, this does reflect or measure the many higher-level competencies achieved in different types of education programs for nurses.

> ### DISCUSSION POINT
> Does having just one NCLEX for multiple levels of educational levels into practice argue that the associate degree in nursing provides an adequate knowledge base for competence in all areas of professional nursing practice?

Despite this flaw, licensure by examination continues to be a highly regarded strategy for assuring competence levels of health care professionals such as nurses. Indeed, some professional organizations and regulatory bodies suggest that RNs should be required to repeat the NCLEX periodically or that nurses should be required to take examinations similar in scope to the NCLEX for license renewal.

Efforts to implement mandatory re-examination as a prerequisite for license renewal in nursing, however, have met with minimal success. This is because there is little agreement about what such an examination should look like, how it would be administered, and how often it should be required. Nonetheless, 11 states have introduced legislation with varying approaches from retesting to requiring a provider to demonstrate competence in the workplace, but resistance is high, and there is little hope that periodic re-examinations to assess competence will be a part of nursing's immediate future.

Licensure Processes in Medicine

In contrast to the NCLEX, U.S. medical licensure examinations are developed using a competence-based process that requires examinees to be cognizant of practice changes, the evidence required for practice, and the knowledge necessary to be competent into the future. In addition, to achieve full authority to practice independently, physicians are required to pass three licensure examinations (United States Medical Licensing Examination, 2007). Furthermore, a clinical skills examination was implemented in 2004.

In addition, although periodic re-examination was recommended in 1967 by the Bureau of Health Manpower of the U.S. Department of Health for licensure of physicians as of 1971, the decision regarding whether to do so has been left to the discretion of individual states, and "In most states, physicians can maintain their licenses just by having no disciplinary actions against them and by completing a minimum number of hours of continuing medical education" (Adams, 2007, para 2).

As a result, a committee of the Federation of State Medical Boards (FSMB) recommended in 2007 that

> Boards require doctors applying for relicensure to participate in self-evaluation and practice assessment, show continued competence in areas such as patient care and medical knowledge, and complete an exam in their practice areas. The process, committee members said, would be similar to maintenance of certification, a voluntary program used by specialty boards to ensure lifelong learning as a part of board certification. Members said most medical boards likely would accept recertification as meeting the maintenance of licensure requirements (Adams, 2007, paras 3–4).

Licensure Processes in Pharmacy

Pharmacists have also been reluctant to embrace the IOM's *To Err Is Human* recommendation that periodic re-examination of key providers is critical to resolving health care quality problems, especially medical errors. Pharmacists take a licensing exam on graduation, known as the North American Pharmacist Licensure Examination (NAPLEX). The NAPLEX is a computer-adaptive examination that consists of 185 multiple-choice test questions. Of these, 150 questions are used to calculate the test score, and the remaining 35 items serve as pretest questions (National Association of Boards of Pharmacy [NABP], 2008).

In addition, states require a Multistate Pharmacy Jurisprudence Examination (MPJE), which

> combines federal- and state-specific law questions to serve as the state law examination in participating jurisdictions. The MPJE is based on a national blueprint of pharmacy jurisprudence competencies; however, the questions are tailored to the specific laws in each state. The MPJE consists of 90 multiple-choice test questions. Of these, 60 questions are used to calculate the test score. (NABP, 2008, para 5)

Reciprocity is then granted between states by an electronic licensure transfer program. At present, pharmacists are not required to retake the NAPLEX at any point for license renewal.

DISCUSSION POINT

Why are professional health care organizations reluctant to support re-examination as a means of assuring continuing competence? Who are the stakeholders involved? What are some ramifications of adopting such a mandate?

CONTINUING EDUCATION

Instead of requiring health care providers to periodically repeat their initial licensure examinations, many professional associations and states have mandated continuing education (CE) for license renewal. This has been done in an attempt to promote continued competence and is less controversial than periodic reexamination for licensure.

Continuing Education in Nursing

Taft and Sparks (2008) suggested that about 60% of the states in the United States have some kind of requirements for CE for professional nurse license renewal. These requirements typically vary from a few hours to 30 hours every 2 years (Box 18.2). Some states—Colorado, for example—required CE at one time but removed that requirement because it felt that CE did not guarantee competence. Similarly, Hawaii discontinued CE requirements for many professions, including nursing and physical therapy, because of high costs of these courses to the individual practitioner, considerable costs to the state to administer the legislation, and the inability to demonstrate positive outcomes.

BOX 18.2 | **SAMPLE STATE CONTINUING EDUCATION (CE) REQUIREMENTS FOR NURSES**

Arkansas: 15 practice focused contact hours every 2 years, or certification or recertification during the renewal period by a national certifying body or an academic course in nursing or related field (Arkansas Board of Registered Nursing, 2005).

California: 30 hours every 2 years (California Board of Registered Nursing, 2007).

Florida: 24 hours every 2 years with 2 hours dedicated to prevention of medical errors. In addition, HIV/AIDS is now a one-time, 1-hour CE requirement to be completed prior to the first renewal and Domestic Violence CE is now a 2-hour requirement every third renewal (Florida Board of Registered Nursing, 2007).

Iowa: 36 hours for a 3-year license and 24 hours for licenses less than 3 years (Iowa Board of Nursing, 2007).

Michigan: Not less than 25 hours of continuing education, with at least 1 hour in pain and symptom management (Michigan Nurses Association, 2007).

New Jersey: 30 hours every 2 years (Continuing Education Requirements, 2008).

New York: 3 contact hours infection control every 4 years and 2 contact hours child abuse (one time) (Continuing Education Requirements, 2008).

North Dakota: 12 contact hours every 2 years (Continuing Education Requirements, 2008).

Ohio: 24 hours every 2 years (LaWriter Ohio Laws and Rules, 2007).

Oregon: One-time, 7-hour course on pain management (Continuing Education Requirements, 2008).

Texas: 20 hours every 2 years (Texas Board of Nursing, 2008).

DISCUSSION POINT

Is the need for continuing education greater for one type of health care professional than another? When required, should the minimum number of mandated hours be the same for all health care professionals? If not, how many should be required for each health care specialty?

Continuing Education in Medicine

Forty-three states plus Guam, Puerto Rico, and the Virgin Islands require some form of continuing medical education (CME) for relicensure of medical doctors (MDs) and for doctors of osteopathy (DOs), although the requirements frequently differ for the two groups (Medscape Today, 2007).

The number of required hours also varies dramatically by state. For example, Montana, Colorado, Indiana, New York, Oregon, South Dakota, and Vermont require no CME hours for either MDs or DOs. North Carolina, Illinois, and New Hampshire require 150 hours every 3 years, whereas Alabama requires only 24 hours every 2 years, and Arkansas requires only

20 hours each year (Medscape Today, 2007). It should be noted, however, that some medical specialty societies, specialty boards, hospital medical staffs, the Joint Commission, and insurance groups require physicians to demonstrate continuing education, even if the state does not require this for reclicensure (American Medical Association, 2008).

In addition, many states have laws that direct the format of the CME. Miller et al. (2008, p. 95) stated that 17 of the 68 medical and osteopathic licensing boards "require physicians to participate in legislatively mandated topics that may have little to do with the types of patients seen by the applicant physician." Required topics include pain management, acquired immunodeficiency syndrome (AIDS), and domestic violence. Other states require that physicians renewing their licenses must receive instruction on ethics and professional responsibility.

Furthermore, unlike nursing CE, which is typically monitored by the state boards of nursing, there is no central repository of CME (American Medical Association, 2008). Instead, accredited CME providers are required to keep records of CE credits awarded to physicians who participate in their activities for 6 years, and physicians are responsible for maintaining a record of their CME credits from all sources.

Miller et al. (2008) argued that using CME to ensure continued competence is flawed, and that CME for physicians must evolve from counting hours of course time to recognizing physician achievement in knowledge, competence, and performance. In addition, Miller et al. advocated that "state medical boards should require valid and reliable assessment of physicians' learning needs" and that "CME planners should create learning activities on the basis of the assessed practice needs of physicians" (p. 97), rather than having a CME system that encourages coursework based on interest alone.

CONSIDER

"To provide the best care to patients, a physician must commit to lifelong learning, but continuing education and evaluation systems in the United States typically require little more than records of attendance for professional association memberships, hospital staff privileges, or reregistration of a medical license" (Miller et al., 2008, p. 95).

Continuing Education in Other Health Care Professions

Almost all states require CE for pharmacists, and most require the CE be from approved sources such as the American Counsel on Pharmacy Education. Sometimes carryover is allowed, and sometimes the type is proscribed.

In addition, many states require acupuncturists, audiologists, and occupational therapists to have CE for license renewal. Physician Assistants (PAs) must log 100 hours of continuing medical education every 2 years and sit for a recertification every 6 years to maintain their national certification (American Academy of Physician Assistants, 2008).

In addition, 45 states and the District of Columbia mandate CE for relicensure for dentists, with the average being 20 hours per year (Schleyer & Dodell, 2005). Ten states have specified a minimum number of clinical hours for dentists, 17 states have limited nonclinical hours, and 7 states have placed constraints on both clinical and nonclinical CE (Schleyer & Dodell).

DISCUSSION POINT

Continuing education is mandated in most states for certified public accountants, optometrists, real estate brokers, nursing home administrators, and insurance brokers. Why are there fewer states mandating continuing education for health care professionals? What rationale can be given for why these occupations have a greater need for continuing education than health care professionals?

Does Requiring Continuing Education Ensure Competence?

The CE approach to continuing competence continues to be very controversial because there is limited research demonstrating correlation among CE, continuing competence, and improved patient outcomes. In addition, many professional organizations have expressed concern about the quality of mandated CE courses and the lack of courses for experts and specialists. Likewise, there is no agreement on the optimal number of annual credits needed to ensure competence. Until consensus can be reached regarding how CE should be provided and how much is needed, and until research findings show an empirical link between CE and provider competence, it is difficult to tout CE as a valid and reliable measure of continuing competence. Taft and Sparks (2008) summarized the pros and cons of mandating continuing education for nurses (see Box 18.3).

CERTIFICATION

As defined by the American Board of Nursing Specialties (ABNS) (2005, para 1), certification is "the formal recognition of the specialized knowledge, skills, and experience demonstrated by the achievement of standards identified by a nursing specialty to promote optimal health outcomes."

Certification does not, however, include a legal scope of practice. The ANCC suggested, however, that it "does protect the public by enabling anyone to identify competent people more readily; aids the profession by encouraging and recognizing professional achievement; recognizes specialization, enhances professionalism and, in some cases, serves as a criterion for financial reimbursement" (ANCC, 2008a, para 2). Organizations offering specialty certifications for nurses include the

BOX 18.3 | PROS AND CONS OF CONTINUING EDUCATION REQUIREMENTS FOR NURSES

Pros

- Demonstrates professionalism.
- Demonstrates commitment to maintaining competence.
- Demonstrates attention to patient safety and a reduction in medical errors.
- Motivates employers to support continuing education needs of RN employees.
- Raises the standard for continuing education for all nurses.
- Research supports the conclusion that continuing education positively affects nursing practice.

Cons

- Seat time does not guarantee learning.
- Difficult to agree on competence standards.
- Administrative and monitoring costs.
- Concerns about the cost, access, quality, and relevance of continuing education offerings.
- Research is inconclusive about the benefits of mandatory continuing education over voluntary continuing education.
- Difficult to measure outcomes of mandatory continuing education on patient care due to the many variables that influence patient outcomes; including the individual nurse, the choice of the continuing education program, the continuing education program itself, learning styles, professionalism, and accountability.

Source: Taft, L., & Sparks, R. K. (2008). *Nursing matters. Continuing education for nurses.* Available at: **http://www.nursingmattersonline.com/nursingmattersonline/studentdetail.asp?newsid=1782.** Accessed August 21, 2008.

ACCN, the American Association of Critical Care Nursing, the American Association of Nurse Anesthetists, the American College of Nurse Midwives, the Board of Certification for Emergency Nursing, and the Rehabilitation Nursing Certification Board.

Becoming Certified

To achieve professional certification, nurses must meet eligibility criteria that typically include years and types of work experience, as well as minimum educational levels, active nursing licenses, and successful completion of a nationally administered examination. Certifications normally last about 5 years.

The American Board of Nursing Specialties

There are approximately 500,000 nationally certified nurses in the United States and more than 70 certifications at the RN and advanced practice nurse (APN) lev-

els (Ridge, 2008). This translates to 15% to 17% of all practicing nurses certified in at least one specialty (Ridge).

In addition to the large numbers of certified nurses, there are many different types of nursing certification credentials, and certification programs often have very different standards. This makes it difficult for providers and consumers to determine the value of a particular nursing certification. For this reason, the American Board of Nursing Specialties (ABNS) was created in 1991. The ABNS comprises 28 nurse-certifying organizations, some which offer only one specialty, such as the Orthopaedic Nurses Certification Board, whereas others offer more, such as the ANCC, which offers 26 specialty certifications (Ridge, 2008).

The ABNS seeks to create uniformity in nursing certification, advocate for consumer protection by establishing specialty nursing certification, and increase public awareness of the value of quality certification to health care. Member organizations of ABNS are located around the world. As the only accrediting body specifically for nursing certification, the Accreditation Council provides a peer-review process for accrediting nursing certification programs that demonstrate compliance with ABNS standards. The 5-year program approval is renewable for both members and nonmember organizations (ABNS, 2005).

The American Nurses Credentialing Center

The ANCC calls itself "the largest and most prestigious nurse credentialing organization in the United States" (ANCC, 2008b). The ANA established the ANA Certification Program in 1973 to provide tangible recognition of professional achievement in a defined functional or clinical area of nursing. The ANCC, a subsidiary of the ANA, became its own corporation in 1991, and since then it has certified more than a quarter million nurses and approximately 75,000 advanced practice nurses (ANCC, 2008a). The ANCC administers nearly 30 specialty and advanced practice certification examinations each year at authorized testing agencies across the country.

Certification and the Advanced Practice Nurse

Advanced practice nurses were the first nurses to use professional certification as a means of documenting advanced knowledge in practice. In 1946, the American Association of Nurse Anesthetists began certifying nurse anesthetists. The American College of Nurse Midwives soon followed.

Many states now use certification as an indicator of entry-level competence in advanced practice nursing, which includes clinical nurse specialists (CNS) and nurse practitioners (NPs). Fitzgerald (2008) noted, however, that nine states do not mandate national certification as a requirement for NP practice, including the three states with the highest number of NPs—California, Florida, and New York. She cautioned, however, that many third-party insurers and other entities are now requiring it, so that the pressure for an APN to be certified will only increase.

Even the NCSBN, which originally proposed second licensure for NPs, now recognizes the certification examination as the regulatory mechanism for advanced nursing practice. A master's degree is required to take the certification examinations for advanced practice

nurses. Certification, then, in the case of the advanced practice nurse is not really voluntary; it is required to ensure public safety and enhance public health.

> **DISCUSSION POINT**
> The ANCC currently does not allow educational waivers for the CSN or NP certifying examination (all applicants must have at least a master's degree). Do you support this decision to not "grandfather" advanced practice nurses who completed their educations through certifying programs (no master's degree) and who are currently practicing in an advanced role? Why or why not?

> **DISCUSSION POINT**
> Physician assistants must pass a national certification examination for licensure. Why is this not also required for nurse practitioners?

The Effect of Professional Certification

A great deal of research has been completed the last decade regarding the use of certification to ensure competence and its inherent value. Most of these studies suggest that certification does have an effect on both the creation of a positive work environment and improved patient outcomes.

For example, Piazza, Donahue, Dykes, Griffin, and Fitzpatrick (2006) found that certification enhanced nurses' autonomy, allowed them to have more control over their work, and facilitated collaboration in the workplace. This research also validated that nurses with national certification feel more empowered than nurses who are not certified and that specialty certification often results in recognition of the nurse throughout the organization. In addition, certification increases nurses' informal power on their work units because it indicates knowledge and expertise in their specialty (Piazza et al.).

Similarly, Grief (2007) reported that Certified Emergency Nurses (CENs), Certified Flight Registered Nurses (CFRNs), noncertified nurses, and nurse managers showed a high level of agreement (90% and greater) on value statements that specialty certification validates specialized knowledge, indicates attainment of a practice standard, enhances professional credibility, and enhances a feeling of personal accomplishment and confidence in clinical abilities. Grief concluded that the attainment of specialty certification provides external validation of criteria for job performance and ensures consistency in knowledge.

Finally, the *2006 ABNS White Paper on Nursing Certification* showed that "certification is perceived by nurses and the public as influencing accountability, professional accomplishment and growth, and specialized knowledge in a particular specialty (ABNS, as cited in Ridge, 2008, p. 50). In addition, nurses who pursue and obtain national specialty certification "perceive themselves as having a higher level of commitment to the profession" (Ridge, p. 50).

Creating Work Environments That Value Certification

According to Ridge (2008, p. 50), "Strategic support of nursing specialty certification is a vital element of an effective workforce development program." It is middle- and top-level nurse managers who play the most significant role in creating work environments that value and reward certification. For example, nurse managers can grant tuition reimbursement and cash incentives to workers who seek certification, or they can purchase and make available certification prep books for review by nurses interested in taking such exams (Healthy Work Environments, 2008).

Managers can also show their support for professional certification by displaying posters about its benefits in the workplace and by giving employees paid time off to take the certification exam. In addition, managers can publicly recognize employees who have earned professional certification or recertification because this recognition tends to encourage others to emulate the behavior (Healthy Work Environments, 2008).

This importance of managerial support in encouraging staff to complete professional certification was evident in research completed by Niebuhr and Biel (2007). In this large study of 11,427 nurses, "managers bolstered the positive perceptions of certification and had a correspondingly high rate of agreement on certification value statements" (p. 179), such as "certification enhances feelings of personal accomplishment" and "certification validates specialized knowledge." In fact, 77.3% of nurse manager respondents were certified themselves. Yet, staff nurses reported that a lack of institutional reward and institutional support were two of the top three barriers to becoming certified, although the cost of the examination was the barrier cited most often in the study. (See Research Study Fuels the Controversy.)

This lack of institutional reward or recognition for professional certification was also apparent in research completed by Bekemeier (2007) of 655 public health nurses (PHNs). The PHNs in this study perceived that credentialing had a high personal value but suggested that it provided less value in terms of extrinsic recognition or reward.

Research Study Fuels the Controversy: Validation of Certification

This Web-based survey of 11,427 certified nurses examined respondent perceptions, values, and behaviors related to professional certification. The Perceived Value of Certification Tool (PVCT) was used as the survey tool.

STUDY FINDINGS
Seventy-five percent of the respondents identified themselves as certified nurses. Both certified and noncertified nurses showed a high level of agreement with the value statements on certified practice. Nurse managers demonstrated correspondingly high values as well. Of the 18 certification value statements, only one statement ("Certification increases salary"), did not receive a majority of respondent agreement.

Although certification was positively received, respondents did suggest that barriers to obtaining and maintaining certification remain. Cost coupled with lack of institutional reward and support kept some nurses from pursuing certification. The effect of certification on absenteeism and retention was unclear.

The researchers concluded that certification continues to be a valuable method for nurses to differentiate themselves in the workplace and that health care organizations typically offer incentives to attract and retain professional certified nurses. Cost and lack of recognition were, however, major reasons nurses did not become certified.

Source: Niebuhr, B., & Biel, M. (2007). The value of specialty nursing certification. *Nursing Outlook, 55*(4), 176–181.

REFLECTIVE PRACTICE

Reflective practice is defined by the NCBN (2008, para 7) as "a process for assessing one's own practice to identify and seek learning opportunities to promote continued competence." Inherent in the process is the evaluation and incorporation of this learning into one's practice. Such self-assessment is gaining popularity as a way to promote professional practice and maintain competence. Perhaps that is why nursing is moving away from a continuing education model to a reflective practice/professional portfolio model for competence assessment (O'Malley, 2008).

For example, North Carolina now requires RNs to use a reflective practice approach to carry out a self assessment of her or his practice and develop a plan for maintaining competence (NCBN, 2008a). This assessment is individualized to the licensed nurse's area of practice. RNs seeking license renewal or reinstatement must attest to having completed the learning activities required for continuing competence and be prepared to submit evidence of completion if requested by the Board on random audit (NCBN).

Similarly, the Nurses Association of New Brunswick (NANB) developed a mandatory continuing competence program for implementation in 2008 that requires registered nurses to demonstrate on an annual basis how they have maintained their competence and enhanced their practice (NANB, 2007). The three steps of the NANB mandatory Continuing Competence Program (CCP) are as follows:

1. Self-assessment of nursing practice to determine learning needs.

2. Development and implementation of a learning plan to meet the identified learning needs.

3. Evaluation of the effect of learning activities.

CONSIDER

"Reflective practice, or the process of continually assessing one's own practice to identify learning needs and opportunities for growth, is the key to continuing competence" (NANB, 2007, para 4).

The College of Registered Nurses of British Columbia (CRNBC) also has a mandatory CCP in place. This program was created in 2000 in response to the Health Professions Act, which required the establishment and maintenance of a CCP to promote high practice standards among registered nurses. In the year before license renewal, registrants are expected to

complete a self assessment using CRNBC's Professional Standards for Registered Nurses and Nurse Practitioners, and where relevant, review the practice standards and the Scope of Practice Standards to identify learning needs; obtain peer feedback; develop and implement a learning plan based on their self assessment and peer feedback; and evaluate the impact of last year's learning on their practice (Winslow, 2008, p. 17).

Of the just more than 2,900 CRNBC registered nurses audited in 2008, only 177 received "conditions" on their licensure for noncompliance with the continuing competence requirements (Winslow, 2008). Registrants are allowed to practice only for an additional 3 months before requirements must be met.

Peer feedback, such as that described by the CRNBC, is increasingly becoming a part of reflective practice and continuing competence assessment. Mantesso, Petrucka, and Bassendowski (2008) suggested that in addition to self-evaluation, collegial feedback is one of the strategies within reflective practice that enables nurses to enhance professional performance and to work toward continuing professional competence. Such a process, however, must be formalized, and participants must be educated about how to use peer review and collegial feedback to promote growth in others.

Portfolios and Self-Assessment

Portfolio development is another strategy the individual RN can use to be both reflective about his or her practice and/or to assess or demonstrate competence: "While the standards for portfolio organization and type remain undecided, the literature reveals the critical elements for the nursing portfolio" (O'Malley, 2008, p. 24). For example, Sherrod (2007) suggested that the professional portfolio typically contains a number of core components, such as biographical information; educational background; certifications achieved; employment history; a one- to two-page resume; a competence record or checklist; personal and professional goals; professional development experiences, presentations, consultations, and publications; professional and community activities;

honors and awards; and letters of thanks from patients, families, peers, organizations, and others.

O'Malley (2008) suggested that the portfolio should not, however, just be a collection of certificates nor a diary or logbook. Instead, she suggested that it be a "living document" that demonstrates critical thinking, values, skills, and perhaps most important, reflection. O'Malley suggested that the writer and the reader of the portfolio should experience a nursing career journey with diverse sources of evident and written reflections.

McColgan (2008) agreed, suggesting that portfolios allow nurses to assess their competence, complete work-based reflection, pursue lifelong learning, create career paths, and pursue professional development. McColgan concluded that for portfolios to work effectively, nurses and their employers must have a working partnership and jointly appreciate the value and the opportunities that exist through personal portfolio development.

Similarly, a literature review by McCready (2007) suggested that having clear guidelines for portfolio construction and assessment, as well as for qualitative assessment, were imperative for their successful use. The literature review also suggested that when the portfolio process is well developed, there are clear links to competence in practice.

> CONSIDER
> Future research in the area of professional portfolios "should focus on qualitative methodologies in keeping with the holistic nature of the portfolio itself" (McCready, 2007, p. 149).

WHO IS RESPONSIBLE FOR COMPETENCE ASSESSMENT IN NURSING?

Who, then, has the responsibility for competence assessment in nursing? Should it be the individual, the employer, the regulatory board, or the certifying agency? Is it a shared responsibility? If so, are these entities willing to work together to create an integrated and systematic approach to promoting continuing competence in nursing?

Certainly, an individual responsibility for maintaining competence is suggested by the *ANA Code of Ethics for Nurses with Interpretive Statements* in its assertion that nurses are obligated to provide adequate and competent nursing care (ANA, 2001). State nurse practice acts also hold nurses accountable for being reasonable and prudent in their practice. Both standards require

the nurse to have at least some personal responsibility for continually assessing his or her professional competence through reflective practice.

> CONSIDER
> The individual registered nurse has a professional obligation to maintain competence.

The role of the professional association also lacks clarity. Although professional associations develop and promote standards, there is no oversight function of either initial or continuing competence.

Employers also play a role in assuring competence of employees by performing periodic performance appraisals and by carrying out the requirements of the accrediting bodies to ensure the ongoing competencies of employees. Yet employers are often among the first to argue that "a nurse is a nurse is a nurse" when it comes to meeting mandatory staffing or licensure requirements.

Regulatory boards, such as the state boards of nursing, regulate initial licensure, monitor compliance with requirements for license renewal, and take action when professional standards are breached. Yet, clearly, licensure and relicensure per se do not guarantee competence, particularly in a discipline as broad in scope and practice as nursing.

Finally, certifying organizations do help to identify those individuals who have an expertise in a specific area of practice; however, knowledge expertise does not always translate into practice expertise. A lack of professional certification does not necessarily mean that the nurse lacks continuing competence. Recertification does not ensure continued expertise, because recertification is usually a product of meeting CE requirements rather than re-examination.

CONCLUSIONS

The challenge in assuring competence in nursing is that nursing practice is dynamic, and thus best practice must be continually redefined as a result of new discoveries. Licensure, continuing education, and professional certification can only ensure provider competence if they reflect the latest thinking, research, and clinical practice needs. In addition, each of these three strategies is limited in its effectiveness as a competence assessment strategy.

Clearly, the NCLEX, as it currently exists, assures only minimum entry-level competence for professional nursing practice. Given that NCLEX content derives from a retrospective model and that technological changes and the rate of knowledge acquisition are increasing exponentially in the 21st century, the knowledge base of the newly licensed nurse has a great likelihood of being dated even before examinations are scored. In addition, as long as a single NCLEX exists and there are multiple levels of educational entry into practice, the examination will continue to have to meet educational content directed at the lowest educational level of entry.

In addition, health care professionals, professional organizations, and regulatory bodies are reluctant to implement mandatory reexamination for licensure. One must at least question whether this is because of the fear that many providers would be unable to demonstrate the continuing competence necessary for relicensure.

CE has similar limitations for assuring provider competence. Some states do not require nurses to complete CE. Those that do demonstrate wide variation in how much CE is required, what content can be included, and how that CE can be provided. In addition, there is no guarantee that completing CE courses results in a change in the provider's knowledge level or practice or even that the content provided in the CE course is current and relevant.

Finally, professional certification does ensure that the nurse has some specialized area of knowledge and practice expertise. The reality, however, is that many nurses perform outside of the area of their certification expertise each and every day in their jobs, particularly if their area of specialty certification expertise is narrow. In addition, there are multiple certifying bodies and numerous types of certification. Determining the exact value of that certification in terms of improving patient care has not completely been ascertained.

How best to ensure provider competence cannot yet be answered. Efforts that address the need to do so are under way, but these efforts have not been coordinated or integrated by the professional associations, regulatory bodies, and stakeholders that are affected. In addition, most professional entities involved in ensuring continuing competence are reluctant to mandate interventions for fear of alienating stakeholders. Individual practitioners also seem reluctant to embrace reflective practice or to put the thought and effort into creating portfolios that identify continuing competence in concrete and measurable ways. Until the focus rests solely on the need to protect patients and improve the quality of health care, mandated interventions for continuing competence are likely never to occur and provider competence will not be assured.

FOR ADDITIONAL DISCUSSION

1. Who should be responsible for the cost of ensuring provider competence—the provider, the employer, the clients that are served, or some other entity?

2. How likely is it that states, professional organizations, professional certifying organizations, and employers will be willing to agree on standardized measures for assessing professional competence?

3. Would most RNs support mandatory development of a portfolio? Are most RNs actively engaged in reflective practice in an effort to assess their ongoing competence?

4. Why should the entry-level examination for nursing be broad and general in scope, whereas continuing competence is arguably demonstrated by professional certification in specialty areas?

5. Are cost and access deterrents to professional certification? If so, how can these barriers be overcome?

6. Do most nurses view continuing education coursework as a reliable and valid tool for increasing provider competence?

7. Should nurses be required to complete mandated continuing education hours in the area of nursing practice in which they work?

8. Are there core competencies all licensed nurses must achieve regardless of the setting in which they practice?

REFERENCES

Adams, D. (2007). *Stricter requirements sought for relicensure as medical boards draft proposal.* Amednews. com. Available at: http://www.ama-assn.org/ amednews/2007/12/24/prl21224.htm. Accessed August 22, 2008.

American Academy of Physician Assistants (2008). *Information about PAs and the PA profession.* Available at: http://www.aapa.org/geninfo1.html. Accessed August 24, 2008.

American Board of Nursing Specialties (ABNS) (2005). *Promoting excellence in nursing certification. A position statement on the value of specialty nursing certification.* Available at: http://nursingcertification.org/ pdf/value_certification.pdf. Accessed August 21, 2008.

American Medical Association (2008). *Physician frequently asked questions.* Available at: http://www. ama-assn.org/ama/pub/category/16340.html. Accessed August 25, 2008.

American Nurses Association (ANA) (2001). *Code of Ethics for Nurses with Interpretive Statements.* Washington, DC: American Nurses Association.

American Nurses Association (ANA) (2007). *Position Statement on Competence and Competency [Draft].* Available at: http://www.cc-institute.org/docs_ upload/anaCompetency.pdf. Accessed January 23, 2009.

American Nurses Credentialing Center (ANCC) (2008a). *Certification FAQs.* Available at:http:// www.nursecredentialing.org/FunctionalCategory/ FAQ/CertiticationFAQs.aspx. Accessed August 25, 2008.

American Nurses Credentialing Center (ANCC) (2008b). *Certification.* Available at: http://www. nursecredentialing.org/Certification.aspx. Accessed August 25, 2008.

Arkansas Board of Registered Nursing (2005). *Chapter two licensure: R.N., L.P.N, and L.P.T.N.* Available at: http://www.arsbn.org/pdfs/rules_regs/2004/ RR_Chapter2.pdf#page=9. Accessed August 23, 2008.

Bekemeier, B. (2007). Credentialing for public health nurses: Personally valued . . . but not well recognized. *Public Health Nursing, 25*(5), 439–448.

Boards of nursing in the United States state-by-state Web links (2008). Available at: http://www.

medscape.com/viewarticle/482270. Accessed August 21, 2008.

California Board of Registered Nursing (2007). *Continuing education for license renewal.* Available at: http://www.rn.ca.gov/licensees/ce-renewal.shtml. Accessed August 24, 2008.

Canadian Nurses Association and Canadian Association of Schools of Nursing (2004). *Joint position statement. Promoting continuing competence for registered nurses.* Available at: http://www.cnanurses.ca/_frames/search/searchframe.htm. Accessed May 5, 2005.

Carliner, S., Ally, M., Zhao, N., Bairstow, L., Khoury, S., & Johnston, L. (2006). *A review of the state of the field of workplace learning: What we know and what we need to know about competencies, diversity, e-learning and human performance improvement.* Canadian Society for Training and Development. Available at: http://www.cstd.ca/networks/ FldRev_WLP_0606.pdf. Accessed August 21, 2008.

Continuing education requirements by state: New Hampshire-Oregon (2008). *Advance for Nurses.* Available at: http://nursing.advanceweb.com/Article/ Continuing-Education-Requirements-by-State. aspx?CP=5. Accessed August 24, 2008.

Fitzgerald, F. A. (2008). *Certification after years of NP practice.* Fitzgerald Health Education Associates Inc. Available at: http://www.fhea.com/certificationcols/cert_ after_years.shtml. Accessed August 27, 2008.

Florida Board of Registered Nursing (2007). *Continuing education.* Available at: http://www.doh.state.fl.us/ mqa/nursing/nur_ceu.html. Accessed August 26, 2008.

Grief, C. L. (2007). The perceived value of BCEN certification. *Journal of Emergency Nursing, 33*(3), 214–216.

Healthy work environments promote specialty certifications (2008). *AACN News, 25*(6), 5.

Iowa Board of Nursing (2007). *Continuing education: The basic requirements.* Available at: http://www.iowa.gov/ nursing//continuing_ed/basic_requirement.html. Accessed August 25, 2008.

LaWriter Ohio Laws and Rules (2007). *4723-14-03 Continuing education requirement for licensed nurses.* Available at: http://codes.ohio.gov/oac/4723-14-03. Accessed August 24, 2008.

Mantesso, J., Petrucka, P., & Bassendowski, S. (2008). Continuing professional competence: Peer feedback success from determination of nurse focus of control. *Journal of Continuing Education in Nursing, 39*(5), 200–207.

McColgan, K. (2008). The value of portfolio building and the registered nurse: A review of the literature. *Journal of Perioperative Practice, 18*(2), 64–69.

McCready, T. (2007). Portfolios and the assessment of competence in nursing: A literature review. *International Journal of Nursing Studies, 44*(1), 143–151.

Medscape Today (2007). State CME requirements. Available at: http://www.medscape.com/pages/cme/staterequirements. Accessed August 25, 2008.

Michigan Nurses Association (2007). *Continuing education requirements for Michigan nurses.* Available at: http://www.michigan.gov/documents/cis_fhs_bhser_nurse_cebroc_67748_7.pdf. Accessed August 26, 2008.

Miller, S., Thompson, J., Mazmanian, P., Aparicio, A., Davis, D., Spivey, B. E., & Kahn, N. B. (2008). Continuing medical education, professional development, and requirements for medical licensure: A white paper of the Conjoint Committee on Continuing Medical Education. *Journal of Continuing Education in the Health Professions, 28*(2), 95–98.

National Association of Boards of Pharmacy (NABP) (2008). *Examinations: North American Pharmacist Licensure Examination (NAPLEX).* Available at: http://www.nabp.net/. Accessed August 21, 2008.

National Council State Boards of Nursing (NCSBN) (2005). *Fast facts about the continued competence practice analysis.* Available at: https://www.ncsbn.org/07_25_05_continued_comprtencyt_faq.pdf. Accessed August 21, 2008.

National Council State Boards of Nursing (NCSBN) (2008a). *What boards do.* Available at: https://www.ncsbn.org/126.htm. Accessed August 22, 2008.

National Council State Boards of Nursing (NCSBN) (2008b). *NCLEX examinations.* Available at: https://www.ncsbn.org/nclex.htm. Accessed August 22, 2008.

Niebuhr, B., & Biel, M. (2007). The value of specialty nursing certification. *Nursing Outlook, 55*(4), 176–181.

North Carolina Board of Nursing (NCBN) (2008). *Continuing competence.* Available at: http://www.ncbon.com/content.aspx?id=664. Accessed August 22, 2008.

Nurses Association of New Brunswick (NANB) (2007). *Continuing competence program: Learning in action.* Available at: http://www.nanb.nb.ca/pdf_e/CCP/Section%201%20-%20Continuing%20Competence%20Program%20(English).pdf. Accessed August 28, 2008.

O'Malley, P. A. (2008). Profile of a professional. *Nursing Management, 39*(6), 24–27, 48.

Piazza, I., Donahue, M., Dykes, P., Griffin, M., & Fitzpatrick. J. (2006). Difference in perceptions of empowerment among nationally certified and noncertified nurses. *Journal of Nursing Administration, 36*(5), 277–283.

Ridge, R. (2008). Nursing certification as a workforce strategy. *Nursing Management, 39*(8), 50–52.

Schleyer, T. K. L., & Dodell, D. (2005). Continuing dental education requirements for relicensure in the United States. *Journal of the American Dental Association, 136*(10), 1450–1456.

Sherrod, D. (2007). Professional portfolio: A snapshot of your career. *Nursing, 2007*(37), 18.

Taft, L., & Sparks, R. K. (2008). *Nursing matters. Continuing education for nurses.* Available at: http://www.nursingmattersonline.com/nursingmattersonline/studentdetail.asp?newsid=1782. Accessed August 21, 2008.

Texas Board of Nursing (2008). *The 1-2-3s of CE understanding and complying with the continuing education requirements for nurses in Texas.* Available at: http://www.bon.state.tx.us/nursingeducation/ceu.html. Accessed August 24, 2008.

The Free Dictionary by Farlex (2008). *Licensure. Definition.* Available at: http://medical-dictionary.thefreedictionary.com/licensure. Accessed August 22, 2008.

Tilley, S. (2008). Competency in nursing: A concept analysis. *Journal of Continuing Education in Nursing, 39*(2), 58–64.

United States Medical Licensing Exam (2007). Available at: http://www.usmle.org/General_Information/bulletin/2007/overview.html. Accessed August 22, 2008.

Winslow, W. (2008). Personal practice review inspires RNs to be lifelong learners. *Nursing BC. College of Registered Nurses of British Columbia, 40*(3), 16–19.

BIBLIOGRAPHY

Advantages of certification (2007). *Critical Care Nurse Supplement, 27,* 36–38.

American Board of Nursing Specialties (2006). *Specialty nursing certification: Nurses' perceptions, values and behaviors.* Available at www.nursingcertification.org/pdf/white_paper_final_12_12_06.pdf. Accessed January 23, 2009.

Baghi, H., Panniers, T. L., & Smolenski, M. (2007). Description of practice as an ambulatory care nurse: Psychometric properties of a practice-analysis survey. *Journal of Nursing Measurement, 15*(1), 62–74.

Biel , M. (2007). Infusion nursing certification—Identification of stakeholders and demonstration of the value of certification. *Journal of Infusion Nursing, 30*(6), 332–338.

Byrne, M., Delarose, T., King, C. A., Leske, J., Sapnas, K. G., & Schroeter, K. (2007). Continued professional competence and portfolios. *Journal of Trauma Nursing, 14*(1):24–31.

Clarke, S. (2007). Changing paediatric orthopaedic education and certification for the RN in Northern Ireland ? *Orthopaedic Nursing, 26*(2), 126–129.

DeSilets, L. D. (2007). Nursing professional development certification. *Journal of Continuing Education in Nursing, 38*(1), 12–13.

Ericsson, K. A., Whyte, J., & Ward, P. (2007). Expert performance in nursing—Reviewing research on expertise in nursing within the framework of the expert-performance approach. *Advances in Nursing Science, 30*(1), E58–E71.

Fulton, J. S. (2007). The value of professional certification for Clinical Nurse Specialists. *Clinical Nurse Specialist, 21*(3), 137–138.

Gladfelter, J. (2006). Nursing certification: Why it matters. *Plastic Surgical Nursing, 26*(4), 208–210.

Goudreau, K. A., Baldwin, K., Clark, A., Fulton, J., Lyon, B., Murray, T., Rust, J. E., & Sendelbach, S.; National Association of Clinical Nurse Specialists (2007). A vision of the future for Clinical Nurse Specialists. *Clinical Nurse Specialist, 21*(6), 310–320.

Lamonte, M. K. (2007). Test-taking strategies for CNOR certification. *AORN Journal, 85*(2), 315.

Lazarus, J. B., & Lee, N. G. (2006). Factoring consumers' perspectives into policy decisions for nursing competence. *Policy, Politics & Nursing Practice, 7*(3), 195–207.

Miracle, V. A. (2007). Thinking about certification. *Dimensions of Critical Care Nursing, 26*(2), 72–75.

Prowant, B. F., Niebuhr, B., & Biel, M. (2007). Perceived value of nursing certification—Summary of a national survey. *Nephrology Nursing Journal, 34*(4), 399–402.

Sechrist, K. R., & Berlin, L. E. (2006). Psychometric analysis of the Perceived Value of Certification Tool. *Journal of Professional Nursing, 22*(4), 248–252.

Sechrist, K. R., Valentine, W., & Berlin, L. E. (2006). Perceived value of certification among certified, non-certified, and administrative perioperative nurses. *Journal of Professional Nursing, 22*(4), 242–247.

Wendt, A., & Alexander, M. (2007). Toward a standardized and evidence-based continued competence assessment for Registered Nurses. *JONA's Healthcare Law, Ethics, and Regulation, 9*(3), 74–86.

Wolf, P. (2008). Specialty certification organizations. *Nursing, 2008*(January/Supplement Career Directory), 20–21.

WEB RESOURCES

Alberta Association of Registered Nurses, Continuing Competence Bibliography	http://www.nurses.ab.ca/Carna-Admin/Uploads/cc_bibliography_cont_comp.pdf
American Board of Nursing Specialties	http://www.nursingcertification.org/
Canadian Nurses Association and Canadian Association of Schools of Nursing, Joint Position Statement, Promoting Continuing Competence for Registered Nurses	http://www.cna-nurses.ca/CNA/documents/pdf/publications/PS77_promoting_competence_e.pdf

Competency and Credentialing Institute, Continued Competence Reading Library	http://www.cc-institute.org/tt07_reading.aspx
Nurses Association of New Brunswick, Continuing Competence Program: Learning in Action	http://www.nanb.nb.ca/pdf_e/CCP/Section%201%20-%20Continuing%20Competence%20Program%20(English).pdf
Nursing Council of New Zealand, Health Practitioners Competence Assurance Act 2003	http://www.nursingcouncil.org.nz/hpca.html

CHAPTER 19

The Nursing Profession's Historic Struggle to Increase Its Power Base

• CAROL J. HUSTON •

Learning Objectives

The learner will be able to:

1. Explore factors that have led to nursing's relative powerlessness as a profession.
2. Examine characteristics of oppressed groups and analyze whether the nursing profession displays those characteristics.
3. Identify driving forces in place to increase the nursing profession's power base.
4. Examine factors that led to the divergence of the nursing profession and feminism in the 1960s and 1970s and then subsequently to their convergence in the mid 1980s as part of second-wave feminism.
5. Analyze the influence of gender in how many nurses view policy and politics, the willingness of nurses to work together collectively to achieve common goals, and the mentoring opportunities available to the profession's future leaders.
6. Identify partners/external stakeholders that the nursing profession could seek in forming

alliances or coalitions to strengthen its position in the national and global policy arenas.
7. Name nurses currently holding elected office in Congress and state legislatures, as well as the significant committees they serve on or positions they hold.
8. Identify issues being debated in the legislature that affect nursing and health care.
9. Explore individual, organizational, and professional responsibilities for succession planning to ensure that an adequate number of highly qualified nursing leaders exist in the future.
10. Create a plan, appropriate for his or her energy level, time constraints, and interest, for increasing the nursing profession's power base.
11. Reflect on whether the need to be politically competent should be internalized by nurses as a moral and professional obligation.

P ower is an elusive concept. The word "power" is derived from the Latin verb *potere*, meaning "to be able"; thus, power may be appropriately defined as that which enables an individual or a group to accomplish goals. Power can also be defined as the capacity to act or the strength and potency to accomplish something (Marquis & Huston, 2009). Having power then gives an individual or a group the potential to change the attitudes and behaviors of others.

How individuals view power varies greatly. Indeed, power may be feared, worshipped, or mistrusted, and it is frequently misunderstood (Marquis & Huston, 2009). Many women (and thus nurses) have traditionally demon-

strated ambivalence toward the concept of power and until fairly recently have even eschewed the pursuit of power.

This may have occurred because women traditionally were socialized to view power differently from men. As a result, many women believed that they did not inherently possess power (formal or informal) or authority. In addition, rather than feel capable of achieving and managing power, many women felt that power managed them. These gender-based perceptions are changing, yet women still have much ground to make up in terms of learning to use power as a tool for personal and professional success.

Similarly, the nursing profession has not historically been the powerful force it could have been in dealing with issues directly affecting health care and the profession. Indeed nurses are often thought of as an apolitical group. As a result, nursing has more often than not, been reactive (rather than proactive) in the policy arena, addressing proposed legislation after its introduction rather than drafting or sponsoring legislation that reflects nursing's agenda. As a result, external forces (typically male dominated and medically focused) have often controlled nursing.

All of these factors have contributed to the nursing profession having a relatively small power base in the political arena and its historical invisibility as a force in health care decision making. This chapter explores six factors that historically led to nursing's relative powerlessness as a profession. It also identifies five driving forces that are in place to increase nursing's professional power. The chapter concludes with an action plan to increase nursing's power base so that the profession is recognized as an increasingly significant force in health care decision making in the 21st century.

DISCUSSION POINT

Why is it that nurses, the largest group of health professionals, with perhaps the greatest first-hand knowledge of the health care problems faced by consumers, have not historically been an integral part of health care policy decision making?

FACTORS CONTRIBUTING TO POWERLESSNESS IN NURSING

Many factors have contributed to the nursing profession's relative powerlessness in health care policy setting. Six factors are discussed here (Box 19.1).

BOX 19.1

FACTORS CONTRIBUTING TO POWERLESSNESS IN NURSING

1. The oppression of nurses as a group.
2. Nursing's failure to fully align with the feminist movement.
3. Limited collective action by nurses.
4. The socialization of women to view power and politics negatively.
5. The inadequate recognition of nursing as an educated profession with evidence-based practice.
6. The nursing profession's history of being reactive (rather than proactive) in national policy setting.

Oppression of Nurses as a Group

Nursing historically has been controlled by outside forces with greater prestige, power, and status. Generally, these forces were patriarchal and male dominated, such as medicine and hospital administration. For example, historically, physicians attempted to exclude women from knowledge emerging from the basic sciences, and their refusal to let nurses use new instrumentation sustained women's subordination in nursing, although many nurses continually and actively sought greater scientific knowledge and techniques and incorporated these into their education.

Twenty-first century nurses continue, however, to report what they perceive as "disrespectful behavior from physicians." Many new nurses in Deppoliti's (2008, p. 260) study reported that they "felt humiliated, debased, and devalued by physicians and described disrespect. They coped with this perceived abuse through increasing knowledge, maturity, experience, and observing more experienced nurses."

When a group is oppressed, it tends to have value confusion and low self-esteem. This occurs because the dominant groups identify their norms and values as the "right ones" and use their initial power to enforce them as the status quo. Oppressed groups accept these norms, at least externally, in an effort to gain some power and control. For example, nursing's oppressors have not always held the same values as nursing (i.e., caring, nurturance, and advocacy). This has led to confusion for some nurses and even, at times, contempt for their own profession and what it represents.

CONSIDER

"As a profession, nurses do not have a very positive self-image nor do they think highly of themselves" (Fletcher, 2007, p. 207).

Failure to Align Fully with the Feminist Movement

A second factor contributing to nursing's relative powerlessness in national policy setting is the profession's failure to align fully with the feminist movement. Although both nurses and women have improved their status in the last four decades, nursing has not kept pace with the progress women have made in other areas. This has occurred, because, at least in part, nurses have not been fully engaged in the feminist movement.

This occurred for several reasons. One was that many feminists in the 1960s and 1970s were influenced by a more radical feminist perspective and, as a result, spoke out against women becoming nurses because it suggested that female nurses were in subordinate, caregiving roles. In addition, many nurses feared public identification with feminism.

The reality, however, is that nursing continues to be a profession composed of approximately 94% women, and this figure has changed very little over time. This is noteworthy, given that there have been major gender shifts in virtually all of the other traditionally female-dominated professions (such as social workers, librarians, K-to-12 teachers) since the 1970s.

DISCUSSION POINT

Many nursing leaders in the early 1900s were political activists, actively involved in social issues such as women's suffrage and public health. At what point did nursing diverge from a sociopolitical agenda and why?

CONSIDER

"The ground that nursing has developed in is gendered ground that is a reflection of a broader societal devaluation of women and the work they do" (C. Davies, as cited in Fletcher, 2007, p. 210).

Although having female dominance in the profession may have some benefits, it also poses some liabilities. Indeed, some nursing leaders have suggested that nursing will never attain greater status and power until more men join the ranks (see Chapter 9). Others think that adding men to nursing's ranks is not the answer. Instead, nurses need to accept the responsibility for addressing the problems that have historically plagued the profession and take whatever steps are necessary to proactively build a power base that does not depend on gender.

CONSIDER

Being a female professional in a male-dominated health care system brings to mind the "Ginger Rogers syndrome." Both Ginger Rogers and her dancing partner, Fred Astaire, were known as wonderful dancers, but Fred Astaire's name always came first, and he always received the greater recognition. In reality, Ginger Rogers danced the same steps as Fred Astaire, but she did them backward and in high heels. So, who deserved the greater recognition?

Susan Malka (as cited in Irvine, 2008) suggested, however, that nursing's divergence from feminism has changed. She noted that in the mid 1960s through the mid 1980s, the nursing profession was focused on defining the profession and was out of step with the feminist movement. From the mid 1980s to the present, however, nursing became more compatible with *second-wave feminism*, in that the profession began actively lobbying for greater rights and recognition, more men joined the profession, and women became nurses by choice, not because it was one of the few career choices open to them. Feminist issues such as pay equity and equal opportunities for advancement are now widely espoused by nurses.

In addition, recognition that assertive, independent nurses cannot exist if they have been socialized to be dependent women is growing. Similarly, it is improbable, if not impossible, for female nurses to implement expanded roles in advanced practice if they are unaware of or unwilling to recognize the social constraints imposed on them because they are women. Clearly, the battles between the American Medical Association (AMA) and advanced practice nurses about scope of practice, reimbursement, and the need for medical oversight are likely related as much to gender as they are to competition over patients (see Chapter 21).

Nurses need then to continue to examine the progress women have made in other professions and work with them inside and outside of nursing to strengthen power for women everywhere. This holds true for the men in nursing as well because the relative powerlessness of the profession transfers to them too, despite gender differences. Both male and female nurses must solve problems, exchange current literature, network to increase nursing's knowledge base and power, and provide mutual support.

Limited Collective Representation of Nurses

A third factor limiting the development of the nursing profession's power base is the limited collective representation of nurses by groups, such as collective bargaining agents and professional nursing organizations. Only about 16% to 22% of the 2.9 million nurses in the United States belong to collective bargaining units (Marquis & Huston, 2009), and less than 6% of nurses belong to the American Nurses Association (ANA), the recognized professional association for all U.S. nurses [the ANA (2008) shows 165,000 individual registered nurse members as of 2008]. This relatively small membership number directly reflects the money that is available for lobbyists to represent nursing in the political arena. In contrast, the AMA has one of the most powerful lobbying organizations in the United States.

There are many reasons for the small representation of nurses in the ANA. The dual and often conflicting role of the ANA as both a professional organization for nurses and a collective bargaining agent is certainly one reason (see Chapter 17). In addition, some nurses think that state nurses associations have been burdened with the task of collective bargaining under the federation model of the ANA and that other programs have suffered as a result of funds being used for collective bargaining. Other nurses have expressed concerns about the cost of membership in the ANA or argued that the ANA is not responsive enough to the needs of the nurse at the bedside. Other nurses look on nursing as a job and not as a career and have little interest in professional issues outside of their immediate work environment.

DISCUSSION POINT

Do you belong to a professional nursing organization? Why or why not? Do contemporary nursing leaders espouse this as a value? Is it encouraged in the workplace? In the academic world?

Whether these issues are valid or not is almost immaterial. The reality is that as long as such a small percent-

age of nurses belong to the ANA, the economic power of the ANA will be limited, as will its ability to significantly influence policy setting and legislation. Perhaps even more important, until nurses are willing to work together collectively in some form, they will be unlikely to increase either their personal or their professional power.

CONSIDER

At times, nurses have lacked pride in their collective groups and have viewed alignment with other nurses as alignment with other powerless persons, something that does little to advance an individual's professional power.

Unfortunately, more often than not, nurses in this country have not acted cohesively, whether at the local level fighting for wage increases or at the national level attempting to influence health policy. Even the various professional nursing organizations to which nurses belong have not historically worked together cooperatively. The reality is that nurses continue to be widely divided on basic issues such as entry into practice, mandatory staffing ratios, and collective bargaining.

Thupayagale-Tshweneagae and Dithole (2007) agreed, suggesting that the nursing profession's numerical strength should give it power over other health professionals, if only it could unite: "However, unity has remained elusive to nurses and, hence, programs geared toward improving their welfare have never succeeded" (Thupayagale-Tshweneagae and Dithole, 2007, p. 143). Strategies to promote greater nurse unity are shown in Box 19.2.

BOX 19.2 | STRATEGIES FOR PROMOTING UNITY WITHIN THE NURSING PROFESSION

1. Nurses must respect each other's specialties and work toward enriching each other's job and work environments.
2. Nurses must acknowledge the different expertise that will help promote the quality care expected of them.
3. Nurses need to be self-aware regarding their behaviors that lead to disunity.
4. Nurses need to examine and learn from the nursing legacy that has negatively affected their behavior individually and collectively.
5. Accommodation of new vibrant views should be encouraged. This could be done through proper mentoring of the newly graduated nurses.
6. Collaboration among nursing organizations and working collectively, as in a union, would strengthen nursing.

Adapted from: Thupayagale-Tshweneagae, G., & Dithole, K. (2007). Unity among nurses: An evasive concept. *Nursing Forum, 42*(3), 143–146.

> ### CONSIDER
> A metaphor for increasing nursing's power base through collective action would be a snowball. Individual snowflakes are fragile, but when they stick together, they become a force to be reckoned with.

Socialization of Women to View Power and Politics Negatively

A fourth factor contributing to powerlessness in the nursing profession has been the socialization of women to view power and politics negatively. Women in particular, and thus most nurses, often hold negative connotations of power and never learn to use power constructively (Marquis & Huston, 2009). Nurses must recognize that power and politics provide opportunities for change—the chance to make things better for both nurses and clients. Therefore all nurses should seek skill in being able to appropriately intervene in political processes.

> ### CONSIDER
> Changing nurse's view of both power and politics is perhaps the most significant key to proactive rather than reactive participation in policy setting.

Blass and Ferris (2007, p. 6), incorporating a number of definitions, defined political skill as "managing interactions with others in influential ways that lead to organization goal accomplishment amid rapidly changing contexts." The politically skilled individual is focused outward (toward others) and is able to maintain a balance on accountability to others, as well as to self.

Similarly, Marquis and Huston (2009) defined political skill as the art of using legitimate power wisely and suggested that it requires clear decision making, assertiveness, accountability, and the willingness to express one's views. It also requires being proactive rather than reactive and demands decisiveness.

Nurses therefore must perceive a need not only to be more knowledgeable about power, negotiation, and politics, but also to be more involved in broad social and political issues. This requires becoming politically astute. Nurses need to understand what politics means, and they need to become experts in using politics to help nursing achieve both its professional goals and the needs of their clients.

Inadequate Recognition of Nursing as an Educated Profession with Evidence-Based Practice

A fifth factor contributing to the nursing profession's relative powerlessness is the inadequate recognition of nursing as a profession driven by research and the pursuit of higher education. Although nurses should value highly the caring, intuitive, nurturing part of nursing practice, the nursing profession has been negligent about equally emphasizing their extensive scientific knowledge base and the high level of critical thinking and analysis professional nurses use every day in their clinical practice.

Both the art and the science of nursing require highly developed skills and a well-developed knowledge base. The nurse of the 21st century has an incredible knowledge base in the sciences, as well as in the arts. In addition, nurses must be expert critical thinkers, as they continually look for and analyze subtle clues in their client data, make independent nursing diagnoses, and create plans of care. Constant assessment and adjustment to the plan of care are almost always necessary, so that nurses must be highly organized and know how to set priorities. In addition, nurses must have highly refined communication skills, well-developed psychomotor skills, and sophisticated leadership and management skills. This is the image nurses must promote to the public.

> ### DISCUSSION POINT
> If the public was asked to list five adjectives to describe nursing, what would they be? Would the art or the science of nursing be recognized more? Would nurses use different adjectives?

The Nursing Profession's History of Being Reactive in National Policy Setting

The last factor discussed here as contributing to a relative lack of professional power in nursing is the profession's history of being reactive rather than proactive in national policy setting regarding nursing practice. *Reactive* means waiting until there is a problem and then trying to fix it. *Proactive* is more anticipatory; it means developing appropriate policy before taking action or a problem occurs.

This was especially apparent in a study by Deppoliti (2008) of new nurses (1 to 3 years out of school). Nurse respondents reported that "they felt the nursing profession was disorganized and did not vocalize the needs of nurses" (p. 261). In addition, several nurses "commented on a sense of discontinuity in the profession that negatively influenced their sense of themselves as a nurse." In fact, the negative comparison of professional unity in nursing with that in other professions, particularly education, was prevalent in the data.

Unfortunately, these feelings are more accurate than not, given that the nursing profession has been far from proactive in shaping its own course or that of the health care system. In the 1990s, health care became big business. Managed care proliferated, and gatekeepers, not providers and consumers, began deciding who needed care and how much care was needed. Hospitals lost their place as the center of the health care universe as client care shifted from inpatient hospital stays to outpatient and ambulatory health care settings. Physicians lost much of their autonomy to practice medicine as they saw fit as insurers increasingly placed restrictions not only on which physicians patients could see, but also what services the physician was authorized to prescribe.

Patients found themselves with limited choices of providers, longer wait times for care, more rules to follow, and more confusion about what would and would not be a covered expense. At the same time, registered nurses (RNs) in record numbers, for the first time in history, were downsized, restructured, and often replaced by a cheaper counterpart in an effort to reduce costs.

Many nurses felt both overwhelmed and helpless with this degree of change. However, these changes did not happen overnight. Many of them were incremental and insidious, and the health care system changes occurred with little concerted effort by nurses to stop them.

There is a brief parable that Peter Senge (1990) wrote about in *The Fifth Discipline* that nurses should keep front and foremost when they think about the need to be proactive, even with incremental change. It's called "The parable of the boiled frog" and it goes like this:

If you place a frog in a pot of boiling water, it will immediately try to scramble out. But if you place the frog in room temperature water, and don't scare him, he'll stay put. Now, if the pot sits on a heat source, and if you gradually turn up the temperature, some-thing very interesting happens. As the temperature rises from 70 to 80 degrees F., the frog will do nothing. In fact, he will show every sign of enjoying himself. As the temperature gradually increases, the frog will become groggier and groggier, until he is un-able to crawl out of the pot. Though there is nothing restraining him, the frog will sit there and boil. He will boil to death, oblivious to what is happening to him.

CONSIDER

Gradual but constant change may be even more dangerous than cataclysmic change because resistance is less organized.

In responding to the profession's trend toward passivity, Pierce (2004) argued that nursing can no longer afford to be reactive in the policy arena. Instead, she stated that, collectively, the nursing profession must decide what the significant priorities are and then construct a legislative agenda based on these priorities. The priority list cannot be an exhaustive laundry list to combat all the profession's issues and woes. It must be strategic and timely relative to the debates taking place at the national level.

Sorensen, Iedema, and Severinsson (2008) agreed, arguing

Nurses are not universally powerless to confront the inequities that they (and thereby the patients they care for) experience. Nursing complacency may itself be a barrier to nurses recognizing and acting upon the opportunities that exist and that arise in the organization to intervene and transform the ways in which nurses engage with their professional and managerial roles (Sorensen et al., p. 542).

DRIVING FORCES TO INCREASE NURSING'S POWER BASE

So what is the likelihood that the nursing profession will ever be a powerful force in health care decision making and the political arena? The answer is unclear, although the likelihood of this happening is increasing because of several driving forces in place. This chapter discusses six of these forces (Box 19.3).

BOX 19.3 | DRIVING FORCES TO INCREASE NURSING'S POWER BASE

1. The timing is right.
2. The size of the nursing profession.
3. Nursing's referent power.
4. The increasing knowledge base and education for nurses.
5. Nursing's unique perspective.
6. The desire for change among consumers and providers.

Timing Is Right

Timing is everything. The political ferment regarding health care reform continues to escalate, and issues of cost and access are paramount in this country. There are more than 45 million uninsured individuals in the United States and likely tens of millions more who are underinsured. In fact, the fastest-growing segment of the uninsured population in the last 10 years in the United States has been middle- and upper-income families (Herrick, 2008):

> From 1998 to 2007, the number of uninsured among households earning more than $50,000 annually actually increased by more than five million, the ranks of the uninsured in households earning $50,000 to $75,000 increased 27 percent, while the number of uninsured households earning above $75,000 increased 65 percent (Herrick, 2008, para 11).

This alone should draw a crowd of interested parties to the policy table.

Furthermore, as a result of publications like *To Err is Human*, consumers, health care providers, and legislators are more aware than ever of the shortcomings of the current health care system, and the clamor for action has never been louder (see Chapter 14). Clearly the public wants a better health care system, and nurses want to be able to provide high-quality nursing care. Both are powerful elements for change, and new nurses are entering the profession at a time when their energy and expertise will be more valued than ever.

CONSIDER

"When they choose to take on the role of policy advocate to change the system, nurses often have to move out of the comfort zone of their practice arena and into less familiar arenas where the laws and regulations impacting patient care are developed, and the battles for scarce resources are negotiated and decided" (Abood, 2007, para 4).

Size of the Nursing Profession

The second driving force for increasing nursing's professional power base is the size of the profession itself. There are almost 2.9 million RNs in the United States. Numbers are the lifeblood of politics. The nursing profession's size is its greatest asset, and its potential for a collective voting block is increasingly being recognized as a force to be dealt with.

CONSIDER

Involvement of only a fraction of the nation's 2.9 million registered nurses in even the smallest way could become a force for change for the nursing profession and for the health care system and the patients it serves (Artz, 2006).

DISCUSSION POINT

Have nurses ever made a concerted effort to vote collectively? What positions have professional organizations such as the ANA taken on recent election issues or candidates for office? Have endorsements by professional nursing organizations influenced how you vote?

Nursing's Referent Power

A third driving force for increasing the power of the profession is the referent power nurses hold. *Referent power* is the power one has when others identify with you or what you symbolize; therefore you have their admiration or respect (Marquis & Huston, 2009). Abood (2007) suggested that the nursing profession has a great deal of referent power as a result of the high degree of trust and credibility the public places in them. Indeed, nurses have placed number one every year in the Gallup Organization's annual poll on professional honesty and ethical standards since nurses were first included in the survey in 1999, with the exception of 2001, when firefighters ranked first (Jones, 2007). According to Abood, "This trust is valuable and is transferable into action to improve what is failing in today's modern health care delivery system" (Abood, 2007, p. 5). As a result, Abood calls on nurses to be stewards in pushing an agenda that calls for quality health care for all and to use their referent power to open the door to the offices of power brokers and decision makers.

An Increasing Knowledge Base and Education for Nurses

A fourth driving force for increasing the power of the profession is nursing's increasing knowledge base. Fortunately, more nurses are being prepared at the master's and doctoral level than ever before. More nurses are also stepping into advanced practice roles as nurse practitioners, clinical nurse specialists, certified nurse midwives, registered nurse anesthetists, or clinical nurse leaders. In addition, between 15% and 17% of all nurses now hold a specialty certification (Ridge, 2008) (see Chapter 18).

Furthermore, leadership, management, and political theory are increasingly a part of baccalaureate nursing education, although the majority of nurses still do not hold baccalaureate degrees. These are learned skills, and, collectively, the nursing profession's knowledge of leadership, politics, negotiation, and finance is increasing. This can only increase the nursing profession's influence outside the field.

Nursing's Unique Perspective

A fifth driving force for increasing the nursing profession's power base is the unique philosophical perspective nursing brings to the health care arena. Nursing's perspective is unique as a result of its blending of art and science—a blending of "caring" and "curing," so to speak. The caring part of the nursing role is better known and better understood by the public. It is what historically has defined nursing. It is important that nurses not forget or underappreciate the unique values nursing represents because these are the values that make the profession different from all the others. These same values will make nursing irreplaceable in the current health care system.

Manthey (2008, pp. 4–5) agreed, stating that as nursing matures as a profession, she is "more convinced than ever that the choice to care, and to express that care and compassion by our behavior, is the absolutely correct

choice nurses must make in order to continue serving society." She went on to say that "this covenant between nursing and society is truly nursing's power base; the invisible power of nursing."

It truly is a privilege for nurses to care, because it allows them to intimately enter so many lives, helping in very ordinary and yet extraordinary ways. It is important to remember, however, that important work does not always mean that the work is extraordinary. It simply means making a difference in someone's life.

The "science" part of nursing is less understood by the public. Nursing has an extensive scientific knowledge base, and the high level of critical thinking and analysis professional nurses use everyday in their clinical practice is enormous. Nursing practice is increasingly becoming *evidence based*, meaning that nursing practice reflects what the literature says is "best practice." That is, the practice of nursing is research based and scientifically driven (see Chapter 2). Unfortunately, consumers, legislators, and sometimes even other health care professionals fail to recognize this. Nursing then must do a better job of both explaining and emphasizing both the art and the science of nursing practice.

Consumers and Providers Want Change

Finally, health care restructuring and downsizing are resulting in unrest for health care consumers, as well as providers. Limited consumer choice, hospital restructuring, the downsizing of registered nursing, and the Institute of Medicine (IOM) medical errors reports were the sparks needed to mobilize nurses, as well as consumers, to take action. Nurses began speaking out about how downsizing and restructuring were affecting the care they were providing and the public began demanding accountability. The public does care who is caring for them and how that affects the quality of their care. The good news, then, is that the flaws of the health care system are no longer secret and nursing has the opportunity to use its expertise and influence to help create a better health care system for the future.

ACTION PLAN FOR THE FUTURE

Based on these driving forces, an action plan can be created to increase the power of the nursing profession in the 21st century. This chapter identifies seven possible strategies to achieve this goal (Box 19.4).

BOX 19.4 | ACTION PLAN FOR INCREASING THE POWER OF THE NURSING PROFESSION

1. More nurses must be placed in positions that influence public policy.
2. Nurses must stop acting like victims.
3. Nurses must become better informed about all health care policy efforts.
4. Coalition building must occur within and outside of nursing.
5. More research must be done to strengthen evidence-based practice.
6. Nursing leaders must be supported.
7. Attention must be paid to mentoring future nurse leaders and leadership succession.

Place More Nurses in Positions That Influence Public Policy

First, more nurses must be placed in positions that influence public policy. For example, there is a significant effort underway to establish an Office of the National Nurse in the United States. The proposal first came forward in 2005 in a letter to the Editor of the *New York Times* by Teri Mills, a nurse practitioner and nurse educator in Oregon (Office of the National Nurse, 2006). The desired end result is the appointment of a full-time Chief Nurse Officer (CNO) of the U.S. Public Health Service within the Office of the Surgeon General (currently there is a half-time CNO). This National Nurse would serve as an assistant to the Surgeon General and would officially be titled the National Nurse for Prevention (The National Nurse, 2008).

As a result of this grassroots movement, legislation HR 4903 IH, proposing the establishment of such a position, was introduced into the 109th Congress in March 2006. Although the legislation had not been reintroduced as of August 2008 into the 110th Congress, the grassroots effort is continuing, seeking support from legislators, nursing and public health organizations, and individual nurses (ANA, Tri-Council Members Send Letter, 2008).

Proponents of the idea suggest that such a position would raise the profile of nursing and assist in a nationwide cultural shift to prevention and health promotion.

Opponents suggest that this might not be the best way to effect change both within nursing and in the health care system. In addition, the Tri-Council on Nursing (the ANA, the American Association of Colleges of Nursing [AACN], the American Organization of Nurse Executives [AONE], and the National League for Nursing [NLN]) opposed the idea, arguing that creating such an office would divert scarce resources away from providing quality health care to patients. Instead, opponents argue that legislation is needed that promises more immediate and tangible advances for nurses, their patients, and public health overall (ANA, Tri-Council Members Send Letter, 2008).

Not all positions that influence public policy, however, occur on the national level. McLaughlin and McLaughlin (2008, p. 391) suggested that "having the professional power to participate effectively in the political process is earned through leadership in one's profession, one's institution, and in one's community." In other words, few leaders burst on to the national scene directly. Instead, they assume leadership roles in entities such as medical centers, community hospitals, government agencies, and insurance companies.

McLaughlin and McLaughlin (2008) went to say

Leadership career paths often overlooked in the health policy arena are those in corporations and entrepreneurs. A number of very influential health professionals have stopped delivering care directly and have moved into the management of health institutions, insurance companies, occupational health, medical device and supply companies, pharmaceutical companies, and government agencies (p. 391).

Running for and holding elected office is, however, the ultimate in political activism and involvement. As of 2006, the U.S. Surgeon General was a nurse, and three nurses were serving in the U.S. Congress: Rep. Lois Capps (D-CA), Rep. Carolyn McCarthy (D-NY), and Rep. Eddie Bernice Johnson (D-TX) (Office of the National Nurse, 2006). Many more nurses hold elected office in state legislatures.

In fact, nurses are uniquely qualified to hold public office because they have the greatest first-hand experience of problems faced by patients in the health care system, as well as an ability to translate the health care experience to the general public. As a result, more nurses need to seek out this role. In addition, because the public respects and trusts nurses, nurses who choose to run for public office are often elected. The problem then is not that nurses are not being elected . . . the problem is that not enough nurses are running for office.

Stop Acting Like Victims

A second part of the action plan to increase the power of the nursing profession in the 21st century is that nurses must stop acting like victims. This is not to say that some nurses have not been victimized. The reality, however, is that nursing, like any other profession, has its good points and its bad points. It is important that nurses enjoy what they do for a career because this affects everyone around them. If a nurse is unhappy in nursing, he or she needs to address what is wrong rather than whine about nursing and act like a victim. Doing so just demoralizes everyone around them. There are too many other opportunities within nursing that can be explored; nurses unhappy with their career choice either need to fix what is wrong or leave and find a job that fulfills their expectations.

In addition, it is critical that each nurse never lose sight of his or her potential to make a difference. Some legislators and nursing employers have argued that "a nurse is a nurse is a nurse." This is wrong. Nurses can be whatever they want to be in nursing, and they can achieve that goal at whatever level of quality they choose. The bottom line, however, is that the profession will only be as smart, as motivated, and as directed as its weakest link. If the nursing profession is to be the powerful force it can be, it needs to be filled with bright, highly motivated people who want to make a difference in the lives of the clients with whom they work, as well as in the health care system itself.

> CONSIDER
> Individuals may be born average, but staying average is a choice.

Become Better Informed about All Health Care Policy Efforts

The third step of the action plan is that nurses must become better informed about all health care policy efforts—especially those that influence their profession. This is difficult because no one can do this but nurses. This means grass roots knowledge building and in-

volvement. Nurses need to be better-informed consumers and providers of health care.

For example, McLaughlin and McLaughlin (2008, p. 394) suggested that nurses must "experience and participate in change processes undertaken by groups involving payers, providers, public health agencies, and patient organizations in the community." In addition, they "need to understand the limits of community-based cooperation and planning in a market-driven health care system" (pp. 394–395). In doing so, they are able to step back from a narrower professional role and think in terms of what is best for society and to examine health care changes over the sweep of time (McLaughlin & McLaughlin).

> CONSIDER
> Nurses who do not understand the legislative process will not be able to influence the policymaking process.

Each nurse, then, needs to decide how directly or indirectly he or she will be involved in politics and policy setting. Fortunately, nurses are in the enviable position of having great credibility with legislators and the public. For nurses who choose to be directly involved in politics and policy setting, they can seek public office or become more involved in lobbying legislators about issues pertinent to health care and nursing. Such lobbying can be done either in person or by writing, and there are many good sources on how to do both (see Chapter 22). The legislator needs to understand why this is an issue that is critical to not only the nursing profession, but also to his or her constituents. It is important, then, to create a need for the legislator to listen to what is being said.

Nurses can also give freely of their time and money to support nursing's position in the legislative arena. This can be done indirectly by contributing to professional associations such as the ANA, which have lobbyists in the legislative arena to protect nursing's interests, or by giving money directly to a political campaign. In this case, nurses should try to give early and to make as large a contribution as possible. It is the early and significant contributions that are remembered most.

Nurses interested in a more indirect contribution to policy development may work to influence and educate the public about nursing and the nursing agenda to reform health care. Either role is helpful—at least the nurse will have made a conscious decision to be involved.

Build Coalitions Inside and Outside of Nursing

The fourth step of the action plan to increase professional power in the 21st century is for the nursing profession to look within itself, as well as beyond its organizations for coalition building. McLaughlin and McLaughlin (2008) suggested that health policy takes place in a virtual network of participants, professions, and organizations, both locally and nationally.

Belonging to professional nursing organizations is one way in which nurses can network for coalition building. For example, the International Council of Nurses (ICN) is a federation of national nurses' associations representing nurses in more than 128 countries: "Founded in 1899, ICN is the world's first and widest reaching international organisation for health professionals" (ICN, 2008, para 1). The ICN works to ensure quality nursing care worldwide, sound health policies globally, the advancement of nursing knowledge, and the presence worldwide of a respected nursing profession and a competent and satisfied nursing workforce (para 1).

Coalitions also exist in the United States, such as the Health Professions and Nursing Education Coalition (HPNEC). This informal alliance of more than 50 organizations represents a variety of schools, programs, and individuals dedicated to educating professional health personnel and advocating for adequate and continued support for the health professions and nursing education programs authorized under Titles VII and VIII of the Public Health Service Act (HPNEC, 2008).

Coalitions have been formed within nursing groups as well. The Tri-Council for Nursing is an alliance of four autonomous nursing organizations: the AACN, the ANA, the AONE, and the NLN. The Tri-Council focuses on leadership for education, practice, and research.

The Council for the Advancement of Nursing Science (CANS) is another example of coalition building among nursing groups. The Council is composed of representatives from the four major regional research societies; the Honor Society of Nursing, Sigma Theta Tau International; the American Academy of Nursing; and the National Institute of Nursing Research (CANS, 2008).

Similarly, the National Federation for Specialty Nursing Organizations and the Nursing Organizations Liaison Forum, an entity of the ANA, merged in 2001 to become the Nursing Organizations Alliance (NOA), also known as The Alliance. The Alliance "provides a forum for identification, education, and collaboration building on issues of common interest to advance the nursing profession" (The Alliance, 2005, para 1).

CONSIDER

More collaboration among nursing organizations would strengthen nursing (Thupayagale-Tshweneagae & Dithole, 2007).

Nurses have not done as well, however, in building political coalitions with other interdisciplinary professionals with similar challenges. Pierce (2004), a nurse and congressional detailee in 2003, stated that she saw first-hand other professions that were struggling with professional issues similar to those in nursing, such as scope of practice, critical provider shortages, use of technology, and services for the poor and underserved. Pierce urged nursing to build coalitions with these other professions and not to restrict problem solving and strategizing "to our professional silo" (p. 115).

DISCUSSION POINT

All too frequently, the AMA and the ANA stand in opposition to each other in the legislative arena. Are there health care issues on which they could partner? Are there issues on which the ANA and the American Hospital Association could partner?

Nurses have also not done well in building political coalitions with legislators. Most legislators have a great deal of respect for nurses but know little about their qualifications to speak with authority about the health care system. Nurses need to become experts at political networking, making tradeoffs, negotiating, and coalition building. They also need to see the bigger picture of health care. This is not to say that nurses should lose sight of client needs, but that they must do a better job of seeing the bigger picture and of building and strengthening alliances with others before they will be seen as powerful and capable.

Conduct More Research to Strengthen Evidence-Based Practice

Another critical strategy for increasing nursing's power base is to continue to develop and promote evidence-based practice in nursing. Great strides have been made in researching what it is that nurses do that makes a difference in patient outcomes (research on *nursing sensitivity*), but more needs to be done. Nursing practice must reflect what research has identified as best practices, and a better understanding of the relationship between nursing practice and patient outcomes is still needed.

CONSIDER

Only relatively recently has research been able to prove that patients get better because of nurses and not in spite of them.

Building and sustaining evidence-based practice in nursing will require far greater numbers of master's and doctorally prepared nurse researchers, as well as entry into practice at an educational level similar to that of other professions. Social work, physical therapy, and occupational therapy all now have the master's degree as the entry level into practice. Nursing cannot afford to continue debating whether or not a bachelor's degree is necessary as the minimum entry level into professional practice (see Chapter 1).

Support Nursing Leaders

Another part of the action plan to increase the profession's power is that nurses must support their nursing leaders and recognize the challenges they face as visionary change agents. Nurses have often viewed their leaders as rule breakers, and this has often occurred at a high personal cost to innovators. In fact, Thupayagale-Tshweneagae and Dithole (2007, p. 145) went so far as to say "the enemy of nursing is inside the profession."

In addition, nurses often resist change and new ideas from their leaders and instead look to leaders in medicine and other health-related disciplines. Some of this occurs as a result of nurse leaders being discounted, at least in part, because most of their female majority, but also in part to the low value placed on nursing expertise.

It is important to remember that typically, it is not outsiders that divide nursing followers from nursing leaders. Instead, the division of nursing's strength often comes from within. Nursing leaders must be perceived as its best advocates. Differing viewpoints should not only be acknowledged, they should be encouraged.

There is a proper arena for conflict and argument, but the outward force presented must be one of unity and direction.

Mentor Future Nurse Leaders and Plan for Leadership Succession

Finally, and perhaps most important, before nursing can become a powerful profession, nurses must actively plan for leadership succession and care for younger members by providing mentoring opportunities. It is the future leaders who face the task of increasing nursing's power base in the 21st century.

Female-dominated professions have a history of exemplifying what is known as the *queen bee syndrome.* The queen bee is a woman who, after great personal struggle, becomes successful in her career. Her attitude, however, is that because she had to make it on her own with so little help, other novices should have to do the same. Thus, there has been inadequate empowering of young nurse leaders by older, more established nurse leaders.

Deppoliti (2008) noted that a disparity continues to exist between the idealism and professionalism of the educational process and the actuality of the practice environment. She suggested that this disparity plays a key role in the development of professional identity. In her qualitative study of new nurses (graduated less than 3 years), she found that they experienced various passage points as they joined the nursing profession. Within all of these passages, relationships were identified as paramount to a successful transition. (See Research Study Fuels the Controversy on page 333.)

DISCUSSION POINT

Is the nursing profession proactive in planning its leadership succession, or is it a change that occurs by drift?

It is the young who hold not only the keys to the present, but also the hope for the future. The nursing profession is responsible for ensuring leadership succession and is morally bound to do it with the brightest, most highly qualified individuals. According to Pierce (2004, p. 115),

Leaders chart the direction, facilitate communication, inspire others, and perhaps, most importantly, provide hope. For the nursing profession to flex its collective

Research Study Fuels the Controversy: Shaping Professional Identity

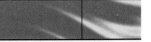

This qualitative study of 16 U.S. hospital nurses at 1 to 3 years after graduation from nursing school, used in-depth interviewing and open-ended questions with a semistructured format to describe and explore the experiences that contribute to the construction of professional identity. The researcher analyzed the data through the lens of symbolic interactionism.

STUDY FINDINGS

The study identified various passage points as nurses progressed in establishing their professional identity in the first 1 to 3 years after graduation. These points required adaptation to stress to accomplish successful negotiation and included finding a niche, orientation, the conflict of caring, taking the licensure examination, becoming a charge nurse, and moving on. A sense of responsibility and the need for continual learning and perfection were inherent in all passage points. The researcher concluded that the significance of the study rests in situational influences on the construction of identity, the need for balance and support in the practice environment, passage points in the first 3 years of practice, and the organizational need to support nursing empowerment and voice.

Source: Deppoliti, D. (2008). Exploring how new registered nurses construct professional identity in hospital settings. *Journal of Continuing Education in Nursing, 39*(6), 255–262.

political muscle and get involved with the redesign of the nation's health care system, we have to use our leadership to get the professional organizations to think and act collaboratively and to deliver a clear and strategic message to lawmakers. As nurses, as voters, and as constituents, we must be part of the solution.

CONCLUSIONS

Nursing, as a female-dominated profession, will have to work harder and fight longer than male-dominated professions to have a strong voice in health care policy. Nursing lobbyists in the nation's capitol are influencing legislation on quality, access to care, patient and health worker safety, health care restructuring, reimbursement for advanced practice nurses, and funding for nursing education. Representatives of professional nursing organizations regularly attend and provide testimony at government agency meetings to be sure that the "nursing perspective" is heard on health policy issues.

The United States spends more than $2 trillion on health care annually, with 60% of this being paid through taxes (Harrison, 2008). In fact, the United States spends more than any other industrialized country in the world (two to three times that of many industrialized countries), and yet its rankings in terms of life span, infant mortality, and teenage pregnancy are much lower than many countries that spend significantly less on health care. The elderly in this country cannot afford prescription coverage, and too many people lose their life savings trying to pay for catastrophic medical bills.

To make things worse, future projections are not encouraging. McLaughlin and McLaughlin (2008) suggested that the health care sector will comprise 20% of the U.S. economy by 2015, up from 17% in 2008. Those without insurance are projected to spend $30 billion out of pocket on health care in 2008, and the government is expected to chip in another $56 billion to cover their costs (Zhang, 2008). Even more alarming is the projection that the tab to cover all the uninsured in 2008 is expected to be $208.6 billion (Zhang).

Clearly, nurses, as health care professionals, need to have greater input into and control over how the health care system evolves in this country. We need a health care system that will guarantee basic, affordable health care coverage for all citizens and in which all the members of the multidisciplinary health care team work together to create policy and provide care based on what is best for the patient. We also need a health care system that is accountable for its outcomes—that recognizes that individuality, autonomy, quality, and basic human dignity are essential components of health care services and that the bottom line is not always a number.

The nursing profession must be held accountable for being an integral force in shaping such a health care system. Indeed, nursing has a moral and professional obligation to do so.

FOR ADDITIONAL DISCUSSION

1. Should the nursing profession target the recruitment of men into nursing in an effort to increase professional power?

2. What partners/external stakeholders should the nursing profession seek in terms of alliances or coalitions to strengthen its position in the policy arena?

3. What are the priority issues the nursing profession should identify in creating a proactive legislative agenda?

4. Will nursing ever be able to increase its power base if it does not increase its educational entry level to a level similar to that of other health care professions?

5. Do nursing schools provide enough content on politics, policy, and leadership for nurses to develop some degree of political competence? If not, what is missing?

6. Do most nurses internalize the need to be politically competent as a moral and professional obligation?

7. What legislature issues being debated have the greatest potential effect on nursing and health care?

REFERENCES

Abood, S. (2007). Influencing health care in the legislative arena. *Online Journal of Issues in Nursing, 12*(1), 5.

American Nurses Association (ANA) (2008). *Frequently asked questions.* Available at: http://www. nursingworld.org/FunctionalMenuCategories/FAQs. aspx#about. Accessed August 29, 2008.

ANA, Tri Council members send letter opposing Office of the National Nurse (2008). *Capitol Update, 6*(6). Available at: http://www.capitolupdate.org/Newsletter/ index.asp?nlid=206&nlaid=1022. Accessed August 29, 2008.

Artz, M. (2006). The politics of caring: Ask not what nursing can do for you. *American Journal of Nursing, 106*(9), 91.

Blass, F. R., & Ferris, G. R. (2007). Leader reputation: The role of mentoring, political skill, contextual learning, and adaptation. *Human Resource Management, 46*(1), 5–19.

Council for the Advancement of Nursing Science (CANS) (2008). *Home page.* Available at: http:// www.nursingscience.org/i4a/pages/index.cfm? pageid=1./. Accessed August 30, 2008.

Deppoliti, D. (2008). Exploring how new registered nurses construct professional identity in hospital settings. *Journal of Continuing Education in Nursing, 39*(6), 255–262.

Fletcher, K. (2007). Image: Changing how women nurses think about themselves. Literature review. *Journal of Advanced Nursing, 58*(3), 207–215.

Harrison, J. A. (2008). Paying more, getting less. *Dollars & Sense. The Magazine of Economic Justice.* Available at: http://www.dollarsandsense.org/archives/2008/ 0508harrison.html. Accessed August 28, 2008.

Health Professions and Nursing Education Coalition (HPNEC) (2008). *Home page.* Available at: http:// www.aamc.org/advocacy/hpnec/start.htm. Accessed August 28, 2008.

Herrick, D. (2008). *Crisis of the uninsured: 2008. Brief analysis. No. 626.* National Center for Policy Analysis. Available at: http://www.ncpa.org/pub/ba/ba626/. Accessed August 26, 2008.

International Council of Nurses (2008). *About ICN. ICN's mission.* Available at: http://www.icn.ch/abouticn.htm. Accessed August 29, 2008.

Irvine, H. (2008). Review: *Daring to Care: American Nursing and Second-Wave Feminism* [by Susan Gelfand Malka]. *Feminist Review,* February 17, 2008. Available at: http://feministreview.blogspot.com/2008/02/ daring-to-care-american-nursing-and.html. Accessed August 29, 2008.

Jones, J. M. (2007). *Lobbyists debut at bottom of honesty and ethics list. Nurses again perceived as having highest honesty and ethical standards.* Available at: http://www.gallup.com/poll/103123/Lobbyists-Debut-Bottom-Honesty-Ethics-List.aspx. Accessed August 29, 2008.

Manthey, M. (2008). The invisible power of nursing. *Creative Nursing, 14*(1), 3–5.

Marquis, B., & Huston, C. (2009). *Leadership Roles and Management Functions in Nursing* (6th ed.). Philadelphia: Lippincott Williams & Wilkins.

McLaughlin, C. P., & McLaughlin, C. D. (2008). *Health Policy Analysis. An Interdisciplinary Approach.* Sudbury, MA: Jones & Bartlett.

Office of the National Nurse (2006). *New Mexico Nurse.* Bnet. Available at: http://findarticles.com/p/articles/mi_qa4086/is_200604/ai_n17175701. Accessed August 29, 2008.

Pierce, K. M. (2004). Insights and reflections of a Congressional nurse detailee. *Policy, Politics, & Nursing Practice, 5*(2), 113–115.

Ridge, R. (2008). Nursing certification as a workforce strategy. *Nursing Management, 39*(8), 50–52.

Senge, P. (1990). *The Fifth Discipline.* New York: Doubleday/Currency.

Sorensen, R., Iedema, R., & Severinsson, E. (2008). Beyond profession: Nursing leadership in contemporary healthcare. *Journal of Nursing Management, 16*(5), 535–544.

The Alliance (2005). *Home page.* Available at: http://www.nursing-alliance.org/. Accessed August 28, 2008.

The National Nurse (2008). *Official site of the National Nursing Network Organization.* Available at: http://nationalnurse.org/. Accessed August 29, 2008.

Thupayagale-Tshweneagae, G., & Dithole, K. (2007). Unity among nurses: An evasive concept. *Nursing Forum, 42*(3), 143–146.

Zhang, J. (2008). Uninsured to spend $30 billion, study says. *Wall Street Journal* (online). Available at: http://online.wsj.com/article/SB121963245880668193.html?mod=hpp_us_whats_news. Accessed August 28, 2008.

BIBLIOGRAPHY

Ballard, K. A. (2008). Environments and health. Nurses as environmental health activists. *American Journal of Nursing, 108*(5), 69–72.

Bradbury-Jones, C., Sambrook, S., & Irvine, F. (2008). Power and empowerment in nursing: A fourth theoretical approach. *Journal of Advanced Nursing, 62*(2), 258–266.

Clark, C. (2008). Student perspectives on faculty incivility in nursing education: An application of the concept of rankism. *Nursing Outlook, 56*(1), 4–8.

Georges, J. M., & Benedict, S. (2008). Nursing gaze of the eastern front in World War II: A feminist narrative analysis. *Advances in Nursing Science. Violence, Injury, and Human Safety, 31*(2), 139–152.

Jansen, L. (2008). Collaborative and interdisciplinary health care teams: Ready or not? *Journal of Professional Nursing, 24*(4), 218–227.

Jasper, M. (2008). Valuing and empowering nurses. *Journal of Nursing Management, 16*(3), 225–226.

Leavitt, J. K. (2008). Making a difference: Why perianesthesia nurses must be involved in the policy and political process. *Journal of PeriAnesthesia Nursing, 23*(3), 157–162.

Mills, T., & Schneider, A. (2007). The Office of the National Nurse: Leadership for a new era of prevention. *Policy, Politics & Nursing Practice, 8*(1), 64–70.

Morrisey, M. A., & Cawley, J. (2008). Health economists' views of health policy. *Journal of Health Politics, Policy & Law, 33*(4), 707–724.

Reeves, S., Nelson, S., & Zwarenstein, M. (2008). The doctor–nurse game in the age of interprofessional care: A view from Canada. *Nursing Inquiry, 15*(1), 1–2.

Sirota, T. (2008). Nursing 2008 nurse/physician relationships survey report. *Nursing, 38*(7), 28–31.

Sumner, J. (2008). Is caring in nursing an impossible ideal for today's practicing nurse? *Nursing Administration Quarterly, 32*(2), 92–101.

Udod, S. A. (2008). The power behind empowerment for staff nurses: Using Foucault's concepts. *Nursing Leadership (Toronto, Ontario), 21*(2), 77–92.

Vesely, R. (2008). 'Unleash the energy': Activists, professors try to use their own sphere of influence to affect U.S. healthcare policy and improve patient care. *Modern Healthcare, 38*(17), 6–7, 16.

Volp, K. (2008). Let's talk nursing. Your decision power. *Queensland Nurse, 27*(3), 8–9.

WEB RESOURCES

American Nurses Association	http://www.nursingworld.org/
Center for Health Outcomes and Policy Research, University of Pennsylvania	http://www.nursing.upenn.edu/chopr/research.asp
Government Affairs, ANA in Action	http://www.nursingworld.org/gova/
National Council of State Legislatures	www.ncsl.org/programs/health/health.htm
Office of Nursing Policy, Health Policy Branch, Health Canada	http://www.hc-sc.gc.ca/ahc-asc/branch-dirgen/hpb-dgps/onp-bpsi/index-eng.php
Petition to Establish an Office of the National Nurse	http://www.petitiononline.com/rnusa1/petition.html
RN Activist Tool Kit	http://www.nursingworld.org/MainMenuCategories/ANAPoliticalPower/Election2008/ToolKit.aspx
The National Nurse	http://nationalnurse.org/
Tips—Contacting Members of Congress	http://www.nursingworld.org/MainMenuCategories/ANAPoliticalPower/Election2008/ToolKit/ContactCongress.aspx
U.S. Congress	http://www.congress.org/congressorg/home/

CHAPTER 20

Professional Identity and Image

• CAROL J. HUSTON •

Learning Objectives

The learner will be able to:

1. Explore the roots and prevalence of historical and contemporary nursing stereotypes, including nurse as angel of mercy, love interest (particularly to physicians), sex bombshell/naughty nurse, handmaiden to the physician, and battle axe, as well as the stereotype of the male nurse as being gay, effeminate, or sexually predatory.

2. Identify common public portrayals or descriptions of nurses in terms of gender, dress, and role responsibilities

3. Examine the role that the Center for Nursing Advocacy has assumed in addressing inaccurate or negative portrayals of nursing in the media and the process they use to raise public and professional awareness of the issues surrounding nursing's public image.

4. Explore findings and recommendations from the Woodhull Study on Nursing and the Media that speak to nursing's invisibility as a profession.

5. Analyze the effect of inaccurate nursing stereotypes on the profession's ability to recruit the best and brightest students to nursing, as well as on the collective identity and self-esteem of all nurses.

6. Name well-known fictional nurse characters depicted in contemporary media (radio, television, movies) and identify the nursing stereotypes that they best represent.

7. Discuss the challenges inherent in attempting to change deeply ingrained stereotypes about nursing that are likely instilled very early in childhood.

8. Analyze how a lack of uniformity in dress and the way in which nurses introduce themselves to patients have contributed to the public's confusion about who is a nurse.

9. Explore the roles and responsibilities that individual nurses, employers, professional associations, and the media have to see that nurses are portrayed accurately and positively to the public

10. Assess the effect of strategies undertaken by professional coalitions and corporations such as Johnson & Johnson to improve recruitment and retention in nursing.

11. Reflect on the premise that every nurse controls the image of nursing.

12. Reflect on what image he or she would like the public to have of the nursing profession.

An *image* can be defined as a reproduction or an imitation of something or as a mental picture or impression of something (Merriam Webster Online Dictionary, 2008). In other words, an image is often an unknown reality because it depends on the subjective perception of others. Perhaps that is why the public image of the nursing profession is typically one dimensional and inaccurate.

If asked to describe a nurse, most of the public would use such terms as *nice*, *hardworking*, or *caring*. They would also use the terms *ethical* and *honest*. There is little question that the public trusts and respects nurses. In fact, since they were added to the list in 1999 nurses have ranked number 1 on every Gallup poll on honesty and ethics (with the exception of 2001) (Jones, 2007). Few people, however, would use the terms *highly educated, bright, powerful, well-educated, professional,* or *independent thinker* to describe a nurse. Even fewer would call the nursing profession *prestigious.*

CONSIDER

Nursing continues to lag considerably behind the medical profession in terms of occupational prestige and status (Seago et al., 2006).

DISCUSSION POINT

If the nursing profession is so well thought of and so highly recommended, why are there persistent concerns that not enough people are becoming RNs? (Donelan et al., 2008, p. 143).

Many people would, however, describe a nurse as a caring young woman, dressed in a white uniform dress, cap, and shoes, altruistically devoted to caring for the ill ("angel of mercy"), under the supervision of a physician. Common job functions would be identified as making beds, passing out pills, emptying bedpans, giving shots, and helping doctors. Some people, however, would allude, at least subtly, to a lustier image of sexy young females dressed in provocative attire and seeking sexual gratification from both patients and physicians. Still others might depict stern, aged "battle axe" females thrusting hypodermic needles into recalcitrant patients and seemingly enjoying the discomfort they cause and the power that they hold.

What do these portrayals have in common? Almost nothing and yet everything. All are part of the convoluted, often conflicting stereotypical images of nurses. In addition, all of these images demean the true nature and complexity of nursing, and most are based almost entirely in fiction. Yet these stereotypes are pervasive, and efforts to change them have yielded only limited progress.

Clearly, public perceptions about the nursing profession are mixed and even contradictory at times. The public trusts and admires nurses, but this does not necessarily equate with respect. Nor does the public consider the profession prestigious or understand what nursing is all about.

The end result of this public image confusion is that old stereotypes of nurses as overbearing, brainless, sexually promiscuous, and incompetent women are perpetuated, as are images of nurses as caring, hardworking, altruistic, and selfless. This image conflict is an enduring issue for nursing, and the profession's efforts to address the problem have been fragmented and largely unsuccessful. Indeed, many nurses believe nursing's image to be one of the most important and enduring issues they face as a profession.

This chapter explores common historical and contemporary nursing stereotypes. The effect of these inaccurate stereotypes on recruitment into the profession and the collective self-esteem and identity of nurses is examined. In addition, strategies for improving the public image of nursing are presented, as are the challenges inherent in trying to change stereotypes that are ingrained in the profession's history and even in how nurses view themselves.

NURSING STEREOTYPES

Of the many nursing stereotypes, the most common ones are shown in Box 20.1: the nurse as an angel of mercy; the nurse as a love interest (particularly to physicians); the nurse as a sex bombshell or "naughty nurse"; the nurse as a handmaiden to physicians; the nurse as a battle axe; and the male nurse as a gay, effeminate, or sexually predatory man. All of these stereotypes are profiled in this chapter. In addition, contemporary nursing images as depicted in movies and on television are profiled in an effort to better identify what images of nursing are before the public, especially the young people who represent the potential future nursing workforce.

Angel of Mercy

One of the oldest and most common nursing stereotypes is that of the nurse as an angel of mercy. Some individuals suggest that the image of the nurse angel with

---

BOX 20.1 | COMMON NURSING STEREOTYPES

- Angel of mercy.
- Love interest (particularly to physicians).
- Sex bombshell/naughty nurse.
- Handmaiden to the physician.
- Battle-axe.
- Male nurses as homosexual, effeminate, or sexually predatory.

BOX 20.2 | THE NIGHTINGALE PLEDGE

I solemnly pledge myself before God and in the presence of this assembly, to pass my life in purity and to practice my profession faithfully. I will abstain from whatever is deleterious and mischievous, and will not take or knowingly administer any harmful drug. I will do all in my power to maintain and elevate the standard of my profession, and will hold in confidence all personal matters committed to my keeping and all family affairs coming to my knowledge in the practice of my calling. With loyalty will I endeavor to aid the physician, in his work, and devote myself to the welfare of those committed to my care.

Source: *Florence Nightingale. "The Nightingale Pledge."* (n.d.). Available at: **http://www.countryjoe.com/nightingale/pledge.htm.** Accessed September 6, 2008.

wings actually comes from the capes nurses historically wore as part of their uniforms.

When most people think of nurses as angels of mercy, the saintly image of Florence Nightingale bringing comfort to maimed soldiers during the Crimean War comes to mind. Clearly, Florence Nightingale's legacy of caring is beyond remarkable; however, few individuals outside of nursing would recognize Nightingale as a politically astute, assertive change agent who used her knowledge of epidemiology and statistics to document the effectiveness of nursing interventions. Both images are equally important parts of her legacy.

A more contemporary depiction of a nurse as an angel of mercy occurred in the 1996 movie *The English Patient*. In this film, a man injured in a plane crash is cared for by a nurse named Hana. Hana, at risk to herself, did everything she could to save this man's life. She also demonstrated supreme emotional strength as she watched her patient die, a quality that nurses often learn and gain through practicing their profession (Nursing Stereotypes, n.d.).

The nurse "angel of mercy" stereotype persists even as the second decade of the 21st century begins. Indeed, a book published by Harlequin in 2008 entitled *Single Dad, Nurse Bride* details the fictional life of an orthopedic doctor, Dr. Dane Hendricks, "who is every nurse's dream—handsome and a take charge kind of guy when it comes to medicine but also warm and humorous" (Amazon.com, 2008, para 2). He is also wealthy. Rikki Johansen, "a conscientious nurse, taking to heart all the lessons she learned in nursing school, . . . always puts others before herself and as a result, she must drive a car that doesn't always start right away" (para 4). "When Dane's brother is diagnosed with cancer and Rikki turns out to be the only bone marrow match, there is never any doubt what her choice will be"(para 8).

The Center for Nursing Advocacy (n.d.-a) concluded that such images of the nurse as an "angel" or "saint" are generally unhelpful to the profession because they "fail to convey the college-level knowledge base, critical thinking skills, and hard work required to be a nurse. They also suggest that nurses are supernatural beings who do not require decent working conditions, adequate staffing, or a significant role in health care decision-making or policy" (para 1).

Some individuals argue that the angel of mercy stereotype is unconsciously promoted by nurses even today—in the Nightingale Pledge, for instance (see Box 20.2). When one looks closely at the Pledge, which originated in 1893 but is still cited frequently in nursing graduation ceremonies, it speaks of nurses forgoing their personal wants and needs for the good of others. Being giving and caring in nature is a wonderful thing, but to suggest that it should be done to the extent of self-neglect is likely not the desired message.

It is important to remember, however, that being an angel of mercy is not all bad. It does encompass behaviors that many nurses typify, such as caring and dedication. Unfortunately, the angel of mercy image all too often also carries with it the idea that pay is never an issue and that suffering must be a part of the nurse's life if the role is to have value. This intrapersonal conflict between the values of altruism and pay befitting a professional is still experienced by many nurses.

Love Interest (Particularly to Physicians)

Another historical stereotype of nurses is that of a love interest, particularly to physicians. Doctor/nurse romance novels first appeared in the 1930s and 1940s, when becoming a nurse was one of the few career opportunities available to women besides secretarial work and child care (Ryan, n.d.). Nurses in these novels were cast as intelligent, strong women who felt fulfilled in their careers until they met the physician who would eventually become their husband. Then their career would end and the nurse would live happily ever after, caring for her spouse and children.

With the women's rights movement of the 1970s, women's career opportunities expanded and fewer books were devoted to women as nurses. In addition, readers' interest in medical romances dwindled. This is not to say that there are not still doctor/nurse romance novels. There are, but the characters typically are different from what they were in decades past. The female character in contemporary books is often now a physician or at least a charge nurse of a critical care unit in a large, urban medical center who is beautiful. Her strongest personality trait is "determination tempered by compassion" (Clichés Abound, 2007). The male character, however, continues to be a physician, coping with a tragedy in his past, who is "brilliant, tall, and muscular" and "with chiseled features, working in emergency medicine" (Lovesick Doctors and Lovelorn Nurses, 2007).

Romantic relationships between nurses and doctors abound on contemporary television shows as well, such as ER, Scrubs, House, and Gray's Anatomy. It could be argued, however, that most of these relationships are not so much love interests as sexual liaisons.

Romantic relationships between nurses and doctors are also depicted in the movies. In 2000, the movie Nurse Betty depicted a waitress from Kansas who witnessed violence perpetrated by hit men. As a result of her trauma, she became disoriented and transformed into Nurse Betty—convinced that her favorite soap opera nurse character was real and that she was romantically involved with its lead character, Dr. David Ravell. The point of the movie is that Nurse Betty cannot distinguish medical soap operas from reality, and the implication is that nurses actively seek personal relationships with physicians.

Sex Bombshell/Naughty Nurse

Another common nursing stereotype is that of the nurse as a sex bombshell or "naughty nurse." Use of the word "naughty" probably is not powerful enough, however, given that the depiction of nurses in the sex and pornography industry is even more rampant that the general sexual stereotyping of nurses in the media. In fact, for at least 40 years, nurses have been portrayed as sex objects both on television and in the movies. Indeed, movies in the 1960s, 1970s, and 1980s, were filled with images of nurses garbed in miniskirts, sleazy, low-cut tops, and high heels, who spent all of their time fulfilling sexual fantasies and virtually no time providing care to patients.

One of the most famous portrayals of a lusty nurse during the 1970s was the character "Hot Lips" Houlihan in the movie M*A*S*H (1970). Hot Lips was, at least at times, a positive role model for nursing, although her sexual weaknesses were highlighted at least as much as her skills as a nurse. Hot Lips was also a key character in the television series (1972–1983), in which, however, her sexual exploits were less of an issue.

More recently, in the spring of 2004, a 10-week series entitled No Angels depicting the lives of four young nurses appeared on television in the United Kingdom. Three nurses who reviewed the show said the characters were "all smoking, all drinking, sexed up independent women, sashaying through the wards en route to another wild night of clubbing or a steamy clinch in the linen cupboard" (Allen, 2004, para 2). In fact, the press release for the show stated that No Angels was about the life, death, and lunacy inherent in nursing and the antics that nurses indulge in when they want to let off steam (Allen).

Nurses are even depicted as sex objects in contemporary television commercials. In 2003, Clairol Herbal Essences shampoo launched a commercial that showed a nurse abandoning her patient to wash her hair in his bathroom and then tossing her hair sensually at the patient as she left the room. Many nurses and nursing organizations, including the Center for Nursing Advocacy, condemned the unprofessional stereotype perpetuated in the ad and asked sponsor Procter & Gamble to discontinue it (Procter & Gamble Pulls Offending Ad, 2003). Procter & Gamble did issue an apology to nurses and pull the ad, stating that the company "holds the nursing profession in the highest esteem" (p. 35). The company declined, however, to make a contribution to a nursing image campaign to counteract the damage that had been done.

DISCUSSION POINT

Do you think that the public truly believes that a nurse would abandon patient care duties to wash her hair in a patient's bathroom and then sensually shake her hair at the patient? If not, does the commercial still cause harm?

Another commercial sexualizing nurses was launched in September 2007 by Cadbury Schweppes Canada for Dentyne gum (Center for Nursing Advocacy, 2007a). The Cadbury Schweppes ads showed female nurses being lured into bed with male patients the instant the male patients popped Dentyne into their mouths. The tag line for the commercial was "Get Fresh" and the message was that when hospitalized patients used Dentyne products, there would be an instant, erotic reaction from the "always available" bedside nurse (para 1).

More than 1,000 protest letters were sent from the Web site of the Registered Nurses Association of Ontario (RNAO) in response to the Cadbury Schweppes commercial (Center for Nursing Advocacy, 2007b). Another 500 supporters from the Center for Nursing Advocacy wrote letters to top Cadbury Schweppes executives, "leaving long messages explaining that such imagery reinforces a stereotype of workplace sexual availability that contributes to the global nursing crisis" (para 1).

Initially, the company responded that its ads were causing no harm. On October 6, 2007, however, the company told the Center and RNAO that it would pull the ads and consult nurses in creating its future U.S. and Canadian ads involving nurses (Center for Nursing Advocacy, 2007b).

Another recent example of the perpetuation of the naughty nurse stereotype became apparent when the Heart Attack Grill, a theme restaurant in Arizona, began dressing their waitresses in naughty nurse uniforms, which included "skimpy, cleavage-baring outfits, high heels and thigh-high stockings" (Waitresses Dressed as Naughty Nurses, 2006, para 3). Because nurses are already the most sexually fantasized profession (Nurses and Fireman Top Fantasy Poll, 2006), the Center for Nursing Advocacy asked the Heart Attack Grill to reconsider their uniform choice. The Grill's owner, Jon Basso, responded that he felt it "glorified nurses to be thought of as a physically attractive and desirable individual instead of as some old battle ax who changes

bedpans for a living" (Waitresses Dressed as Naughty Nurses, para 7).

In addition, the state Board of Nursing filed a complaint with the Arizona Attorney General's office that Basso was using the illegally using the term "nurse" in advertising for his restaurant (Arizona Statute A.R.S. 32-1636 states only someone who has a valid nursing license can use the title "nurse"). In response, Basso, who refused to remove the term "nurse" from his advertising, did put an asterisk on his Web site and in his ads suggesting that the use of the word "nurse" was only intended as a parody (Waitresses Dressed as Naughty Nurses, 2006).

DISCUSSION POINT

Heart Attack Grill owner John Basso referred to critics of his waitress uniform choice as "prudes, cranks and lunatics" (Waitresses Dressed as Naughty Nurses, 2006, para 6). Do you feel that the uniform policy at Heart Attack Grill is simply good fun, or does it truly denigrate the nursing profession and sexualize nursing?

Handmaiden to the Physician

Perhaps the most pervasive stereotype of nurses is that of handmaiden to physicians. In the handmaiden role, the nurse simply serves as an adoring backdrop to the omnipotent physician, demonstrating little, if any, independent thought or action.

CONSIDER

Nursing care is frequently perceived by the public as simple and unskilled.

This same view of nurses as a handmaiden to physicians in the 1950s and 1960s was reported in classic research by Philip and Beatrice Kalisch, pioneering students of nursing images in the 1970s. Indeed, during the 1970s, nurses generally had no substantial role in television stories, and were a part of the hospital background in programs that focused on physician characters. When nurses were the focus of a program, the storyline frequently involved the nurse's personal problems rather than his or her role as a nurse, and attributes such as obedience, permissiveness, conformity, flexibility, and serenity were emphasized.

Many of the commercial representations of nurses today continue to represent the stereotype of nurse as a handmaiden. For example, in spring 2008, the Angela Moore jewelry catalog featured "Nurse Nancy" bracelets and necklaces. According to the Center for Nursing Advocacy (2008), the jewelry was composed of four different types of balls; one ball featured a smiling, rosy-cheeked nurse in white uniform and cap giving a balloon to a girl; the second ball had a ladybug next to a stethoscope; the third ball featured a nurse's cap with a thermometer; and the fourth ball had a stuffed bear holding flowers next to a lollipop. The text in the catalog "asked readers to buy the Nurse Nancy jewelry to "celebrate the ladies who give lollipops and band aids a whole new meaning" (para 1).

In response to letters of concern from nurses, the jewelry maker did agree to modify the description of the jewelry. According to the Center for Nursing Advocacy (2008, para 3), however, what they changed it to, was "Here's a special theme to celebrate the wonderful women who promote health and make us feel so much better. Talented, terrific and leaders to love!" The Center (para 4) suggested that "while this was probably an improvement over lollipops and band aids," it was still problematic in that it suggested that only women are nurses. In addition, the Center argued that "statements such as 'makes us feel so much better,' 'leaders to love,' and 'wonderful women' sound like adoration for someone's loving mom who makes them feel so much better by making them soup or tea" (para 5), not that nurses are highly trained health care professionals who use both science and art to make a difference in their patient's outcomes.

Battle Axe

Few stereotypes in nursing are as dark or demented, however, as that of the nurse as a battle axe. The battle axe stereotype often depicts an overbearing, unhappy, mean senior nurse who intimidates both patients and staff. The movie *One Flew over the Cuckoo's Nest* (1975) provides a perfect example of the battle-axe nurse (Nursing Stereotypes, n.d.). Nurse Ratched, a nurse in a mental hospital, fits the description of a battle-axe in almost every way. She craves power and control over others and forces patients to obey her every whim or suffer the repercussions.

Nurse Diesel, in the movie *High Anxiety* (1978), was another stereotypical battle-axe nurse, with the addition of enormous prosthetic breasts. As an overbearing, evil

charge nurse, Nurse Diesel continually displayed a dark sneer and a love of domination. Finally, Annie Wilkes from the novel and movie *Misery* gave new meaning to the sociopathic battle-axe nurse as she kidnapped, maimed, and held hostage a writer she admired and wanted to be close to.

Battle-axe stereotypes of nurses have always existed; however, they seemed to hit their peak in the 1970s and 1980s. There are, however, still multiple images of battle-axe nurses available on the Internet. Perhaps this reflects "society's continuing discomfort with powerful women, and its inability to reconcile the apparently conflicting ideas of nursing and assertive conduct" (Center for Nursing Advocacy, 2005a, para 4). It is also of interest that the battle-axe counterpart of male physicians in medicine is viewed less negatively. For example, the television show *House* stars a prickly male physician specialist whose hostility is often viewed as a by-product of an intense professional commitment rather than as a sign of dangerous psychosis or sexual frustration (Center for Nursing Advocacy, 2005a).

The Male Nurse: Gay, Effeminate, and Sexually Predatory

Female nurses are not the only ones who are stereotyped. Male nurse stereotypes are at least as prevalent as those for females, and the stereotypes for male nurses are virtually all negative, which only adds to the difficulty of recruiting men to the profession (see Chapter 9).

Male nurses are frequently stereotyped as being homosexual (or at least feminine). They may even be stereotyped as being hypersexual and, as a result, the intent of their actions may be questioned as being either sexual in nature or, in some cases, even sexually predatory. This makes it very difficult for male nurses to demonstrate the caring, therapeutic interactions that are such an important part of nursing.

Woldt (2008), a male nurse, stated that while some individuals perceive that male nurses are less sensitive, they might, in fact, be holding back on reaching out to patients physically, in fear that their actions might be perceived in the wrong manner. He concluded that the "greatest consequence of stereotyping male nurses is the impact on their ability to give adequate patient care" (para 4).

CONSIDER
Many male nurses live in fear of how their caring actions might be interpreted.

Another popular stereotype for male nurses is that they are nonachievers for going into nursing rather than more traditionally male occupations. This was certainly the case in the most recent effort to depict a male nurse in a major motion picture: the 2000 movie *Meet the Parents*. Unfortunately, despite the protestations of Greg Focker, the male Registered Nurse (RN) in the movie, that he loves nursing and became a nurse by choice, his future in-laws and other relatives constantly questioned his sexual orientation and manliness. They also clearly implied that Greg must have become a nurse because his test scores were not high enough for him to qualify for medical school.

Woldt (2008) concluded that it is not easy when patients or other staff members ask male nurses about their sexuality or suggest that their career choice implied that they were incapable of succeeding in a traditional male occupation. He argued that the public owes male nurses the same degree of care in actions and words as patients deserve from their care providers.

CONTEMPORARY NURSING STEREOTYPES ON TELEVISION

Television medical dramas currently provide the greatest number of visual images of nurses at work. In fact, a recent study by Donelan, Buerhaus, Desroches, Dittus, and Dutwin (2008) revealed that 60% of the general public watched television shows and news stories in 2007 that included nurses or had seen advertisements about nursing. Although most suggested that fictional television shows made no difference in their level of respect for registered nurses, some respondents stated that such depictions increased their respect for nurses and others reported less as a result.

There is little doubt, however, that television medical dramas build on traditional stereotypes of nurses, as well as suggest new ones. One of the best-known medical dramas in the last decades, with strong nurse figures, was *ER* (1994—2009). This medical drama focused on the lives and events of the emergency department staff at County General Hospital in Chicago, a level I trauma center.

The character Carol Hathaway was perhaps the best-known nurse on *ER*. After surviving the September 1994 pilot episode in which she tried to commit suicide, Hathaway became the charge nurse of the emergency department. She went on to have a sexual relationship with a physician and bore twins out of wedlock. Nurse Hathaway left the show in 1999—to join her physician love interest in another state. Of interest, in a survey of 1,800 children in grades 2 through 10 in 10 cities conducted by the health care group of JWT Specialized Communications (Sherman, 2000), Carol Hathaway was cited as the strongest image of a nurse. The students, however, felt that she was more defined by her romantic involvements than her profession.

Even with the departure of Nurse Hathaway, *ER* continued to provide probably the most influential portrayals of nurses on television. One of the highest profile nurses remaining on the show was Abby Lockhart, an alcoholic, former maternity nurse from a family afflicted with bipolar disorder. She started on the show as a medical student, dropped out of medical school, worked as a nurse, and then became a doctor. Abby had sexual relationships with several doctors on the show and eventually married one of them.

In addition, Samantha Taggart, a nurse who joined the *ER* cast in 2003, was a tough, free-spirited, single mother of an emotionally troubled child, who almost immediately entered into a sexual relationship with one of the physicians. In her introductory scene, "Sam" (who had come to the hospital inquiring about employment), grabbed a syringe and leaped to sedate an unruly patient through a central vessel in his neck. This behavior not only earned her a job, but the respect of her soon-to-be coworkers.

One of the newest TV shows to stir nurses to action, however, is *Grey's Anatomy* (2005–present). Reviews by the Center for Nursing Advocacy (2005b) suggested that nurses are simply invisible on this show and that the physician characters do all of the patient monitoring, patient emotional support, family relations, patient advocacy, and virtually all supportive and therapeutic care. When nurses are seen, they are focused on administration and care tasks that are trivial, like changing bedpans, handing things to physicians, minor hand-holding, and tracking little patient quirks. Indeed, it could be argued that the only truly visible nurse on the show has been the one who gave sexually transmitted diseases to the male physicians.

THE IMAGE OF NURSING ON THE INTERNET

The Internet is also filled with images of nurses, some accurate and some very stereotypical. A recent review of nurse images on Google found numerous inappropriate images of nurses. Many were sexually suggestive, as well as demeaning. Some were in caricature, but many were of young women dressed in cleavage-baring uniforms and wearing fishnet stockings, high heels, and garter belts.

Unprofessional images of nurses on the Internet do not always come from external sources, however. Sometimes, they come from health care professionals. Lagu, Kaufman, Asch, and Armstrong (2008) looked at how health care professionals (physicians and nurses) communicated through blogs on the Internet. In the 271 medical blogs reviewed, patients were described in 114 blogs (42.1%), and 45 blogs (16.6%) included sufficient information that patients would be able to identify their doctors or themselves. Three blogs showed recognizable photographic images of patients. The researchers concluded that whereas the Internet offers health care professionals the opportunity to share their narratives, revealing confidential information reflects poorly on blog authors and their professions.

Finally, in a review of 144 Web sites in 2001 and 152 Web sites in 2004, Kalisch, Begeny, and Neumann (2007) found that 70% of the Internet sites showed nurses as intelligent and educated and 60% as respected, accountable, committed, competent, and trustworthy. Nurses were also shown as having specialized knowledge and skills in 70% (2001) and 62% (2004) of the Web sites. However, images of the nurse as sexually promiscuous increased between 2001 and 2004, whereas images of the nurse as a committed, attractive/well-groomed, and authoritative professional decreased during the same time period. The researchers concluded that the Internet provides important opportunities for improving the image of the nurse.

HOW INGRAINED ARE NURSING STEREOTYPES?

Increasingly, researchers are concluding that inaccurate and negative stereotypes of nurses are not only well ingrained, but also are instilled early in life. Indeed, gender stereotyping about career opportunities begins at a very early age. By the age of 3 years, most children already have firmly rooted gender-based ideas about the roles they can and should hold when they grow up.

This was borne out in research by Teig and Susskind (2008) of first-graders (age 6 to 8 years), who had already identified nursing as a high-status feminine occupation. This research suggested that boys attend to both gender roles and status when considering occupations, but that boys are willing to consider high-status "feminine" occupations as much as the low-status "masculine" jobs. Girls, however, focused primarily on the gender role of occupations and only attended to status within the less desirable masculine occupations. Teig and Susskind (p. 861) concluded that "if the social status of nurses is promoted during elementary school, it may enhance young boys' perceptions of the profession," and "if boys do not eliminate nursing from future consideration during childhood, the percentage of men entering these vocations may increase."

The reality, then, is that by the end of middle school, most students report having their minds made up about desirable and undesirable careers. An unpublished study by Huston (*Nursing Stereotypes Engrained by Second Grade*; see Research Study Fuels the Controversy on page 345) suggested that basic beliefs and stereotypes about professions such as nursing may be ingrained at a far younger age, and that waiting until fifth, sixth, or even seventh grade to address inaccurate or negative images of nursing might be too late.

This has been clearly borne out in studies of high school students. In the JWT Specialized Communications study (Sherman, 2000), the older students—those in ninth or tenth grade—already had firmly entrenched ideas about nursing. They said that they thought of nursing "as being technical as opposed to professional" (para 9). They also reported that they thought nursing was "more like shop, than a college degree" (para 9) and that they were unsure of career advancement opportunities and job security for nurses. In addition, the students were quick to point out that nursing is a "girls' job" (para 10), and this belief crossed all age and ethnic groups. Indeed, male students had to be asked directly about their thoughts on nursing because many automatically responded as if the discussion did not involve them (Sherman, 2000).

The students also said "they had no compelling reason to be a nurse" (Sherman, 2000, para 7). Most knew at least one nurse, and some had had an extraordinary experience

Research Study Fuels the Controversy: Second-Graders' Image of Nurses

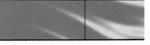

This unpublished study examined stereotypes held by 25 second-graders regarding "important" nursing roles and functions. In an effort to introduce students to nonhospital nursing roles, which students stated they already knew, a 30-minute slide show and discussion was held showing nurses actively engaged in less traditional nursing roles such as cardiac rehabilitation, primary care, flight nursing, education, management, and public health. In addition, nurse practitioners were introduced as primary care providers. Students were shown photos of nurses in all types of garb, except for white uniforms. Efforts were made to assure ethnic and gender diversity in all presentation materials. At the conclusion of the presentation, students were asked to draw a picture of what they thought was the most exciting role that had been presented for nurses.

STUDY FINDINGS

The caption on the first drawing was "the nurse is doing surgery on a real important disease." In the second, the nurse, with a red cross on her white uniform, was noted to be "rushing" into the hospital. In the third, the nurse, in her white starched cap, was making up a hospital bed.

In the fourth drawing, the nurse was giving a hospitalized patient a backrub. In another, a dour nurse, as denoted by a capital N on her starched white cap with red cross on it, was entering a hospital nursery. In the sixth, a patient in a bed was hooked up to an intravenous line, expressing pain. The smiling nurse was walking away from him.

In the seventh drawing, the nurse was helping the child in the hospital bed, and it included a caption that the "nurse is in a rush." In another drawing, nurses were scurrying to patients in their hospital beds. Rushing, for nurses, seemed to be a recurrent theme.

In the eighth drawing, the most exciting role for a nurse was noted as transporting a cot from room to room. Similarly, another student noted that the most important thing a nurse did was to transport people to the operating room, and yet another student noted that transporting patients in wheelchairs to their car was the most important thing that nurses did.

Several drawings included stern nurses in white uniforms and caps and with red crosses on their chests making patients take medicine that tasted bad. Others depicted nurses working in nurseries or teaching mothers how to care for a crying baby. Another depicted a flight nurse taking an injured patient to the hospital, and yet another showed a nurse, in a white uniform with a red cross on her chest and wearing a cap, taking blood pressures.

All of the nurses in the drawings were female and white. The overwhelming majority wore white uniforms and caps and had red crosses on their chests. All but one drawing depicted nurses in hospital settings. Many associated the nurse with pain or an unpleasant experience. Despite the educational intervention, these second-graders already held deeply ingrained stereotypes about nursing and nursing roles, which were resistant to change. This suggests that if stereotypes are this difficult to modify in second-graders, the challenges in changing the image of nursing with the greater public will likely be very difficult.

Source: Huston, C. (n.d.). *Nursing stereotypes ingrained by second grade.* Unpublished.

within the health care system, but the nurses did not stand out in their experience or affect what profession they would choose to enter. Overwhelmingly, the students said they had been "drilled on what was good about becoming a medical doctor as opposed to virtually *no* positive talk about becoming a nurse" (Sherman, para 8).

Erickson, Holm, and Chelminiak (2004) reported that the young people surveyed in their focus groups, without exception, stated they had clear mental images of a nurse as "a young, sexy woman in a traditional nurse's uniform with a short skirt, white hat, and white shoes" (Erickson et al., 2004, p. 83). This unflattering image of nurses created a perception that nurses were unprofessional and that their role in health care was trivial (Erickson et al.). Clearly, an early positive image for students is important if this is the population group the profession hopes will solve the current shortage.

Why the Stereotypes Persist

The domination and pervasiveness of nursing stereotypes is due, at least in part, to what has been called "nursing's invisibility as a profession." In 1997, the Honor Society of Nursing, Sigma Theta Tau International (STTI), commissioned the Woodhull Study on Nursing and the Media, which was conducted by the University of Rochester School of Nursing. This study analyzed 1 month of health care media coverage (2,000 health-related articles published in September 1997) to determine how often and in what context nursing was mentioned. The study found that nurses were mentioned in only 3% of health-related articles found in 16 major news publications and in only 4% of the 7 newspapers surveyed (Honor Society of Nursing, 1997–2007). In 4 news magazines, nurses were referenced in 5% of the health-related articles. In 5 trade publications that focused on the health care industry, nurses were referenced in only 1% of the articles. When nursing was mentioned, it was mostly just in passing; in many of the stories, nurses and nursing would have been more appropriate for the story's subject matter than the sources used (Honor Society of Nursing). Recommendations from the study are shown in Box 20.3.

CONSIDER

"The media will continue to miss major elements of health care news if it continues to disregard the contributions of nurses. By the same token, if nurses merely wait for the media to discover their emerging roles as researchers, educators, problem solvers, and practitioners, they are doing the public—whom they seek to serve—a disservice" (Honor Society of Nursing, 1997–2007, para 9).

Finally, nurses should recognize that media stereotypes are not limited to nonprofessional sources. Even advertisements in medical and nursing journals often included stereotypical and demeaning nursing images, with frequent depictions of nurses as dependent, passive minor figures on the health care scene. If nurses are not depicted accurately in their own trade publications, how can they expect representation in other types of media to be better?

CONSEQUENCES OF INACCURATE OR NEGATIVE IMAGES

Inaccurate or negative public images of nursing have many consequences, particularly because these images influence the attitudes of patients, other health care providers, policy makers, and politicians. Perhaps even more critical, given the current, severe nursing shortage, is that negative attitudes about nursing might discourage capable prospective nurses who will instead choose another career that offers greater appeal in stature, status, and salary.

Recruitment Challenges

One significant consequence of the public not understanding both the scope of practice and the skill level required to be a nurse is that it may limit the profession's ability to recruit the best and brightest students. Whereas 30 years ago, a significant number of young people would have chosen to be nurse when they grew

---

BOX 20.3 | RECOMMENDATIONS FROM THE WOODHULL STUDY

1. Both media and nursing should take a more proactive role in establishing dialogue.
2. The often-repeated advice in media articles and advertisements to "consult your doctor" ignores the role of nurses in health care and needs to be changed to "consult your primary health care provider."
3. Journalists should distinguish researchers with doctoral degrees from medical doctors to add clarity to health care coverage.
4. To provide comprehensive coverage of health care, the media should include information by and about nurses.
5. It is essential to distinguish health care (the umbrella) from medicine or subject matter in the media.

Source: Honor Society of Nursing, Sigma Theta Tau International (1997–2007). *Woodhull study on nursing and the media.* Available at: **http://www.nursingsociety.org/Media/Pages/woodhall.aspx.** Accessed September 5, 2008.

up, less than 5% of students responded so in a 2004 study (Erickson et al., 2004).

As with other predominantly female professions, the literature suggests that many clients and their families undervalue nursing and do not understand what it is that nurses do that makes a difference in patient outcomes. Indeed, many nurses will honestly admit that they had little factual basis for what nursing would be like when they chose it as a profession. Instead, what drove them to become a nurse were actually images that emphasized the caring, nurturing, and personal rewards associated with the profession.

Still, newer research is encouraging. Donelan et al. (2008) found that nursing, along with several other health/science careers, was viewed positively as a career choice by 70% of the public. Women were more likely than men to give nursing a positive rating (74% vs. 64%), as were those already employed in health care versus those who were not (80% vs. 68%). Finally, Donelan et al.'s research revealed that one in four Americans had personally considered a career in nursing, although only 15% identified it as a serious consideration.

Similarly, a study by Seago, Spetz, Alvarado, Keane, and Grumbach (2006) of more than 3,000 college students in California found that students generally had favorable perceptions of nursing, with two thirds agreeing that nursing had good income potential, job security, and interesting work. However, nursing lagged behind the other occupations in perceptions of independence at work and was more likely to be perceived as a "women's" occupation.

Self-Concept and Self-Esteem

Another consequence of inaccurate nursing stereotypes is that they can threaten the collective identity and self-esteem of all nurses. Fletcher (2007) argued that public image is intimately intertwined with nurse self-image, and that nurses frequently do not think highly of themselves or have a positive self-image.

In an effort to explore how nursing student perceptions of the public image of nursing affected their self-concept and academic performance in nursing school, Wallace (2007) completed a quantitative descriptive study of 63 students enrolled in an associate degree nursing program. The study found a positive relationship between participants' perception of the public image of nursing and their self-concept. There was no relationship between participants' self-concept and grades earned in nursing school. Wallace concluded that because the public image of nurses and nursing can have a critical effect on nurses' self-concept, it has the potential to affect whether nursing is chosen as a career, as well as how effectively nurses function in a wide array of situations.

THE CENTER FOR NURSING ADVOCACY

Most nurses are upset about their depiction in contemporary media, but their efforts to respond to and change the situation have been fragmented. A more unified voice has been possible since the creation of the Center for Nursing Advocacy in 2001. The Center was created when Sandy Summers and seven other graduate nursing students at the Johns Hopkins University in Baltimore joined forces to address the media's disrespectful portrayal of nursing.

As a 501c(3) corporation, the Center "seeks to increase public understanding of the central, front-line role nurses play in modern health care" (Center for Nursing Advocacy, n.d.-b, para 1). They do this by promoting "more accurate, balanced and frequent media portrayals of nurses and by increasing the media's use of nurses as expert sources" (para 1). Moreover, "The Center's ultimate goal is to foster growth in the size and diversity of the nursing profession at a time of critical shortage, to strengthen nursing practice, teaching and research, and to improve the health care system" (para 1). The Center's work is funded by individual memberships and donations.

CHANGING NURSING'S IMAGE IN THE PUBLIC EYE

Changing nursing's image in the public eye will not be easy. Nor will there be a silver bullet. Instead, multiple strategies are needed, including active interaction with the media and restriction of the term "nurse" to licensed nurses. In addition, nurses must increase their efforts to publicly praise and value nursing in addition to emphasizing how nursing uniquely contributes to patients achieving their desired health outcomes. Finally, nurses will need to become even more involved in the political processes that shape their profession.

Accomplishing this will take time and resources, including the time, energy, and funding of coalitions, foundations, and professional nursing organizations. Perhaps most important, it will take a concerted effort by individual nurses that will come only by first recognizing that there is a need to take action and then by doing what is necessary to achieve that goal. Gonzales (2005, para 12) agreed, arguing that nurses must "get involved in changing the media's portrayal of nurses because each time our image is harmed, our nation's healthcare is harmed."

Finding a Voice in the Press

One of the most important strategies needed to change nursing's image is to change the image of nursing in the mind of the image-makers. That means proactively seeking positive and accurate media exposure of what nursing really is and what nurses really do. This job cannot be left to professional nursing organizations or to the image-makers. Nurses' self-worth needs to be recognized and proclaimed.

CONSIDER

Knowing how to interact with the media is not intuitive for most nurses. Media training should always be provided to give nurses the skills and self-confidence to be effective in this role.

Unfortunately, many nurses feel ill prepared or lack the self confidence to interact with the media. Indeed Kemmer and da Silva (2007) found that communications professionals working in radio, television, the written press, and advertising and events expressed ignorance about nurses' field of work, job market, and profession categorization. They also suggested that nurses were invisible in media and the society and argued that it is nursing's responsibility to obtain professional recognition and visibility.

This cannot be emphasized enough. Nurse are uniquely qualified to speak with editors, reporters, and media producers on topics related to health care because they have a view from the front lines and are able to localize national health care issues. Nurses are also well qualified to simplify medical gibberish, explain the latest health care research, and identify current trends. Nurses, then, must be taught the basic skills necessary to self-confidently interact with the media. Nurses must also never pass up the opportunity to work with the media and should always view the media as playing a critical role in changing nursing's image.

CONSIDER

Nurses are experts in health care. Their invisibility in the media is likely a result of nurses lacking the basic skills and self-confidence to get involved, not that the media does not want to talk to nurses.

Gordon (2004) suggested that public relation (PR) departments in hospitals also have a responsibility in terms of journalistic coverage of nurses. Journalists generally must call hospital PR departments to find out whom to talk to when covering a particular topic and to get permission for interviews. Yet, according to Gordon, many hospital PR departments conceal the contributions of nurses. In fact, hospital PR departments "are sometimes described as 'nurses' worst enemies,' and when PR staff direct journalists to the 'real' experts on, say, diabetes they are invariably doctors" (Gordon, para 10).

Gordon (2004) concluded that if the media are to inform the public about nursing, senior nurses must teach their hospital PR staff why nursing is important and what nurses really do—and then direct them to spread the message outside their institutions. Crucially, they must ensure that nurses feel comfortable talking to journalists.

Reclaiming the Title of "Nurse"

Another strategy needed to improve the image of nursing is to assure that use of the term "nurse" is limited to licensed nurses. The International Council of Nurses (ICN) stated in 2004 that the term "nurse" "should be protected by law and applied to and used only by those legally authorised to practice the full scope of nursing" (ICN, 2004, para 1). In addition, all state boards of nursing have passed legislation restricting unlicensed personnel from using the title of "nurse." Unfortunately, on a regular basis, nursing aides and attendants either intentionally or unintentionally misrepresent themselves as nurses.

With the increased use of unlicensed assistive personnel and cross-training in the 1990s, a blurring of titles, roles, and responsibilities occurred among RNs, licensed vocational nurses, and unlicensed support staff.

Nametags increasingly recognized all staff as "care partners" or "associates," and some hospitals went so far as to prohibit the listing of RN on a name tag. At the same time, a loss of differentiated uniforms further added to the public's confusion about who truly was caring for them.

In addition, RNs often contribute to the confusion by how they introduce themselves to patients. Nurses are often very casual about how they introduce themselves to patients, rarely identifying their specific role as the leader of the health care team. Nor do they differentiate how the roles of other members of the health care team differ. This may be due in part to typical female role socialization, which encourages women not to promote themselves, or it may be part of a team-building effort. Either way, patients end up confused about who the leader of the team is or how their roles differ. In addition, the media frequently perpetuates the misappropriate use of the term "nurse" by referring to all nurse's aides, volunteers who do health-related work, and medical assistants as "nurses."

Dressing Like Professionals

Nurses in this country began shedding their white uniforms in the 1960s as part of the anticonformist movement. As a result, the identity of the RN has blurred. Whereas nursing caps and white starched uniforms were often impractical in caring for acutely ill patients, 30 years ago the public knew who the nurse was by the uniform he or she wore. Today, many patients are unable to tell the members of the health care team apart, a problem that has become worse as the result of widespread adoption of scrubs as work uniforms.

Skorupski and Rea (2006), in their analysis of how uniforms affect nursing's public image, found that older patients consistently identified white uniforms as essential for nurses to be considered both professional and approachable. Members of Generation X and Baby Boomers, however, said nurses in print uniforms were approachable, although they did not associate them with being professional. The authors concluded that the lack of a standardized uniform leaves patients confused about who is caring for them.

Some nurse leaders have suggested that a return to white uniforms would restore the public respect that was lost when "nurses stopped dressing like professionals." However, nurses are split on the issue of whether uniforms are essential to maintaining professionalism in nursing. They argue that comfort and uniformity of dress are equally important and that uniforms are not a requirement for professional trust and respect.

> **DISCUSSION POINT**
> Is it the white uniform that makes the professional, or is it the actions nurses take that define what a nurse is?

Positive Talk by Nurses about Nursing

Another strategy for improving the image of nursing is to change how nurses talk about nursing to others. Some nurses bad-mouth the profession and discourage young adults from considering nursing as a profession, yet go on to bemoan the current nurse shortage. The effect of these comments by nurses to the general public should not be underestimated in terms of their effect on the recruitment of young people into the profession.

Donelan et al.'s (2008) research found that the public is significantly more likely to recommend a career in either nursing or medicine than are either doctors or nurses. In fact, Donelan et al. found that one in three Americans have discussed nursing as a career choice with a family member or friend, and so how nurses talk about nursing affects the perception of nursing by the general public.

The reality is that every nurse controls the image of nursing. Nursing, like any other profession, has strengths and weaknesses. It is important, however, that nurses enjoy their work, whatever it might be. Nurses should not stay in jobs that make them unhappy, because it demoralizes everyone around them. Whining and acting like a victim does little to improve the situation.

The bottom line is that nurses must tell the public that nursing is an essential service with equal worth to other professions; that it can provide many services better than other health care disciplines; and that nursing is often more cost-effective than other disciplines. The public's demand for nursing likely rests on the demand nursing creates for itself in the public's eye.

In addition, Erickson et al. (2004) suggested that nurses must go beyond just positive talk about nursing; nurses must be ambassadors for the profession. Erickson et al. suggested that this can be done by making classroom visits as nurse "ambassadors," by allowing young people interested in nursing to job-shadow an empowered nurse, and by participating in "bring your child to work days." All of these activities allow nurses to be positive role models for their profession. In addition, Erickson et al. suggested that nurses should visit youth clubs and organizations such as Boy Scouts, Girl Scouts, and the Boys and Girls Clubs to talk with young people about the benefits and rewards of a nursing career.

Emphasizing the Uniqueness of Nursing

Another tactic nurses can use to improve nursing's image is not only to emphasize the profession's unique combination of "caring" and "curing," but also to underscore the depth and breadth of the scientific perspective that underlies its practice. Evidence-based practice and the application of best practice principles are an expectation for contemporary professional nursing practice. Nurses, then, must emphasize how clinical research and the use of current best evidence affect their decision making and the care they provide.

In addition, newer research on nursing sensitivity and nursing outcomes is able to clarify what it is that nurses do that makes a difference in patient outcomes; there is increasing recognition that patients get better as a result of nursing interventions, not despite them. Generally speaking, however, the public knows very little about the research base that drives high-quality, evidence-based practice, and it is nurses who are in the best position to tell them about it.

CONSIDER
The efforts of individual nurses can multiply to create a critical mass that change the stereotypes held by not only the public, but also by nurses (Fletcher, 2007).

Participating in the Political Arena

The political process can influence nearly everything nurses do and every problem they confront each day. In addition, public opinion is often based on inaccurate images, and nursing is no exception. Participating in the political arena, then, becomes a powerful strategy for changing the public's image of nursing.

The reality, however, is that although the nursing profession has some strong professional organizations, of the approximately 2.9 million RNs, only a small percentage are members of national nursing organizations. This limits the profession's ability to be a force in the political arena. In addition, many nurses know little about the political process or feel too overwhelmed by the daily demands of their job to become involved in addressing larger professional issues in the political arena. Some nurses just assume that the best interests of the profession are being guarded by some unknown force out there. Legislators wonder whether inactivity means simply not caring or not having an opinion. The end result is that nurses are inadequately represented in the political arena, and another opportunity for nurses to be represented as knowledgeable, active participants in the health care system is lost.

Because the underlying causes of the profession's political inactivity are numerous, just as the strategies needed to address this issue are complex, it is only discussed briefly here. Instead, a separate chapter has been dedicated to more fully discussing the issue (see Chapter 22).

CONCLUSIONS

Fletcher (2007) suggested that the problem of image has been a struggle for nurses since the 1800s. From a sociological perspective, conflicting stereotypes of nursing have not served the nursing profession well, and a disconnect continues to exist between reality and public image. The greater public clearly does not understand what professional nursing is all about, and the nursing profession has done a poor job of correcting long-standing historically inaccurate stereotypes. Gonzales (2005, para 14) suggested that "as long as the public only sees nurses through mass media stereotypes our messages will fall on deaf ears and our nation's healthcare will continue to crumble."

The responsibility for changing nursing's image lies squarely on the shoulders of those who claim nursing as their profession. Until such time as nurses are able to agree on the desired collective image and are willing to do what is necessary to both tell and show the public what that image is, little will change. Derogatory stereotypes are likely to continue to undermine public confidence in and respect for the professional nurse.

FOR ADDITIONAL DISCUSSION

1. Historically, images of physicians in the media have been more positive than those of nurses. Why? What factors have led to this difference?

2. Some nurses feel that no longer wearing white uniforms and caps has reduced the professionalism of nursing. Is how nurses dress an important part of public image? Would reverting to more traditional nursing attire improve nursing's public image?

3. Would you want your son or daughter to be a nurse? What have you told them about nursing that would either encourage or discourage them from doing so?

4. Who are the best-known nurses currently depicted in the media (radio, television, movies) you access on a regular basis? Do their characters represent nursing stereotypes that have been discussed in this chapter?

5. What do you believe to be the greatest restraining forces that discourage nurses from interacting with the media? Is media training the answer?

6. The contributions of Johnson & Johnson to improve the image of nursing and increase recruitment into the nursing profession are unparalleled. Why would a corporation such as Johnson & Johnson be interested in this pursuit? Why did such an initiative not originate with a professional nursing organization?

7. Are nurses confused about what shared image they want the U.S. public to have of their profession?

REFERENCES

Allen, D. (2004). No holds barred. *Nursing Standard, 18*(24), 24–26.

Amazon.com (2008). *Single Dad, Nurse Bride.* Reader reviews. Available at: http://www.amazon.com/Single-Nurse-Harlequin-Medical-Romance/dp/037319904X. Accessed September 4, 2008.

Center for Nursing Advocacy (n.d.-a). *Are nurses angels of mercy?* Available at: http://www.nursingadvocacy.org/faq/nf/are_nurses_angels.html. Accessed September 3, 2008.

Center for Nursing Advocacy (n.d.-b). *Mission statement.* Available at: http://www.nursingadvocacy.org/about_us/mission_statement.html. Accessed September 4, 2008.

Center for Nursing Advocacy (2005a). *Helen Wheels, RN—Compu Caddy pulls battleaxe ad.* July 25, 2005. Available at: http://www.nursingadvocacy.org/news/2005jul/compucaddy.html. Accessed September 3, 2008.

Center for Nursing Advocacy (2005b). *Grey's Anatomy—2005 to present.* March 27, 2005. Available at: http://www.nursingadvocacy.org/media/tv/2005/greys.html. Accessed September 6, 2008.

Center for Nursing Advocacy (2007a). *Don't you think I'm so sexy—I'm just so fresh, so clean!* September 27, 2007. Available at: http://www.nursingadvocacy.org/news/2007/sep/27_dentyne.html. Accessed September 4, 2008.

Center for Nursing Advocacy (2007b). *Getting fresher.* October 6, 2007. Available at: http://www.nursingadvocacy.org/news/2007/oct/06_dentyne.html. Accessed September 4, 2008.

Center for Nursing Advocacy (2008). *Let's "celebrate the ladies who give lollipops and band aids" with a Nurse Nancy bracelet!* Available at: http://nursingadvocacy.org/news/2008/mar/18_angela_moore.html. Accessed September 5, 2008.

Clichés abound in medical romance novels. (2007). Available at: http://www.6minutes.com.au/articles/z1/view.asp?id=133899. Accessed September 2, 2008.

Donelan, K., Buerhaus, P., Desroches, C., Dittus, R., & Dutwin, D. (2008). Public perceptions of nursing careers: The influence of the media and nursing shortages. *Nursing Economics, 26*(3), 143–150, 165.

Erickson, J. I., Holm, L. J., & Chelminiak, L. (2004). Keeping the nursing shortage from becoming a nursing crisis. *Journal of Nursing Administration, 34*(2), 83–87.

Fletcher, K. K. F. (2007). Image: Changing how women nurses think about themselves. Literature review. *Journal of Advanced Nursing, 58*(3), 207–215.

Florence Nightingale. "The Nightingale Pledge." (n.d.). Available at: http://www.countryjoe.com/nightingale/pledge.htm. Accessed September 6, 2008.

Gonzales, L. (2005). *Nursing and the media: A mission for the Center for Nursing Advocacy.* NevadaRNformation. Available at: http://findarticles.com/p/articles/mi_qa4102/is_200511/ai_n15744770. Accessed September 4, 2008.

Gordon, S. (2004). Coast to coast media friendly. *Nursing Management—UK, 10*(10), 9. Honor Society of Nursing, Sigma Theta Tau International (1997–2007). *Woodhull study on nursing and the media.* Available at: http://www.nursingsociety.org/Media/Pages/woodhall.aspx. Accessed 9/5/08.

Huston, C. (n.d.). *Nursing stereotypes ingrained by second grade.* Unpublished.

International Council of Nurses (ICN) (2004). *Position statement. Protection of the title "nurse."* Available at: http://www.icn.ch/pstitle99rev.htm. Accessed September 5, 2008.

Jones, J. M. (2007). *Lobbyists debut at bottom of honesty and ethics list.* Available at: http://www.gallup.com/poll/103123/Lobbyists-Debut-Bottom-Honesty-Ethics-List.aspx. Accessed September 2, 2008.

Kalisch, B. J., Begeny, S., & Neumann, S. (2007). The image of the nurse on the Internet. *Nursing Outlook, 55*(4), 182–188.

Kemmer, L. F. & da Silva, M. J. P. (2007). Nurses' visibility according to the perceptions of the communication professionals. *Revista Latino-Americana de Enfermagem, 15*(2), 191–198.

Lagu, T., Kaufman, E., Asch, D., & Armstrong, K. (2008). Content of weblogs written by health professionals. *Journal of General Internal Medicine, 23*(7). Available at: *http://www.springerlink.com.mantis.csuchico.edu/ content/k7r6123g4x776q5l/fulltext.html. Accessed* September 4, 2008.

Lovesick doctors and lovelorn nurses (2007). *Nurse Ratched's Place.* Available at: http://nurseratcheds.

blogspot.com/2007/11/lovesick-doctors-and-lovelorn-nurses.html. Accessed September 2, 2008.

Merriam-Webster Online Dictionary (2008). *Image—Definition.* Available at: http://www.merriam-webster.com/dictionary/image. Accessed September 1, 2008.

Nurses and firemen top fantasy poll. (2006). The Age Company, LTD. Fairfax Digital. London. Available at: http://www.theage.com.au/news/world/nurses-and-firemen-top-fantasy-poll/2006/08/23/1156012609767.html. Accessed September 5, 2008.

Nursing stereotypes: Images that underestimate the profession. (n.d.). Available at: http://www.english.iup.edu/eaware/nursing/. Accessed September 2, 2008.

Procter & Gamble pulls offending ad. (2003). *Nursing, 33*(8), 35.

Ryan, K (n.d.). *Doctors and nurses.* Available at: http://www.romantictimes.com/books_themes.php?theme=69. Accessed September 2, 2008.

Seago, J., Spetz, J., Alvarado, A., Keane, D., & Grumbach, K. (2006). The nursing shortage: Is it really about image? *Journal of Healthcare Management, 51*(2), 96–108; discussion 109–110.

Sherman, G. (2000). *Memo to Nurses for Healthier Tomorrow Coalition Members.* St. Louis, MO: JWT Specialized Communications Healthcare Group.

Skorupski, V. J., & Rea, R. E. (2006). Patients' perceptions of today's nursing attire: Exploring dual images. *Journal of Nursing Administration, 36*(9), 393–401.

Teig, S., & Susskind, J. (2008). Truck driver or nurse? The impact of gender roles and occupational status on children's occupational preferences. *Sex Roles, 58*(11/12), 848–863.

Waitresses dressed as naughty nurses. (2006). MSNBC, December 8, 2006. Available at: http://www.msnbc.msn.com/id/16112393/. Accessed September 4, 2008.

Wallace, C. B. (2007). *Nursing students' perceptions of the public image of nursing.* Dissertation. Capella University, Minneapolis, MN.

Woldt, M. (2008). *Nurse perspective. Male nurses and the caring touch.* Healthcare POV. Available at: http://community.advanceweb.com/blogs/nurses7/archive/2008/07/22/male-nurses-and-the-caring-touch.aspx. Accessed September 5, 2008.

BIBLIOGRAPHY

Better public image wanted. (2007). *Nursing Times, 103*(31), 2.

Changing views: Influencing how the public sees nursing. (2007). *ISNA Bulletin, 33*(3), 17–21.

Culp, M. L. (2008). *Stereotypes down for male nurses.* NYDailyNews.com. Available at: http://www.nydailynews.com/money/2008/05/12/2008-05-12_stereotypes_down_for_male_nurses.html. Accessed September 4, 2008.

Hanchett, M. (2008). Please, no love or kisses. A reflection on the image of nurses. *Journal of Gerontological Nursing, 34*(6), 3–4.

Harding, T. (2007). The construction of men who are nurses as gay. *Journal of Advanced Nursing, 60*(6), 636–644.

Image matters. (2007). *Nursing Standard, 22*(6), 26–27.

Kennedy, M. (2007). *Angel of mercy or power-crazed meddler? Unseen letters challenge view of pioneer nurse.* Available at: http://www.guardian.co.uk/uk/2007/sep/03/health.healthandwellbeing. Accessed September 4, 2008.

Leathem, C. (2007). Stereotypes belittle us, but we are now taking ourselves too seriously . . . Petra Kendall-Raynor, Nurse Stereotypes (News December 6). *Nursing Standard, 21*(17), 32–39.

Malchau, S. (2007). 'Angels in nursing': Images of nursing sisters in a Lutheran context in the nineteenth and twentieth centuries. *Nursing Inquiry, 14*(4), 289–298.

Meadus, R.J., & Twomey, J. C. (2007). Men in nursing: Making the right choice. *Canadian Nurse, 103*(2), 13–16.

Newland, J. (2007). Editor's memo. Tinseltown nurses and public perception. *Nurse Practitioner, 32*(2), 5.

Reyes, S. (2007). Male nurses stitching stereotypes. *The Lantern—The Student Voice at Ohio State University,* May 26, 2007. Available at: http://media.www.thelantern.com/media/storage/paper333/news/2007/04/26/Campus/Male-Nurses.Stitching.Stereotypes-2883200.shtml. Accessed February 20, 2009.

Salvage, J. (2006). More than a makeover is needed to improve nursing's image. *Journal of Advanced Nursing, 54*(3), 259–260.

Scarrow, J. (2007). Challenging the stereotypes. *Registered Nurse Journal, 19*(3), 24.

Spragley, F., & Francis, K. (2006). Nursing uniforms: Professional symbol or outdated relic? *Nursing Management, 37*(10), 55–58.

WEB RESOURCES

American Nurses Association, Considering Nursing	http://nursingworld.org/EspeciallyForYou/StudentNurses.aspx
A Positive Image Right From the Top (2008)	http://include.nurse.com/apps/pbcs.dll/article?AID=/20080616/NJ02/106160067
Center for Nursing Advocacy	http://www.nursingadvocacy.org/news/news.html
Discover Nursing, The Johnson and Johnson Campaign for Nursing's Future	http://www.discovernursing.com/
Job Opportunities for Nurses 2005-2020	http://www.discovernursing.com/job-opportunities
Looking for a Few Good Men	http://www.minoritynurse.com/features/nurse_emp/05-03-02a.html
Media Training Programs for Nurses (Donna Cardillo and the Center for Nursing Advocacy)	http://www.nursingadvocacy.org/action/media_training.html

Nurses Do Research? How Nursing's Public Image Obscures Nursing Science (2007)

http://videos.med.wisc.edu/videoInfo.php?videoid=244

Nursing Dean Courtney Lyder shatters stereotypes (2008)

http://spotlight.ucla.edu/faculty/courtney-lyder-nursing/

Nursing Stereotypes, Images That Underestimate the Profession

http://www.english.iup.edu/eaware/nursing/

One Hundred Networks and Resources for Male Nurses (July 2008)

http://www.nursingschoolsearch.com/blog/2008/07/100-networks-and-resources-for-male-nurses/

The In/Visbility of Nurses in Cyberculture

http://www.visiblenurse.com/visiblenurse7.html

CHAPTER 21

Advanced Practice Nursing: The Latest Issues and Trends

• MARGARET ROWBERG •

Learning Objectives

The learner will be able to:

1. Differentiate among the definition of and roles commonly assumed by certified nurse-midwives (CNMs), clinical nurse specialists (CNSs), nurse practitioners (NPs), and certified registered nurse anesthetists (CRNAs).
2. Explore reasons why so few nurses seek doctoral education preparation, particularly the PhD.
3. Describe the impetus for and controversies associated with the granting of the Doctor of Nursing Practice (DNP) degree.
4. Describe the driving and restraining forces for increasing the entry educational level for advanced practice nursing to that of a practice doctorate.
5. Explore issues surrounding role recognition for APNs, including confusion over educational entry levels, restrictions in scope of practice, and the lack of full prescriptive authority.
6. Identify the current educational entry educational level for each of the four types of advanced practice nurses.
7. Identify the educational preparation and common role expectations of the clinical nurse leader (CNL).
8. Reflect on whether nurses educated at the DNP level should complete a certification exam based on the same test that physicians take to qualify for a medical license.
9. Explore how scope of practice and reimbursement in advanced practice nursing have been influenced by organized medicine.
10. Analyze evidence-based literature that compares outcomes for patients cared for by APNs with those of other health care providers.
11. Identify local, state, and national task forces that are working to remove the barriers to practice for APNs.
12. Reflect on his or her interest in exploring advanced practice nursing as a career choice.

According to the American Association of Colleges of Nursing (AACN) (2004a, para 17), "The health system's increasing demand for front-line primary care, and the accelerating drive toward managed care, prevention, and cost-efficiency are driving a need for nurses with advanced practice skills in this country." Although increasing numbers of advanced practice registered nurses (APRNs) are skilled clinical practitioners, inadequate numbers have the knowledge and expertise to address persistent professional issues arising in the health care system.

In 2002, the AACN requested that a group of nurse leaders study an evolving discussion about developing a clinical or practice doctorate. Several nursing schools had existing practice doctorate programs, and many more were assessing whether to develop such a program (AACN, 2004b). The AACN thought it would be appropriate to develop a position about this degree. The AACN (2007) believed that nursing had the "unparalleled opportunity and capability to address the critical issues that face the nation's current health care system" (p. 3). They also believed that nursing "has the answers to the predominant health care dilemmas of the future" (p. 3) and that "each of the prevailing health problems is suited to the nursing paradigm. Their amelioration is what nursing students are educated to do" (p. 4). Consequently, the AACN (2007), after a task force recommendation, also proposed the development of the Clinical Nurse Leader role.

There have been many articles written and documents published that address the recommendations of the AACN task forces. This chapter discusses the development of the Doctor of Nursing Practice (DNP) and the Clinical Nurse Leader (CNL) and offers some insight into the current trends, issues, and concerns surrounding these evolving new roles.

ROLE DEFINITION

There are more than 240,000 APRNs in the United States (National Sample Survey of Registered Nurses [NSSRN], 2004). Four categories of nurses are considered to be APRNs: nurse practitioners (NPs), clinical nurse specialists (CNSs), certified nurse midwives (CNMs), and certified registered nurse anesthetists (CRNAs).

Approximately 141,000 of the APRNs in the United States are NPs, including 14,600 who are both NPs and CNSs. More than 72,500 are CNSs, 13,600 are CNMs, and 32,500 are CRNAs (NSSRN, 2004, paras 34–36). These numbers represent a 22.5% increase since 2000, when the previous survey was completed (NSSRN, para 34). The survey further reported that three of four APRNs, or more than 179,000, are master's prepared, with another 18,000 stating that they received a post-master's certificate in their advanced practice education (NSSRN, para 34). Although all advanced practice roles require specialization of knowledge and a high degree of practice autonomy, the roles and their associated scope of practice differ greatly.

Nurse Practitioners

According to the American College of Nurse Practitioners (ACNP) (n.d.),

> Nurse practitioners are registered nurses who are prepared, through advanced education and clinical training, to provide a wide range of preventive and acute health care services to individuals of all ages. NPs take health histories and provide physical examinations; diagnose and treat common acute and chronic problems; interpret laboratory results and x-rays; prescribe and manage medications and other therapies; provide health teaching and supportive counseling with an emphasis on prevention of illness and health maintenance; and refer patients to other health professionals as needed (para 1).

Clinical Nurse Specialists

The National Association of Clinical Nurse Specialists (NACNS) (n.d.) defines CNSs as

> licensed registered nurses who have graduate preparation (Master's or Doctorate) in nursing as a Clinical Nurse Specialist. Clinical Nurse Specialists are expert clinicians in a specialized area of nursing practice, be it a population or setting, disease or medical subspecialty, a type of care or problem. Clinical Nurse Specialists practice in a wide variety of health care settings. In addition to providing direct patient care, Clinical Nurse Specialists influence care outcomes by providing expert consultation for nursing staffs and by implementing improvements in health care delivery systems. Clinical Nurse Specialist practice integrates nursing practice, which focuses on assisting patients in the prevention or resolution of illness, with medical diagnosis and treatment of disease, injury and disability (para 1).

Certified Nurse-Midwives

The American College of Nurse-Midwives (ACNM) (n.d.) states

> The word midwife describes a woman who is "with women" at birth. Midwives practice under a philosophy of care that focuses on the specific needs of women, empowers women to actively participate in their health care, and minimizes unnecessary intervention. Certified nurse-midwives and certified midwives (CM) are highly educated professionals who work collaboratively with physicians (para 1).
>
> All CMs and CNMs have earned at least a bachelor's degree, and more than 80 percent hold a master's degree or higher (para 3).
>
> Today's CNM/CM is a skilled healthcare professional who provides primary healthcare to women. This includes evaluation, assessment,

treatment, and referral to a specialist, if required. CNMs and CMs emphasize health promotion, education, and disease prevention. CNMs and CMs provide preconception counseling, care during pregnancy and childbirth, normal gynecological services, and care of the peri- and post-menopausal woman. With health education as a primary focus, CNMs and CMs help prevent problems and assist women in developing and maintaining good health habits. Midwives can prescribe medications including methods of contraception and treatment for common infections" (para 5).

Certified Registered Nurse Anesthetists

According to AllNursingSchools (n.d.),

A Nurse Anesthetist, or Certified Registered Nurse Anesthetist (CRNA), is a licensed professional nurse who provides the same anesthesia services as an anesthesiologist (MD). After completing extensive education and training with a completion of a master's degree, CRNAs become nationally certified . . . . Working closely with other health care professionals such as surgeons, dentists, podiatrists and anesthesiologists, a CRNA takes care of a patient's anesthesia needs before, during and after surgery or the delivery of a baby. CRNAs practice in a variety of settings in the private and public sectors and in the U.S. military (paras 1–7).

BACKGROUND OF ADVANCED PRACTICE NURSING IN THE UNITED STATES

APRNs have been making significant contributions to the health of the nation and around the world for more than 40 years, but they function in a health care system in the United States that is in need of change. In 1999, the Institute of Medicine (IOM) published a report titled *To Err is Human: Building a Safer Health System* that stated that as many as 98,000 people die each year due to errors that occur while receiving health care (IOM, 1999). The IOM further reported in 2001 that "research on quality of care reveals a health care system that frequently falls short in its ability to translate knowledge into practice, and to apply new technology safely and appropriately" (IOM, 2001, p. 3).

Although these reports have been in existence for nearly a decade, an unacceptable high number of errors continue to be reported. New safeguards have been put in place in most institutions, but nursing can and should be a key profession in leading the way to significant change to the health care system. It will require nurses, however, who have advanced degrees and who plan to remain in clinical practice: "The necessity for practitioners who focus on promotion of health and wellness and the prevention of disease has emerged as not only a good and wholesome thing to do in society, but also as a means of addressing escalating medical costs" (AACN, 2007, p. 4).

Part of the problem in achieving that goal is that nursing has so few nurses with doctoral degrees. According to the NSSRN (2004), of almost 3 million nurses, only slightly more than 40,000 obtained a doctorate after becoming a nurse, and only 5.8% of these nurses focused their study on clinical practice (paras 31–33). By comparison, there were more than 57,000 engineering doctorates awarded in the last 10 years alone (National Science Foundation [NSF], 2007). It was further discovered in the NSSRN survey that only 8,600 of more than 220,000 nurses pursuing further education in 2004 were studying to obtain a doctorate (para 33). According to the NSF (2007), however, only slightly more than 1,700 people were pursuing doctorates in a health-related field in 2004, although the number did increase to more than 1,900 by 2006.

> ### DISCUSSION POINT
> Why do you think so few nurses are willing to pursue a doctoral degree?

There are many reasons why nurses have not pursued advanced degrees, but Apold (2008) suggested the following:

Nursing has fallen short in mentoring nurses for research career trajectories. The requirement of the "one year of med/surg" after graduation, the development of boring and pedantic introductory research courses, the invention of language for nursing theory, and general failure to create learning environments that celebrate the development of the discipline has resulted in the valuing of practice and the dread of research (p. 104).

It is also believed that nurses avoid master's and doctoral education because salaries for people with these degrees have not kept pace with salaries in the clinical setting. Many associate or baccalaureate degree nurses are making more than $73,000 a year, whereas faculty members who hold a master's degree or higher may only be making about $58,000 a year (AACN, 2005b).

These issues have contributed to a lack of appropriately prepared nurses who are willing to accept the challenge of the health care system and work toward effecting the needed changes. Research by PhD-prepared nurses is essential, but clinically active professionals who have a background in policy, leadership, and organizational behavior are vital to making needed changes. Others agree and suggest a possible solution. The National Academy of Sciences recommended that nursing should "develop a new nonresearch clinical doctorate, similar to M.D. and Pharm.D. in medicine and pharmacy respectively" to help fill the need for practitioners and faculty (National Research Council, 2005, p. 74).

About the same time as these reports were released, reports from the American Hospital Association Commission on Workforce for Hospitals and Health Systems (2002), the Joint Commission on Accreditation of Healthcare Organizations (JCAHO) (2002), and the Robert Wood Johnson Foundation (Kimball & O'Neill, 2002) appeared that discussed the issues surrounding the nursing shortage and the need for health professionals to be educated with an emphasis on evidence-based practice. The United States is faced with several major problems: a health care system in need of reform, an ever-increasing nursing shortage, and an insufficient number of practicing nurses who are educationally prepared to address these problems.

DISCUSSION POINT

Do you think the United States can recover from its severe nursing shortage? If so, how long will it take?

Because of these problems, the AACN initiated several task forces to assess these issues. In 2002 one expert group was asked "to examine the current status of clinical or practice doctoral programs, compare various models, and make recommendations regarding future development" (AACN, 2004b, p. 1). The group was to determine whether a practice doctorate would be an appropriate degree for advanced practice registered nurses. Another task force was asked to assess how

nursing could provide the kind of leadership needed in light of the issues in the health care system and the ever-increasing nursing shortage. Ultimately the Board of the AACN proposed to its members that the DNP degree and the CNL role be developed.

THE DOCTOR OF NURSING PRACTICE

It is important to start the discussion of the DNP with the exact words from AACN to clarify why it recommended that this new degree be developed. In its position statement, the AACN (2004a) stated

Doctoral programs in nursing and other practice disciplines can be categorized into two distinct types: research-focused and practice-focused. The term practice, *specifically nursing practice, as conceptualized in this document refers to any form of nursing intervention that influences health care outcomes for individuals or populations, including the direct care of individual patients, management of care for individuals and populations, administration of nursing and health care organizations, and the development and implementation of health policy. Preparation at the practice doctorate level includes advanced preparation in nursing, based on nursing science, and is at the highest level of nursing practice.*

What distinguishes this definition of practice from others is that it includes both direct care provided to patients by individual clinicians as well as direct care policies, programs and protocols that are organized, monitored, and continuously improved upon by expert nurse clinicians (p. 3).

CONSIDER

The definition of practice has been expanded to include policy and program development with ongoing continuous quality improvement strategies.

It is frustrating for APRNs to learn that despite the fact that the master's degree required many clinical hours and course credits, it often does not provide an education in areas such as leadership, health policy, practice management, information technology, process and outcomes evaluation, and similar topics that are vital to health care. APRNs are finding that they must take continuing education courses to help fill the gap. Schools of nursing have struggled to keep up with the increasing demand for this knowledge while maintaining a reasonable length to their master's degree programs. Consequently, the AACN responded to the need to proactively move forward to develop the practice or clinical doctorate.

Doctoral programs are not new to nursing. Apold (2008) reported that the first doctoral programs in nursing were offered in the 1920s at Columbia University, which awarded a Doctor of Education degree, and the first PhD in Nursing program was established at New York University (p. 102). When the first Doctors of Nursing Science (DNS/DNSc) programs were begun, schools stated that these degrees were "different" from a PhD, but it soon became clear that most of these programs were research-focused much like the PhD, not practice based.

Practice-based doctorates are also not new to nursing. The first program was begun at Case Western Reserve University (CWRU) in 1979 as a Doctor of Nursing (ND) degree. This degree was recently converted to the Doctor of Nursing Practice (DNP), but the focus has always been to "provide an alternative terminal degree to research-focused doctoral programs" (CWRU, 2005, para 1).

There is some confusion over the differences between a research doctorate (PhD or DNS/DNSc) and a practice doctorate (DNP or ND). According to a 2003 report by L. Marion et al. (as cited in AACN, 2004a), the differences are as follows: In a practice doctorate, there is:

- Less emphasis on theory and meta-theory

- Considerably less research methodology content, with the focus being on evaluation and use of research rather than conduct of research

- Different dissertation requirements, ranging from no dissertation to theses or capstone projects (termed dissertations in some programs) that must be grounded in clinical practice and designed to solve practice problems or to inform practice directly

- An emphasis on practice in any research requirement

- Clinical practica or residency requirements

- Emphasis on scholarly practice, practice improvement, innovation and testing of

interventions and care delivery models, evaluation of health care outcomes, and expertise to inform health policy and leadership in establishing clinical excellence

One of the major issues that supported the move to the practice doctorate was the need for APRN programs to frequently increase the "number of didactic and clinical clock hours far beyond the requirements of master's education in virtually any other field. . . . Many NP master's programs now exceed 60 credits and cannot be completed in less than three years" (AACN, 2004a, p. 7). As a result, AACN (2004a) suggested that

> In response to changes in health care delivery and emerging health care needs, additional knowledge or content areas have been identified by practicing nurses. In addition, the knowledge required to provide leadership in the discipline of nursing is so complex and rapidly changing, that additional or doctoral level education is needed (p. 7).

Based on the work of the task force, the AACN (2004a) endorsed the Position Statement on the Practice Doctorate in Nursing where it recommended that all advanced practice education change from graduating APRNs with master's degrees to doctoral degrees by 2015. Then AACN (2006) continued its work in this area and approved a document titled "The Essentials of Doctoral Education for Advanced Practice Nursing." This document provided schools of nursing with the key content areas that should be included in the DNP curriculum. It is intended not to be prescriptive of actual courses but to provide guidelines and standards around which faculty can develop the courses that they feel are appropriate to their DNP degree. The "Essentials of Doctoral Education for Advanced Practice Nursing" are given in Box 21.1, as well as on the AACN Web site.

> **DISCUSSION POINT**
> How difficult do you believe it will be for APRN programs to meet the 2015 deadline recommended by the AACN?

In the years since these documents have been published, many changes have occurred. It is interesting to note that schools have adopted the recommendations with much less resistance than has previously been seen in nursing. In early 2008, 75 programs were listed on the

---

BOX 21.1 THE ESSENTIALS OF DOCTORAL EDUCATION FOR ADVANCED PRACTICE NURSING

1. Scientific underpinnings for practice.
2. Organizational and systems leadership for quality improvement and systems thinking.
3. Clinical scholarship and analytical methods for evidence-based practice.
4. Information systems/technology and patient care technology for the improvement and transformation of health care.
5. Health care policy for advocacy in health care.
6. Interprofessional collaboration for improving patient and population health outcomes.
7. Clinical prevention and population health for improving the nation's health.
8. Advanced nursing practice.

Source: American Association of Colleges of Nursing (AACN) (2006). *The essentials for doctoral education for advanced practice nursing.* Available at: **http://www.aacn.nche.edu/DNP/pdf/Essentials.pdf.** Accessed July 1, 2008.

AACN Web site as offering DNP programs, with another 140 stating to the AACN that they will have a program in the near future (AACN, 2008b). The programs that are most quickly moving to the DNP seem to be the ones that provide nurse practitioner education.

This change has created some controversy. Because nursing historically has been unwilling to adjust in a timely manner, it has created an environment in which there is resistance to change. As discussed in Chapter 1, it has been more than 40 years and yet nursing still cannot agree on what degree is appropriate for entry into practice. This fact helps to explain the current reticence to adopt the DNP as entry for APRNs, but movement toward the DNP has occurred in a fairly short time period. This rapid change may be reflective of a better understanding by nursing leaders that, due to the persistent health care system issues, nursing must be the leader in change.

What Do the APRN Organizations Think?

Some of the APRN organizations were fairly quick in responding to the recommendation to adopt the DNP degree as the entry into practice for APRNs by 2015. The National Organization of Nurse Practitioner Faculties (NONPF) began work on the practice doctorate in 2001 and held a national meeting in partnership with the AACN in 2003 to gain input from its members and key stakeholders from practice, education, regulation,

certification, and accreditation (NONPF, 2008). It then published recommendations for nurse practitioner education and practice at the doctoral level and developed entry-level competencies. In the end, the NONPF decided that it could not support the 2015 deadline for NP programs to prepare graduates at the doctoral level (NONPF, 2006) but acknowledged that the DNP is a worthwhile goal for NP programs to attain.

DISCUSSION POINT

Should the NONPF establish a new deadline for making the change to doctoral-level education of nurse practitioners?

The other three advanced practice specialties (CNS, CNM, and CRNA) have taken a more conservative approach to the DNP recommendation. Their representative associations have published position statements that offer different views on the topic.

The National Association of Clinical Nurse Specialists (NACNS) (2005a) believes that there are seven key areas of concern: issues about the nursing profession, education, patient safety, economic issues, development and implementation of the DNP, and regulatory issues. The NACNS decided to remain neutral about the recommendation and requested ongoing dialogue to tackle these lingering questions. The association did state that the "NACNS will partner with other national organizations to develop a doctoral level CNS curriculum and to identify additional competencies that could emerge from the additional coursework" (para 13).

The nurse-midwives stated that though they see the DNP as an option, it "should not be a requirement for entry into midwifery practice" (American College of Nurse Midwives [ACNM], 2007, para 1). One must keep in mind though that this group also resisted master's-level preparation as entry into practice, and is only enforcing that mandate beginning in 2010 (ACNM, 2006). The ACNM (2007) believes that midwives, for decades, "regardless of terminal degree, are safe, cost-effective providers of maternity and women's health care" (para 3).

The nurse anesthetists support mandating the DNP but believe that the timeline should be extended to 2025 (American Association of Nurse Anesthetists [AANA], 2007, p. 9). This decision was not made lightly. In an effort to thoroughly examine the issues and arrive at a logical decision, AANA commissioned a task force that did an extensive study of this issue and in 2007 published a 266-page report with another almost 200 pages of exhibits about the DNP.

It is interesting to note that along with this effort, the AANA commissioned a study that took a detailed look at practice doctorates. A communication plan that included many focus groups and surveys was developed. Several issue papers, including a comprehensive literature review, history of educational requirements, existing data, credentialing and faculty issues, and barriers to doctoral education, were requested. Curricular models and competencies were assessed, as were legislative and regulatory concerns. In the end, AANA is to be commended on its approach and this level of detail about its decision to support this requested change. It is understandable why the CRNAs decided that it should aim for a different timeline.

CONSIDER

All advanced practice nursing organizations have established their own guidelines for changing to doctoral education.

Issues and Concerns

Some have challenged the need to even have the DNP and have raised some important questions (Fulton & Lyon, 2005; Meleis & Dracup, 2005; Milton, 2005). Much of the initial concern over the DNP seems to have been resolved with the AACN's clarification of

the role and its release of the DNP Essentials document (J. Stanley, personal communication). However, some issues persist. These uncertainties include the timing of this recommendation; a feeling of insufficient dialogue and input; concern that the DNP does not include theory; the effect of the DNP on nursing education, particularly PhD programs; concern that DNP graduates who become faculty members cannot attain tenure; concern about whether DNP programs will have the same amount of rigor as other doctoral programs; and the use of "DNP" as a title.

DISCUSSION POINT

Do the concerns mentioned above seem logical and reasonable questions to raise?

Timing

Meleis and Dracup (2005) argued that the timing for introduction of the DNP is inappropriate because this recommendation "is detracting from other pressing matters related to quality and safe care" (para 20). That statement alone is an argument *for* the DNP because nursing with its focus on health promotion and disease prevention is fundamental to effecting the needed changes in the health care system. Having nurses prepared at the doctoral level is vital for that change to occur. The main focus of the PhD nurse is the development of research, which does not always include implementation of that research. DNP student projects focus on implementation for change and improvement. Consequently, the timing is right for introducing the DNP degree. Those issues of quality can be addressed by these graduates in that they will have the needed coursework and clinical practice preparation to implement change.

In addition, there is evidence to support that the timing is right for professional doctorates such as the DNP. As cited in a literature review by J. G. Weisbrod, B. J. Horton, and C. Saavedra, the Australian government is funding professional doctorates at its universities because it is "believed that the professional doctorate provides advanced preparation for practicing professionals who need formal preparation in solving problems or need the credential for advancement" (AANA, 2007, p. 105).

Insufficient Dialogue and Input

In their argument against the DNP, Fulton and Lyon (2005) expressed concern that there had been insufficient dialogue and input from key stakeholders. Chase and Pruitt (2006) also expressed their concerns that AACN had not included others in this process. The NACNS, of which both Fulton and Lyon are past presidents, questioned the exclusion of major stakeholders such as the National League for Nursing (NLN). A review of the NLN Web site, however, found that the NLN has developed an opinion paper on the DNP (NLN, 2007). Even though this organization may not have been at some of the initial meetings, it is indeed involved in the discussion.

The mission of the AACN is to set standards for nursing education. On its Web site, the AACN states "The American Association of Colleges of Nursing is the national voice for baccalaureate and graduate-degree nursing education (2008c, para 1). A unique asset for the nation, AACN serves the public interest by providing standards and resources, and by fostering innovation to advance professional nursing education, research, and practice."

It is well within the purview of the AACN to make a recommendation without "asking approval" of all stakeholders. It did make a concerted effort, however, to inform all interested parties and obtain their feedback through its regional meetings and multiple presentations following the release of its position statement.

Effect of the DNP on Nursing Education

Important questions are raised over the effect of the DNP on nursing education. One such concern is how schools that do not offer doctorates will approach the DNP recommendation. Chase and Pruitt (2006) suggested creating partnerships with other universities but noted that the issues surrounding "credit allocation, admission and curriculum, and faculty preparation make these partnerships extremely difficult" (p. 157).

For example, in the state of California there is a two-tiered classification of higher education—the University of California (UC) system and the California State University (CSU) system. The CSU system by design was not meant to award doctoral degrees because this role was designated for the UC system. There has been extensive discussion about the DNP at the chancellor level for both systems. Jack Scott, chairman of the State Senate Education Committee, introduced a bill that would allow schools of nursing in the CSU to independently grant the DNP. The doctoral barrier was previously broken when an earlier bill passed that allowed schools within the CSU system to award educational doctorates (EdD) (Goulette,

2008, p. 8). Although Scott proposed that the bill will increase the number of faculty and advanced practice registered nurses, these programs are already graduating APRNs at the master's level, and the DNP is not focused on teaching pedagogy. It is expected that any state with similar issues will watch this bill closely.

Another concern expressed about the effect of the DNP on nursing education relates to the actual content of each DNP program. Fulton and Lyon (2005) commented that "confusion is created when there is one degree proposed with varied outcomes and the functional role is not well articulated" (para 20). They also suggest that degree focus varies from program to program. As noted in the DNP Essentials (AACN, 2006) document, eight areas of content have been identified. These areas explain the key elements without being prescriptive of actual courses. These essentials are similar in focus to the Essentials of Baccalaureate Education for Professional Nursing Practice (AACN, 2008e). Each of these documents is designed to provide a framework that allows each program to interpret the documents so individual program needs and accreditation requirements are met. This framework permits flexibility in program focus but defines the critical components of the education.

In further discussion regarding the effect of the DNP on nursing education, Meleis and Dracup (2005) stated that "all doctoral education must be designed to help define, generate, develop, translate and test the substantive base of knowledge in nursing" (para 12). This statement implies that practice doctorates will not contribute to this knowledge base. The DNP Essentials document describes the requirements of students' final DNP project, which may focus on "manuscripts submitted for publication, systematic review, research utilization project, practice topic dissemination, substantive involvement in a larger endeavor, or other practice project" (AACN, 2006, p. 20).

A review of some outstanding DNP projects found that they met and exceeded these criteria (Rush University, n.d.). These projects have been defining, translating, and testing the research. For example, A. Matos-Pagan (personal communication) developed a coalition of nurses who were trained to respond to disasters on the island of Puerto Rico. Her work has continued and is now expanding to other islands in the Caribbean.

It has also been suggested that the master's degree (MS) and PhD are the only degrees "well understood by our public" (Meleis & Dracup, 2005, para 22). To say that people cannot appreciate and understand that many degrees exist in a university does not give the public enough credit. The real issue is not that terminal degrees confuse the public; it is the conundrum that almost anyone in health care is called a "nurse." As pointed out by Weisbrod et al., "the title 'doctor' is easily recognizable by the general population as being the pinnacle of educational achievement for the prospective fields of study" (AANA, 2007, p. 105).

CONSIDER
Some suggest that the public is incapable of differentiating among the many doctoral degrees offered at universities.

As opposed to worrying about the understanding of degree titles by the public, nursing should be focusing on what the public needs to improve its health. In fact, Weisbrod et al. found that some nurse leaders feel that PhDs "may have been too focused on research while neglecting faculty and nonacademic responsibilities" (AANA, 2007, p.106). It is unclear what is meant by "nonacademic responsibilities," but it might be interpreted as meaning that many PhD nurses do not work in a clinical practice. By not being clinically active, these nurses are doing a disservice to the profession. Their knowledge and expertise could be used to help effect change. The initiation of a doctorate that focuses on clinical practice can only aid in improving the profession and the lives of patients.

There is also the concern that the practice doctorate or DNP will detract from nurses applying to PhD programs (Fulton & Lyon, 2005; Meleis & Dracup, 2005). O'Sullivan, Carter, Marion, Pohl, and Werner (2005) suggested, however, that "the practice doctorate helps to preserve the integrity of the PhD as a true research degree" (para 21) and "because of the limited availability of a practice doctorate degree in nursing, many faculty and other nurses seeking advanced preparation have pursued a PhD or other research degree" (para 22). This comment was found to be true in conversations with several directors of DNP programs. Nurses, particularly APRNs, had previously not considered pursuing a doctorate because their only options were research-based PhD degrees. The rapid growth of DNP programs nationwide supports the idea that nurses indeed would like to obtain doctoral degrees but want them to be relevant to their clinical practice.

CONSIDER
Many nurses never pursued doctoral degrees because the PhD degree was their only option.

Some nurse leaders have expressed concern, however, that the DNP will not increase the number of nursing faculty because there are no teaching courses included in the curriculum (Chase & Pruitt, 2006). The AACN (2004), in fact, stated that the DNP graduates, as well as PhD graduates, would need additional education if their intent was to teach at the collegiate level (p. 13). At the same time, Chase and Pruitt admitted that, "Unfortunately, PhD programs also fail to prepare educators who understand curriculum development and evaluation" (p. 159) and further stated, "On-the-job training will not promote quality educational outcomes" (p. 160). Consequently, all persons who wish to be educators need to understand that neither of these two key nursing doctorates will prepare them adequately to teach at the collegiate level, and they must pursue additional coursework that focuses on teaching.

Concern That DNP Graduates Who Become Faculty Cannot Attain Tenure

Another common concern that arises about DNP graduates is that they may not be able to obtain tenure and equal status with PhDs in academia (Spear, 2006; Meleis & Dracup, 2005). The AACN (2008a) states on its Web site that "Though primarily an institutional decision, AACN is confident that a DNP faculty member will compete favorably with other practice doctorates in tenure and promotion decisions, as is the case in law, education, audiology, physical therapy, pharmacy, criminal justice, public policy and administration, public health, and other disciplines" (para 11).

A small survey of DNP directors found that there would, in fact, be some challenges for DNP-educated faculty in obtaining tenure. One DNP director commented that no faculty at her institution, including her, receives tenure if he or she is not involved in extensive research (K. White, personal communication). This author, however, did not find any barriers to her appointment as a tenure track faculty and was pleased to learn that one university (University of Colorado) in its advertisement for faculty included the DNP as one of the doctorates accepted for appointment as tenure track faculty (HigherEdJobs, 2008a). A review of nursing faculty jobs offered on the Internet also found advertisements for faculty for DNP programs (HigherEdJobs, 2008b).

> ### CONSIDER
> There may be resistance to obtaining tenure for DNP graduates.

Do DNP Programs Have the Same Amount of Rigor as Other Doctoral Programs?

Milton (2005), in her article on ethics and the DNP, commented that because there is no recommended theory and research in the curriculum, DNP graduates would not be able to make decisions based on evidence and best practices and could not "provide optimal nursing services" (p. 115). She cited Sigma Theta Tau International's (STTI) (2005) statement on evidence-based practice, which discusses having "access to the most recent research" (para 4). This comment by Milton seems very short-sighted, in that she implies that DNPs cannot understand the need for an evidence-based focus in their practice when, in fact, evidence-based practice is the third item on the DNP Essential document (AACN, 2006). She contradicts her comments and provides support for the DNP when she later notes "The past, present and future are cocreated (*sic*) anew all-at-once as novel activities and projects in education, research, and practice are offered for advancement and enhancement of the discipline" (p. 155). The AACN-recommended goal and design of all DNP projects is to improve practice, provide better patient outcomes, decrease errors and promote health for individuals and communities, all of which meet the concept of "novel activities and projects."

> ### CONSIDER
> DNP graduates will base their practice on the latest evidence as defined in the third item of the DNP Essentials document.

In response to this question of rigor, the NONPF released a paper on the criteria for scholarly projects (NONPF, 2007). Most programs have written guidelines and requirements of a quality DNP project, which will help dispel this apprehension.

In addition, the Commission on Collegiate Nursing Education (CCNE), the independent accrediting agency for the AACN, released a press report stating, "In a move

consistent with other health professions, . . . [CCNE] has decided that only practice doctoral degrees with the Doctor of Nursing Practice (DNP) title will be eligible for CCNE accreditation" (AACN, 2005a, para 1). This support by the CCNE reinforces that these programs do indeed meet the rigor of any doctoral degree.

Finally, with the development of the DNP Essentials, the AACN (2006) laid the groundwork for a strong and rigorous curricular model for nursing programs to follow. The suggestion that the PhD is the only worthwhile doctoral program and that the DNP could not be as rigorous or as valuable to the profession is discourteous to the many outstanding institutions that have initiated DNP programs.

Concern That the DNP Curriculum Does Not Include Theory

Whall (2005) and Milton (2005) questioned the lack of theory in DNP programs. Theories, however, are often integrated throughout a curriculum depending on the particular course and topic. The fact that these may not be nursing theories may be an issue for some, but nursing in the 21st century does not practice in a vacuum. The profession must consider that nurses are working as part of an interdisciplinary team and need to understand many types of theories. The inability to understand nonnursing theories has been one of the major barriers to nurses effecting significant change. In addition, because the BSN curriculum includes courses that discuss a number of types of theories, professional nurses have the needed theoretical background.

> *The doctor of nursing practice (DNP) is a unique degree taught by nursing professionals who focus on the issues of the health care system. The program allows an intense concentration of study on concerns facing the health care system and nursing. Graduates finish with the ability to influence policy and practice. This degree also provides the tools and knowledge to effect change that will improve the health care system and its related outcomes (Rowberg, 2005, p. 213).*

Business, leadership, and organizational theories are crucial for anyone looking to transform the health care system, making acquisition of this knowledge vital for the DNP. Leaders require knowledge of all conceptual theories, not just those in nursing, if they are to be successful in their attempts at change.

The Use of DNP as a Title

A final area of debate has been the actual use of the title "DNP." The AACN (2004) suggested the use of the title DNP because schools that had begun practice doctorate programs were each coming up with their own acronyms. Chase and Pruitt (2006) believed that these letters are confusing since nurse practitioners already use "NP" as the acronym designating their specialty. However, the AACN is advocating for the use of the "APRN" acronym for all advanced practice registered nurses. In a letter to its members in May 2008, the AACN (2008d), in commenting on the national consensus project with which it had been involved, stated, "The group has agreed to use the protected title 'APRN' to designate all individuals prepared for direct care roles as nurse practitioners (NPs) certified registered nurse anesthetists (CRNAs), certified nurse midwives (CNMs) and clinical nurse specialists [CNS]" (para 2).

As suggested in the first edition of this book (Rowberg, 2006), many nurses feel compelled to list every degree and/or certification after their names. Although this may be an effort to increase credibility, it has only created more confusion for patients and providers. Use of APRN would make it clear to all that the person is a certified and/or graduate-level advanced practice registered nurse. When that APRN obtains a DNP, the degree could be easily added to the title. Consequently, the multiple and sundry acronyms could finally be eliminated.

Recent Developments

Some recent, very disconcerting developments have occurred regarding the DNP. In June 2008, at the American Medical Association (AMA) House of Delegates (HOD) meeting, physicians passed two resolutions about the DNP (Sorrel, 2008): "Citing patient safety concerns, members of the AMA House of Delegates protested the unregulated expansion of doctors of nursing practice and urged organized medicine to ensure transparency on and supervision of their role in medical care" (Sorrel, p. 25). Although this resolution is only a policy statement and not legally binding, it does demonstrate a continued effort by medicine to attempt to control nursing. It is not in the purview of physicians to dictate the role of nursing and the right to practice. Medicine frequently comments about patient safety issues but in this situation has no evidence to support its position. A review of the 1999 IOM report should remind physicians that they have more issues surrounding patient safety than do APRNs.

Another resolution, number 214, was also passed and states, "RESOLVED, That our AMA adopt policy that Doctors of Nursing Practice must practice as part of a medical team under the supervision of a licensed physician who has final authority and responsibility for the patient" (Sorrel, p. 19). Many nursing organizations submitted comments or testified against this resolution to no avail.

It is unfortunate that medicine continues to believe that health care is a pyramid and that it is at the pinnacle with the right to direct all other health care professionals. Medicine has no legal right to attempt to regulate advanced practice registered nurses or to state that they must function under the direct supervision of a physician. Boards of nursing are the legal bodies that regulate nursing and monitor its practice. State nurse practice acts clarify the role and function of a nurse. One can only imagine the backlash if nursing tried to tell physicians how to practice, but unfortunately physicians have a long history of defending what they believe is their turf.

The goal should be to work in collaboration and as a team, given that all health care professionals make significant contributions to the health of the patient. One would think that the medical profession would focus on the issues in the health care system instead of wasting time and energy trying to regulate other providers who have extensive documentation of their worth.

Another AMA resolution had called for limitations on the use of the term "doctor" and suggested that it be restricted to physicians, dentists, and podiatrists. After much discussion, however, the terminology was changed to say that all professionals must clearly identify their qualifications and credentials to patients (National Association of Pediatric Nurse Practitioners [NAPNP], 2008). A floor amendment was approved that AMA will support legislation to "make it a felony for non-physician health care professionals to misrepresent themselves as physicians" (Sorrel, 2008, p. 25). Why some physicians believed it was necessary to make such an amendment is unclear, given that it has always been illegal to misrepresent oneself as a licensed health care professional.

A similar issue came to nursing's attention in the spring of 2008 when the *Wall Street Journal* published an article about the DNP (Landro, 2008). Landro reported that "the Council for the Advancement of Comprehensive Care (CACC) plans to announce . . . that the National Board of Medical Examiners has agreed to develop a voluntary DNP certification exam based on the same test physicians take to qualify for a medical license" (para 3). Within 2 days, the AACN sent an electronic message to its members with its comments on this announcement. The AACN (2008d) then followed up with an official response stating that it had been involved in a process that would "develop a national consensus on issues related to education, certification, licensure, and accreditation for Advanced Practice Registered Nurses (APRNs)" (para 1) and that "a critical element of this consensus is the agreement that all APRNs should be certified through a nationally recognized *nursing* certifying body and that the exams offered by these certification agencies will be used by state boards to grant APRNs the authority to practice" (para 2).

The AACN does not see the exam being developed by CACC as an exam that will be used to certify APRNs. Unfortunately, Dr. Mary Mundinger, Dean and Centennial Professor in Health Policy at Columbia University School of Nursing, has been advocating for DNPs to take this exam. APRNs do not want to be physicians, and do not need to take a medical exam to show that they have the knowledge and expertise to provide quality care. It is disconcerting that a nurse leader feels it necessary to encourage such a movement, because it undermines the current and very effective certification system. A positive note occurred at the 2008 AMA House of Delegates meeting, however, when it opposed the Board of Medical Examiners writing test questions for this exam (NAPNP, 2008).

Nursing must continue to be vigilant about these attempts to encroach on its right to practice. Nurses must be strong advocates of the profession by joining and being actively involved in professional associations that focus on monitoring practice issues and voting for legislators who will support the role. Legislators must be kept informed of nursing practice and its meaning and provide documentation of its outstanding patient outcomes. Nursing must define nursing before others take away the freedom to practice.

> ### CONSIDER
> Nursing must continue to be vigilant about these attempts to encroach on its right to practice.

THE CLINICAL NURSE LEADER

The AACN released its white paper on the CNL in 2007 with the following critical statement:

While there is ample evidence for the need to produce many more nurses to meet the pressing health care needs of society, this is not just a matter of increasing the volume of the nursing workforce. The nursing profession must produce quality graduates who:

- *Are prepared for clinical leadership in all health care settings;*
- *Are prepared to implement outcomes-based practice and quality improvement strategies;*
- *Will remain in and contribute to the profession, practicing at their full scope of education and ability; and*
- *Will create and manage microsystems of care that will be responsive to the health care needs of individuals and families (Batalden et al., as cited in AACN, 2007).*

In addition, unless nursing is able to create a professional role that will attract the highest-quality women and men into nursing, it will not be able to fulfill its covenant with the public. The CNL addresses this call for change (AACN, 2007, p. 5).

The many advances in knowledge in science and technology over the last century have put increased pressure on nursing education to produce graduates who have the educational preparation and expertise to meet the challenges in health care in the 21st century. This effort must occur through collaboration of education and practice. For too many years, nursing education has functioned somewhat in a vacuum without input from the practice setting as to its needs. "Change cannot occur in isolation. Nursing education must collaborate and work in tandem with the health care delivery system to design and test models for education and practice that are truly client-centered, generate quality outcomes and are cost-effective" (AACN, 2007, p. 6).

CONSIDER

Nursing education must collaborate and work in tandem with the health care delivery system to design and test models for education and practice that are truly client centered, generate quality outcomes, and are cost-effective.

According to Tornabeni and Miller (2008, p. 609), "Central and key to the process of developing this role had been a commitment to engage multiple stakeholders in the process." Tornabeni and Miller reported on a task force that monitored the implementation of pilot projects in which schools of nursing partnered with practice partners to initiate the CNL role (p. 609). The projects were able to demonstrate that just adding a CNL did not effect the changes anticipated: "Practice sites needed to redesign their patient care delivery models to center the care around the expertise the CNL

would bring to patient care" (p. 609). It was also decided that the "skills and competencies required in this role" (p. 610) necessitated recommending that the CNL be educated with a master's degree curriculum.

"The CNL is a leader in the health care delivery system across all settings . . . functions within a microsystem and assumes accountability for healthcare outcomes for a specific group of clients" (AACN, 2007, p. 6). In addition, the CNL applies the best evidence to practice and provides or manages at the point of care. He or she designs, implements, and evaluates care by coordinating, delegating, and supervising the care provided by the health care team (p. 6).

In developing this new role for nursing, the AACN (2007) made ten assumptions for preparing the CNL. These assumptions are shown in Box 21.2. Details about the assumptions can also be viewed on the AACN Web site. At first glance, these assumptions seem intuitive to nursing practice, but unfortunately not all are being integrated into the practice of each individual nurse. By making these declarative statements, the AACN is helping to clarify the role of the CNL.

A key area of focus of the CNL is integrating the care of all health care providers. As Tornabeni and Miller (2008) noted, "The goal is to develop strong communication between health professionals through patient-centered care and to create synergy, collaboration, and value for the contributions each discipline brings to patient care" (pp. 610–611).

BOX 21.2 | ASSUMPTIONS FOR PREPARING CLINICAL NURSE LEADERS

1. Practice is at a microsystems level.
2. Client care outcomes are the measure of quality practice.
3. Practice guidelines are based on evidence.
4. Client-centered practice is intra- and interdisciplinary.
5. Information will maximize self-care and client decision making.
6. Nursing assessment is the basis for theory and knowledge development.
7. Good fiscal stewardship is a condition of quality care.
8. Social justice is an essential nursing value.
9. Communication technology will facilitate the continuity and comprehensiveness of care.
10. The clinical nurse leader must assume guardianship for the nursing profession.

Source: American Association of Colleges of Nursing (AACN) (2007). *White paper on the education and role of the clinical nurse leader.* Available at: **http://www.aacn.nche.edu/Publications/WhitePapers/ClinicalNurseLeader07.pdf.** Accessed July 1, 2008.

It is expected that the CNL will:

1. Provide and manage care, including the delegation of tasks and supervision and evaluation of personnel and care outcomes

2. Critically evaluate and anticipate risks to client safety

3. Profile patterns of need and tailor interventions using an evidence-based approach

4. Advocate for clients and community and assume accountability for delivery of high-quality care

5. Assume the role of educator

6. Be responsible for the provision and management of care in and across all environments

7. Be a member and leader of the health care team (AACN, 2007, pp. 11–12).

It has been further defined that the CNL must have "strong critical thinking skills, communication and assessment skills . . . with a strong focus on health promotion, risk reduction and population-based health care" (AACN, 2007, p. 12). The AACN finalized its vision of the CNL by recommending core competencies and a framework of the potential curriculum. The role is being accepted across the country with exciting outcomes. As of mid-2008 "the number of partnerships engaged in the [CNL] initiative have grown to include 92 schools with 192 health care institutions" (Stanley et al., 2008, p. 615).

Unfortunately, controversy usually accompanies any innovation and change. The CNSs believe that the CNL functions in a manner similar to their practice. The NACNS declared that the "proposed competencies of the new nurse duplicate the competencies of the CNS" (NACNS, 2004, para 3). The position statement further states that "continued efforts to implement this new nurse proposal will disenfranchise clinical nurse specialists, a role that has been providing leadership to meet the needs of health care of the public for the past 50 years" (para 4).

DISCUSSION POINT

Does the CNL role overlap with the role of the CNS?

The CNSs continued their commentary in late 2005 with an update on their position (NACNS, 2005b). Their ongoing concern revolves around their belief that the CNL and CNS have overlapping roles and competencies. The NACNS questions how, in light of limited resources, this role could be added when CNSs, case managers, and nurse managers already function in parallel roles: "We believe that the roles that can accomplish the bridging of the chasm already exist in the system" (NACNS, 2005b, para 8), and they requested that AACN continue to "support CNS education and practice" (para 8).

Support for the CNS role is actually coming from nurses who have become CNLs: "The CNL is a master's prepared advanced generalist nurse. This differs from, but compliments, the role of the clinical nurse specialist (CNS), who is a master's prepared APN with a specialty focus" (Poulin-Tabor et al., 2008, p. 624). An excellent example of the collaboration and interdisciplinary approach of the clinical nurse leader is the following:

I consulted the diabetic clinical nurse specialist as well as the heart failure CNS for the best approach for in-hospital and outpatient goals for this patient. As a result of working with the patient, physician assistants, doctors, social worker, dietician and clinical nurse specialists . . . the patient was discharged safely home without readmission (Poulin-Tabor et al., 2008, p. 627).

Although the concern of the NACNs can be appreciated, the CNL is definitely providing a new approach and focus. As the NACNS states in its documents, the clinical nurse specialist helps to improve nursing practice, but the CNL is patient focused, providing care across the care continuum. Patients are followed prior to hospital admission, during their stay, and after discharge. Although it is agreed that case managers work in a similar fashion, the point of the CNL role is that *all* patients receive this special attention, not just ones with certain diagnoses.

Sherman, Clark, and Maloney (2008) made specific note that "what surfaced in the discussion was the need for a consistent figure to act as a point person for staff, physicians, patients, and families" (p. 56). Poulin-Tabor et al. (2008) stated, "we focus on the patients as a whole rather than as a sum of their parts. As this has not been the traditional approach in medicine, it has been a noticeable difference to the patients and families that we touch" (p. 628).

CONSIDER

The CNL acts as a point person for staff, physicians, patients, and families.

Too many stories have been told by patients and their families about the disorganization of and lack of caring by health care professionals. Sitting for an hour after the scheduled time for an outpatient procedure is unfortunately the norm. Discharges get delayed because no planning occurred. Cancellation of procedures wastes staff time and ties up operating/procedure rooms unnecessarily. The cost savings to the health care delivery system can be seen within months of initiating the CNL role. Although there is the added expense of the CNL salary and benefits, the overall costs savings can be significant (Harris & Ott, 2008).

However, before the CNL is employed, the rationale for hiring someone for this role should be made clear. Specific objectives that clarify the expected outcomes should be written. Reasons for and against the initiation of the CNL, as well as the probable costs and benefits, should be identified. Finally, alternatives and consequences should be assessed. All stakeholders need to be aware of "the possibilities to address any issue(s) and any future opportunities" (Harris & Ott, 2008, p. 27).

Nursing at the Veteran Affairs (VA) is being transformed through the use of the CNL: "The CNL initiative supports the transformation of existing organizational nursing practice structures to achieve patient-driven, evidence-based, outcome-oriented nursing practice at all points of care across the continuum" (Office of Nursing Services [ONS], 2007, p. 4). By late 2007 more than 80 VA medical centers had implemented the role.

The nurses who are functioning as CNLs best state the case for the role:

> We humanize and personalize the health care experience and in doing this, have rediscovered the art of nursing. . . . We believe that the role of the CNL will be instrumental as a coordinator and change agent to meet not only the demands of today but to anticipate the demands of tomorrow (Poulin-Tabor, et al., 2008, p. 628).

The role of the CNL will continue to be assessed in the coming years, but it appears that these nurses are making a difference in the lives of their patients. Documentation of CNL outcomes is provided in Research Study Fuels the Controversy.

CONCLUSIONS

The controversy over the clinical practice doctorate will probably continue for many years, but advanced practice registered nursing must consider what level of education is needed to adequately care for patients in today's health

---

Research Study Fuels the Controversy: Effect of the Clinical Nurse Leader

Two case studies were discussed that examined the role of the clinical nurse leader (CNL) and its effect on improving quality and patient safety. One study focused on quality of care by assessing rates of patient falls, the percentage of patients who reported that their pain had been well managed, and the percentage of patients who reported "excellent" to the nurse response to calls and overall care. A final area of evaluation looked at length of stay.

STUDY FINDINGS

Pain management satisfaction went from 82% prior to the residency by the CNL student to 96% during her time on site. This rate fell to baseline rates after her departure (p. 617). Satisfaction with care and response to calls rose from 87% and 58%, respectively, to 99% and 96% (p. 617). Fall rates and injury due to those falls more than doubled during the student CNL's clinical experience: "One reason, supported by the student's journal entries, is that in the process of frequent rounding, patients were found to have fallen" (p. 618).

The other study had some difficulty in assessing the true effect of the implementation of the CNL because data collection was poor prior to initiation of the role. Since that time, "the unit reports no nosocomial pressure ulcer development, 100% compliance with pneumonia and flu vaccine administration, and the implementation of heart failure patient education and smoking cessation counseling" (p. 618). It was also found that the length of stay decreased by almost 1 day on the oncology unit.

Source: Stanley, J. M., Gannon, J., Gabuat, J., Hartranft, S., Adams, N., Mayes, C., Shouse, G. M., Edwards, B. A., & Burch, D. (2008). The clinical nurse leader: A catalyst for improving quality and patient safety. *Journal of Nursing Management, 16,* 614–622.

care system. Of equal importance is that individual APRNs must learn from the lessons of the past and develop the skills needed to survive as a vital constituent of the health care system in the 21st century. The movement to the DNP is a crucial part of that process.

In addition, the CNL role provides exciting new opportunities for nursing and the health care system.

As the number of nurses with these specialties increases, the public will become more aware of the positive outcomes these individuals bring to their care. There is little doubt that advanced practice nursing makes valuable contributions to the health care system. Doctors of nursing practice and CNL will have a significant effect on the health care of tomorrow.

FOR ADDITIONAL DISCUSSION

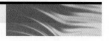

1. Can the public appropriately distinguish among the many doctoral degrees offered by universities?

2. Will offering the DNP decrease the number of PhD candidates?

3. Is it necessary for DNP graduates to have coursework in nursing theory?

4. Should the medical profession be allowed to dictate the scope of practice for DNPs or other nurses?

5. Does the CNL function differently than a clinical nurse specialist?

REFERENCES

AllNursingSchools (n. d.). *What do nurse anesthetists do?* Available at: http://www.allnursingschools.com/faqs/crna.php. Accessed August 14, 2008.

American Association of Colleges of Nursing (2004a). *AACN Position Statement on the Practice Doctorate in Nursing.* Washington, DC: AACN. Available at: http://www.aacn.nche.edu/DNP/DNPPosition Statement.htm. Accessed June 28, 2008.

American Association of Colleges of Nursing (AACN) (2004b). *Your nursing career: A look at the facts.* Available at: http://www.aacn.nche.edu/education/career.htm. Accessed May 5, 2005.

American Association of Colleges of Nursing (AACN) (2005a). *Commission on Collegiate Nursing Education moves to consider for accreditation only practice doctorates with the DNP degree title.* Available at: http://www.aacn.nche.edu/Media/News Releases/2005/CCNEDNP.htm. Accessed January 25, 2009.

American Association of Colleges of Nursing (AACN) (2005b). *Faculty shortages in baccalaureate and grad-*

uate nursing programs: Scope of the problem and strategies for expanding the supply. Available at: http://www.aacn.nche.edu/publications/white papers/facultyshortages.htm. Accessed August 16, 2008.

American Association of Colleges of Nursing (AACN) (2006). *The essentials for doctoral education for advanced practice nursing.* Available at: http://www.aacn.nche.edu/DNP/pdf/Essentials.pdf. Accessed July 1, 2008.

American Association of Colleges of Nursing (AACN) (2007). *White paper on the education and role of the clinical nurse leader.* Available at: http://www.aacn.nche.edu/Publications/WhitePapers/ClinicalNurse Leader07.pdf. Accessed July 1, 2008.

American Association of Colleges of Nursing (AACN) (2008a). *Frequently Asked Questions: AACN Position Statement on the Practice Doctorate in Nursing.* Washington, DC: AACN. Available at: http://www.aacn.nche.edu/DNP/DNPFAQ.htm. Accessed August 12, 2008.

American Association of Colleges of Nursing (AACN) (2008b). *Doctor of Nursing Practice (DNP) Programs*. Washington, DC: AACN. Available at: http://www.aacn.nche.edu/DNP/DNPProgramList.htm. Accessed January 27, 2009.

American Association of Colleges of Nursing (AACN) (2008c). *Mission*. Available at: http://www.aacn.nche.edu/ContactUs/strtplan_mission.htm. Accessed August 14, 2008.

American Association of Colleges of Nursing (AACN) (2008d). *Letter in response*. Available at: http://www.aacn.nche.edu/DNP/pdf/responseletter08.pdf. Accessed July 2, 2008.

American Association of Colleges of Nursing (AACN) (2008e). *Revision of the essentials of baccalaureate education for professional nursing practice (draft)*. Available at: http://www.aacn.nche.edu/education/pdf/BEdraft.pdf. Accessed August 14, 2008.

American Association of Nurse Anesthetists (AANA) (2007). *Report of AANA Task Force on Doctoral Preparation of Nurse Anesthetists*. Park Ridge, IL: American Association of Nurse Anesthetists.

American College of Nurse Practitioners (ACNP) (n.d.). *What is a nurse practitioner?* Available at: http://www/acnpweb/org/i4a/pages/index.cfm?pageid=3479. Accessed August 14, 2008.

American College of Nurse-Midwives (ACNM) (n.d.). *About midwifery*. Available at: http://www.mymidwife.org/midwife.cfm. Accessed August 14, 2008.

American College of Nurse-Midwives (ACNM) (2006). *Mandatory degree requirements for nurse midwives*. Available at: http://www.acnm.org/siteFiles/position/Mandatory_Degree_Requirements_3.06.pdf. Accessed August 11, 2008.

American College of Nurse-Midwives (ACNM) (2007). *Midwifery education and the Doctor of Nursing Practice (DNP)*. Available at: http://www.acnm.org/siteFiles/position/Midwifery_Ed_and_DNP_6_07.pdf. Accessed July 20, 2008.

American Hospital Association Commission on Workforce for Hospitals and Health Systems (2002). *In Our Hands, How Hospital Leaders Can Build a Thriving Workforce*. Chicago: American Hospital Association. Available at: http://www.aha.org/aha/resource-center/Statistics-and-Studies/ioh.html. Accessed July 1, 2008.

Apold, S. (2008). The doctor of nursing practice: Looking back, moving forward. *Journal for Nurse Practitioners, 2008*(February), 101–107.

Case Western Reserve University (CWRU) (2005). *Case Western Reserve University's Bolton School of Nursing establishes Ohio's first Doctor of Nursing Practice degree*. Available at: http://www.case.edu/news/2005/8-05/dnp.htm. Accessed August 6, 2008.

Chase, S. K., & Pruitt, R. H. (2006). *The practice doctorate: Innovation or disruption?* Available at: http://www.apn-dnp.com/UserFiles/File/Chase2006.pdf. Accessed August 7, 2008.

Fulton, J., & Lyon, B. (2005). The need for some sense making: Doctor of nursing practice. *Online Journal of Issues in Nursing*. Available at: http://www.nursingworld.org/MainMenuCategories/ANAMarketplace/ANAPeriodicals/OJIN/TableofContents/Volume102005/Number3/tpc28_316027.aspx. Accessed June 28, 2008.

Goulette, C. (2008). *A look at current state legislation and government-related issues. Doctor nurse*. Available at: http://nursing.advanceweb.com/Article/From-the-Hill-4.aspx. Accessed January 27, 2009.

Harris, J. L., & Ott, K. (2008). Building the business case for the clinical nurse leader role. *Nurse Leader, 6*(4), 25–28, 37.

HigherEdJobs (2008a). *Senior faculty—Loretta C. Ford Endowed Professorship*. Available at: http://www.higheredjobs.com/faculty/details.cfm?JobCode=175327958. Accessed August 18, 2008.

HigherEdJobs (2008b). *Faculty Doctor of Nursing Practice*. Available at: http://www.higheredjobs.com/faculty/details.cfm?JobCode=175319154. Accessed August 18, 2008.

Institute of Medicine (IOM) (1999). *To Err Is Human: Building a Safer Health System*. Washington, DC: National Academy Press.

Institute of Medicine (IOM) (2001). *Crossing the Quality Chasm*. Washington, DC: National Academy Press.

Joint Commission on Accreditation of Healthcare Organizations (JCAHO) (2002). *Health Care at the Crossroads. Strategies for Addressing the Evolving Nursing Crisis*. Chicago: JCAHO. Available at: http://www.jointcommission.org/NR/rdonlyres/5C138711-ED76-4D6F-909F-B06E0309F36D/0/health_care_at_the_crossroads.pdf. Accessed July 1, 2008.

Kimball, B., & O'Neill, E. (2002). *Health Care's Human Crisis: The American Nursing Shortage*. Princeton, NJ: The Robert Wood Johnson Foundation. Available at: http://www.rwjf.org/files/newsroom/NursingReport.pdf. Accessed January 27, 2009.

Landro, L. (2008). Making room for Dr. Nurse. *The Wall Street Journal,* April 2, 2008. Available at: http://online.wsj.com/article/SB120710036831882059.html. Accessed January 27, 2009.

Meleis, A. I., & Dracup, K. (2005). The case against the DNP: History, timing, substance, and marginalization. *Online Journal of Issues in Nursing,* September 30, 2005. Available at: http://www.nursingworld.org/MainMenuCategories/ANAMarketplace/ANAPeriodicals/OJIN/TableofContents/Volume102005/Number3/tpc28_216026.aspx. Accessed June 28, 2008.

Milton, C. L. (2005). Scholarship in nursing: Ethics of a practice doctorate. *Nursing Science Quarterly, 18*(2), 113–116.

National Association of Clinical Nurse Specialists (NACNS) (n.d.). *What is a clinical nurse specialist?* Available at: http://www.nacns.org/faqs.shtml. Accessed August 14, 2008.

National Association of Clinical Nurse Specialists (NACNS) (2004). *NACNS position statement on the clinical nurse leader.* Available at: http://www. nacns.org/NACNS_Positionstatement_CNL_9_05_3_04.pdf. Accessed July 2, 2008.

National Association of Clinical Nurse Specialists (NACNS) (2005a). *White paper on the nursing practice doctorate.* Available at: http://www.nacns.org/nacns_dnpwhitepaper2.pdf. Accessed July 2, 2008.

National Association of Clinical Nurse Specialists (NACNS) (2005b). *NACNS update on the clinical nurse leader.* Available at: http://www.nacns.org/NACNS_Positionstatement_CNL_9_05_3_04.pdf. Accessed July 2, 2008.

National Association of Pediatric Nurse Practitioners (NAPNP) (2008). *AMA House of Delegates report.* Available at: http://www.napnap.org/index.cfm?page=611. Accessed August 5, 2008.

National League of Nursing (NLN) (2007). *Reflections and dialogue: Doctor of Nursing Practice (DNP).* Available at: http://www.nln.org/aboutnln/reflection_dialogue/refl_dial_1.htm. Accessed August 11, 2008.

National Organization of Nurse Practitioner Faculties (NONPF) (2006). *Statement on the Practice Doctorate in Nursing: Response to recommendations on clinical hours and degree title.* Available at: http://www.nonpf.com/NONPF2005/PracticeDoctorate ResourceCenter/PDstatement1006.htm. Accessed July 2, 2008.

National Organization of Nurse Practitioner Faculties (NONPF) (2007). *NONPF recommended criteria for NP scholarly projects in the Practice Doctorate program.* Available at: http://www.nonpf.com/ NONPF2005/PracticeDoctorateResourceCenter/ScholarlyProjectCriteria.pdf. Accessed August 8, 2008.

National Organization of Nurse Practitioner Faculties (NONPF) (2008). *Practice Doctorate Resource Center.* Available at: http://www.nonpf.com/NONPF2005/PracticeDoctorateResourceCenter/PDResourceCenter.htm. Accessed July 2, 2008.

National Research Council (2005). *Advancing the nation's health needs: NIH research training programs.* Available at: http://books.nap.edu/openbook.php?record_id=11275&page=74. Accessed July 2, 2008.

National Sample Survey of Registered Nurses (NSSRN) (2004). Available at: http://bhpr.hrsa.gov/healthworkforce/rnsurvey04/3.htm. Accessed August 4, 2008.

National Science Foundation (NSF) (2007). *U.S. doctoral awards in science and engineering continue upward trends.* Available at: http://www.nsf.gov/statistics/infbrief/nsf08301/. Accessed August 15, 2008.

Office of Nursing Services (ONS) (2007). *Annual Report: VA nursing today.* Available at: http://www1.va.gov/nursing/docs/2007ONSannualRptFNLweb2.pdf. Accessed July 2, 2008.

O'Sullivan, A. L., Carter, M., Marion, L., Pohl, J. M., & Werner, K. E. (2005). Moving forward together: The practice doctorate in nursing. *Online Journal of Issues in Nursing 10*(3). Available at: http://www.apn-dnp.com/UserFiles/File/OSullivan2005.pdf. Accessed January 27, 2009.

Poulin-Tabor, D., Quirk, R. L., Wilson, L., Orff, S., Gallant, P., Swan, N., & Manchester, N. (2008). Pioneering a new role: The beginning, current practice and future of the clinical nurse leader. *Journal of Nursing Management, 16,* 623–628.

Rowberg, M. (2006). *Advanced practice nursing: Challenges of role definition, recognition, and reimbursement.* In: C. J. Huston (Ed.), *Professional Issues in Nursing* (pp. 412–434). Philadelphia: Lippincott Wilkins & Williams.

Rowberg, M. (2005). Why have the Doctorate of Nursing Practice? *Journal for Nurse Practitioners, 1*(4), 212–215.

Rush University (n.d.). *Doctor of nursing (DNP) projects.* Available at: http://www.rushu.rush.edu/nursing/ ND%20Project%20Summaries.htm. Accessed January 27, 2009.

Sherman, R., Clark, J. S., & Maloney, J. (2008). Developing the clinical nurse leader role in the twelve bed hospital model: An education/service partnership. *Nurse Leader, 6*(3), 54–58.

Sigma Theta Tau International (STTI) (2005). *Evidenced based nursing.* Available at: http://www. nursingsociety.org/aboutus/PositionPapers/Pages/ EBN_positionpaper.aspx. Accessed August 11, 2008.

Sorrel, A. L. (2008). *Physicians demand greater oversight of doctors of nursing.* Available at: http://www.ama-assn.org/amednews/2008/07/07/prsd0707.htm. Accessed August 5, 2008.

Spear, H. (2006). Letter to the Editor on "Doctor of Nursing Practice." *Online Journal of Issues in Nursing,* October 27, 2006. Available at: http://www. nursingworld.org/MainMenuCategories/ ANAMarketplace/ANAPeriodicals/OJIN/Letters totheEditor/HilaJSpearLetter.aspx. Accessed August 11, 2008.

Stanley, J. M., Gannon, J., Gabuat, J., Hartranft, S., Adams, N., Mayes, C., Shouse, G. M., Edwards, B. A., & Burch, D. (2008). The clinical nurse leader: A catalyst for improving quality and patient safety. *Journal of Nursing Management, 16*, 614–622.

Tornabeni, J., & Miller, J. F. (2008). The power of partnership to shape the future of nursing: The evolution of the clinical nurse leader. *Journal of Nursing Management, 16*, 608–613.

Whall, A. (2005). "Lest we forget": An issue concerning the Doctorate in Nursing Practice (DNP). *Nursing Outlook, 53*(1), 1.

BIBLIOGRAPHY

Borgmeyer, C. (2008). *AMA delegates oppose DNPs as medical team leaders.* Available at: http://www.aafp. org/online/en/home/publications/news/news-now/ professional-issues/20080625ama-dnp.html. Accessed August 2, 2008.

Broome, M. E. (2005). Constructive debate and dialogue in nursing. *Nursing Outlook, 53*, 167–168.

Brown, M. A., Draye, M. A., Zimmer, P. A., Magyary, D., Woods, S. L., Whitney, J., Acker, M., Schroeder, C., Motzer, S., & Katz, J. R. (2006). Developing a practice doctorate in nursing: University of Washington perspectives and experience. *Nursing Outlook, 53*(3), 130–138.

Draye, M. A., Acker, M., & Zimmer, P. A. (2006). The Practice Doctorate in Nursing: Approaches to transform nurse practitioner education and practice. *Nursing Outlook, 54*(3), 123–129.

Ford, J. (2008). DNP certification exam announced. *Advance for Nurse Practitioners, 16*(6), 16.

Gabuat, J., Hilton, N., Kinnaird, L. S., & Sherman, R. O. (2008). Implementing the clinical nurse leader role in a for-profit environment. *Journal of Nursing Administration, 38*(6), 302–307.

Grindel, C. (2005). AACN presents the clinical nurse leader and the Doctor of Nursing Practice roles: A benefit or a misfortune? *MedSurg Nursing, 14*(4), 209–210.

Hoppel, A. M. (2008). Degrees of latitude: Real issues behind clinical doctorates. *Clinician Reviews, 18*(3), 1, 3, 7, 13.

Maag, M. M., Buccheri, R., Capella, E., & Jennings, P. (2006). A conceptual framework for a clinical nurse leader program. *Journal of Professional Nursing, 22*(6), 367–372.

Magyary, D., Whitney, J. D., & Brown, M. A. (2006). Advancing practice inquiry: Research foundations of the practice doctorate in nursing. *Nursing Outlook, 54*(3), 139–151.

Martin-Sheridan, D., Ouellette, S. M., & Horton, B. J. (2006). Is doctoral education in our future? *AANA Journal, 74*(2), 101–104.

Partin, B. (2008). Update on the DNP degree. *Nurse Practitioner Journal, (4)*3, 7.

Sherman, R., Clark, J. S., & Maloney, J. (2008). Developing the clinical nurse leader role in the twelve bed hospital model: An education/service partnership. *Nurse Leader, (6)*3, 54–58.

Sperhac, A. M., & Clinton, P. (2008). Doctorate of Nursing Practice: Blueprint for excellence. *Journal of Pediatric Health Care, 22*(3), 146–151. Available at: http://www.medscape.com/viewarticle/576073_print. Accessed July 7, 2008.

Spross, J. A., Hamric, A. B., Hall, G., Minarik, P. A., Sparacino, P. S. A., & Stanley, J. M. (2004). *Working statement comparing the clinical nurse leader and the clinical nurse specialist roles: Similarities, differences, and complementarities.* Available at: http://www.

aacn.nche.edu/CNL/pdf/CNLCNSComparisonTable.pdf. Accessed July 2, 2008.

Stringer, H. (n. d.). *Clinical nurse leaders bring problem-solving skills to the bedside.* Available at: http://career-advice.monster.com/career-planning/nursing/Clinical-Nurse-Leaders-Bring-Proble/home.aspx. Accessed July 2, 2008.

Triolo, P. K., & Wood, G. L. (2005). Developing clinical nurse leaders at the unit level. *Nurse Leader, 3*(2), 45–48.

WEB RESOURCES

All Nursing Schools	http://www.allnursingschools.com
American Association of Colleges of Nursing	www.aacn.nche.edu
American Association of Nurse Anesthetists	http://www.aana.com/
American Association of Nurse Practitioners	www.aanp.org
American College of Nurse-Midwives	http://www.midwife.org/index.cfm
American College of Nurse Practitioners	www.acnpweb.org
American Hospital Association	http://www.aha.org
American Nurses Association	www.nursingworld.org
Doctors of Nursing Practice	http://www.apn-dnp.com/
National Association of Clinical Nurse Specialists	www.nacns.org
National Organization of Nurse Practitioner Faculties	www.nonpf.org
Sigma Theta Tau International	www.nursingsociety.org

CHAPTER 22

Nursing and Public Policy: Getting Involved

• CATHERINE J. DODD • CLARILEE HAUSER •

Learning Objectives

The learner will be able to:

1. Define the terms *politics* and *policy* and explore their relationship.
2. Differentiate among defense, domestic, and foreign policy and give health-related examples of each.
3. Differentiate among the problem stream, the political stream, and the policy stream in John Kingdon's three-stream model of policy development.
4. Discuss how ideological "interest groups" shape social change.
5. Identify sequential stages found in most systems models that describe policymaking.
6. Identify nursing leaders who were pioneers in public policy and describe their contributions in effecting social change.
7. Explore the relationships among social inequity, health disparities, and access to health care.
8. Cite examples of actions that nurses might take to increase their influence in public policy.
9. Determine whether his or her values align more closely with the Democratic or Republican Party.
10. Investigate the most significant nursing issues being debated in the policy arena and predict the next "great" policy issues that will be debated as affecting nursing.
11. Lobby a legislator, either in writing or face to face, about an issue related to nursing practice or health care.
12. Reflect on why so many nurses are reluctant to become active in the political arena.

Many of the preceding chapters discussed policy issues affecting the nursing profession. For example, mandatory overtime, staffing ratios, whistle-blower protection, and the treatment of chemically impaired nurses have all been addressed recently in the health care policy arena. Indeed, nurses have long been involved in shaping public policy. Some of the earliest policy debates in nursing were about the "training" of nurses. Subsequent debates centered on both the process for licensing nurses and the appropriate scope of their practice. State legislatures responded and adopted licensure laws relating to the practice of nurses and the protection of the public. Today these laws define the scope of nursing practice as distinctly separate from medicine and inclusive of responsibilities independent of medicine.

> **CONSIDER**
> Nursing's involvement in policy and politics has resulted in state nurse practice acts that allow many things, including autonomy of practice, reimbursement for advanced practice nurses (APNs), and limitations on the ability of hospitals to force nurses to work overtime.

In addition, policy debates regarding nursing shortages and working conditions have occurred every decade of nursing's policy history. Often these debates have centered on whether policy should be shaped by collective bargaining or by legislation and/or regulation.

Participating in shaping public policy is an essential part of professional nursing practice because public policy shapes the environment in which nurses provide care and determines the kind of care nurses are permitted to provide. This chapter defines public policy, explains the policy process and the role of politics in that process, and demonstrates how policy and politics are inextricably linked. John Kingdon's three-streams metaphor, a systems model, stages of nursing's political development, and a continuum of political involvement are introduced to conceptually explore the relationship between politics and policy and to examine how nurses participate in both.

In addition, this chapter identifies nursing leaders who were pioneers in public policy, traces nursing's involvement in key policy/political debates throughout the 20th century, and explores contemporary issues being debated in the political arena. Finally, because politics is part of every organization and a part of government at every level, the political skills necessary for nurses to protect their practice, their profession, and the patients entrusted to their care are identified. In addition, the chapter discusses actions nurses might take to increase their influence in public policy.

DEFINING POLITICS AND POLICY

Defining terms helps to clarify the relationship between politics and policy. Definitions of *politics* stem from the original Greek meaning, which referred to the government of the city-state; the actions of a government, politician or political party; the process by which communities make decisions and govern; or the managing of a state or government. In addition, politics is considered a process that involves power and influence in decision making in social relationships. In governing, politics is an activity that is central to developing policy (*American Heritage Dictionary of the English Language*, 2000; Online Dictionary of Social Sciences, n.d.). Although this chapter focuses on policy and politics as they relate to government, many of the principles are applicable to non-governmental institutions and organizations as well.

Indeed, politics is part of all organized human activity; any group of two or more individuals has to establish how to make decisions that require common action and how to resolve conflicts. Ellis and Hartley (2004, p. 70) defined politics as "the way in which people in any society try to influence decision making and the allocation of resources." Because resources (money, time, and personnel) are limited, it is necessary to make choices regarding their use. There is no perfect process for making optimum choices because whenever one valuable option is chosen, usually some other option must be left out.

In contrast, *policy* refers to a specific plan of action to achieve certain goals, or a deliberate act of government to influence the actions of citizens and society (American Heritage Dictionary of the English Language, 2000; Wikipedia, n.d.; The Free Dictionary.com, n.d.). The word *policy* is Greek in origin and is linked to citizenship. In government, it comes from the relationship of citizens to one another in public. Policy has also been defined as "an authoritative decision made in the legislative, executive, or judicial branches of government that are intended to direct or influence the actions, behaviors, or decisions of others" (Block, 2008, p. 7).

DISCUSSION POINT

How great an effect does politics have on policy at the institutional level? At the governmental level? Are politics typically considered before policy development begins at both levels?

DEFENSE, DOMESTIC, AND FOREIGN POLICY

At the federal level, the U.S. Congress and the president make policy in three major areas: defense, domestic, and foreign. Health-related policies can be found in all three areas. Health-related *defense* policies include what kinds of health care the military and their families will receive and whether weapons of mass destruction (such as nuclear weapons) will be used by the United States. *Domestic* policy refers to policies such as whether children's vaccinations will be paid for in the public health budget or what services are included in Medicare, the health insurance plan for the elderly. Health is also a major part of *foreign* policy. Congress decides whether to assist other nations with preventing HIV/AIDS or in providing family planning and nutrition assistance to developing countries.

CONSIDER

Nurses serving in the military are affected by *defense* policy, nurses working to improve health in developing countries are affected by *foreign* policy, and nurses working within the health care system anywhere in the United States are affected by *domestic* policy. The president and Congress decide how many tax dollars to spend on defense, foreign aid, and domestic health care. If more is spent on one, less is available for the others, unless taxes are increased.

POLICIES AND VALUES

Policy involves the setting of goals and priorities by a society or an organization and the decisions about how and what resources should be used to achieve those goals. Thus, policies reflect the values and beliefs of the leaders of society and/or organizations who make the policies (Mason, Leavitt, & Chafee, 2002).

> CONSIDER
> Policy always has a moral dimension because it relates to decisions about how to act toward others.

Frequently, female policy makers, regardless of their political party, have tended to promote policies that address social issues such as family medical leave, child care, and domestic violence (Freeman, 2008). Mason, Leavitt, and Chafee (2007) posited that women who became involved in political activism were likely to focus on community, collective responsibility and connectedness, in contrast to men, who focused on individual rights. Similarly, policies developed by nurses have frequently shown a strong belief in the importance of assisting people to care for themselves despite their illness or disability, and this belief has distinguished nursing from other professions. Caring, whether it is for families, for patients, or for the environment, is a value central to nursing and to women. Unfortunately, it is not a value that receives much attention from institutions and government policy makers. Nurses have had some success at the state and federal levels at moving such a policy agenda forward; however, if nurses want policies that reflect nursing's values, then nurses must get involved in the policy process that makes decisions on which policies to adopt, and that requires involvement in politics.

> DISCUSSION POINT
> What values are reflected in state nurse practice acts that limit the autonomy of the advanced practice nurse in prescribing? Similarly, what values are

reflected in state policies that allow chemically impaired nurses to participate in diversion programs rather than face disciplinary proceedings?

CONCEPTUALIZING POLITICS AND POLICY DEVELOPMENT

Although there are many models for conceptualizing politics and policy development, only four are presented in this chapter: (1) Kingdon's streams of policy development (Sabatier, 1999), (2) a stage sequential (systems) model of policy making (Hanley & Falk, 2007), and Mason et al.'s (2002) continuum for political development.

Kingdon's Three Streams of Policy Development

Kingdon posited that there are *three streams* that determine why some problems are chosen over others for policy development (Sabatier, 1999) (Box 22.1). The three streams are the *problem stream*, the *policy stream*, and the *political stream*. These three streams often flow endlessly without converging, but when the streams come together, a window of opportunity opens to move an agenda, to legislate, or to regulate policy solutions to problems.

The *problem stream* includes what are defined as problems, indicators of a problem, and the social construction of problems. It also includes how problems come to the attention of policy makers, such as in the form of causal stories or personal experiences. For example, U.S. Representative Caroline McCarthy, a licensed practical nurse, ran for Congress after her husband and son were shot on the Long Island Railroad in New York and she wanted to pass gun control legislation.

Another example of the problem stream coming to the attention of legislators is the current nursing shortage. Legislators have had to take note of the shortage as

---

BOX 22.1 | **THE THREE STREAMS OF JOHN KINGDON'S STREAMS METAPHOR**

1. **Problem:** embodies the process of problem recognition
2. **Policy:** embodies the formulation and refining of policy proposals as responses to problem recognition
3. **Politics:** considers the associated benefits and costs to subgroups of the population and the degree of external pressure the legislator feels to take action

a result of constituent complaints, an increasing number of medical errors, and high nursing vacancy rates. In addition, television and newspaper reports abound with stories of poor patient care due to the shortage of nurses.

Dodd (2008) also emphasized the significance of the problem stream in her Ten Universal Commandments of Politics for Nurses (Box 22.2). The first commandment states that the personal is political, and that each of us is just one personal or social injustice away from being involved in politics (p. 16).

Kingdon's second stream is the *policy stream*. Ideas that are potential policy solutions are considered based on their "technical feasibility and value acceptability" (Sabatier, 1999, p. 76). The reality is that policy makers are presented with many problems, and it is impossible to address all of them. Policy makers, then, must set an agenda that reflects their values and select problems on which to focus legislation or regulatory action that fits their priorities. Because policy makers want to be successful (for re-election and job security), most avoid introducing legislative or regulatory proposals that are unlikely to pass and or to be implemented.

BOX 22.2 | TEN UNIVERSAL COMMANDMENTS OF POLITICS FOR NURSES

1. The personal is political. Each of us is just one personal or social injustice away from being involved in politics.

2. Friends come and go, but enemies accumulate.

3. Politics is the art of the possible, and majority rules.

4. Be polite, be persistent, be persuasive, be polite.

5. Ignore your mother's rule: Do talk to strangers.

6. Money is the mother's milk of politics.

7. Negotiate visibility. Take credit, take control.

8. Politics has a "chit economy." So keep track.

9. Reputations are permanent.

10. Don't let 'em get to ya.

Source: Dodd, C. (2008). Play to win: Know the rules (pp. 15–26). In: C. Harrington & C. Estes (Eds.), *Health Policy: Crisis and Reform in the U.S. Health Care Delivery System.* Sudbury, MA: Jones & Bartlett.

For example, a policy to resolve the nursing shortage by re-establishing hospital-based nursing diplomas is unlikely to be pursued because, technically, hospitals are no longer set up as nursing schools and because nursing education outside the hospital has become more highly valued and accepted by society. Another example might be Rep. McCarthy's failure to ban guns because Americans value the "right to bear arms" as protected by the Second Amendment of the U.S. Constitution. She was successful, however, in leading the fight to at least pass a temporary ban on assault weapons (the legislation passed in 1993 and was made effective for 10 years, expiring in September 2004) because Americans value their safety. Banning assault weapons provided safety and protected the guarantees of the Second Amendment.

DISCUSSION POINT

California is the only state that has enacted minimum licensed staff–to-patient ratios in acute care hospitals, and this passed only after vigorous opposition from the state hospital association. Is this an issue most state legislators would be eager to take on? Is such an issue "technically feasible and value acceptable"?

The political stream is the third and final stream. Politics, according to Kingdon, describes an environment that includes (1) the national mood—what the public sentiment is on issues, (2) support or opposition of *interest groups*, and (3) legislative or executive branch turnover accompanied by a change in political ideology and values (Sabatier, 1999). In other words, the political stream looks at associated benefits and costs to subgroups of the population and the degree of external pressure the legislator feels to take action.

An example of a strong *political stream* occurred when support from the public, professional nursing, and consumer and hospital organizations came together to help fund the Nursing Education Act. In contrast, the ban on assault weapons met with opposition because of the change of national mood, the turnover of Congress and the White House to Republican rule, and the powerful interest group of the National Rifle Association.

The significance of *interest groups* as part of the political stream cannot be overestimated. Indeed, throughout history, ideological interest groups have shaped social change. Interest groups provide politicians with one of three resources essential for their success (i.e., re-election).

The first, and sometimes seemingly most important, is money; the second is the ability to mobilize voters; and the third is image. It is this image enhancement that may be most significant for nurses in terms of legislative interest. Clearly, having the support of nurses improves a candidate's image.

Historically, nurses have ranked high in public opinion polls, and the public believes that the endorsement of nurses demonstrates a candidate's integrity. Nursing is a profession of more than 2 million members nationally. When divided by 435 congressional districts nationally, there are approximately 5,000 registered nurses (RNs) per congressional district who can and have mobilized voters.

A strong political stream, however, is not enough. Convergence of the three streams is required. Nursing and the professional organizations that represent nursing (interest groups) in the legislature at the state and federal levels, then, have repeatedly worked to achieve this degree of stream convergence in public policy decisions related to health care. For example, in the 1990s, during the Clinton Administration, the rising costs of health care, President Bill Clinton's personal respect for nurses (his mother was a nurse anesthetist who worked in rural Arkansas), and pressure from nursing organizations created an opportunity to add nurse practitioners and clinical nurse specialists as providers under Medicare.

Another example of stream convergence relates to medical errors, workplace injuries, and mandatory overtime. Public awareness of rampant medical errors was the subject of the Institute of Medicine report *To Err is Human*, which appeared during the Clinton Administration (Kohn, Corrigan, & Donaldson, 2000). Nursing organizations collected data and proposed that mandatory overtime contributed to medical errors and injuries in the workplace (the idea/policy proposal stream) (American Nurses Association [ANA], 2001b, ANA, 2001c). Combined with public awareness (stream one), ideas/policy proposals (stream two), and the ideological support of the Clinton Administration for nursing combined with nursing and labor interest group pressure (stream three), the Department of Labor promulgated regulations limiting overtime and budgeting funding for occupational health needle safety training. In this instance, the idea/policy stream combined with the political stream comprised the interest groups of nursing and labor combined with an administration (president) whose ideology embraced labor and nursing.

During President George W. Bush's administration, however, the overtime regulations were overturned and needle safety training was curtailed. This was an example of the (third) political stream. The ideological shift and the powerful hospital interest group lobby succeeded in overturning the regulations and cutting the budget.

> **CONSIDER**
> Nursing interest groups have seized the public's frustration with rising health care costs and promoted policies that emphasized the cost effectiveness of advanced practice nurses (stream one—conditions, plus stream two—ideas/policies). President Clinton supported this idea and included APNs in his Medicare budget (stream three—political change in values).

Stage Sequential Systems Approach to Analyzing Policy Making and Interest Groups

A more traditional approach to analyzing policymaking uses a systems-based model that considers policy making in sequential stages. It is much like the nursing process: *assess, plan, implement, evaluate, assess again.* In a policy system, a problem is identified and put on a policy agenda; then a policy is developed, adopted, implemented, evaluated, and extended, modified, or terminated; and the cycle begins again (Hanley & Falk, 2007).

Critics of the systems model approach suggest that the model fails to consider that the elected government's policy agenda rarely, if ever, reflects a consensus. In the last two decades the country has become more and more divided on a partisan and thus philosophical basis of how best to govern (Ferguson, Fowler, & Nichols, 2008). Critics argue that the systems analysis of policy development leaves out the influence of interest groups, whether they are nursing organizations or oil companies. It would be like using the nursing process for diabetic teaching of an adolescent without taking into consideration that the patient might not follow the diet because his or her peer group is eating fast food every day after school.

In contrast, policy development, adoption and implementation, and politics are inextricably linked in Kingdon's model, and the political environment in which policy is formed is considered. Nursing can play a role in all three of Kingdon's policy streams that create windows of opportunity: For example, nursing professional organizations and unions raise public awareness about the quality of care or lack of access to care. Professional nursing organizations and unions develop ideas and propose policies to solve problems of worker safety, health and safety, or quality of care. Nursing professional organizations and unions are interest groups that lobby and engage in political action to influence policy.

In all of these examples, nursing is acting as an interest group. The unique thing about nursing as an interest group is that when nurses advocate for nurses and nursing, patients and the public get better care. Political action is a key part of interest group action. Interest groups do more than support or oppose policies; they help to elect the policy makers by engaging in grassroots campaign activity and raising money for campaigns.

Stages of Political Development

Another model used to explore nursing's development in politics and the policy arena was created by Sally Cohen and colleagues and described by Mason et al. (2007). It includes four stages of political development in nursing:

Stage 1: *Buy-in* occurred when the profession began to promote the political sensitivity of nurses to injustices or changes needed in the policy arena.

Stage 2: *Self-interest* occurred when the nursing profession began to develop its identity as a special interest and crystallized its uniqueness as a political voice.

Stage 3: *Political sophistication* began when nurses began to be recognized by policy makers and health care leaders as having valuable perspectives and expertise in health policy.

Stage 4: *Leadership* indicates that nursing has developed its own political identity as exemplified by setting the agenda for change.

Nursing entered stage 4 during President Clinton's tenure in office but returned to stage 3 during the last decade. Unfortunately, the profession is represented by so many different "specialty organizations" and unions that a single unified voice for nursing has become diluted. Furthermore, until nurses become the initiators of critical health care policy that is broader than nursing, the values of nursing will be left out of reshaping the health care system.

> ### CONSIDER
> Nursing has the potential to hold a significant leadership position in policy and politics. At the national level the profession is represented by the American Nurses Association (ANA), the National League for Nursing (NLN), and many specialty organizations and several different unions.

Continuum of Political Involvement

The final conceptual model used here to explore nursing's involvement in policy and politics is that of a continuum. Continuums for political involvement extend from no involvement in politics to that of extreme activism. Individuals move up and down these continuums throughout their lives in response to intrinsic and external motivators, time and energy resources, and situational opportunities and needs.

Mason et al. (2007) identified such a continuum with their description of *nurse-citizens, nurse-activists,* and *nurse-politicians* (pp. 44–45). This work is similar to that of Kalisch and Kalisch (1982), who described *spectator activities, transitional activities,* and *gladiatorial activities* (p. 316). Another continuum that has been identified is that of people *who make things happen, people who watch what's happening,* and *people who wonder what's happened.* For example, nurses *who wonder what's happened* vote occasionally or not at all; they are not involved in improving the workplace or their community. Nurses *who watch things happen* are spectators; they expose themselves to political stimuli, they are members of their union, they vote, sometimes they wear buttons or put bumper stickers on cars, and they participate in community activities that are important to them such as parent–teacher organizations or homeowners associations.

> ### CONSIDER
> There are people who make things happen, people who watch what's happening, and people who wonder what's happened!

Nurses *who make things happen* fall into three categories: professionals, leaders, and political change agents.

Professional nurses vote in every election and stay informed regarding issues affecting the health care system. They participate in their union or speak out about working conditions and quality of care. They participate in their professional organization, know who their local, state, and federal elected officials are, and communicate with them regarding issues of concern.

Nurse leaders are active members of nursing organizations that are political; they are active members of a political party and attend political meetings, forums, and rallies; they help register people to vote; they contribute and raise money for causes and campaigns and to nurses' *political action committees* (PACs) that are concerned about access to quality nursing care; they lobby elected and appointed officials on issues of concern to the profession; they write letters to the editor of professional journals and newspapers; they participate in coalitions; they encourage the participation of other nurses; they mentor future leaders.

Finally, nurse political change agents are nurse leaders who use their nursing expertise to enact and implement policies that enhance access to quality health care, including nursing care; they seek appointments or assist other nurses and friends of nursing in securing appointments to governing boards in the public and private sectors; they are active members of political parties; they query candidates about their positions on health care and assist with fundraising for candidates that support nurses and nursing; they seek elected and/or appointed office and continue to identify themselves as a Registered Nurse; they work on staffs of elected/appointed officials; and they extend their policy influence beyond the health system to the community and the globe.

ROOTS OF INVOLVEMENT IN POLICY AND POLITICS: EARLY 1900S

Nursing has a long history of involvement in politics and policy development. At the end of the 19th century, nursing alumnae associations, motivated by the need for "standardization in nurse training schools, as well as by the need to protect the public from poorly trained nurses," came together to establish "standards of nursing education and nursing practice and to promote the general welfare of nurses" (Flanagan, 1976, p. 27).

Nursing Alumnae Associations

The ANA was founded by these alumnae associations. Almost immediately after this founding, the United States became engaged in the Spanish American War, requiring a nursing workforce to care for the wounded and those who had yellow fever, typhoid and other communicable diseases. Isabel Hampton Robb, ANA's first president, sought to influence the Secretary of War and the Surgeon General to insist that the nurses needed for the war be trained and offered to organize them, but she was unsuccessful. Both trained and untrained nurses were recruited and sent to the battlefield without any system of care or triage by skilled nurses.

After the war, a special committee of nurses formulated the Army Bill for Nurses. Congress initially failed to enact the legislation; however, the policy/idea had become popular, and in 1901 the Army Reorganization Act included an army nurse corps under the direction of a "graduate nurse" (Flanagan, 1976). Indeed, in 1900, Robb called for a complete system of registration for nurses, and state nurses associations began to lobby for registration.

Nursing Leaders as Public Policy Pioneers

There are numerous nursing leaders who served as pioneers in public policy formation in the early to mid 1900s. Only a few are presented here, as is the area of policy they were most noted for. Yet their stories are similar; all of them shared passion, courage, and perseverance. They also all shared a commitment to collective strength. These same attributes are recognized in nursing policy activists today (see Research Study Fuels the Controversy on page 382).

Lavinia Dock: Organizing Nurses for Social Awareness

At the 1904 ANA convention, Lavinia Dock, a founder of the ANA and the first to donate money to establish the *American Journal of Nursing* that same year, stated that it was essential that nurses exercise social awareness. As a result, delegates to the ANA convention that year considered social (policy) issues of the time, including child labor, women's suffrage, and sex education.

Research Study Fuels the Controversy: Political Competence

This phenomenological study used narratives from six politically expert nurse activists to examine the concept of *political competence*. Political competence was defined as the skills, perspectives, and values needed for effective political involvement within nursing's professional role.

STUDY FINDINGS

Six themes emerged from the analysis of the lived experiences of the six activists. They included nursing expertise as valued currency, opportunities created through networking, powerful persuasion, commitment to collective strength, strategic perspectives, and perseverance. All six themes were represented in almost all of the interviews, and the author concluded that political competence was not about demonstrating one or several of these behaviors. Instead, it appeared to be a "wholistic enterprise requiring the whole package" (p. 142). Each identified theme was a necessary but not sufficient ability in political competence.

The findings, although not generalizable to the total population, concluded that nurses who aspire to be more effective in political contexts should consider the behaviors described in the narratives of these seasoned activists and explicitly explore their use in their practice and professional lives. The author concluded with an assertion that more and more practitioners, educators, and leaders need to hone and express their political competence if nursing's collective political development is to be advanced.

Source: Warner, J. R. (2003). A phenomenological approach to political competence: Stories of nurse activists. *Policy, Politics & Nursing Practice, 4*(2), 135–143.

Lillian Wald: Public Health and Child Welfare

Lillian Wald, one of the founders of the ANA, exemplified involvement in social change, community leadership, and politics. She was born to a family of Jewish scholars and rabbis. She graduated nursing school and entered Women's Medical College in New York to become a doctor. During her first year of medical school, she volunteered to teach hygiene to immigrant women in a school on Henry Street in New York City.

She quit medical school, and, in 1893, she and a classmate, Mary Brewster, moved to the Lower East Side neighborhood to provide nursing care in the community (American Association for the History of Nursing [AAHN], 2004). A friend and philanthropist, Jacob Schiff, and Mrs. Solomon Loeb agreed to fund Wald and Brewster's purchase of a house on Henry Street. This house became the Henry Street Settlement and is considered the founding place for public health nursing. Neighbors came to the house for help with their health, housing, employment, and educational needs.

Wald was also concerned about the living conditions of the neighborhood and the lack of safe places for children to play. She helped found the Outdoor Recreation League, which worked to gain attention for the need for public parks and raised funds for what would become the first municipal playground in New York City.

Fortunately, Wald's concern for children at the time was shared by many wealthy charity leaders. During the 1890s, close to 250 new orphanages were incorporated. Vast numbers of children were working in factories. Wald believed that the government needed to protect children and that child labor should be abolished. In 1904, she participated in a meeting with President Theodore Roosevelt lobbying for the creation of a national Children's Bureau. However, the powerful industrialist lobby made up of the wealthy factory owners who used child labor was successful in tabling the legislation through their lobbying and political support of legislators (Jewish Women's Archive, n.d.).

However, as an example of how Kingdon's first stream (the conditions that are defined as problems sometimes come to the attention of policy makers through personal experiences), one of President Roosevelt's close friends was James West, who was an orphan. West joined Wald and others in 1909 to host a national Conference on Children that drew more than 200 leaders from all over the country. The publicity created a public sentiment largely among women of all classes that child welfare must be put on the national policy agenda.

Kingdon's third stream—politics—resulted in the creation of the Children's Bureau in 1912 (Krain, n.d.). Wald was appointed to New York's Immigration Commission in 1908 by Governor Charles Evans Hughes after he visited the Settlement House. Wald's efforts resulted in a report that called for improved living and working standards for workers and their families. The report led to the formation of a State Bureau of Industries in New York. Kingdon's three streams again appear to hold: conditions—of immigrant workers; idea/policy—need for government regulation; and politics—Wald's relationship with the governor.

By 1909, Wald convinced the Metropolitan Life Insurance Company that protecting the health of employees was good for business, and they funded nurses from the Henry Street Settlement to care for sick employees of companies they insured. The Henry Street Visiting Nurses Society began with 10 nurses in 1893. By 1916, it had 250 nurses and was serving more than 1,300 patients a day in their homes. Wald convinced the New York Board of Education to hire a nurse in 1902 and so began school nursing in the United States. She also lobbied successfully to change divorce laws so that abandoned spouses could sue for alimony, and she assisted the Women's Trade Union League in protecting women from "sweatshop working conditions" (National Association for Home Care and Hospice [NAHC], 2008, para 6).

In 1912, Wald founded the National Organization for Public Health Nursing. She was also part of the peace movement against World War I, and for that was cited as an "undesirable" citizen. In spite of this, she served as chairperson of the Committee on Community Nursing of the American Red Cross and worked with the International Red Cross in the campaign to fight the flu epidemic of 1918 (Jewish Women's Archive, n.d.). Wald was also active in the suffrage movement and believed women should have the right to vote and to be involved in politics.

Wald was active in nursing at the local, national, and international levels. At her insistence, Columbia University appointed the first professor of nursing at a U.S. college or university. She was among the founders of the International Council of Nurses in 1899. Wald's nursing leadership also demonstrated that policy and politics are linked, and that nurses must be active beyond their immediate workplace and also in the community, in business, and in government.

Margaret Sanger: Birth Control

Among the many nurses whose training included a rotation through the Henry Street Settlement was Margaret Sanger. Sanger witnessed maternal and infant mortality resulting from uncontrolled fertility in the neighborhoods of the Lower East Side of New York City. She cared for women suffering from self-induced abortions and was motivated to make birth control available to women. In 1912, she began writing a column on sex education titled "What Every Girl Should Know," but it was soon censored (Steinem, 2004).

In 1914, Sanger was indicted for violating postal "Comstock" laws after disseminating contraceptive information. She jumped bail and fled to England. She returned to the United States and continued to promote access to birth control throughout her life. She opened a clinic in New York with her sister Ethel Byrne and was jailed, only being released after a hunger strike. She smuggled contraceptive diaphragms from Europe, and she founded the National Committee on Federal Legislation for Birth Control and the American Birth Control League, which became the Planned Parenthood Federation of America.

In 1965, after years of effort, the Supreme Court decision *Griswold v. Connecticut* made birth control legal for married couples. Sanger died shortly thereafter (Sanger, Margaret, n.d.). Here again, Kingdon's streams took some time to come together: first conditions had to be compelling—maternal and infant mortality caused by lack of spacing pregnancies and poverty. Then the political stream converged with the women's movement and women demanding that they be able to control their pregnancies. Finally, policy change occurred with the legalization of birth control.

Martha Minerva Franklin: Segregation and Discrimination

Martha Minerva Franklin was another pioneering public policy nurse in the early 20th century. She founded the National Association of Colored Graduate Nurses (NACGN) in 1908 with the fundraising assistance of Lillian Wald and Lavinia Dock, who mailed letters to more than 1,000 nurses (ANA Hall of Fame: Martha Minerva Franklin, n.d.). The NACGN was formed because many states barred black nurses from membership in state nurses associations. Segregation and discrimination kept nursing education and hospitals separate.

The NACGN was instrumental, however, in political lobbying efforts to integrate black nurses into the armed services during World War II. In 1951, the NACGN merged with the ANA (Flanagan, 1976). Today the National Black Nurses Association exists as one of more than 70 national nursing organizations, some organized around clinical issues, some relating to ethnicity, and some relating to religious beliefs.

DISCUSSION POINT
Can you identify nurses today who are demonstrating the same degree of risk taking in attempting to influence nursing/health care policy as Dock, Wald, Sanger, and Franklin did in the early 20th century? If so, who are they, and what causes are they championing? If not, why not?

NURSING, PUBLIC POLICY, AND POLITICS: MID TO LATE 1900S

World War II

War has always affected nursing. In January 1945, President Franklin Roosevelt proposed the induction of every Registered Nurse between the ages of 18 and 45 years into the land and naval forces. The ANA lobbied to amend the legislation to provide for the "commissioning" of nurses and for deferments for teachers and supervisors who were essential on the home front. In addition, the ANA suggested that credit be given to the states for voluntary recruitment, that a commissioned nurse corps be established by the Veterans Administration with the same benefits that were applied to the military, and that the draft be voluntary. The ANA also lobbied for the protection of nursing standards and education at accredited schools and for the prohibition of discrimination based on race, color, creed, or sex.

All of the ANA's conditions were accepted except the voluntary recruitment. Instead, Congress agreed to implement mandatory enlistment only if voluntary enlistment failed to meet needed quotas. Final action on the bill was tabled because of changes in the events of the war (Deloughery, 1998; Flanagan, 1976).

DISCUSSION POINT
Wars have played an important role in nursing history and in nursing's involvement in politics. Are nurses highly visible in any current conflict or war worldwide? Are you aware of any legislative efforts that are being driven by nursing's involvement in such conflicts?

Effecting Social Change

Historically, nursing leaders have participated in many efforts to bring about social change. The efforts of nurse leaders in the suffrage movement have already been discussed. Nurse leaders in the early 20th century were also integrally involved in passing socially focused legislation that outlawed child labor and provided protection for women abandoned by their husbands.

Nursing was also at the forefront of and lent integrity to the civil rights movement. As a result of the civil rights movement, poll taxes and literacy tests were made illegal. In addition, politicians elected with the aid of newly enfranchised blacks passed laws to eliminate discrimination based on race. Nursing was one of the first professions to eliminate segregation. However, educational opportunities remain out of reach for many students of color, and nursing's responsibility to ensure that the face of the profession reflects the faces of those entrusted to its care still requires much work.

Nursing did not formally participate in the "peace movement" against the Vietnam War, but some nursing leaders participated in the women's movement that emerged around that time. Nursing and teaching were professions almost exclusively made up of women, and employment ads at the time were separated for men and women.

In 1974, the ANA set up a special account to help pass the Equal Rights Amendment to the Constitution. The ANA joined a national boycott and moved its convention to a state that had ratified the Amendment. The Amendment failed ratification by a sufficient number of the states. The women's movement continued, and nursing and teaching were often used as examples of professions requiring a significant amount of knowledge and skill for which compensation fell far below male-dominated jobs requiring the same levels of knowledge and skill, or "comparable worth." Nursing also became involved in the effort to establish comparable worth in employment settings during the 1970s. During this time, women were often paid less for the same work that men did. Many states passed "comparable worth laws" during the 1970s, supported by state nurses associations. During the 1980s and beyond, nurses at various places around the country went on strike to achieve wages of comparable worth. Nursing's involvement in the women's movement as its own interest group working in coalition with other women's interest groups strengthened that movement.

National Health Insurance and Recognition of Nursing's Impact

National health insurance and efforts to increase access to health care have also been recurrent political and policy issues for nursing. Indeed, nursing leaders such as Lillian Wald, Lavinia Dock, and Annie W. Goodrich supported the first unsuccessful platform for national health care proposed by Theodore Roosevelt in 1912. In fact, some critics labeled Goodrich and Wald socialists for their efforts.

The next proposal for national health care came during President Franklin Roosevelt's Administration. It was made by Frances Perkins, the first woman to serve in the Cabinet as Secretary of Labor. Perkins headed up a committee on economic security during the Great Depression that recommended both income security (social security) and health security. The American Medical Association (AMA), however, opposed national health care insurance and mounted a successful grassroots campaign to discredit a government-sponsored and -regulated health care system.

Roosevelt abandoned the linkage of health insurance to the social security provisions because he did not want to jeopardize the New Deal programs, which included social security (Corbin, 1993), but he did promise to consider it in his next term. However, Roosevelt died in 1945 and was succeeded by Harry Truman. When Truman ran for his first full term as president, he promoted a prepaid medical insurance plan financed by increasing the social security tax. Again, the AMA opposed these efforts and likened national health coverage to totalitarianism in Nazi Germany (Corbin, 1993). The ANA, the National League for Nursing (NLN), and the National Organization for Public Health Nursing, however, supported Truman's proposals (Kalisch & Kalisch, 1982).

In 1948, Truman won his first full term as president on a platform promoting universal health coverage—a comprehensive benefit package including prescription drugs, dental coverage, and nursing home care. However, just before the 1950 congressional election, the AMA again waged a successful campaign by assessing each of their members $25 to fund a program designed to "educate" physicians and the public throughout the country about the dangers of socialized medicine and

worked against candidates for Congress who supported Truman's plan. The AMA spent more than $4.5 million dollars to defeat this health reform, and there were not enough members elected to Congress in 1950 who supported Truman's plan.

National health insurance was an idea that lost its attraction in the 1950s, despite the fact that families were losing their life savings and being forced into poverty by costly hospitalizations while science and technology were promising to save lives (Families USA, 1993). Again from Kingdon's perspective, this occurred because only one of the three criteria was met: conditions—because of the rising costs of medical care, the idea/policy had significant support; however, the politics—the opposition from powerful interest groups, the AMA, and organized labor who used health coverage as a tool to recruit members—made it impossible to pass national health reform (Families USA). This is an example of grassroots political activity by a group of health professionals (the AMA) directly in the electoral (political) process.

Efforts to create national health insurance did not die. In 1974, the ANA continued its support of national health insurance and adopted a resolution supporting national health insurance with the intent to increase nursing's participation in the policy debate. The resolution stated that a national health insurance program should be implemented that would "guarantee coverage for all people for the full range of comprehensive health services" and that nursing care should "be a benefit of the national health insurance program." The resolution also said that data systems necessary for effective management of the national insurance program should be in place to "protect the rights and privacy of individuals" and that nurses should be designated "as health providers in all pending or proposed legislation on national health insurance" (Flanagan, 1976, pp. 670–671). This was an example of the nursing profession's foresight: to cover all people, to protect privacy, to include nurses as essential providers. Indeed, the legislative agenda of the ANA included all of these principles in subsequent health care legislation.

In 1978, the first black president of the ANA, Barbara Nichols, was asked to testify on behalf of Senator Edward Kennedy's Health Care for All Americans Act. Television coverage of major issues meant that the organizations selected to testify had to have the trust of the public, and nursing was held in high regard. Nichols not only advocated for access to comprehensive health services for all, she also specifically mentioned mental health services and nursing care in all settings. She insisted that we needed a health system and not a medical system. The AMA opposed the measure. It failed by only a few votes, and no major health legislation has passed since that time.

CONSIDER

The ANA was selected to testify at key hearings on national health insurance, amplifying nursing's voice on television to households throughout the country in advocating for comprehensive health coverage, including nursing care in all settings for all Americans.

The ANA has remained active in advocating for access to quality affordable health care. The ANA and the NLN drafted Nursing's Agenda for Health Care Reform (ANA, 2001a), which emphasized the cost-effectiveness of using the appropriate provider in the appropriate place at the appropriate level of care. An example of this tenet was public health nurses providing primary care screening in community-based settings. More than 70 nursing specialty organizations signed onto the agenda so that nursing could speak with one voice about health care reform.

President Bill Clinton was elected in 1992 with the support of the ANA, and he promised to reform the health care system and to include nursing as part of the solution. Nurse leaders were a part of the task force that developed the Health Security Act. This legislative proposal was complex and was opposed by the insurance industry, the pharmaceutical industry, and the AMA.

In 1994, these powerful and well-financed interest groups successfully worked to defeat any member of Congress who supported reform. The proposal was completed and introduced after the 1994 elections, and enough members of Congress who supported it had lost that, like President Truman, President Clinton lost the majority he needed in Congress to pass health care reform.

DISCUSSION POINT
Why would the insurance industry, the pharmaceutical industry, and the AMA work together to defeat the Health Security Act? What motives may they have shared?

Nursing and Collective Bargaining

Another area in which nurses were actively involved in politics and policy in the mid to late 1900s was in determining eligibility for nurses to participate in collective bargaining. For the most part, nurses had little opportunity to participate in the decision making regarding their working conditions in the early to mid 1900s. In 1935, the Wagner–Connery Labor Relations Act passed as part of the New Deal. This act guaranteed the right of employees to organize, form unions, and bargain collectively with their employers. It ensured that workers would have a choice on whether to belong to a union or not, and it promoted collective bargaining as the major way to ensure peaceful industry–labor relations.

The act also created a new National Labor Relations Board to arbitrate deadlocked labor–management disputes, guarantee democratic union elections, and penalize unfair labor practices by employers (National Labor Relations Board, n.d.). Health care workers were not included as protected workers; however, they were permitted to organize under this law (Foley, 2002).

Nursing struggled with whether collective bargaining was consistent with professional ethics and whether collective bargaining should be controlled by professional societies or unions. The ANA asserted that nurses had the "right and responsibility to promote and protect their economic security" and "to participate actively in determining the conditions of employment which directly affect them" and included "the freedom of association" and "unified action through organization." The ANA Board of Directors in 1938 advised that nurses carefully evaluate the benefits of union membership before joining (Flanagan, 1976).

In 1946, the ANA established a Committee on the Employment Conditions of Nurses because of the postwar persistence of poor salaries and difficult working conditions. The ANA House of Delegates endorsed legislation promoting the 8-hour-day, 40-hour workweek for all nurses, and the California Nurses Association negotiated their first hospital contracts. That same year, the ANA affirmed that state nurses associations should represent nurses in collective bargaining. However, in 1947, Congress passed the Taft–Hartley Amendments to the Wagner Act and exempted the nonprofit health care industry from governance under the National Labor Relations Act (NLRA). It was not until 1974 that those amendments were repealed, with the ANA participating in the political debate (Flanagan, 1976).

Today, nursing union activity is centralized around a few unions and state nurses professional organizations, including the United American Nurses, an AFL-CIO affiliate and affiliate of the ANA, several independent state nurses associations still affiliated with the ANA, the California Nurses Association (not affiliated with the ANA), the Service Employees International Union (SEIU), the American Federation of State and Municipal Employees Union (AFSME), and other unions. Many disagree regarding who best represents nurses—professional organizations or unions?

Who best represents nursing's interests? Mary Foley, president of the ANA in 2002, asserted that professional organizations concerned with all aspects of nursing and *only* nursing are best equipped to represent nurses in contrast to unions, who have multiple groups to represent and multiple agendas (Foley, 2002). In contrast, Warino (2007) contended that which union(s) represent nurses matters because it has a major effect on the public's perception of the profession, and state nurses associations affiliated with the ANA are more likely than other unions to negotiate nursing practice issues, as well as wages and working conditions.

Emergence of Medicare and Medicaid

In the early part of the 20th century the cost of medical care was a serious problem impoverishing families throughout the nation. The creation of the Medicare program negotiated through several iterations represented the first two steps in Kingdon's policy process. The legislation that created Medicare, a social health insurance program for all people older than 65 years of age regardless of income, took over a decade to pass Congress. In 1955, the ANA took a position supporting Medicare, which demonstrated a high degree of political sophistication for the organization at that time. The initial hearings on the first Medicare bill were held in June 1958 and were inconclusive. ANA was joined in supporting the legislation by the AFL-CIO, the National Farmers' Union, the American Public Welfare Association, the National Association of Social Workers, and other groups. It was opposed by the AMA, the National Chamber of Commerce, the National Association of Manufacturers, the Health Insurance Association of America (a newly formed organization of some 260 health insurance companies), the Pharmaceutical Manufacturers' Association, and the American Farm Bureau Federation, among others (Social Security Online, n.d.).

The AMA lobbied successfully for compromises to charge "usual" or "customary fees for services," which were included in the final bill. The AMA position changed when doctors realized they would be paid for *all* their care by the government, without government interference. After nearly a decade of debate, along party-line votes because of political advocacy (the third of Kingdon's policy streams), the Medicare Act (officially part of the Social Security Amendments of 1965) passed in 1965 as a two-part insurance program:

> *The "basic" program of hospital and related benefits was financed through social security taxes. Benefits included 90 days of hospital care, 100 days of nursing-home care, 100 home-nursing "visits" in each "spell" of illness, and hospital outpatient service—all subject to "deductibles," "coinsurance," and other features, as well as certain other conditions. The second part consisted of a voluntary program of "supplementary" benefits, covering 80 percent (above an annual deductible of $50) of physicians' fees, additional home-nursing services, in-hospital diagnostic and laboratory work, certain kinds of therapy, ambulance services, surgical dressings, and so forth. This supplementary plan would be financed initially through a $3 monthly premium from each beneficiary, with a matching amount paid by the Government out of the general revenues. In addition, the act provided for a substantially expanded Kerr-Mills program extending "medical indigency" benefits to other age groups besides those over age 65 (Social Security Online, n.d.).*

The "medical indigency" benefits became Medicaid, a federal–state partnership that provides health coverage for the poor based on income eligibility. Not surprisingly, just as Medicare and Medicaid passed, and *before* the terms "usual and customary" were defined, physician fees increased dramatically, so physician fees started out higher in the new government-funded Medicare and Medicaid systems than they were before their passage because the government was paying the bills (Families USA, 1993). These programs were part of President Lyndon Johnson's dream of a Great Society.

Medicare provides coverage to more than 43 million persons who are elderly or disabled. It would be impossible for any but the wealthy to afford to pay out-of-pocket for hospital stays of any length, so Medicare continues to protect Medicare beneficiaries, the elderly, and the disabled from bankruptcy related to hospital costs. Outpatient costs have outpaced inflation and many are covered by Medicare Part B.

NURSING IN CONTEMPORARY POLITICS AND POLICY

There are many contemporary issues that those in nursing are discussing in the political arena and at the policy table. Environmental health, the current nursing shortage, and access to health care are among the most pressing.

Nursing Shortage

Shortages of nurses in the United States occur in cycles. They have recently occurred in the 1950s, 1970s, 1980s, and 1990s. However, today's nursing shortage will be the greatest nursing shortage in history. It has been estimated that the nation will experience a shortage of up to 500,000 nurses by 2025 (Buerhaus, Stainger, & Auerbach, 2008). One often-cited reason for the growing shortage is that the most recent generation of women to enter the profession (the Baby Boomers) will retire between 2015 and 2025. Add to that the aging of their entire generation and one has what has been referred to as a "perfect storm"—a severe shortage of nurses at a time when the demand for nurses is the greatest.

Nursing shortages in the past have been addressed by increasing salaries for nurses; however, there are other factors that affect the current shortage. Among the issues cited for the lack of interest in nursing as a career are poor working conditions, low job satisfaction, and the existence of other, more attractive career opportunities for women. Among the reasons given by working nurses for either leaving the profession entirely or choosing early retirement are shift work, heavy patient loads, mandatory overtime, and lack of responsiveness by supervisors and administrators.

An additional component of the current nursing crisis is that the nursing education system does not have the resources in terms of faculty or funding to replace nurses who are retiring from the workforce. Although there has been an increase in applications to nursing programs, many qualified students have been refused admission due to lack of funding for staff and facilities. A study published in 2005 of trends for 2003 indicated that 33,000 students who were qualified for admission to nursing schools in the United States were turned down because of the lack of available resources to accommodate them. The reason given by 76% of the schools was lack of faculty (Berlin, Wilsey, & Bednash, 2005).

Many of the present nursing faculty are also of the Baby Boomer generation and will be retiring in unprecedented numbers, with few replacements in the process of preparing for an academic career. The Robert Wood Johnson Foundation suggested several approaches for increasing the supply of nursing educators, including the following: (1) stimulate interest in the academic role, (2) combine clinical experience with academic disciplines, (3) provide greater financial assistance, (4) increase salary and faculty support, (5) offer more accessible academic training, (6) increase available faculty positions, (7) offer programs to improve faculty productivity, and (8) support research training (Yordy, 2006, pp. 6–8).

There have been some attempts to address the nursing shortage at the state level. There is a growing movement to establish safe staffing levels, such as those enacted by California in 1999, which became effective in 2003. New York State is expected to enact a law banning mandatory overtime for nurses to take effect in 2009. Other states are attempting similar legislation.

At the federal level, recruitment and retention are addressed by the Nurse Reinvestment Act of 2002, which establishes nurse scholarships, nurse retention and patient safety enhancement grants, comprehensive geriatric training grants for nurses, faculty loan cancellation programs, career ladder grant programs, and public service announcements (American Association of Colleges of Nursing [AACN], 2005, paras 1–6).

To combat the growing shortage of nurses, many hospitals in the United States have begun recruiting from other English-speaking countries around the world that have their own nursing shortage for similar reasons to those in this country (Health Resources and Services Administration, 2000). This practice has been referred to as "poaching," and although to many this might seem a viable solution, it raises serious ethical questions. Instead of increasing funding to nursing schools, training and hiring more faculty, and increasing facilities, the developed nations increasingly look to the impoverished nations of the world to supply nurses. Many argue that nurses have the right, like anyone else, to migrate for a better life; however, they are often "wooed from countries in which serious needs of patients and communities are being left unmet, resulting in even worsening conditions within those countries" (Salmon & Guisinger, 2007, p. 985).

Nurses migrate for the same reasons that others migrate, with economic reasons being the most significant.

However, there are other reasons nurses migrate: to improve the quality of life or the quality or their careers, to escape from armed conflicts in their home country, because of natural disasters, or to follow a spouse (Kingma, 2006). For whatever reason they migrate, they have all been educated in their home country and then migrate to another nation, creating what has been referred to as a "brain drain" in their home country. The poorest nations with the greatest burden of disease and the greatest health disparities have the fewest nurses. For instance, migration away from the African continent has resulted in a severe shortage of medical professionals in the region of the world that has the largest number of persons infected with HIV (Kingma).

In 2000 the United Nations Millennium Summit issued a list of Millennium Development Goals. These include eight goals specifically designed to improve conditions internationally by 2015 (United Nations Development Programme, 2007). They include the following:

1. Eradicate extreme poverty and hunger
2. Achieve universal education
3. Promote gender equality and empower women
4. Reduce child mortality
5. Improve maternal health
6. Combat HIV/AIDS, malaria, and other diseases
7. Ensure environmental sustainability
8. Develop global partnerships for development

Due, in part, to the increasing migration of medical personnel, especially nurses, it is unlikely that the poorest nations will achieve the health-related goals by 2015.

The international nursing shortage is recognized around the world as a crisis that undermines the health care systems of all countries. Worldwide, nations are trying individually to create strategies to improve the recruitment and retention of nurses. What are needed are efforts at all levels—internationally, nationally, and locally—to increase the world's supply of nurses so that nursing can meet the needs of patients.

Environmental Health

Concern for the effects of the environment on health and quality of life is not new to nursing. In fact, Florence Nightingale went so far as to claim that nurses are accountable for managing or changing the environment to improve health: "No amount of medical knowledge will lessen the accountability for nurses to do what nurses do; that is, manage the environment to promote positive life processes" (Nightingale, 1992, p. 71). Today this is as true as it was then.

Environmental health can be defined as freedom from injury or illness due to the effects of the environment. More formally, it is defined as "the state of health that exists as a result of the biological, chemical, physical and social forces and conditions that surround and influence human beings" (Primomo & Salazar, 2005, p. 596).

In the workplace and in everyday life nurses are witness to an increase in illness and disability linked to the environment. An increase in childhood asthma is but one example of the effect of air pollution. Diseases such as breast and lung cancer have been linked to the environment. Arsenic exposure has been associated with cancer of several human organs, and lead exposure has been linked to nervous system disorders (U.S. Environmental Protection Agency, 2007). Increasingly, the newspapers are reporting episodes of *Salmonella* and *Escherichia coli* poisoning from the food and water supply.

Increased awareness about global warming and finite fossil fuel energy resources has helped to launch an international "environmental health" movement. Nurses are involved in efforts to protect the public from harmful human-made toxins, social inequities, and the often resulting civil unrest over scarce resources. Environmental concerns that are global in scope are ozone and energy depletion and global warming, overpopulation, deforestation, wetlands destruction, contaminated and scarce food supplies, water and biologic pollution, waste disposal, rodent and insect control, safety, and terrorist activity (Allender & Spradley, 2005).

A concept of particular importance to nursing is *environmental justice*, a concept that refers to the link between low-income populations and neighborhoods and high exposure to health risks from the environment. Low-income neighborhoods, often populated by minorities, contain a disproportionately high number of hazardous waste incinerators and toxic landfills. The problem of environmental justice has become so serious that Congress passed the Environmental Justice Act in 1993, and Executive Order 12898, Federal Actions to Address Environmental Justice in Minority Populations, was signed in 1994. These policies were intended to reduce the effects of environmental inequality by mandating all federal agencies to act in such a manner as to prevent injuries and illness caused by the environment (Sattler, Afzal, & McPhaul, 2006).

Anderko (2003) claimed that countless human-caused diseases have arisen from declining environmental health conditions and called for political advocacy in uncovering and tracking this health problem. For example, nurses are involved in drafting legislation to decrease the use of polyvinylchlorides (PVCs; soft plastics) in hospitals because of their known carcinogenic effects. Registered Nurse Charlotte Brody was one of the founders of an international organization, Health Care Without Harm (Brody, 2007), that works with health organizations worldwide to eliminate toxins produced by the health industry.

Nurses are working in neighborhoods (like Lillian Wald) to insist on cleaning up toxins and to make safe places for children to play. Nurses are educating the public regarding proper disposal of extra medications to prevent contaminating the water system, as well as decreasing the use of personal care products, household cleaners, and foods that contain chemicals that are hormone disrupters and mimic estrogen. Jeanne Rizzo, a Registered Nurse who has lead the Breast Cancer Fund since 2000, has launched a national online education campaign and has recently successfully lobbied to pass legislation to eliminate phthalates from children's toys (Breast Cancer Fund, 2008).

Nursing must protect the public's health from potential threats in the environment and help to protect and promote the health of the environment so that it can be life and health enhancing. Strategies for nursing action in environmental health include the following (Allender & Spradley, 2005, p. 227; Brody, 2007):

1. Learn about possible environmental health threats.

2. Assess clients' environment and detect health hazards.

3. Plan collaboratively with citizens and other professionals to devise protective and preventive strategies.

4. Assist with implementation of programs to prevent health threats to clients and the environment.

5. Take action to correct situations in which health hazards exist.

6. Educate consumers and assist them to practice preventive measures.

7. Take action to promote the development of policies and legislation that enhance consumer protection and promote healthier environments.

8. Assist with and promote program evaluation to determine the effectiveness of environmental health efforts.

9. Apply environmentally related research findings and participate in nursing research.

Nurses are in a perfect position to promote environmental health because there are more than 2.5 million nurses who live and work in every neighborhood in the country. To the public, nurses are the most trusted and visible representation of health care. Nurses as a powerful, respected, and sophisticated interest group must be a part of future social movements to increase access to quality, affordable health care and to make the world a safer place for all people.

For example, the Luminary Project (n.d.) was formed in 2005 to highlight the work of nurses in environmental health and to engage nurses in actions that will protect the public and the environment. It has tool kits for projects such as eliminating mercury thermometers, reducing hospital and health system waste, phasing out toxic chemicals at home and at work, improving indoor air quality, changing hospital purchasing practices to support safe products, and educating nurses about the links between health and the environment.

Access to Health Care: Health Disparities and Social Justice

The cost of health care increases every year. In 2006, the United States spent $2.1 trillion, or an average of $7,026 per person, on health care. Sixteen percent of the nation's economic resources are spent on health care (Kaiser Family Foundation, 2008). Health insurance provided by employers accounted for coverage for 54% of Americans in 2007, a percentage that dropped from 69% in 2000. People who have health coverage that they pay for themselves have seen their premiums increase by 78% while their wages were going up by 17% (Kaiser Family Foundation, 2007). Some individuals receive it as a benefit of employment (or their spouse's or parent's employment), some are military veterans, and some are covered by Medicare, Medicaid, or the State Children's Health Insurance Program (SCHIP). In recent years local jurisdictions (cities and counties) and states have begun experimenting with health insurance and coverage options for their residents.

The number of people in the United States without health coverage grows annually. Schoen, Collins, Kriss, and Doty (2008) found a 60% increase in the number of uninsured between 2003 and 2007, and estimated that one in four people ages 19 to 64 years was uninsured. The greatest rate of increase was for people above the 200% of poverty level. In 2007, 42% of U.S. adults were uninsured or underinsured (Centers for Medicare and Medicaid Services, n.d.). The high unemployment rate has contributed to the number of uninsured, and the rising cost of care results in employers dropping coverage.

The Institute of Medicine (IOM) found overwhelming evidence that the uninsured receive poor health care, if they receive care at all. The uninsured are less likely to receive preventive and screening services; therefore, serious diseases are detected later. In 2004, the IOM estimated that 20,000 people die each year because they are uninsured (Cutler, 2004). In 2006, the number had increased to 22,000 (Dorn, 2008).

The cost of coverage is increasing, and cost sharing as a measure to save money on the part of insurers has increased. This contributes to income insecurity and is forcing millions of uninsured and underinsured to be at risk of spending large portions of their incomes on health care (Schoen et al., 2008).

People of color comprise a higher percentage of the uninsured mortality statistics. Lack of health insurance is one factor in explaining why people of color rank the lowest on key health status indicators (Lillie-Blanton & Hoffman, 2005). Half of the nation's 47 million uninsured are ethnic minorities (Smedly, 2008). Three fourths of the 23 million uninsured in communities of color in the United States lived below 200 percent of the federal poverty level of $41,300 for a family of four in 2007 (Centers for Medicare and Medicaid Services, 2007).

Health disparities among communities of color are found in the "differences in the incidence, prevalence, mortality and burden of diseases and other adverse health conditions that exist among specific population groups in the U.S." (Almgren, 2007, p. 221). The *mortality* (death) rate of the population in the 45- to 54-year-old group is considered a measure of premature death and of the "burden of disease" (Almgren, p. 224); the latter can also be expressed in terms of *morbidity*, the incidence of disease.

Almgren (2007) cited 2003 data from the National Center for Health Statistics that revealed that there are major differences in the mortality rates of middle-aged persons in the United States by race and Hispanic ethnicity. Between the ages of 45 and 54 years, the highest death rate is among non-Hispanic blacks, and it is nearly twice that of non-Hispanic whites and more than twice that of Hispanics. Native Americans also have mortality rates that are significantly higher than those for both Hispanics and non-Hispanic whites. Health insurance and access to care are important, and systems must be improved to ensure access to convenient, culturally appropriate care that is simple to enroll in; however, access to care alone will not ensure that health disparities will be eliminated (Smedly, 2008).

The burden of disease of a population subgroup can be measured across populations and geography. It reflects the susceptibilities, as well as exposures, to diseases that are linked to biology (genetics) and the environment—both the social and the physical environment. Disparities in access to health care and/or quality of health care have an effect on prevention, early diagnosis, and treatment, which can influence mortality.

Social inequity is directly linked to the burden of disease. Clean air, clean water, open space to play, safe streets, and healthy nutritional options (e.g., access to affordable fresh fruit and vegetables conveniently located in the neighborhood) are social/environmental determinants of health disparity. Social determinants of health, or "upstream predictors" of health status, include education, housing, employment, and poverty (Smedly, 2008, p. 443). According to Smedly, to eliminate health disparities or inequalities, a clinical model is inadequate. A conceptual model that includes income security, jobs that pay a living wage, protection of social insurance programs such as Medicare and Medicaid, housing security, environmental security—including safe, clean neighborhoods—education opportunities, and the elimination of institutional racism must be integral parts of health promotion.

Kimbro, Bzostek, Goldman, and Rodriguez (2008) examined National Health Interview Survey data from 2000 to 2006 and found that education is a more powerful determinant of health behaviors and outcomes for some ethnic groups than for others, and they argued for different interventions based on whether people were born in the United States or were immigrants.

When mortality rates from chronic and noncommunicable diseases (e.g., asthma, diabetes) were examined across level of education, people with 1 year of education beyond high school (12 years education) were found to live longer. Higher social class is also associated with reduced burden of chronic and noncommunicable diseases (Almgren, 2007). Social class and educational attainment are linked, increasing the likelihood that disadvantages associated with poverty increase the likelihood of the incidence of noncommunicable and chronic illness.

DISCUSSION POINT

Children who live near highways and industrial plants have a higher incidence of asthma and are more likely to live in poverty and have lower educational attainment. Should nurses be involved in advocating for better schools and safer neighborhoods for children to play in?

Preserving Medicaid and Medicare

The Kaiser Family Foundation (2008) stated that the projected cost of Medicare in 2009 will be $420 billion, 14% of the total federal budget (for comparison, defense makes up 20% of the budget), and that more than 44 million Americans, 16% of whom are younger than 65 years or have disabilities, will receive coverage through Medicare. Medicaid—the joint federal–state program that provides health coverage and long-term care assistance to more than 45 million children and adults in low-income families and 14 million elderly persons and people with disabilities—makes up 7% of the federal budget (Kaiser Family Foundation, 2008).

Federal Medicaid funds to states have been cut every year since 2002. Since 2005, the national economic downturn causing state funding reductions has required states to limit provider payments, implement copayments for services, and reduce benefits (such as vision, dental, and pharmaceutical formulary choices) and limit eligibility (Rudowitz & Marks, 2008). Twenty-eight states are projecting budget shortfalls for fiscal year 2009 as the U.S. braces for continued financial hard times.

During economic downturns, the number of people who lose their health coverage grows as the number of unemployed people increases. This causes an increased demand for Medicaid. As of this writing, year 2008 Medicaid and SCHIP cuts have already been proposed

in 13 states. A 2008 Kaiser Family Foundation analysis produced by the Urban Institute found that for every.

1 percentage point rise in the national unemployment rate, Medicaid and SCHIP enrollment would increase by 1 million (600,000 children and 400,000 non-elderly adults) and cause the number of uninsured to grow by 1.1 million. That would increase Medicaid and SCHIP costs by $3.4 billion, including $1.4 billion in state spending. This represents a 1 percent increase in total Medicaid and SCHIP expenditures. Further: at the state level, a 1 percentage point increase in the unemployment rate causes state General Fund revenue to drop by 3 to 4 percent below expected levels. If states must balance their budgets and all state spending is reduced proportionally, a 1 percentage point increase in unemployment would therefore entail a 3 to 4 percent reduction in Medicaid and SCHIP spending (Dorn, Garrett, Holahan, & Williams, 2008, p. 5).

More than 39 million Americans rely on Medicaid for their health care (Rowland, 2008). The greatest number of people relying on Medicaid are poor families with children; however, the majority of Medicaid dollars are spent on the elderly and persons with disabilities. In 2006, 36% of Medicaid funds were spent on long-term care for the elderly. Skilled nursing facilities received $48,638,435,956, and another $45,471,600,985 was spent on home and personal care (Kaiser Family Foundation, 2009). The number of people requiring long-term care will increase every year, and cuts in Medicaid funding will result in less care for the most frail in nursing homes.

The AMA and other health care PACs have continued to strongly support Medicare and Medicaid because these programs reimburse physicians and other health services. Physicians and the health insurance industry spend significant amounts of money on lobbying Congress and Executive Branch agencies and make substantial contributions to congressional campaigns. Steinbrook (2007) noted that in 2004, the "health sector" contributed $123.9 million to presidential and congressional campaigns. In 2006 the sector contributed $98.6 million. These contributions made up more than 7% of all contributions; more than three fifths of these contributions were to Republicans. In 2006 the health sector spent $351.1 million on lobbying costs, the second highest in such spending. Health sector lobbying costs made up 13.8% of all lobbying spending.

When elements of the health sector lobbying spending were ranked, pharmaceuticals came in on top, then hospitals and nursing homes, then health professionals, followed by health service systems and health management organizations (HMOs) (Steinbrook, 2007). Among the top spending organizations, the AMA ranked third at $19.9 million in 2006.

Over the opposition of the ANA and a broad array of health care organizations, in 2003, Medicare Part D was added to the Medicare benefit package by President Bush and passed by a narrow margin in Congress; it covers some prescription drug costs to the elderly and persons with disabilities as part of the Medicare Modernization Prescription Drug, Improvement and Modernization Act (MMA).

The MMA actually weakened the Medicare program by increasing costs to Medicare beneficiaries and the government and failed to improve coverage for needed health care. The 73 health care companies approved to administer the new Medicare drug discount card programs gave President Bush and congressional conservatives a total of more than $5 million in hard money, soft money, and PAC contributions between 2000 and 2004. The Center for American Progress (2004) suggested that the Bush Administration overlooked the fact that 20 of the 73 contributors had been involved in fraud charges because of their financial ties to the Bush presidential campaign.

The MMA (Public Law 108-173) contains provisions that include financial benefits for Medicare Advantage plans (largely for profit managed care plans) over traditional Medicare and allows for unequal benefit packages among insurance options. It increased costs to beneficiaries (increased Part B by "means testing," adding a new "premium support pilot project," and cost-sharing copays), and it also limits needed occupational and physical therapy benefits. The MMA imposes cost sharing for home health, hospitalization, durable medical equipment, and inpatient mental health services. It exempts Medicare Advantage plans from being required to report quality data, making comparisons based on quality difficult, and it places an arbitrary limit on spending designed to limit the federal government's commitment to Medicare while doing nothing to address the rising cost of health care. In order to entice private insurance and drug companies into the Part D program, the MMA provides billions in subsidies to the private sector to participate. Both the rising cost of drugs and the private sector subsidies provide little or no benefit to Medicare enrollees (National Committee to Preserve Social Security and Medicare, 2008).

The MMA Part D created confusion and locked beneficiaries into a drug plan for an entire year while the plans were allowed to change formularies at any time. Most formularies cover the cost of male performance drugs such as Viagra and Cialis but lack of coverage for mental health medications, such as benzodiazepines, that are often needed by the elderly. The plan also prohibits purchasing medications from Canada and prohibits negotiating bulk pricing.

In 2008 the ANA House of Delegates passed a resolution supporting the elimination of the parts of the MMA just described. It also urged that Medicare be strengthened by ensuring that the essential care provided by nurses and nurse practitioners be adequately reimbursed, ensuring that palliative and hospice care are adequately reimbursed, and urging that drugs commonly prescribed in the elderly population not be excluded from coverage (Protection and enhancement of Medicare, 2008).

Nursing Political Action Coalitions

The year 1974 brought new election laws allowing for contributions by PACs. The laws limited the amount an individual could contribute to a campaign, and allowed groups to contribute up to $5,000 per election. Contributions from nurses giving small amounts individually could not compare to what physicians gave; however, together, they could contribute to a PAC and give $5,000. The Nurses Coalition for Action in Politics (N-CAP; the precursor of the ANA PAC) was created by the ANA to establish political power through the endorsement of candidates and political contributions. The slogan "1 in 44" was worn on buttons when nurses visited their legislators to point out that 1 in 44 registered women voters was a Registered Nurse.

When President Gerald Ford vetoed the Nurse Training Act of 1974 and attempted to eliminate the scholarship and student loan programs for nursing, the ANA lobbied Congress, which passed legislation extending the Nurse Training Act, which included, for the first time, funding for advanced practice nursing. President Ford vetoed the bill, and the ANA mounted a nationwide lobbying effort. Congress overrode the veto with many more than the two thirds votes required (Kalisch & Kalisch,

1982). Again, a convergence of Kingdon's streams can be identified: a problem of not enough nurses and a powerful political interest group of nurses!

The proliferation of nursing specialty organizations and unions all claiming to represent "nursing" sometimes jeopardizes nursing's effectiveness because different nursing organizations bring different messages to elected officials. Elected officials tend to listen to the people who help elect them, so whichever nursing organizations are most active in political campaigns through contributions and through grassroots activity (usually only important in an official's first few elections because of the power of incumbency) are the organizations that will be heard.

As more and more nurses are represented by unions, unions are often the voice of nurses in the nation's capital. It is essential for nurses to be involved in all organizations that represent nurses, especially those with PACs, because "money talks." Contributing to candidates that promote nursing's agenda to improve the quality of health care is important. It is unfortunate that campaigns are expensive, but it costs money to buy television ad time and to mail literature to people's homes. Professional nurses must make things happen or they will find themselves not only wondering what happened, but also complaining about it.

The ANA PAC has grown over the years through contributions of members. The PAC considers the voting records of incumbent candidates for re-election and the relationships with the state constituent member of the ANA for candidates running for open seats. Keeping track of voting records is important, and PAC contributions are essential for successful re-election campaigns of friends of nursing (ANA, 2006).

CONSIDER

Of the 252 candidates endorsed by ANA PAC for election to the 106th Congress, 88% won their elections (ANA, 2000). Do all Registered Nurses benefit from the contributions and work of the members of the ANA who make monetary contributions to the ANA PAC and help to elect "nurse-friendly" members of Congress?

Aligning with a Political Party

Nurses naturally work to affect policy in the workplace but often fail to realize that the work they do and the environment in which it is done are controlled by the government. So, nurses must be involved beyond the private sector if they are to bring about change. To do so requires nurses to examine their values and pick a political party that reflects their views and become involved.

From a health perspective, the primary difference between the two major parties in the United States is that Democrats typically favor "public" systems with taxpayers funding access to health services with a guaranteed benefit package and price controls. Criticism of this philosophy is that price regulation will stifle innovation and quality and that taxpayers should not have to pay for the ills of others.

Republicans tend to favor a market strategy in which consumers will make choices based on cost and quality within private systems, and that with consumers making market choices, competition will keep prices down. The major criticisms of this strategy are that education and health do not behave like traditional market systems and that market mechanisms in health care yield an advantage to the more affluent and healthier people, as well as for providers, suppliers, and insurers. In this system, the financial burden for the sick, disabled, and uninsured is left to the public (government) sector. The public risk pool—or the group of people being cared for by the public sector—is more costly than if the risk were spread among the entire population (Evans, 2003). The reality is that nurses are not born Republicans or Democrats, and party affiliation is often a reflection of core personal values. It is important, then, to have nurses as leaders in both political parties.

DISCUSSION POINT

Do your beliefs about health care align more closely with traditional Democratic or Republican Party values?

Getting Involved

The message throughout this chapter has been that nurses need to be increasingly involved in both politics and public policy. A good way for most nurses to increase their involvement is to join a professional organization that is politically active. Nurses can also become better informed about current issues by consulting the Web sites of these professional organizations (see Web Resources at the end of this chapter). Nurses can also check the status of federal and state legislation online.

BOX 22.3 | ACTIONS NURSES CAN TAKE

To Influence Politics

- Be knowledgeable and get involved in campaigns (the earlier the better).
- Assist candidates in winning the endorsement of key organizations that you may be involved in, such as nursing organizations, parent–teacher organizations, and neighborhood organizations.

To Influence Policy

- Be a member of a nursing organization that influences policy at the local, state, and federal levels.
- Be informed. Subscribe to electronic listservs of elected officials that you agree with and compare the records of your officials.
- Get to know your elected officials.
- Write lobbying letters.
- Write letters to the editor.
- Participate in coalitions of organizations.

Other actions that nurses can take to increase their influence in politics and health care policy are shown in Box 22.3. The first of these is to get more involved in electing candidates they want to win. This requires that nurses be knowledgeable regarding the candidates and their values. It is politically smart for nurses to pick candidates that have a good chance of winning and who share nursing's values. The nurse who works for a losing candidate risks alienating the winner. In races in which the candidate is an incumbent and is in a district in which her or she is likely to be reelected, the candidate still needs help. Specific activities that might be undertaken to support such a candidate include telephone banking, precinct walking, fundraising, writing letters to the editor, and supporting the candidate in public forums, including other organizations in which one participates.

> ### CONSIDER
> Working together, speaking with one strong voice, nurses are a powerful political force.

Actions that nurses can take to increase their influence in the policy setting are also shown in Box 22.3. Again, becoming involved in a professional nursing organization and being informed head the list. Nurses must also know the legislator who represents them. District office staff usually handle constituent case work dealing with local, state, or federal agencies. For example, if someone has a problem with the Post Office or is a veteran and cannot get benefits, they can seek help from their congressional representative's district office. The district chief of staff is often the only "policy person" in the district. The office in the Capitol deals with legislation and policy issues. Staff members are key in getting access to a legislator, so the politically astute nurse is polite and respectful in dealing with these individuals.

Finally, nurses who want to increase their influence in policy should write their legislative representatives regarding health care issues (Box 22.4). Letters should arrive before any proposed legislation is heard in committee because key decisions on proposed legislation are made in committee. Bills that have a financial impact are heard in a policy committee and a financial committee. Some bills are assigned to two or more committees. This is often a tactic used to defeat the bill before it comes to the floor. If your legislator is not on the committee, write to the Committee Chair at the committee office address. If you write to legislators who do not represent you (you do not reside in their district), however, they are unlikely to respond to your communications because you are not one of their constituents. It is a good idea to send a copy of the letter with a brief cover letter to your legislator urging his or her support when the bill comes to the floor (if bills pass out of committee, they go to the "floor" or the entire house of the legislature). If your legislator supports your position on legislation,

BOX 22.4 | SAMPLE LOBBYING LETTER

[1]Lillian Wald, RN, BSN
Henry Street
New York, New York 00251

[2]The Honorable Harry Nemo
Member, U.S. House of Representatives
House Office Building
Washington DC, 20015

[3]RE: SUPPORT for HR 1435

[4]Dear Representative Nemo,

[5]I am a Registered Nurse and I have worked in the area of home health care for over five years. In the past two years more and more of the elderly patients I care for have had to be readmitted to the hospital shortly after being discharged from the hospital because they are not taking their prescribed medications.

As you know, H.R. 1435 would provide a guaranteed, affordable prescription drug benefit within the Medicare program. Currently, despite many drug coverage programs for seniors, many remain unaffordable.

[6]It will save costly hospitalizations to provide needed prescription drugs at affordable costs to seniors. Please support H.R. 1435 and please advise me of your current position on this bill. Sincerely,

[7]Lillian Wald, RN, BSN

Legend:

1: Include your address.

2: Use the proper form of address (most elected and appointed officials are addressed as "the Honorable").

3: State what the letter is regarding.

4: Use the office title in the salutation.

5: State your credentials and experience/belief/position.

6: Urge support/opposition, and *ask* for a response with the official's position.

7: Sign letter.

send a thank you note! Thank you notes tell legislators that you are watching what they are doing.

CONCLUSIONS

What would Lillian Wald do about health care coverage for children and access to health care? What would Minerva Franklin do about racial health inequalities? What would Florence Nightingale do to elevate nursing in the policy debates? Not since 2001, when the ANA called together all the nursing specialty organizations in a Call to the Profession to begin a dialogue on collaboration and to develop Nursing's Agenda for the Future, has

progress been made on speaking with one voice in the policy arena. The ANA argued that it is essential that nursing speak with one voice (ANA, 2003), but how does nursing come together to do so?

So the question is "What should nursing say?" At a time when the country is deeply divided along party lines, nurses must speak for the clients they serve. Nurses are stakeholders in what happens in health care (access, insurance coverage, cost, research), in the workplace (staffing levels, safety, scope of practice, autonomy, working conditions), in the economy (unemployment's effect on mental and physical health and access to care, funding for Medicare and Medicaid), in international trade issues (foreign nurse licensure, importation of less expensive prescription drugs), and in the environment (preventing illness caused by pollution). That is, nurses are directly affected by the outcome of countless policies that are enacted or regulated.

There are many levels of political involvement and many spheres in which nurses can be influential, both public and private. Nurses can influence policies in the workplace (both public and private) and the community (both public and private). They can also influence policy within professional organizations (private) and within the government (Mason et al., 2002). The bottom line is that they must accept a responsibility to be involved in some way.

Pierce (2004, p. 115) perhaps said it best:

For the nursing profession to flex its collective political muscle and get involved with the redesign of the nation's health care system, we have to use our leader-ship to get the professional organizations to think and act collaboratively and to deliver a clear and strategic message to lawmakers.

As nurses, as voters, and as constituents, we must be a part of the solution. Our elected officials truly want to know what nurses think and it is our obligation as professionals and as citizens to let them know. Our patients and the American public trusts nurses and are counting on us to advocate on their behalf.

Per capita, the United States has the most expensive health care system in the world, yet it ranks next to last on five dimensions of a high-performance health system: quality, access, efficiency, equity, and healthy lives (Davis et al. 2007). Nurses must be involved in policy debates to ensure that health care reform addresses cost, quality, and access simultaneously and preserves the notion that health care is a right and not a privilege.

FOR ADDITIONAL DISCUSSION

1. Are nongovernmental and governmental politics more alike than not? If not, how do they differ? If so, how are they alike?

2. Why do you believe nursing was the first profession to eliminate segregation?

3. What are the most significant nursing issues being debated in the policy arena?

4. With such limited membership in the ANA, will nurses ever have a political power base that is representative of the size of their voting block?

5. Why are so many nurses reluctant to become active in the political arena? Do they lack the skills to do so? The confidence? Do nurses perceive a lack of congruity between professional behavior and politics?

6. With the AMA typically being far better represented than the ANA in legislative lobbying, is nursing's risk of being dominated by medicine greater than ever?

7. How well informed are most legislators about contemporary health care and professional nursing issues?

8. What do you believe will be the next major policy issue affecting nursing to be debated in the political arena?

ACKNOWLEDGMENT

This research was supported by a grant from the Robert Wood Johnson Foundation to the Association of Academic Health Centers.

REFERENCES

Allender, J., & Spradley, B. (2005). Environmental health and safety (pp. 226–261). In: J. Allender & Spradley, B. (Eds.), *Community Health Nursing: Promoting and Protecting the Public's Health*, 6th ed. Lippincott: Philadelphia.

Almgren, G. (2007). *Health Care Politics, Policy and Services: A Social Justice Analysis.* New York: Springer, pp. 221–257.

American Association of Colleges of Nursing (AACN) (2005). *Nurse reinvestment act at a glance.* Available at: http://www.aacn.nche.edu/media/nraataglance.htm. Accessed July 1, 2008

American Association for the History of Nursing (AAHN) (2004). *Gravesites of prominent nurses: Lillian D. Wald.* Available at: http://www.aahn.org/gravesites/wald.html. Accessed June 10, 2008.

American Heritage Dictionary of the English language (2000). Policy: Definition. Available at: http://dictionary.reference.com/search?q=politics. Accessed June 27, 2005.

American Nurses Association (ANA) (2000). *ANA-PAC endorses Hillary Clinton for U.S. Senate.* Available at: http://www.ana.org/pressrel/2000/pr0208.htm. Accessed June 27, 2005.

American Nurses Association (ANA) (2001a). *Nursing's Agenda for Health Care Reform.* Washington, DC: ANA.

American Nurses Association (ANA) (2001b). *Analysis of American Nurses Association Staffing Survey.* Available at: http://www.nursingworld.org/MainMenu Categories/ThePracticeofProfessionalNursing/work place/Workforce/ShortageStaffing/Staffing/Satffing Survey.aspx. Accessed January 28, 2009.

American Nurses Association (ANA) (2001c). *Health and safety survey.* Available at: www.nursingworld.org/surveys/hssurvey.pdf. Accessed June 27, 2005.

American Nurses Association (ANA) (2003). *Nursing's Agenda for the Future.* Washington, DC: ANA.

American Nurses Association (ANA) (2006). *Voting score card.* Available at: http://www.nursingworld.org/MainMenuCategories/ANAPoliticalPower/VoteScorecard.aspx. Accessed July 30, 2008.

ANA Hall of Fame: Martha Minerva Franklin (n.d.). Available at: http://www.nursingworld.org/Functional MenuCategories/AboutANA/WhereWeCome From_1/HallofFame/19761982/franmm5536.aspx. Accessed August 17, 2008.

Anderko, L. (2003). Protecting the health of our nation's children through environmental health tracking. *Policy, Politics & Nursing Practice, 4*(1), 14–21.

Berlin L, Wilsey S., & Bednash G. (2005). *2004–2005 Enrollments and Graduations in Baccalaureate and Graduate Programs in Nursing.* Washington, DC: American Association of Colleges of Nursing.

Block, L. E. (2008). Health Policy: What it is and how it works (pp. 4–14). In: C. Harrington & C. L. Estes (Eds.), *Health Policy; Crisis and Reform in the U.S. Health Care Delivery System.* Sudbury, MA: Jones & Bartlett.

Breast Cancer Fund (2008). *Victory is sweet. Protecting kids from toxic phthalates is sweeter.* Available at: http://breastcancerfund.typepad.com/bcfblog/2008/08/victory-is-swee.html. Accessed August 15, 2008.

Brody, C. (2007). Regulating industrial chemicals to protect the environment and human health (pp. 947–953). In: D. J. Mason, J. K. Leavitt, & M. W. Chafee (Eds.), *Policy and Politics in Nursing and Health Care* (5th ed.). St. Louis, MO: Saunders/Elsevier.

Buerhaus, P., Stainger, D., & Auerbach, D. (2008). *The future of the nursing workforce in the United States: Data, trends and implications.* Jones and Bartlett: Maine.

Center for American Progress (2004). *Paying to play: Health care companies, campaign contributions and Medicare drug discount cards.* Available at: http://www.americanprogress.org/issues/2004/06/b84766.html. Accessed January 28, 2009.

Centers for Medicare and Medicaid Services (n.d.). *2007 federal poverty levels.* Available at: http://www.cms.hhs.gov/MedicaidEligibility/Downloads/POV07ALL.pdf. Accessed July 30, 2008.

Corbin, D. (1993). *A History of Health Care Reform: Six Decades of Debate.* Washington, DC.

Cutler, D. M. (2004). *Your Money or Your Life.* Oxford: Oxford University Press.

Davis, K., Schoen, C., Schoenbaum, S. C., Doty, M. M. Holmgren, A. L., Kriss, J. L., & Shea, K. K. (2007). *Mirror, mirror on the wall: An international update on* the comparative performance of American health care. Available at: http://www.commonwealthfund.org/publications/publications_show.htm?doc_id=482678. Accessed September 19, 2008.

Deloughery, G. (1998). *Issues and Trends in Nursing.* St. Louis, MO: Mosby.

Dodd, C. (2008). Play to win: Know the rules (pp. 15–26). In: C. Harrington & C. Estes (Eds.), *Health Policy: Crisis and Reform in the U.S. Health Care Delivery System.* Sudbury MA: Jones & Bartlett.

Dorn, S. (2008). *Uninsured and dying because of it: Updating the Institute of Medicine analysis on the impact of uninsurance on mortality.* Available at: http://www.urban.org/url.cfm?ID=411588. Accessed July 30, 2008.

Dorn, S., Garret, B., Holahan, J., & Williams, A. (2008). *Medicaid, SCHIP and economic downturn: Policy challenges and policy responses.* Kaiser Commission on Medicaid and the Uninsured. Available at: http://www.kff.org/medicaid/upload/7770ES.pdf. Accessed July 30, 2008.

Ellis, J. R., & Hartley, C. L. (2004). *Nursing in Today's World: Trends, Issues and Management* (8th ed.). Philadelphia: Lippincott Williams & Wilkins.

Evans (2003).

Families USA (1993). *a.s.a.p.* Washington, DC: Families USA.

Ferguson, C. C., Fowler, E. J., & Nichols, L. M. (2008). The long road to health reform requires bipartisan leadership. *Health Affairs, 27*(3), 711–717.

Flanagan, L. (1976). *One Strong Voice.* Kansas City, MO: American Nurses Association.

Foley, M. (2002). Collective action in health care (pp. 387–397). In: D. J. Mason, J. K. Leavitt, & M. Chaffee (Eds.), *Policy and Politics in Nursing and Health Care.* Philadelphia: Saunders.

Freeman, J. (2008). *We Will Be Heard: Women's Struggles for Political Power in the United States.* New York: Rowman & Littlefield.

Hanley, B., & Falk, N. L. (2007). Policy development and analysis: Understanding the process (pp. 75–93). In: D. J. Mason, J. K. Leavitt, & M. W. Chaffee (Eds.), *Policy and Politics in Nursing and Health Care* (5th ed.). St. Louis, MO: Saunders/Elsevier.

Harrington, C., & Estes, C. (Eds.). *Health Policy: Crisis and Reform in the U.S. Health Care Delivery System* (5th ed.). Sudbury MA: Jones & Bartlett.

Health Resources and Services Administration (HRSA) (2000). *The Registered Nurse population: Findings from the National Sample Survey of Registered Nurses.* Available at: http://bhpr.hrsa.gov/healthworkforce/reports/nursing/samplesurvey00/default.htm. Accessed January 28, 2009.

Jewish Women's Archive (n.d.). *Exhibit: Women of valor. Lillian Wald.* Available at: http://jwa.org/exhibits/wov/wald/lwbio.html. Accessed May, 10, 2008.

Kaiser Family Foundation (2007). *2007 Employer health benefits survey.* Available at: http://www.kff.org/insurance/7672/. Accessed July 30, 2008.

Kaiser Family Foundation (2008). *Fast facts.* Available at: http://facts.kff.org/?CFID=34882754&CFTOKEN=68369851. Accessed July 30, 2008.

Kaiser Family Foundation (2009). *Distribution of Medicaid Spending on Long Term Care, FY2006.* State HealthFacts.org. Available at: http://www.statehealthfacts.org/comparebar.jsp?ind=180&cat=4&sb=47&yr=29&typ=2. Accessed January 28, 2009.

Kalisch, B., & Kalisch, P. (1982). *Politics of Nursing.* Philadelphia: Lippincott.

Kingma, M. (2006). *Nurses on the Move: Migration and the Global Health Care Economy.* Ithaca, NY: Cornell University Press.

Kimbro, R. T., Bzostek, S., Goldman, N., & Rodriguez, G. (2008). Race, ethnicity and the educational gradient in health. *Health Affairs, 27*(2), 361–372.

Kohn, L., Corrigan, J., & Donaldson, M. (2000). *To Err Is Human: Building a Safer Health System.* Washington, DC: National Academy Press.

Krain, J. B. (n.d.). *Lillian Wald.* Available at: http://www.jewishmag.co.il/51mag/wald/lillianwald.htm. Accessed May, 10, 2008.

Lillie-Blanton, M., & Hoffman, C. (2005). The role of health insurance coverage in reducing racial/ethnic disparities in health care. *Health Affairs, 24*(2), 398–408.

Luminary Project (n.d.). *The Luminary Project: Nurses lighting the way to environmental health.* Available at: http://www.theluminaryproject.org/article.php?id=42. Accessed July 30, 2008.

Mason, D. J., Leavitt, J. K., & Chaffee, M. W. (Eds.) (2002). *Policy and Politics in Nursing and Health Care* (4th ed.). Philadelphia: Saunders.

Mason, D. J., Leavitt, J. K., & Chaffee, M. W. (Eds.) (2007). *Policy and Politics in Nursing and Health Care* (5th ed.). St. Louis: Saunders/Elsevier.

National Association for Home Care and Hospice (NAHC) (2008). *Why the U.S. should celebrate the birthday of Lillian Wald on March 10*. Available at: http://www.nahc.org/media/mediaPR_031008b. html. Accessed September 17, 2008.

National Committee to Preserve Social Security and Medicare (2008). *Fact Sheet: Medicare Provisions in the President's FY 2009 Budget*. Available at: http://www.ncpssm.org/pdf/medicare-provisions-2009. pdf. Accessed August 17, 2008.

Nightingale, F. (1992). *Notes on Nursing: What It Is and What It Is Not* [1859]. Commemorative Edition. Philadelphia: JB Lippincott.

National Institutes of Health (n.d.). *What are health disparities?* Available at: www.http://healthdiaparities. nih.gov/whatare.html. Accessed July 30, 2008.

National Labor Relations Board (n.d.). *National Labor Relations Act*. Available at: http://www.nlrb.gov/about_us/overview/national_labor_relations_act. aspx. Accessed July 21, 2008.

Online Dictionary of Social Sciences (n.d.). *Politics*. Available at: http://bitbucket.icaap.org/dict.pl? alpha=P. Accessed September 18, 2008.

Pierce, K. M. (2004). Insights and reflections of a congressional nurse detailee. *Policy, Politics & Nursing Practice, 5*(2), 113–115.

Primomo, J., & Salazar, M. (2005). Environmental health risks: At home, at work, and in the community (pp. 596–620). In: F. Maurer & C. Smith (Eds.), *Community/Public Health Nursing Practice: Health for Families and Populations* (3rd ed.). St. Louis, MO: Elsevier/Saunders.

Protection and enhancement of Medicare (2008). *Action Report to the American Nurses 2008 Association House of Delegates*. Available at: http://nursesrev.advocateof fice.com/vertical/Sites/%7B41671038-B8D0-4277-90A9-50B10F730CBD%7D/uploads/%7BB0D88BDC-7288-43A6-86F1-388ECABEC2F9%7D.PDF. Accessed January 28, 2009.

Rowland, D. (2008). Medicaid at 40 (pp. 291–299). In: C. Harrington, & C. L. Estes (Eds.), *Health Policy: Crisis and Reform in the U.S. Health Care System* (5th ed.). Sudbury MA: Jones & Bartlett.

Rudowitz, R., & Marks, C. (2008). *Few options for states to control Medicaid spending in a declining economy*. Kaiser Commission on the Uninsured. Available at: http://www.kff.org/medicaid/upload/7769.pdfid/upload/7769.pdf. Accessed July 30, 2008.

Sabatier, P. A. (Ed.). (1999). *Theories of the Policy Process*. Boulder, CO: Westview Press.

Salmon, M., & Guisinger, V. (2007). Global migration of nurses: Managing a scarce resource. (pp. 982–991). In: D. J. Mason, J. K. Leavitt, & M. W. Chaffee (Eds.), *Policy and Politics in Nursing and Health Care* (5th ed.). St. Louis, MO: Saunders/Elsevier.

Sanger, Margaret (n.d.). *Encylopaedia Britannica profiles: 300 women who changed the world*. Available at: http://search.eb.com/women/article-9065508. Accessed January 28, 2009.

Sattler, B., Afzal, B., & McPhaul, K. (2006). Environmental health (pp. 93x113). In: M. Stanhope, & J. Lancaster (Eds.), *Foundations of Nursing in the Community: Community Oriented Practice* (2nd ed.). St. Louis, MO: Mosby Elsevier.

Schoen, C., Collins, S. R., Kriss, J. L., & Doty, M. M. (2008). How many are uninsured? Trends among U.S. Adults, 2003–2007. *Health Affairs, 27*(4), 298–309.

Smedly, B. D. (2008). Moving beyond access: Achieving equity in state health care reform. *Health Affairs, 27*(2), 447–455.

Social Security Online (n.d.). *History*. Available at: http://www.ssa.gov/history/corningchap4.html. Accessed July 30, 2008.

Steinbrook, R. (2007). Election 2008: Campaign contributions, lobbying, and the U.S. health sector. *New England Journal of Medicine, 357*(8),736–739.

Steinem, G. (2004). *Margaret Sanger*. Available at: http://www.time.com/time/time100/leaders/profile/sanger3.htm. Accessed July 30, 2008.

Syme, S. L. (2008). Reducing racial and social-class inequalities in health: The need for a new approach. *Health Affairs, 27*(24), 459.

The FreeDictionary.com (n.d.). *Policy*. Available at: http://www.thefreedictionary.com/policy. Accessed September 17, 2008.

United Nations Development Programme (2007). *Millennium development goals*. Available at: www.undp.org/mdg/basic.shtml. Accessed July 2, 2008.

U.S. Environmental Protection Agency (2007). *Report on the Environment 2007*. Available at: http://yosemite.epa.gov/sab/SABPRODUCT.NSF/81e39f4c09954fcb85256ead006be86e/2457aac81d2003a98525701900616b47!OpenDocument&TableRow=2.2. Accessed January 29, 2008.

Warino, L. (2007). Collective action in the workplace: The role of unions (pp. 589–601). In: D. J. Mason, J.

K. Leavitt, & M. W. Chaffee (Eds.), *Policy and Politics in Nursing and Health Care* (5th ed.). St. Louis, MO: Saunders/Elsevier.

Warner, J. R. (2003). A phenomenological approach to political competence: Stories of nurse activists. *Policy, Politics & Nursing Practice, 4*(2), 135–143.

Wikipedia (n.d.). *Policy.* Available at: http://en.wikipedia.org/wiki/Policy. Accessed September 17, 2008.

Yordy, K. (2006). *The nursing faculty shortage: A crisis for health care.* Available at: www.rwjf.org/files/publications/other/NursingFacultyShortage071006.pdf. Accessed July 30, 2008.

BIBLIOGRAPHY

Barry, M., & Hughes, J. M. (2008). Talking dirty—The politics of clean water and sanitation. *New England Journal of Medicine, 359*(8), 784–787.

Bauer, J. C. (2008). Health reform and payment trends: Don't wait for politicians. *Healthcare Financial Management, 62*(4), 40–42.

Beall, F. (2007). Overview and summary: Power to influence patient care: Who holds the keys? *The Online Journal of Issues in Nursing, 12*(1). Available at: http://nursingworld.org/MainMenuCategories/ANAMarketplace/ANAPeriodicals/OJIN/TableofContents/Volume122007/No1Jan07/tpc32ntr16088.aspx. Accessed September 20, 2008.

Borrell, C., Espelt, A., Rodriguez-Sanz, M., & Navarro, V. (2008). Politics and health. *Journal of Epidemiology and Community Health, 61*(8), 658–659.

DeMoro, R. (2008). Lessons learned: The healthcare reform battle in California taught the public the differences between health insurance and healthcare. *Registered Nurse: Journal of Patient Advocacy, 104*(1), 9.

Hacker, J. S. (2008). Speaking truth to power—The need for, and perils of, health policy expertise in the White House. *New England Journal of Medicine, 359*(11), 1085–1087.

International Council of Nurses (2008). *Delivering quality, serving communities: Nurses leading primary health care.* Available at: http://www.icn.ch/indkit2008.pdf. Accessed September 19, 2008.

Judge, K. (2008). Politics and health: Policy design and implementation are even more neglected than political values? *European Journal of Public Health, 18*(4), 355–356.

Nickitas, D. M. (2008). Policy and politics: It's time for a deliberative discussion. *Nursing Economics, 26*(4), 225, 249.

Rubin, R. J. (2008). Healthcare, ideology, and politics. *Journal of Medical Practice Management, 23*(4), 207–208.

The priority is politics. Funding for healthcare is just one victim of partisan warfare in Washington (2007). *Modern Healthcare, 37*(50), 22.

Vesely, R. (2008). "Unleash the energy." Activists, professors try to use their own sphere of influence to affect U.S. healthcare policy and improve patient care. *Modern Healthcare.* Available at: http://nurseweb.ucsf.edu/public/080428-mdhc.htm. Accessed September 20, 2008.

What is your power to influence healthcare policy? (2008). *Colorado Nurse, 108*(1), 13.

WEB RESOURCES

Academy of Medical Surgical Nurses, Official Position Statement on Political Awareness for the Registered Nurse	http://www.medsurgnurse.org/cgi-bin/WebObjects/AMSNMain.woa/wa/viewSection?s_id=1073744079&ss_id=536873229&tName=positionsPoliticalAwarenessForTheRN
American Nurses Association	http://www.needlestick.org/gova/federal/legis/109/legreg109.pdf

American Nurses Association, Government Affairs	http://www.nursingworld.org/gova/
American Nurses Association, State Government Relations	http://www.nursingworld.org/gova/state.htm
American Public Health Association	http://www.apha.org/
Federal Election Commission, Pacronyms	http://www.fec.gov/pages/pacronym.shtml
How a Bill Becomes a Law (narrative)	http://thomas.loc.gov/home/lawsmade.toc.html
How a Bill Becomes a Law (pictorial)	http://www.leginfo.ca.gov/bil2lawd.html
Kaiser Family Foundation, Resources on Medicare/Medicaid	http://www.kff.org/
Letters to a Legislator (Tips)	http://www.arcwa.org/hottipsletterstolegislators.html
Letters to Legislators (Adapted from League for Women Voters, American Nurses Association Voter materials)	http://nursing.boisestate.edu/nursb434spring/letters.htm
Library of Congress, Meta-Indexes for State and Local Government Information	http://www.loc.gov/global/state/stategov.html
Nurses for a Healthier Tomorrow	http://www.nursesource.org/members.html
Nurses: Money to Congress	http://www.opensecrets.org/industries/summary.asp?Ind=H1710
Nursing World, Reading and Reference Room	http://www.nursingworld.org/readroom/
Registered Nurses Association of Ontario (RNAO), Comparison of the Platforms of the Three Main Political Parties to RNAO's Commitment to Health, Health Care, and Nurses	http://www.rnao.org/policy/platform_comparison.asp
Society of Gastroenterology Nurses and Associates, Understanding and Influencing the Legislative Process	http://www.sgna.org/Resources/guidelines/guideline10.pdfsearch='Understanding%20and%20Influencing%20the%20Legislative%20Process%20nursing'

CHAPTER 23

Nursing's Professional Associations

• MARJORIE BEYERS •

Learning Objectives

The learner will be able to:

1. Examine how professional nursing associations such as the American Nurses Association, the National League for Nursing, the International Council of Nurses, and Sigma Theta Tau International have affected the development of nursing as a profession.
2. Identify driving and restraining forces for membership in professional associations.
3. Describe the organizational structure of a typical professional association.
4. Explore the multiple professional associations that exist in nursing and assess them for redundancy of functions.
5. Describe various types of membership in professional associations, including *full*, *associate*, *affiliate*, *honorary*, *organizational*, and *liaison*.
6. Explore the challenges faced by professional associations, including sustaining membership, ensuring adequate financial resources, dealing with the short life cycle of information, dealing with calls for a more interdisciplinary approach, and responding to the need for membership diversity.
7. Identify common sources of non-dues revenue for professional associations.
8. Explore the effect of the short life cycle of information on the need for professional associations to adopt new technologies to communicate with and between members and to promote networking.
9. Explore the role professional associations can assume in shaping the future culture of professional nursing.
10. Reflect on the need for professional associations to become more flexible and better integrated to accommodate anticipated changes in member preferences.
11. Question the future viability of associations and explore how professional associations may need to recreate themselves to remain viable in a rapidly changing world.
12. Debate whether professional nursing associations are the appropriate venue for sustaining the profession of nursing in the future.
13. Complete a self-evaluation regarding professional association involvement and reflect on whether greater involvement is desired.

Like many things in our lives, nurses often take professional associations for granted. For some nurses, professional associations are a vital part of their professional lives. Other nurses, although they may know about their professional associations, are not members and are not involved in the work of those associations. Nonetheless, nursing's professional associations affect every nurse's practice. This chapter begins with an overview of nursing's professional associations. The influence of these professional associations on the profession of nursing over time is then explored. The chapter ends with an examination of the future of professional associations and ways in which these associations continue to be of value to the profession.

Nursing is often referred to as a "pluralistic" profession—a label earned by the variety of educational programs and the myriad of job types nurses fill. It is not surprising that there is a wide variety of nursing associations. The *Encyclopedia of Associations* lists more than 300 national nursing associations. Although the vast majority of these associations represent Registered Nurses, a few of them represent nurse aides and Licensed Practical Nurses. Some of the nursing associations are international, and others have international counterparts. The American Nurses Association represents all nurses, but most nursing associations are named for a clinical specialty group or a type of service, such as long-term care or policy interests. Others are named for the function of the members, such as education, administration, or clinical practice. Yet others are named to represent a cultural or ethnic background, such as the National Alaska Native American Indian Nurses Association or the Black Nurses Association. It is interesting to note that most of these nursing associations have fewer than 5,000 members. A limited number of nursing associations have more than 150,000 members. A listing of many of these nursing associations is given in the Web Resources section at the end of this chapter.

DISCUSSION POINT

Why are there so many nursing associations? Is the large number of nursing associations a value or a hindrance to the profession?

Associations are typically founded to further the work of the group they represent. Individuals are drawn to the association by a common cause. An important role of professional associations is to protect the public interest, as well as to protect the interests of the professionals. The Internal Revenue Service (IRS) (2008) officially defines an association as a group of persons banded together for a specific purpose. Technically, professional associations must have a written document that shows their creation. Each state, however, has its own definition of associations. Most association are nonprofit, and many qualify under Section 501(c)(3) of the IRS code (IRS, 2008).

In some respects, associations are like a business, with a mission, philosophy, vision, and strategic plan that must be financed through the work of the association. To serve their members, associations must remain viable, not only to their membership, but also in the public venues of economics, government, and regulation and in public support for their work. The common cause that brings members together to form and sustain an association must also be valued by the public served by the members.

Consider the influence and work of nursing professional associations. Each association has a valued history, and many have unique traditions. Typically, nursing associations work to advance the profession by adopting a code of ethics, developing and updating the scope of practice, standards of behavior and practice, and definitions of competency important to protect the public. Membership and certification are the venues most frequently used to recognize individuals who meet the criteria for being an active member of the association. Associations provide services and resources for the members and may provide these services to the public and nonmembers. Often they serve as a source of information for the public about the practice. Services and resources include education, mentoring, leadership development, and opportunities to become involved in shaping the association, the practice, and the profession. Members may serve as volunteer leaders through positions as elected offices or by participating in projects, committees, or other initiatives designed to sustain the association and to explore, further, or develop the work of the professionals.

Most nursing associations hold conventions, annual meetings, or both, provide educational programs, and develop tools and resources to support and advance the practice of nursing. Some associations have research agendas. Another function of associations is to advocate for the practice of nursing with the public, government, and within health care. Major categories of professional association services are shown in Box 23.1.

THE PUBLIC AND PROFESSIONAL ASSOCIATIONS

Professional associations serve members whose common bond is their profession and are formed, at least in part, to enhance the professional status of members. The public depends on associations as a way to reach members, to learn about practice, or to become informed about matters within the association's expertise. The mutual interdependency of professional associations and the public is grounded in trust. The professional association, through the collective work of its members, is expected to define and promote standards of behavior and practice.

BOX 23.1 | MAJOR CATEGORIES OF PROFESSIONAL ASSOCIATION SERVICES

Professional development, including opportunities for networking; publications such as newsletters, journals, and multimedia materials; educational programs; conferences and conventions; information and resources such as tools and issue papers; and credentialing and socialization.

Advancing the profession through activities including research, standards of practice, designations, and productivity, and a code of ethics for the profession.

Policy and advocacy, including government relations, liaisons with related and influential groups, legislative advocacy to provide the resources and support for professional practice, and the appropriate environment for practice.

CONSIDER

Given that the public expects the association to be informed about practice, why do some nurses choose to become members of their professional association, whereas others do not seek membership?

Disseminators of Information

As a source of information about standards of practice and qualifications of persons engaged in the practice, associations are viewed as credible sources of information about services needed by the public. They advocate for the public served, identifying and resolving issues surrounding practice, which can be raised by members, leaders, or the public. When called for, the association takes action to enhance the profession by establishing, revising, or updating relevant standards, laws, rules and regulations. These actions may involve changing or eliminating practices that are harmful or no longer useful and involve cooperation with other groups that affect or influence the practice and the relevant laws and regulations. The focus on the action is to protect the public safety and welfare. Associations also conduct research and participate in programs to advance the knowledge of the profession, which is particularly important, given current emphasis on evidence-based professional decision making.

Advocacy, Integrity, and Competency

Nurses, as members, also have expectations from their professional nursing associations. The fact that there are

so many nursing associations is evidence that they are of value to nurses who form them, establish the mission, and participate in the association activities. Associations advocate for their members. Some view this advocacy role as protecting the "property rights" of members to practice their profession. A counterview is that associations enhance the ability of members to fulfill their professional role with integrity. Generally, their mission is to identify issues and resolve problems affecting the profession, to promote professional development, and to provide services useful to members. Joining a professional nursing association enables nurses both to provide input and to use the services that the association provides to enhance their ability to practice with integrity and competency. They provide valuable resources for both nurses and the public, and they serve as forums for communication with consumers, business, industry, and government on matters affecting nursing and nursing practice.

Clearly, professional nursing associations are an integral part of the culture of nursing, as evidenced by the number of associations. There is a dearth of scientific information, however, about the numerous professional nursing associations, what populations they serve, how their purposes overlap and differ, and what benefits result from that membership. One could speculate that there is a nursing association for almost every purpose; the American Board of Nursing Societies, formed in 1991, which has 25 members responsible for national nursing certification boards and nursing organizations that work with credentialing issues. Another example of an association founded for a particular purpose is the American Assembly for Men in Nursing, founded in 1971. Initially formed to interest men in the nursing profession and to decrease prejudice about the selection of nursing as a profession for men, this association works to further the professional growth of its members and now acts as a clearinghouse for men in nursing and promotes positive health care.

DISCUSSION POINT

Could one nursing association represent all of the diverse interests of nurses, or is having focused multiple nursing associations more effective to promote the profession and to protect the public?

One must question whether professional associations in nursing are more alike than different and what criteria separate one from the other. Most associations have a written history of their origin, their founders, and the initial purposes of the association. Little is known about why so many nursing associations were formed in the first place, what sustains them over time, and how these associations are being affected by changes in society, as well as by the contemporary economic and political environment. Each association tends to its own sustenance. It appears that systematic thinking about the future needs of the nursing profession and of nurses individually for professional association membership and work is lacking. This information is essential to shaping the future of professional nursing associations.

DISCUSSION POINT

What is the rationale for the professional association's continuing existence?

Associations are an organizational entity and are imbedded in the culture of the profession. The future role professional associations should play to support the nursing profession may be very different in the future from that in the past. Several societal forces affect nursing professional associations. Among these forces are the societal trends, changing values, and turbulence in organizations and institutions, the rapid acceptance and use of technology in both health care and in communications, and unique forces such as those related to the gender, age, and affiliation of nurses. It is debatable whether history can be used to predict the future. There is, however, much to be learned about how nurses in the past used their potential to shape nursing as we know it. This learning can be applied to help nurses to use their potential to become a significant force in shaping the

future of the profession. Members have a vital role in this work.

THE GROWTH OF PROFESSIONAL ASSOCIATIONS

Nursing associations, like other types of professional associations, evolved over hundreds of years. Their history reflects the natural tendency of people to join together for a common purpose, the development of commerce and industry, and the political and societal realities of achieving public recognition and prestige. The impetus for the development of many professional associations of all types was and continues to be public safety and welfare. The growth of professional associations reflects the often chaotic progress toward recognition of a given profession by society.

CONSIDER

The professions of law, medicine, and the clergy were among the first to be recognized by professional associations, followed over time by a multitude of other groups.

Professional associations began to take shape during the Industrial Revolution. This time was characterized by the emergence of trade associations, guilds, and professional associations that reflected changes in society. Essentially these groups served a dual but interrelated purpose of recognition; people were concerned about the quality of the goods and services they consumed, and "professionals" were seeking public recognition for their work. Professional associations recognized and met both of these needs.

THE FORMATION AND WORK OF NURSING'S EARLY PROFESSIONAL ASSOCIATIONS

There are some accounts of the role professional nursing associations have played in the development of nursing as a profession, and there have been depictions of the lives and work of nurses who made a difference in nursing. Few research studies have been conducted to examine how nurses, nationally and internationally, have achieved and continue to work to achieve recognition

BOX 23.2 | MILESTONES FOR PROFESSIONAL NURSING ASSOCIATIONS

1893: American Society of Superintendents of Training Schools for Nurses—forerunner to the National League for Nursing (NLN)—is chartered.

1897: Nurses Associated Alumnae of the United States and Canada—forerunner to the American Nurses Association (ANA)—is chartered.

1899: International Council of Nurses is chartered.

1900: American Journal of Nursing is chartered.

1903: First nurse practice acts are passed in the United States.

1908: National Association of Colored Graduate Nurses is founded (became part of the ANA in 1951, making the ANA one of the first national associations to declare membership open to all ethnic groups).

1911: Nurses Associated Alumnae of the United States and Canada is renamed the ANA.

1912: Society of Superintendents of Training Schools for Nurses is renamed the National League for Nursing Education (NLNE). It assumes functions of other associations and becomes the organization known as the National League for Nursing in 1952.

1922: Sigma Theta Tau is founded; it becomes the International Honor Society of Nurses in 1985.

Source: Adapted in part from Cherry, B., & Jacob, S. R. (2002). *Contemporary Nursing. Issues, Trends, and Management* (2nd ed.). St. Louis, MO: Mosby, p. 4.

for nursing as a profession. Such studies would be valuable to provide understanding of how these leaders worked together through the structure of associations in the late 19th and early 20th centuries to achieve their goals (Box 23.2).

Associations have long been integral to world cultures and societies, as evidenced by historical texts, historical novels, family legend, and lore. In the late 18th and 19th centuries, associations generally served the interests of the elite—the landowners, wealthy merchant, and other influential people. A wealth of information on "secret societies" and private clubs further illustrates how people with common interests and affluence joined together to set their own agenda. In the period from the end of the 18th century to the beginning of the 19th century, associations flourished. Associations were the vehicle used by the growing number of scholars, trade groups, and individuals with common economic interests to advance their work within the social structure. Nursing associations in the United States have their roots in this movement, which was closely tied to the emancipation of women.

Reading the history of professional nursing associations engenders respect for the nursing leaders who shaped the profession of today. There is ample evidence that nursing leaders were driven by a common cause, clear direction for action, and passion for achieving the goals to advance the profession for the benefit of the public and of nurses. The work of what we know now as the National League for Nursing, the American Nurses Association, and the International Council of Nurses resulted from collaboration toward a common goal. A brief overview of the origins of each follows.

National League for Nursing

The National League for Nursing (NLN) began its legacy as the Society of Superintendents of Training Schools for Nurses, formed in 1893. Renamed the National League for Nursing Education in 1912, a new association, the National League for Nursing, was formed in 1952 as a result of the reorganization of nursing's major professional associations (Spaulding & Notter, 1965, p. 335; Henderson & Nite, 1978, p. 73). From the outset, NLN's mission has been to advance nursing education.

American Nurses Association

The history of the American Nurses Association (ANA) began with a convening of alumnae groups led by nurses from Bellevue, the Illinois Training School, and Johns Hopkins in the 1880s. These alumnae groups adopted the constitution and bylaws for a new organization, the Nurses Associated Alumnae of the United States and Canada, in 1897. Charter alumnae groups included the Bellevue Hospital Training School; the New York Hospital Training School and the Brooklyn Hospital Training School in New York City; the Farrand Training School; Harper Hospital, Detroit; the Garfield Hospital Training School in Washington, D.C.; the Illinois Training School; Cook County Hospital, Chicago; the Johns Hopkins Training School, Baltimore; the Massachusetts General Hospital Training School, Boston; the Philadelphia Training School and the University of Pennsylvania Training School in Philadelphia; and two schools from Canada.

The *American Journal of Nursing* was established in 1900 as the official journal of the association. In 1911, the association was renamed the American Nurses Association (ANA), which continues to be the official name. The ANA began its collective bargaining activities in the 1940s.

International Council of Nurses

The early development of the ANA and the NLN was influenced by the women's movement at the end of the 19th and beginning of the 20th century. The June 1899 meeting of the *International Congress of Women*, held in London, was particularly notable for nurses. At this meeting, nurses from around the world attended, and American nurse leaders, along with leaders from Great Britain and Germany, founded the International Council of Nurses (ICN). What is now the ANA is both a charter member and constituent member of the ICN. The ICN focused its energy on the organizational development of nurses throughout the world.

Ethel Gordon Fenwick, the first president of the ICN, strongly believed that nurses should step forward to guide their own destiny. Her tireless work for the profession is documented in the literature. Typical of her addresses is this excerpt from the public address she presented in Buffalo, New York, in 1901: "Every country needs practice curriculum, examinations, a uniform system of nursing education and uniform statement of qualification . . . registration essential to practice ... to protect the public" (Fenwick, 1901).

SHAPING THE NURSING PROFESSION

Nurse leaders in the United States, led by the National Associated Alumnae of the United States and Canada and the Society of Superintendents of Training Schools for Nurses, created the template for nursing's development in the United States. The three main prongs for development of the profession were uniform education, standards of practice, and regulation of the profession. In keeping with the spirit and strategy of the ICN, to achieve a legal basis for nursing in every country throughout the world, nurse leaders in the United States began work to achieve licensure for nurses in every state. This work to develop nurse practice acts in every state took place concurrently with similar development in many countries throughout the world. Nursing was not alone in this effort. Many other professional groups were also seeking licensure in the United States and the District of Columbia.

> CONSIDER
>
> The connection between professional competence and licensure in the early 20th century was considered a modern notion.

It took great passion and energy to convince members of the nursing profession, the public, and legislators that licensure was important for the profession and the public. It took almost 20 years for all of the states to pass nurse practice acts. The first was passed in North Carolina in 1903. All states had a nurse practice act by 1923. Nurse leaders collaborated on defining the profession, achieving legal recognition of the profession, and establishing a culture for professional nursing that has continued to the present time. Nursing continues to benefit from this work to establish nurse practice acts, mandatory licensure, the development of standards for nursing education and practice, and the promulgation of nursing's *Code of Ethics*.

Early nursing associations not only worked together to build the base for recognition of nursing as a profession, but they also acted as stewards of the profession. Nursing's professional associations were viewed as resources to advance the profession. In addition to the ANA and the NLN, several other nursing associations were formed by the 1940s. Nurse leaders, cognizant of the role of associations to serve nurses, commissioned

Raymond Rich Associates to study what nurses needed from their professional associations. Changes in society and in health care delivery were considered.

The *Rich Report* recommendations led to reorganization of the professional nursing associations formed between 1892 and 1949. The rationale for the reorganization was that larger associations with more assets and capability could advance the profession better than any one of the participating associations and groups could working singly. In this reorganization, the ANA continued with its mission to advance and support the profession. The National League for Nursing Education (NLNE) became a new organization, the National League for Nursing (NLN). The new NLN absorbed the education functions and related functions of the National Organization for Public Health Nursing, the Association of Collegiate Schools of Nursing, the Joint Committee on Practical Nurses and Auxiliary Workers in Nursing Services, the Joint Committee on Careers in Nursing and the National Committee for the Improvement of Nursing Service, and the National Nursing Accrediting Service (Raymond Rich Associates report, 1946; Henderson & Nite, 1978). The reorganization of nursing's professional associations is testimony to the wisdom and vision of the early leaders as they focused on how best to advance nursing practice and the environment for practice.

DISCUSSION POINT

Imagine a world without any professional nursing associations. In this world, how are standards of education and practice, regulation of the practice, and advancement of nursing knowledge achieved?

DEVELOPMENT OF SPECIALTY NURSING PROFESSIONAL ASSOCIATIONS

While the ANA and NLN concentrated on shaping the nursing profession as a whole, a number of nurses formed associations to meet their practice related needs. The American Association of Industrial Nurses, which traces its origins to 1915, is one of the oldest specialty nursing professional associations. Many other specialty nursing groups established professional nursing associations in the 1950s. Among these were the American Association of Nurse Anesthetists, established in 1952; the Association of Operating Room Nurses, formed in 1957;

the American College of Nurse Midwifery, formed in 1955; the National Association for Practical Nurse Education and Service (NAPNES), established in 1941; the National Federation of Licensed Practical Nurses, formed in 1949; and both the Catholic and Lutheran Nursing Groups (Spaulding & Notter, 1965).

Nursing Professional Associations in the Last 50 Years of the 20th Century

During the early years of the 20th century, most nurses could name the professional nursing associations and could articulate their mission, services to members, and contribution to the nursing profession. The focus was on establishing nursing as a profession. The number of nursing professional associations continued to grow. By the 1950s, there was some concern about how to bring these associations together in an effort to strengthen nursing and to unify the voice of nursing. Virginia Henderson observed the "proliferation of organizations is so marked that only through some federation of organizations could unity be achieved" (Henderson & Nite, 1978, p. 73). However, the focus had changed from concentration on the nursing profession to advancing nursing and nurses.

The proliferation of nursing associations has occurred naturally. Reasons for this proliferation have not been studied, but it can be speculated that contributing factors were the development of specialization in health care following World War II, the growing number of nurses, and the expansion of hospitals. The value of associations to the public may also have been a factor. By the second half of the 20th century, associations were an accepted way for professional, business, and industry related groups to gain recognition and acceptance of their work by the public. It stands to reason that nurses would develop and use professional nursing associations for this purpose.

DISCUSSION POINT

How important are relationships among professional associations within health care to the work of nurses in health care?

It would be informative to study the patterns of association development in nursing, the reasons why nurses seem to establish new specialty nursing associations as practice changes, and how these many associations add value to their members and to the profession.

Why did nurses move to establish separate associations for specialties? Were their reasons tied to the growing complexity of nursing practice, the expanded and more differentiated knowledge base for each nursing specialty, the influence of collegial relationships with physicians and other health professionals, and the growing demand for ensuring practice qualifications through certification? A few specialty nursing professional associations had their origins as nursing sections in physician associations, such as the Association of Women's Health, Obstetric and Neonatal Nurses, which evolved as a separate association to provide education, certification, and support for nursing practice in collaboration with other health professionals. Others have been and continue to be formed as a new area of practice emerges. It can be posited that the proliferation of nursing associations reflects the culture of the United States.

In this culture, the public looks to professional associations as a source of authority and expertise. Leaders in an association relate to the public, to colleagues, and to other professional associations. For individual nurses, membership in their professional association is valued because it conveys professional status, a willingness to uphold the standards of the profession, and a vested interest in the issues and concerns the professional association takes on for benefit of the members. Credentials are valued in a culture that emphasizes the quality of health care. For nurses, the credentials include licensure, certification, formal and continuing education, experience, and participation in community or professional activities. Resumes often include a section for "professional development" or "professional accomplishments." Health care consumers now have technological resources to check credentials, such as professional membership credentials, and reputation when seeking services. Membership may serve as a seal of approval or as a mark of professionalism.

The Vital Role of Members

Associations exist because of members. Those nurses who want to participate in their professional associations have many opportunities for leadership development within associations. They can become members of task forces, which accomplish much of the work of associations; they can become members of committees and groups that work to carry out the mission of the association; and they can serve as experts who inform the association about trends in practice, changes in competencies, and other aspects of the practice role. Members have great influence in the direction associations set for their work. To be an effective member, one must know about the association, understand the issues and concerns the association faces, keep informed about new events and happenings, participate in association programs and projects, and contribute to the association through volunteer activities.

The first step is the decision to join an association. A self-evaluation regarding professional association involvement is given in Box 23.3. Once a decision is made to join an association, members must then decide their level of involvement in the selected association.

Traditionally there have been four ranges of member involvement. *First-level* involvement includes becoming a member and participating in meetings, conventions, and educational programs or using products and services. *Second-level* involvement entails engagement in projects or programs. *Third-level* involvement requires a time commitment, such as appointment to committees or a leadership role in a major activity. *Fourth-level*

BOX 23.3 | SELF-EVALUATION: PROFESSIONAL ASSOCIATION INVOLVEMENT

- Do you belong to one or more professional associations? In nursing? In other areas?
- Do you participate in activities or use services of professional nursing associations? Do you ever visit the Web sites?
- Do you subscribe to e-news?
- Do you attend meetings, conventions, or educational programs?
- Do you behave as a loyal member by being informed regarding issues?
- Do you share your opinions and concerns with leaders?

involvement engages members in leadership roles as an officer, committee chair, spokesperson, or other type of engagement that relies on the member's expertise and talent as a leader. The Internet may be changing the way members are involved in their associations because nurses now can join chat rooms, subscribe to e-mail newsletters, and access information from a number of Web sites. Associations now use the Internet to engage members in several types of activities, such as participating in surveys for member input, selection of leaders, and information or networking important to member recruitment and retention.

Recruitment and retention of members is guided by member input. Most associations routinely survey members to learn why they joined the association, what motivates their continued membership, what type of programs and services they need to support and advance their practice, and whether their expectations of the association are being met. Such surveys inform association leaders in the process of strategic planning. Member participation in these surveys is essential to the development of realistic future goals. Being informed about the survey results also helps members to understand how their association is responding to member needs and values. Many associations now reach out to former members to learn why they discontinued their membership and what factors would influence their return to full membership in the association.

One of the most important roles of members is to understand what associations are, how they function, and how to participate in ways that make a difference. Members seek value from professional associations but have a role to ensure that the association has the capability to produce that value. Typically nursing professional associations are voluntary, not-for-profit organizations formed to advance the profession. The key relationships of these associations are between and among members and between the association and external groups such as other nursing associations, related health care associations, and the public. The following section presents key aspects of associations important to volunteer members who are active in associations.

The Organization of an Association

Associations are legal entities and as such are "democratic" organizations. The organizational structure of associations embodies volunteer leadership and, depending

on the size and resources, paid staff to manage the association's business. The size of the association influences the level of staff and volunteer involvement. Larger associations typically have more staff structure than smaller associations. Both volunteer leadership and staff manage the business of the association, work with members to identify issues, develop positions and insights about the issues for public discussion, conduct meetings, engage members in forming and adopting resolutions that affect practice, plan and provide programs and services, and are accountable to the members.

> ### CONSIDER
> Member involvement is critical to maintaining relevant agendas for associations.

Associations continually work to sustain sufficient numbers of members to represent their interests and influence within the profession and in the public arena. Monitoring membership numbers, trends in membership, and member demographics is essential. Members are also asked about their perceptions of the association's services and resources as a way to keep in contact with members and to learn about the utility of the services and resources. Increasingly, Web sites are used to communicate with members to provide current information and resources. Some Web sites are interactive and provide opportunities for give and take about proposed or needed changes. Maintaining interaction with members is more complex for associations with chapters or other forms of local or regional divisions that may be separate but related associations. In this situation, the interaction has two focal points—the chapter and the member. Ensuring trust between the association and members also requires that associations identify, select, and elect leaders capable of visioning the future and leading the association.

Most associations establish membership requirements in keeping with their mission to define eligibility and types of membership. Multiple categories of membership enable an association to engage more people in association activities. Types of membership categories may include *full, associate, affiliate, honorary, organizational,* and *liaison.* Each association defines criteria for the rights and responsibilities of each type of membership. Generally, full members have access to all programs and services and can vote. Associate members might have access to selected programs and services, as

BOX 23.4 | MEMBERSHIP STRUCTURE OF THE AMERICAN NURSES ASSOCIATION

- Functioned as the Nurses Associated Alumnae before 1887
- Founded as the Nurses Associated Alumnae of the United States and Canada in 1887
- The *American Journal of Nursing* was founded in 1900
- Renamed, The American Nurses Association in 1911
- Established the American Nurses Foundation in 1955

About ANA

The ANA is the only full-service professional organization representing the nation's 2.7 million Registered Nurses (RNs) through its 54 constituent-member associations. The ANA advances the nursing profession by fostering high standards of nursing practice, promoting the rights of nurses in the workplace, projecting a positive and realistic view of nursing, and by lobbying the Congress and regulatory agencies on health care issues affecting nursing and the public.

Members

ANA Constituent Members

There are 54 constituent nurses associations, which include the 50 states, the District of Columbia, Guam, the Virgin Islands, and the Federal Nurses Association.

Organizational Affiliates (a listing of these organizations can be found on the nursingworld.org Web site)

Subsidiaries

- American Nurses Credentialing Center
- American Nurses Foundation
- American Academy of Nursing

Adapted from American Nurses Association (2008). *Home page*. Available at: http://nursingworld.org/. Accessed October 1, 2008.

might affiliate members. Honorary members are selected and recognized for their contributions to the association and to the profession. Organizational members might represent a partnership or relationship tied into the core functions of the association. Liaison members might have access to information and no or limited member privileges.

Associations with chapters or other types of localized constituents might have dual membership. The point of joining the association might be the local association (chapter), the national or international association, or both. In some cases members have the option of joining only the national or only the local association.

Membership categories are tied to the association's revenue base and to the association's public agenda to foster working partnerships with companies and related businesses with mutual concerns and interests. Boxes

23.4 to 23.6 identify types of membership for three professional nursing associations.

CONSIDER

Associations achieve power that is more than the sum of members, but they depend on collective action of members and respected leaders to gain recognition and influence.

The work of associations is similar to the work of most businesses, in that each association has a charter, a mission, and a legal status in the state in which it resides. Because most associations are not-for-profit organizations and are eligible for tax-exempt status, they must carefully separate the not-for-profit activities from revenue or for-profit ventures. Associations do pay tax on their for-profit ventures. There are different types of

BOX 23.5 | MEMBERSHIP STRUCTURE OF SIGMA THETA TAU INTERNATIONAL, HONOR SOCIETY OF NURSING

Established in 1922 by six students from the Indiana University Training School for Nurses in Indianapolis, Indiana, the honor society's charter members were Mary Tolle Wright, Edith Moore Copeland, Marie Hippensteel Lingernan, Dorothy Garrious Adams, Elizabeth Russell Belford, Elizabeth McWilliams Miller, and Ethel Palmer Clarke, advisor.

The Sigma Theta Tau International (STTI) Foundation of Nursing was created in 1993. Its purpose is active fundraising and conscientious stewardship to promote honor society programs and initiatives.

Mission and Vision

The mission of the Honor Society of Nursing, Sigma Theta Tau International is to support the learning, knowledge, and professional development of nurses committed to making a difference in health worldwide. The vision is to create a global community of nurses who lead in using knowledge, scholarship, service, and learning to improve the health of the world's people.

Membership

Baccalaureate and graduate student nurses who have demonstrated excellence in scholarship and nurse leaders who demonstrate exceptional achievements in nursing are invited to become members. There are more than 130,000 active members, residing in 86 different countries, and there are nearly 500 chapters of honor society located on college campuses worldwide.

Nursing Knowledge International

A subsidiary of the honor society, founded in 2002 to serve the knowledge needs of the global nursing community. More than 20,000 nurses worldwide are members of this community.

Source: Reprinted with permission from Honor Society of Nursing, Sigma Theta Tau International (2008). *Organizational fact sheet.* Available at: **http://www.nursingsociety.org/aboutus/mission/Pages/factsheet.aspx.** Accessed October 1, 2008.

tax-exempt codes that determine what the association may or may not do, such as accepting grants and becoming involved in political campaigns, to retain its tax-exempt status. Associations may create separate organizations such as foundations for these purposes.

The Internal Revenue Service provides information about criteria for each of the different types of tax-exempt status (Internal Revenue Service, 2008). Generally, nursing professional associations have 501(c)(3) status, which includes religious, charitable, educational, scientific, and literary associations or those with selected social missions. Labor organizations engaged in educational activities to improve conditions of work and to improve products and efficiency have the 501(c)(5) designation. Tax-exempt status generally prohibits involvement in political action and campaigning, but it does allow associations to engage in lobbying or advocacy related to their exempt purposes (Internal Revenue Service, 2008). Many states also have requirements for

registration by associations to maintain their tax-exempt status. Oversight of not-for-profit organizations and associations is increasingly scrutinized. Criteria for associations are periodically revised; for example, in 2008, not-for-profit organizations must submit Form 990, which lists members of the governance structure.

Bylaws establish the governance structure, including board membership, committees and meetings, and staff accountabilities. Governance responsibilities are set forth in job descriptions. Board members are stewards of the association, and their functions typically include oversight of performance, including audits, decision making regarding membership eligibility, dues structure, policy, strategic direction, budget approval, and board development. Accountability of the board for keeping the association's bylaws up to date, ensuring financial stability with appropriate investment plans and budgets, and developing and implementing the strategic plan for the work of the association is shared with the staff.

BOX 23.6 | MEMBERSHIP STRUCTURE OF THE NATIONAL LEAGUE FOR NURSING

Formed in 1893 as the American Society of Superintendents of Training Schools for Nursing for the purpose of establishing and maintaining a universal standard of training.

- Named the National League for Nursing Education in 1912
- Renamed the National League for Nursing in 1952
- Established the National League for Nursing Accrediting Commission in 1997

Mission

The National League for Nursing promotes excellence in nursing education to build a strong and diverse nursing workforce.

Membership

The National League for Nursing's membership structure and benefits are designed to serve the needs of our principal stakeholders—nurse faculty and leaders in nursing education in all types of nursing programs. Our quality programs and services offer significant educational and leadership opportunities and a voice in the local, state, national, and global arenas.

Membership is open to all individuals, education agencies, health organizations, and other agencies committed to advancing excellence in nursing education. There are three membership categories; individual membership, education agency membership (Schools of Nursing), and associate membership.

Source: Adapted from National League for Nursing (2008). *Home page.* Available at: http://nln.org/. Accessed October 1, 2008.

The mission and goals of the association affect the type of member eligibility established. Nursing associations range from the most exclusive membership to the most inclusive membership. Sigma Theta Tau International and the American Academy of Nursing are examples of exclusive honor societies or associations that limit membership to those selected through an established process. Some nursing associations limit membership to Registered Nurses with credentials in a specialty field of practice. For others, like state nurses associations, the only limitation is that one is a Registered Nurse. Some associations with broad-based membership have subsidiaries or sections dedicated to nurse members. Professional nursing associations vary in the degree of inclusivity or exclusivity regarding membership. The NLN is an example of an association with a more inclusive membership eligibility. In the reorganization of the professional associations in the 1950s, the NLN was designated as the association with personal membership open to the public. As shown in Box 23.6, one of the NLN membership categories is personal membership, which does not require the Registered Nurse credential.

Members of the association also have a responsibility to be informed about the association's activities and to participate in keeping the association up to date. Nursing associations, like all types of organizations, are dynamic and influenced by internal and external forces. The development of many associations over time is marked by structural changes, renaming, or reorganization. Many of these changes are driven by member concerns and actions.

For example, in early 2000, the ANA restructured the organization in response to member perceptions about internal conflict within the ANA. Two organizations emerged in the restructuring, the Center for American Nurses (CAN) and the United American Nurses (UAN), AFL-CIO. CAN, formed as an ANA affiliate to promote and support nurses and nursing in the workplace through non-collective bargaining, is now in the mainstream of the ANA and fulfills much of its collaborative advocacy through the Congress of Nursing Practice and Economics (CPNE). Almost 20 nursing associations are organizational affiliate members of the CPNE (ANA, 2008). The UAN became a chartered affiliate of the AFL-CIO in 2001 and is the national voice for Registered Nurses in hospitals, the public, and the media (UAN United American Nurses, AFL-CIO, 2008). Its fifth anniversary as a national union of, by, and for staff nurses was celebrated in 2005.

Some associations are long-standing, and others have a shorter life cycle. Nursing specialty associations formed because of a shared common bond in practice and are most likely to be affected by changes in care such as new knowledge or technology that significantly affects the practice. Like many businesses, nursing associations may also merge with others, form alliances with associations and groups with similar purposes, or change their mission and focus. As nurses fill positions in related health care fields, they often join associations relevant to the new field, and often they develop new arrangements to bridge nursing and the expertise in the related field. As practice changes, some associations find new partners for collaboration.

DISCUSSION POINT
Will the majority of professional health-related associations begin to merge and partner in significant ways in the next 20 years? If so, what is the potential effect on the nursing profession?

Many health care organizations that work to identify and disseminate best practices involve nurses as members of health care teams to participate. An example is the Institute for Healthcare Improvement, which works with health care institutions to improve the quality and safety of patient care. Some practice areas, especially technologically dependent ones, may be eliminated because of new technology or new modes of treatment. Others, such as space nursing, emerge in accordance with new discoveries and new practice venues.

CHALLENGES FOR CONTEMPORARY PROFESSIONAL ASSOCIATIONS IN NURSING

Key among the future challenges nursing professional associations face are sustaining and increasing membership, financing association programs and services, keeping information current, and changing practices to adapt to or shape nursing in a complex global environment.

Perhaps the greatest challenge is preparing for an unknown future.

Membership
Membership is a particular challenge in a world increasingly dominated by cyberspace. A pertinent question for associations is, How does an association use technology to ensure the continued valuing of membership in the professional association? Many of the services formerly provided exclusively by associations are now available to nurses through the Internet, which may be perceived as competition for nursing associations. Entrepreneurs have found the critical mass of nurses and employers of nurses to be customers for their Web-based products and services. Nurses can access newsletters, informational materials, chat rooms, message boards, and other venues to interact with colleagues. Some of these resources are short lived, whereas others tend to have longer life spans. With all of these resources, why do they need professional associations?

DISCUSSION POINT
With all of the available resources for information and interaction, why do nurses need or why should they value professional associations?

Another membership challenge for associations is finding ways to meet the needs of diverse members. The varying behaviors and styles of the generations have been studied and often discussed in forums about membership. In their book *The New Breed*, Jonathan McKee and Thomas McKee discussed the changing expectations of individuals as related to their generation (McKee & McKee, 2008). The importance of time-honored association structural aspects, including mission, vision, written documents of formation, and governance structure, as well as a charter, continue to be essential. These authors recommended that associations should design their approaches to the age and motivation of members and potential members to engage both their initial interest and sustained involvement in the association. Young people today tend to rally around an urgent or important cause and find traditional scheduled commitments off-putting.

There are similarities between behaviors of early nursing leaders and emerging knowledge of why people today become involved in associations. If we were to examine why early nursing leaders were successful in advancing the profession, we would probably agree that they shared a passion for a common cause. McKee and McKee (2008) considered passion to be the foundation for effective action in associations. Another similarity is that the passion must be focused to accomplish the mission. The early leaders were focused on their goals. Today, it is believed that focus channels the power of passion. Examining these similarities is helpful to associations moving toward the future. Passion is good, but it is powerful when applied to a focused cause. Consequently, the association with a sound strategic plan based on a vision of the future must translate its actions to achieve the vision concerning causes for which members can be passionate.

CONSIDER

Conventional wisdom derived from previous studies indicates that there are "joiners" and "nonjoiners," but the reality is that the majority of Registered Nurses are not dues-paying members of one or more professional associations.

Associations need members. The association's credibility and influence are related to the numbers and representation of its members. Does the association actually represent the field? Some associations seek large numbers of members especially when the potential membership is large. Associations establish membership criteria. For example, one must be a nurse to join the ANA. Membership in the ANA is inclusive for all Registered Nurses. Some associations or societies limit membership by establishing criteria that only a few satisfy. Membership in these associations is exclusive. Membership in exclusive associations is often limited by invitations to join or by peer-reviewed applications. Most associations work to attract eligible members through membership campaigns, aggressive marketing, and member-to-member interactions. Some associations strive to increase membership by changing eligibility requirements, taking care to gain member input and support for the changes. Associations need members to serve members and to be influential in practice and effective in public relations. The integrity of associations is threatened when membership numbers decline.

Some experts, referring to the "new social order," argue that professional associations have declining membership numbers because they tend to be traditional, bureaucratic organizations that are preoccupied with sustaining the status quo, which tends to limit the capability to relate to changing member needs. The American Society of Association Executives (ASAE) serves leaders of member associations (ASAE and the Center for Association Leadership, n.d.). Among the services provided are studies of the future, publications, association assessment and recommendations, and current information about matters related to association viability and management. Some doomsday predictors see the end of the association. The ASAE, however, envisions viable associations as essential to professional life and urges associations to develop realistic plans for a new future. In addition to futures studies and visioning materials, the association provides Web-based information about how to meet future challenges (ASAE). For example, a recent feature article, *Associations Must Get Real*, published in July 2008, emphasized the importance of authenticity in all aspects of association work to satisfy members (Gilmore & Pine, 2008).

In a changing world, one expects increasing diversity from all sources—ethnic, gender, age, geographic location, type of function or specialty, and others. Each nursing association is challenged to relate its programs and services to a diverse membership. Many members value the traditions and rituals of their associations and enjoy the heritage and past practices of the association. Other members may seek the new and different and may be drawn to nontraditional programs, services, and events. Associations now segment their approaches for both members and potential members. Retiring Baby Boomers are expected to have different priorities than young adults who are growing up with cyberspace. Associations must continue to nurture visionary leadership and to find new ways to meet the needs of diverse members. Most people, despite their age group, tend to seek community, colleagues, and support.

Finance

Membership is directly related to an association's finances. Many professional nursing associations are stretched to sustain resources for programs and services. Some associations have begun to partner in sharing services, products, costs, and revenues. Many are seeking financial support of vendors to support new programs and services, including Web-based programs and interactive venues. It can be expected that associations will continue to develop sources of revenue, often finding unlikely partners in nonrelated businesses and industries or groups that may share a common interest in health care or a specific topic. Increasing dues has not been considered a useful option for raising money to finance the association's work, for several reasons. Members tend to balk at paying increased dues but may willingly make contributions to a foundation or special fund. Ways to accomplish work with minimum financing may also be sought. Stretching resources by joining coalitions or groups to promulgate policy, to develop services, or to initiate projects are some of the ways association's link with others to accomplish work.

Many associations seek non-dues revenue, fulfilling the resource needs through investments, fees for services, and margins on major events such as conventions and educational programs. Advertising fees for promotions on Web sites and in journals and participation of vendors in meetings and conventions are another source of revenue. Development of foundations and solicitation of funding for member services is yet another approach, as is embarking on earned revenue ventures. The technology required in the current environment is often a major expenditure for associations but an essential one if the association is to be successful now and in the future. Seeking creative ways to finance these essential changes requires creativity and innovation.

Continued association effectiveness requires that members and leaders explore and pursue sources of funding and projects carefully. Decisions should be based on the mission, vision, values, strategic goals, and focused purpose of any activity. Retaining trust of members and the public is essential, especially in a turbulent environment. This trust is the core of any membership organization and is critical to effective advocacy and legislation. Valued as among the most important services that associations provide for members and nonmembers, advocacy and legislation do not produce revenues. Maintaining a balance between emphasis on revenue-producing activities and essential advocacy is yet another challenge for associations.

> ### DISCUSSION POINT
> What business approaches would be most effective for professional nursing associations to ensure continuation of essential services and to develop useful innovations?

Communication: The Short Life Cycle of Information

Associations have historically been valued for their thoughtful and reliable communications on important matters requiring expertise, peer review, and testing for reliability. This professional communication is threatened by two sources. One is the short life cycle of knowledge, which sometimes taxes the association's capability to maintain up-to-date information. Another is the increasing accessibility to knowledge on the Internet. People have multiple sources for information. They also have high expectations for rapid communication, immediate feedback, prompt resolution of problems and issues, and customization of information.

Web Sites, online directories, chat rooms, message boards, online resources, links, Webinars, and other Internet venues are now used to facilitate member interaction online. Many associations are working to limit the use of traditional print products and use CDs, online downloads, and other technology. These resources are also used to share proceedings of meetings and conventions. During the time of transition from print to Internet access, some associations provide choices. Methods used to disseminate information influence the way knowledge is produced and packaged. To incorporate technology in their work, associations often require large capital expenditures for research and development, costly production and staff training, or the addition of more staff.

In an era of instant messaging, on-the-spot global reporting, and unfettered transmittal of information, associations are challenged to keep up with ever-changing communication strategies. Technology is a tool. It might change the way an association communicates and produces association issue papers, educational materials, and other information, but it does not change the importance of involving members to provide input and review and to ensure reliability. Generating new knowledge and managing instant transmission of knowledge are important for associations to retain their position as expert sources of knowledge.

Members will seek the most convenient, reliable source of information. As members increasingly have access to communications from many sources, it is possible that some nurses may find these new sources to be just as or more effective than their association and may drop their membership. Those who have successfully used a search engine to rapidly and independently obtain reliable information on a multitude of topics may also be open to finding new networks with immediate entry that do not entail paying dues or attending to the requirements of professional associations for membership.

> ### DISCUSSION POINT
> Associations looking to the future must ask whether members will value their associations if they continue along the path of traditional rules of order, procedures, and protocols.

Changes in Nursing Practice

Nursing practice is changing. Many nurses now participate in multidisciplinary care teams. Their practice colleagues are more diverse. Their practice issues now extend beyond the nursing component of care, and they value networking with team members from a variety of disciplines. Chat rooms and new types of affinity groups and even new associations are forming around issues and topics of common concern that go beyond a given profession. The American Association of Critical Care Nurses recognized this phenomenon early and expanded their membership beyond nurses.

> ### CONSIDER
> Associations of the future are challenged to respond to the complex issues of multidisciplinary practice and issues surrounding the new environment for practice.

This challenge involves concurrently supporting the domain of nursing practice and interprofessional interchange in a straightforward manner. Interdisci-

plinary groups now work together to deal with issues and resolve problems they experience with regard to today's integrated management and clinical systems, regulation, and legislation. They are joining in research. One can speculate whether this phenomenon of interdisciplinary teams will lead to an eventual merging of professional associations so that new, interdisciplinary associations will supplant existing discipline-specific associations. Nursing's professional associations are challenged to deal directly with the new reality of partnerships, alliances, membership eligibility, and services.

As society and nursing practice change, so do nurses' preferences for networking. Networking through meetings and conferences has been a mainstay of associations. Meeting colleagues, listening to respected leaders, and exchanging business cards are networking devices related to educational programs, conventions, and association gatherings. The Internet now allows nurses to exchange ideas and meet colleagues at any time without travel expenses from the comfort of the computer. Some associations, anticipating that networking practices have changed the way people communicate, are now incorporating interactive Internet communication and Internet resources in their member services. Will members continue to value the association for personal contacts, or will they be drawn to the increasing number of Web sites for this interaction and communication? Associations have many questions about how people are learning to network and share and about the value of networking to members. Will members want to come to meetings, when they can review the proceedings online after the meeting? Will they want informal groups and small convenings along with Internet access?

Association literature suggests that associations must become more flexible and more integrated to accommodate these anticipated changes in member preferences. Traditional associations may have difficulty adjusting to the new environment, in which distinction among official meetings, conferences, and journals (all traditional marks of an effective association) is blurred by instant communication systems and rapid exchange of information in cyberspace. Associations find that they have less control over communication and intellectual knowledge in the cyberspace environment. (See Research Study Fuels the Controversy on page 419.)

Research Study Fuels the Controversy: Why Nurses Join Specialty Organizations

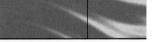

This descriptive research study, with a convenience sample of 81 participants from the Association of Rehabilitation Nursing and four other specialty nursing organizations, used mailed surveys, telephone surveys, and questionnaires to examine why nurses join specialty nursing organizations and what changes would be necessary to increase membership. Herzberg's motivational theory was applied as the conceptual framework.

STUDY FINDINGS

The most frequent reasons given by study participants for joining a professional organization were to increase knowledge, benefit professionally, network, and earn continuing education units. Reasons given for not choosing to participate were family responsibilities, lack of information about these organizations, and lack of time.

Source: White, M. J., & Olson, R. S. (2004). Factors affecting membership in specialty nursing organizations. *Rehabilitation Nursing, 29*(4), 131–137.

To remain viable, associations must focus on understanding member needs, on balancing traditional attitudes and practices with contemporary ways of managing and interacting, and on prioritizing the use of resources. As society changes and as nursing roles change and expand, member needs will change. Balancing current programs and services with emerging expectations involves establishing a new way of approaching the business of associations. Some associations are enlisting participation of members with particular expertise to create the vision and plan for the future. Others are reaching out to other associations to share learning and to fill in gaps. Many associations have already begun to refocus services, becoming brokers for communication, mentoring, and professional dialogue.

The new demands on nursing's professional associations are beginning to change the perspective of what constitutes a "competitor." Previously, competitors have been other nursing and practice-related associations. Competitors, instead of having name recognition and elegant structure, may be flexible, open to experimenting with new approaches and focused on member loyalty to services rather than to associations. Members and association leaders are now challenged to remain focused on their mission, their membership, and their services to make wise decisions about how to use and shape their resources for now and the future.

> ### DISCUSSION POINT
> What should professional nursing associations do now to better understand networking, the motivation to network. and methods for effective networking? What steps should professional nursing associations take to keep pace with changing networking needs of members?

Diversity

As the population becomes increasingly diverse, associations are challenged to ensure that their membership is representative of the cultural diversity of members. Representation of current and potential members is an aspect of an association's mission. It is also a strategic imperative. Definitions of diversity include age, gender, ethnicity, race, physical ability, religion, socioeconomic status, and geographic distribution.

Outreach to potential members to increase the association's diversity, may appear on the surface to be a simple task, but often it is more complex than expected. To be effective, the association's policies and practices must reflect the diversity of its members. Staff and volunteer leadership, member involvement, programs, and services often need to be changed or adapted to reflect the diversity of the membership. For some associations, movement toward greater diversity is a giant step, whereas for others it is a natural evolution. Some of the

BOX 23.7 STRATEGIES FOR ACHIEVING DIVERSITY IN PROFESSIONAL ASSOCIATIONS

- Governing boards' commitment to diversity demonstrated in behaviors
- Allocation of funds to support activities to increase diversity
- Policy statements encompassing the vision and goals for diversity
- Goals and objectives for achieving diversity in the association's strategic plan
- Materials and tools to promote diversity among members
- Staff selection and staff development to promote diversity
- Management practices to promote involvement of diverse staff in all activities
- Outreach to diverse groups to gain support and mentors for diversity
- Evaluation and measurement of objectives to increase diversity

strategies commonly used by professional associations to increase diversity are shown in Box 23.7.

THE ASSOCIATION FOR THE FUTURE

Associations are thoughtful organizations that follow structured patterns to elect officers, develop agendas, study problems and issues, obtain member responses to findings and recommendations, and then transmit the final draft of the information to members and to the public. As cultures evolve and societal, economic, and political structures and more changes, it is inevitable that associations will play a role in either leading change or evolving to support people in a new society. Clearly, technology, the increasing complexity of issues, innovation, and societal changes are forces that affect professional associations. Associations are challenged to be relevant to changing member needs. Those associations that remain understandable to members and dedicated to meeting members' needs will find ways to implement innovations while upholding their values. The relevant associations will be the ones that are most likely to survive in the face of generational gaps and changing values.

Reinvention for Relevance

To remain relevant, it is predicted that many associations will recreate themselves to be viable organizations in a rapidly changing world. These recreated associations will be characterized by the ability to identify and resolve issues with a short life cycle and to change from a structured control and command pattern to become flexible organizations able to meet demands in a changing world. The culture and work of the association may change dramatically to reflect emerging cultures of work and of the profession, as well as changes in organizations. For example, Web 2.0 is a generative force that enables associations to focus on relationships rather than on transactions (Principled Innovation, 2008). Immediate access to information that can be shaped by people outside and inside the association is valued.

Culture of the Future

Associations are part of nursing's culture, which is shaped through relationships, shared traits, and common purpose to achieve unity. Associations that build trust and communication among members are capable of defining ways to move the agenda, achieve support toward change, and have the potential to influence. Building on the legacy of early leaders, nursing associations have the capability to influence the cultures in which nurses function. Great strides have been made to achieve recognition of nursing as a profession and of nurses as professionals. The first half of the 20th century focused on solidifying the profession in society. The second half of the 20th century focused on expanding nursing capability to provide patient care. Which association or group of associations will step forward to identify the focus and lead the journey of the 21st century?

It is difficult to imagine a future so different from the present experience. However, change is inevitable, and forecasting the direction of change is difficult. A first step is collaboration among nursing's professional associations to develop an awareness of forces that affect future nursing practice and the profession. Nursing associations have already established collaboration, as exemplified by the associations that have formed The Alliance: Nursing Organizations Alliance (NOA), which has a growing number of members, reaching 70 in 2008 (The Alliance: Nursing Organizations Alliance, 2008). Any nursing organization or structural component of a multidisciplinary organization may join The Alliance. Initially formed by vote of two nursing coalitions—the National Federation of Specialty Nursing Organizations and the Nursing Organizations Liaison Forum—The Alliance has developed its own bylaws. The history of The Alliance's founding organizations and their relationship to the American Nurses Association is of interest to those wishing to study the evolution of nursing organizations. This history depicts the complex relationships among nursing's professional associations.

The ANA is the inclusive association with membership open to Registered Nurses in the United States, with Constituent Member Associations (CMAs) in each state. It is the U.S. member of the ICN and is generally considered the representative of the nation's nurses in matters affecting the solidarity of the profession and professionalism. As such, the ANA has the public recognition essential to shape the future. Consider how powerful the ANA could be if all of the nation's nurses supported common policy initiatives for the future of the profession (ANA, 2008).

Public Involvement

Because nursing is integral to society, the public must be involved in shaping nursing's future. Creating an agenda to inform the public and to gain support for the future is critical to advancing the profession. Nursing's influence relies on the support of every nurse and on the capability for effective communication between nursing and the public. Each nursing association has its circle of influence within health care and in the public arenas. The Internet is proving to be an effective way to communicate with many audiences and may be an important link in nursing's communication with the public, but it must be managed. As an experiment, put "nursing" in a search engine and analyze the results. The number of results is overwhelming. A first step in

preparing for the future could be codification of references about nursing to facilitate effective Web searches. A collaborative Web site called, say, "All About Nursing" could explain the codes and could be linked to all associations, schools of nursing, and related sites.

> **DISCUSSION POINT**
> What would an integrated professional nursing association look like? What resources would be needed to create a new association that could attract members and sustain member loyalty?

Associations of the future can be expected to evolve from changes in practice. In nursing, these associations would find ways to support nurses in maintaining their strong professional identity and their understanding and commitment to the profession while also supporting their capability to practice in integrated management and clinical patient care services. This association would grow from one that formerly concentrated on nursing to concentrate on building teamwork, bridging territorial domains, and recognizing issues and challenges of integrated systems.

> **DISCUSSION POINT**
> How can professional nursing associations develop services and programs for members that continue to support the nursing identity while also supporting participation in integrated systems?

Recreating professional associations can be considered undertaking a journey to the future. This journey begins with creating and sharing a vision of the future that is then continuously reinterpreted to evolving realities as change takes place. Once a vision is in place, other steps fall into place more naturally but not always easily.

New Initiatives

Types of initiatives associations will undertake on this journey include evaluation of the complexity of nursing practice, needs of nurses, the environment for practice, and nursing roles in health care delivery. Involvement of key stakeholders to grapple with key issues, make recommendations, and deliberate on action plans is important to the success of the endeavor. Preparing nurses and others for potential changes paves the way for action, especially when changes involve experimentation and some risk taking. Intentional outcomes center on serving members within the constraints of the available resources through increasingly flexible and adaptable associations.

The journey is fueled by communication among members and between the association and the public. Understanding the nature and intent of change facilitates participation and support. Keeping in touch with members and the public paves the way for difficult decisions or radical change. If nurses examined their needs for nursing associations of the future, would they recommend radical change? Some might believe that steps should be taken to reduce the redundancy of association functions. For example, does the profession need more than one association to accredit nursing programs or to provide certification for nurses? Or would one strong association better serve the profession and the public? Others believe that the "redundancy" provides necessary competition and responsiveness to members.

Unification: A Radical Change?

Yet another radical change would be creating a manageable unifying body that engenders cooperation of all nursing associations to identify issues for the profession as a whole and to develop an action plan involving all. The proliferation of nursing associations in the 20th century might be viewed as strength. Each of these associations must, of necessity, focus on its own mission but has an important role to play in shaping the nursing profession. To create a unifying body of nursing associations, nursing must transcend some of the current issues. For example, because the ANA is perceived as a union, employers of nurses often see membership in the ANA as a conflict of interest. The ANA has responded to this concern, as well as its internal issues presented by state nurses associations with non-collective bargaining, by restructuring the organization. Will the ANA or the CAN emerge as the national leader toward the future of nursing?

> **DISCUSSION POINT**
> Would it make any difference to you personally and professionally if the multitude of professional nursing associations did not exist?

Many association experts predict that a new social order for professional associations is inevitable. Nursing's professional associations would be affected by a new social order. Members aware of the importance of value will look for evidence of performance outcomes, the effectiveness of political and legislative advocacy, and collaboration to advance the profession and patient care. Demonstrating value is a key to future success of any association. This value is demonstrated by the design of future plans and initiatives, enhanced capability to meet new demands, and elegant communication on issues, change, and outcomes.

> **DISCUSSION POINT**
> What steps should professional nursing associations take now to develop new approaches to become associations that provide evidence-based performance reports to demonstrate value to members?

Research Needed

There is a dearth of information, however, about nursing's professional associations. Nursing would be well served by establishing a research agenda to investigate the role of associations now and in the future to inform initiatives to shape the future of the profession. Some starting points for developing research questions follow:

- What populations are served by nursing associations?
- To what extent are the purposes of the associations the same or different?
- What are the benefits of associations to nurses? To the profession?
- What factors influenced the proliferation of nursing associations?
- What sustains associations over time?
- How are associations affected by societal, economic, and political forces?
- What factors influence changes such as merging or disbanding associations?
- What are the future needs of the profession for association work?
- How should the profession structure itself to meet these needs?
- What role should associations have to advance the future of the profession?

To shape the future of nursing associations, there is a need to establish an evidence base for nursing associations. As mentioned previously, associations are shaped and sustained by societal, political, and economic forces. Nursing associations are influenced by these forces and particularly by changes in health care, where change is now the norm. Research is needed to understand how these forces will affect the nursing profession and nursing associations. At issue is designing the most appropriate venue to advance nursing, to protect the public, to sustain the public recognition for the practice of nursing, and to sustain the profession. Strategies for continuing to advance the profession of nursing, whether led by associations or others, take time to formulate and longer to implement. Research is needed to inform these strategies.

DISCUSSION POINT

Are professional nursing associations the appropriate venue for sustaining the profession of nursing in the future?

CONCLUSIONS

Associations are integral to the cultures of work and society as we know them today. Associations serve members by engaging them in leadership initiatives and providing member services such as education and credentialing, initiatives to advance the profession, and advocacy for the profession and the health needs of the public. Legislative advocacy and policy development entail strong ties with influential persons and groups. Association work is informed by interaction with members and the public and by research. Support is facilitated by public relations to transmit information to members.

Nursing leaders are challenged by future demands and current resources. More than 100 years ago, nurses with vision and passion were defining professionalism for nurses and designing strategies to achieve public recognition for nursing practice, to protect public safety and welfare, and to improve health. Is it time to re-examine their work to develop nursing, to evaluate the relevance of current definitions and strategies, and to reflect on what nursing's professional associations contribute to the profession? Have nursing's professional associations become so embedded in the culture that nurses find it difficult to look beyond the present to envision and shape the future?

A century ago, nurse leaders struggling to gain recognition for nursing as a profession created associations that served the profession. Their passion has been relegated to the history books. The profession they shaped has become pluralistic and diffuse and faces an uncertain future. The profession is being affected by an emerging new social order. The new environment is replete with opportunities and venues for nurses with energy and commitment to meet their needs for professional development, support, and networking. One hundred years from now, what will nurse leaders write about the nurse leaders and the professional nursing associations of this century?

FOR ADDITIONAL DISCUSSION

1. Do most registered nurses relate more directly to their work place than to professional nursing associations on matters pertaining to the advancement of the nursing profession and protection of the public?

2. Some people join professional associations, whereas others do not. What motivates Registered Nurses to participate in and become active in their professional association?

3. Should nurses, through professional associations, take responsibility for regulating the profession? Or is regulation a matter for the public domain?

4. What measures would be effective to engage every Registered Nurse in activities that protect the public welfare and ensure quality nursing care in the policy and legislative arenas? Can this effort be accomplished without professional nursing associations?

5. What alternatives are there to professional nursing associations to provide professional nurses with opportunities to network, socialize, and grow in their profession outside the workplace?

6. Are associations so embedded in society that they will continue to exist even in the new social order? Will associations with redundant functions join to provide accreditation of educational programs and certification for nurses?

7. If you were to establish a professional nursing association today, what would you state as the mission and strategic direction for that association?

8. What research is imperative to better understand the role of professional nursing associations designed to meet member needs in the future? Who should conduct this research, and how should the findings be used?

9. How can nurses keep the profession alive? How can they capitalize on their resources to examine the nursing profession of the future from a global perspective to develop approaches and strategies to sustain nursing in the future? Can professional nursing associations play a part in this activity?

10. How can professional nursing associations become flexible and responsive to changing member values and needs? To new ways of providing members with information and resources to support their work?

REFERENCES

American Nurses Association (ANA) (2008). *Nursing World*. Available at: www.nursingworld.org/Functional MenuCategories/AboutANA/WhoWeAre/CMA. Accessed October 1, 2008.

ASAE and the Center for Association Leadership (n.d.). *Membership FAQ*. Available at: http://www.asaecenter. org/AboutUs/content.cfm?ItemNumber=16273& navItemNumber=16274#who2008. Accessed October 1, 2008.

Cherry, B., & Jacob, S. R. (2002). *Contemporary Nursing. Issues, Trends, and Management* (2nd ed). St. Louis, MO: Mosby.

Fenwick, E. G. (1901). The organization and registration of nurses. In: *Proceedings, 3rd Quinquennia Meeting of the International Council of Nurses Held in Buffalo, New York*, p. 336.

Gilmore, J. H., & Pine, B. J. (2008). *Associations must get real*. Item Number 35090. Available at: www.asaecen ter.org/PublicationsResources. Accessed July 30, 2008.

Henderson, V., & Nite, G. (1978). *Principles and Practice of Nursing* (6th ed.). New York: Macmillan.

Internal Revenue Service (2008). *Facts about operating as an exempt organization*. Available at: http://www. irs.gov/charities/article/0id=96584,00.html. Accessed October 1, 2008.

McKee, J., & McKee, T. (2008). *The New Breed, Understanding and Equipping the 21st Century Volunteer*. Loveland, CO: Group.

National League for Nursing (NLN) (2008). *History*. Available at: www.nln.org/aboutnln/info-history. Accessed October 1, 2008.

Principled Innovation (2008). *Web 2.0 as a generative force*. Available at: http://www.principledinnova tion.com/blog/2008/02/17/web-20-as-a-generative-force/. Accessed July 30, 2008.

Raymond Rich Associates report on the structure of organized nursing (1946). *American Journal of Nursing, 46*(10), 648–661.

Sigma Theta Tau International, Honor Society of Nursing (2008). *Organizational fact sheet*. Available at: http://www.nursingsociety.org/aboutus/ mission/Pages/factsheet.aspx. Accessed October 2, 2008.

Spaulding, E. K., & Notter, L. (1965). *Professional Nursing*. Philadelphia: Lippincott.

The Alliance. Nursing Organizations Alliance (2008). *Home page*. Available at: http://www.nursing-alliance.org/. Accessed October 1, 2008.

UAN United American Nurses, AFL-CIO (2008). *UAN: The power of nurses*. Available at: http://www. uannurse.org/who/history.html. Accessed October 2, 2008.

White, M. J., & Olson, R. S. (2004). Factors affecting membership in specialty nursing organizations. *Rehabilitation Nursing, 29*(4), 131–137.

BIBLIOGRAPHY

Alotaibi, M. (2007). Factors affecting nurses' decisions to join their professional association. *International Nursing Review, 54*(2), 160–165.

ASAE and the Center for Association Leadership (2008). *Publications and resources.* Available at: http://www.asaecenter.org/publicationsresources/index.cfm. Accessed October 1, 2008.

Baldwin, K. M., Lyon, B. L., Clark, A. P., Fulton, J., Davidson, S., & Dayhoff, N. (2007). Developing Clinical Nurse Specialist practice competencies. *Clinical Nurse Specialist, 21*(6) 297–303.

Banschbach, S. K. (2008). Making the most of our association's opportunities. *AORN, 87*(5) 895–898.

Betz, C. L. (2008). Pediatric nursing scope and standards of practice: A unified professional effort. *Journal Rehabilitation Nursing, 23*(2), 79–80.

Gardner, E. A., & Schmidt, C. K. (2007). Implementing a leadership course and mentor model for students in the National Student Nurses' Association. *Nurse Educator, 32*(4), 178–182.

Harper, K. A. (Ed.) (2008). *Encyclopedia of Associations, Vol. 3. Supplement: National Organizations of the U.S.* (46th ed.). Farmington Hills, MI: Gale Cengage Learning.

IPL, The Internet Public Library (2009). *Nursing.* Available at: http://www.ipl.org/div/searchresults/?searchtype=traditional&words=nursing. Accessed January 29, 2009.

Resnick, B. (2007) A call to all nurses working in geriatrics: Make 2007 a great year by joining the campaign, advancing excellence in America's nursing homes. *Geriatric Nursing, 28*(2), 69–71.

Tunajek, K. K. (2006). Professional standards and public accountability. *AANA Journal, 74*(1), 25–27.

Wikipedia (n.d.). *Professional body.* Available at: http://en.wikipedia.org/wiki/Professional_Associations. Accessed July 30, 2008.

Yoder-Wise, P. S. (2006). State and certifying boards/associations: CE and competency requirements, *Journal of Continuing Education in Nursing, 37*(1), 3–11.

WEB RESOURCES

Academy of Medical-Surgical Nurses	http://www.medsurgnurse.org/
Academy of Neonatal Nursing	http://www.academyonline.org/
Aerospace Nursing Association	http://www.Aerospacenursing.org/
Air and Surface Transport Nurses Association	http://www.astna.org/
American Academy of Ambulatory Care Nursing	http://www.aaacn.org/
American Academy of Nursing	http://www.aaanet.org/
American Academy of Nurse Practitioners	http://www.aanp.org/
American Academy of Pain Management	http://www.aapainmanage.org/
American Assembly for Men in Nursing	http://www.aamn.org/
American Assisted Living Nurses Association	http://www.alnursing.org/
American Association for the History of Nursing	http://www.aahn.org/
American Association of Colleges of Nursing	http://www.aacn.nche.edu/
American Association of Critical Care Nurses	http://www.aacn.org/
American Association of Legal Nurse Consultants	http://www.aalnc.org/

American Association of Managed Care Nurses	http://www.aamcn.org/
American Association of Neuroscience Nurses	http://www.aaan.org/
American Association of Nigerian Nurses	http://www.nannm.com/
American Association of Nurse Anesthetists	http://www.aana.com/
American Association of Nurse Assessment Coordinators	http://www.aanac.org/
American Association of Nurse Attorneys	http://www.taana.org/
American Association of Occupational Health Nurses	http://www.aaohn.org/
American Association of Office Nurses	http://www.aaon.org/
American Association of Spinal Cord Injury Nurses	http://www.aascin.org/
American College of Nurse Midwives	http://www.acnm.org/
American College of Nurse Practitioners	http://www.acnpweb.org/
American Forensic Nurses	http://verbaljudo.tripod.com/
American Health Information Management Association	http://www.ahima.org/
American Heart Association Council on Cardiovascular Nursing	http://www.americanheart.org/
American Holistic Nurses Association	http://www.ahna.org/
American Medical Informatics Association	http://www.jamia.org/
American Nephrology Nurses Association	http://www.anna.nurse.com/
American Nurses Association	http://www.nursingworld.org/
American Nursing Informatics Association	http://www.ania.org/
American Organization of Nurse Executives	http://www.aone.org/
American Pediatric Surgical Nurses Association	http://www.apsna.com/
American Psychiatric Nurses Association	http://www.apna.org/
American Radiological Nurses Association	http://www.arna.net/
American Society of Heart Failure Nurses	http://www.aahfn.org/
American Society of Ophthalmic Registered Nurses	http://www.webeye.ophth.uiowa.edu/asorn/
American Society of Pain Management Nurses	http://www.aspmn.org/
American Society of PeriAnesthesia Nurses	http://www.aspan.org/
American Society of Plastic and Reconstructive Surgical Nurses	http://www.aspsn.org/
American Surgical Nurses Association	http://www.pdcnet.com/APSNA.html

Anthroposophical Nurses Association of America	http://www.artemisia.net/anaa/
Association for Child and Adolescent Psychiatric Nurses	http://www.acapn.org/.
International Society of Psychiatric-Mental Health Nurses	http://www.ispn-psych.org
Association of Black Nursing Faculty in Higher Education	http://www.abnf.net/
Association of Clinicians for the Underserved	http://www.clinicians.org/
Association of Community Health Nurse Educators	http://www.achne.org/
Association of Legal Nurse Consultants	http://www.aalnc.org/
Association of Neonatal Nurses	http://www.nann.org/
Association of Nurses in AIDS Care	http://www.anacnet.org/
Association of Pediatric Oncology Nurses	http://www.aphon.org/
Association of periOperative Registered Nurses	http://www.aorn.org/
Association of Rehabilitation Nurses	http://www.rehabnurse.org/
Association of State and Territorial Directors of Nursing	http://www.astdn.org/
Association of Women's Health, Obstetric and Neonatal Nurses	http://www.awhonn.org/
Commission on Graduates of Foreign Nursing Schools	http://www.cgfns.org/
Council on Graduate Education for Administration in Nursing	http://www.cgean.org
Dermatology Nurses Association	http://www.dnanurse.org
Developmental Disabilities Nurses Association	http://www.ddna.org/
Emergency Nurses Association	http://www.ena.org/
Home Health Care Nurses Association	http://www.hhna.org/
Hospice and Palliative Nurses Association	http://www.hpna.org/
Infusion Nurses Society	http://www.insl.org/
Interagency Council on Information Resources in Nursing	http://www.icim.org/
International Academic Nursing Alliance	www.nursingalliance.org
International Association of Forensic Nurses	http://www.forensicnurse.org/
International Nurses Society on Addiction	http://www.intnsa.org/
International Society of Nurses in Genetics	http://www.isong.org/

International Society of Psychiatric Mental Health Nurses	http://www.ispn-psych.org/
Intravenous Nurses Society	http://www.ins1.org/
Midwest Nursing Research Society	http://www.mnrs.org/
Minority Nursing Associations	http://www.minoritynurse.com/
National American Arab Nursing Association	http://www.n-aana.org
National Alaska Native American Indian Nurses Association	http://www.nanainanurses.org/
National Association for Associate Degree Nursing	http://www.noadn.org/
National Association for Practical Nurse Education and Service	http://www.napnes.org/
National Association of Clinical Nurse Specialists	http://www.nacns.org/
National Association of Directors of Nursing Administration/Long Term Care	http://www.nadona.org/
National Association for Home Care and Hospice	www.nahc.org
National Association of Hispanic Nurses	http://www.thehispanicnurse.org/
National Association of Neonatal Nurses	http://www.nann.org/
National Association of Nurse Massage Therapists	http://www.nanmt.org/
National Association of Nurse Practitioners in Women's Health	http://www.npwh.org/
National Association of Orthopaedic Nurses	http://www.orthonurse.org/
National Association of Pediatric Nurse Associates and Practitioners	http://www.napnap.org/
National Association of Pediatric Nurse Practitioners	http://www.napnap.org/
National Association of Pro-life Nurses	http://www.nursesforlife.org
National Association of School Nurses	http://www.nasn.org/
National Organization of Nurse Practitioner Faculties	http://www.nonpf.com/
National Black Nurses Association	http://www.nbna.org/
National Coalition of Ethnic Minority Nurse Associations	http://www.ncemna.org/
National Conference of Gerontological Nurse Practitioners	www.ncgnp.org
National Council of State Boards of Nursing	http://www.ncsbn.org/
National League for Nursing	http://www.nln.org/

National Nurses in Business Association	http:www.nnba.net
National Nurses Association	http//www.nationalnurses.org
National Nursing Staff Development Organization	http://www.nnsdo.org/
National Organization of Nurse Practitioner Faculties	http://www.nonpf.com/
National Student Nurses Association	http://www.nsna.org/
Navy Nurse Corps Association	http://www.nnca.org/
North American Nursing Diagnosis Association International	http://www.nanda.org/
Nurse Healers Professional Association International	http://www.therapeutic-touch.org/
Nurse Organization of Veterans Affairs	http://www.vanurse.org/
Nursing Organizations Alliance	http://www.nursing-alliance.org/
Nurses Christian Fellowship International	http://www.ncfi.org/
Oncology Nursing Society	http://www.ons.org/
Pediatric Endocrinology Nursing Society	http://www.pens.org/
Philippine Nurses Association of America	http://www.phillipinenurses.org/
Preventive Cardiovascular Nurses Association	http//www.pcna.net
Respiratory Nursing Society	http://www.respiratorynursingsociety.org/
Sigma Theta Tau, the International Honor Society of Nursing	http://www.nursingsociety.org/
Society of Gastroenterology Nurses and Associates	http://www.signa.org/
Society of Pediatric Nurses	http://www.pedsnurses.org/
Society of Urologic Nurses and Associates	http://www.suna.org/
Society for Vascular Nursing	http://www.sunnet.org/
Society of Trauma Nurses	http://www.traumanurses.org/
Space Nursing Society	http://www.geocities.com/
The Alliance: Nursing Organizations Alliance	http//www.nursing_alliance.org
Transcultural Nursing Society	http://www.tcns.org/
Uniformed Nurse Practitioners Association	http://www.guidestar.org
Visiting Nurse Association of America	www.vnaa.org
Wound, Ostomy & Continence Nurses Society	http://www.wocn.org/

National Nurses in Business Association	http://www.nnba.net
National Nurses Association	http://www.nationalnurses.org
National Nursing Staff Development Organization	http://www.nnsdo.org/
National Organization of Nurse Practitioner Faculties	http://www.nonpf.com
National Student Nurses Association	http://www.nsna.org/
Navy Nurse Corps Association	http://www.nnca.org
North American Nursing Diagnosis Association International	http://www.nanda.org/
Nurse Healers Professional Association International	http://www.therapeutic-touch.org/
Nurses Organization of Veterans Affairs	http://www.vanurse.org
Nursing Organizations Alliance	http://www.nursing-alliance.org/
Nurses Christian Fellowship International	http://www.ncf.org
Oncology Nursing Society	http://www.ons.org
Pediatric Endocrinology Nursing Society	http://www.pens.org
Philippine Nurses Association of America	http://www.philippinenursesusa.org/
Preventive Cardiovascular Nurses Association	http://www.pcna.net
Respiratory Nursing Society	http://www.respiratorynursingsociety.org/
Sigma Theta Tau, the International Honor Society of Nursing	http://www.nursingsociety.org/
Society of Gastroenterology Nurses and Associates	http://www.sgna.org
Society of Pediatric Nurses	http://www.pedsnurses.org
Society of Urologic Nurses and Associates	http://www.suna.org
Society for Vascular Nursing	http://www.svnnet.org/
Society of Trauma Nurses	http://www.traumanurses.org/
Space Nursing Society	http://www.spacenursing.com
The Alliance, Nursing Organizations Alliance	http://www.nursing-alliance.org
Transcultural Nursing Society	http://www.tcns.org/
Uniformed Nurse Practitioners Association	http://www.gotadutch.org
Visiting Nurse Association of America	www.vnaa.org
Wound, Ostomy & Continence Nurses Society	http://www.wocn.org/

INDEX

A

Abandonment, 185, 186*b*
  employee, 186
  employment, 186
  patient, 185–186, 186*b*
Absenteeism, of unlicensed assistive personnel, 125
Academic careers, 75–76. *See also* Faculty, nursing
AcademyHealth project, on ethical recruitment of
      foreign nurses, 103
Acceptance, 297
Access to health care
  contemporary issues in, 390–392
  nurses' work for, 385–386
Accommodation, 297
Activism. *See also* Public policy
  female role in, 377
  union, 295
Administration, nursing. *See also specific positions
      and titles*
  ethnic diversity in, 150–152
Adult developmental stages, mentoring and, 138–139
Advanced cardiac life support (ACLS), simulation
      training in, 62–63
Advanced practice nurse (APN) certification, 311
Advanced practice nursing (APN), 355–369. *See also
      specific types*
  AANA study on, 361
  background on, 357–358
  certified nurse-midwives in, 356–357
  certified registered nurse anesthetists in, 357
  clinical nurse leader in, 366–370 (*See also* Clinical
      Nurse Leader (CNL))
  clinical nurse specialists in, 356
  Doctor of Nursing Practice in, 358–366 (*See also*
      Doctor of Nursing Practice [DNP])
  history of, 355–356, 358
  need for, 355
  nurse practitioners in, 356
  role definition in, 356
Advanced practice registered nurse (APRN). *See also*
      Advanced practice nursing
  categories of, 356

vs. DNP, 358–359
  titles of, 365
Adverse events
  definition of, 237
  mandatory reporting of, 247–248
Advocacy
  patient, in whistle-blowing, 263, 267
  by professional associations, 405
Affirmative action, for male nurse recruiting, 156–157
Agency for Healthcare Research and Quality (AHRQ), 26
Aging
  of nurses, 78–79
    retention strategies for, 84, 85*t*
    workplace design for, 83–84
  of nursing faculty, 80, 388
Alliance: Nursing Organizations Alliance (NOA), 421
Alliance for Nursing Accreditation (AACN)
  on distance education, 43, 43*b*
  on diversity, 158
Alumnae associations, nursing
  on nursing profession, 408
  public policy work of, 381
Ambassadors, nurse, 349–350
Ambulatory care, simulation training for, 59
American Association of Colleges of Nursing (AACN)
  on clinical nurse leaders, 366 (*See also* Clinical nurse
      leader (CNL))
  on Doctor of Nursing Practice, 365 (*See also* Doctor
      of Nursing Practice (DNP))
  on impaired nursing practice, 278
  mission of, 362
  practice nurse doctorate development by, 355–356
American Association of Critical Care Nurses
      Protocols for Practice (2006), 26, 26*b*
American Association of Industrial Nurses, 409
American Association of University Professors
      (AAUP), collective bargaining by, 297–298
American Board of Nursing Specialties (ABNS),
      310–311
American Hospital Association Committee on Health
      Professions, on simulators, 64
American Journal of Nursing, establishment of, 381